EDHF 2000

EDHF 2000

Edited by
Paul M. Vanhoutte
Institut de Recherches Internationales Servier
Courbevoie
France

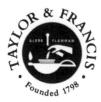

London and New York

First published 2001
by Taylor & Francis
11 New Fetter Lane, London EC4P 4EE

Simultaneously published in the USA and Canada
by Taylor & Francis Inc,
29 West 35th Street, New York, NY 10001

Taylor & Francis is an imprint of the Taylor & Francis Group

© 2001 Taylor & Francis

Every effort has been made to ensure that the advice and information
in this book is true and accurate at the time of going to press. However,
neither the publisher nor the authors can accept any legal responsibility
or liability for any errors or omissions that may be made. In the case of
drug administration, any medical procedure or the use of technical
equipment mentioned within this book, you are strongly advised to
consult the manufacturer's guidelines.

British Library Cataloguing in Publication Data
A catalogue record for this book is available
from the British Library

Library of Congress Cataloging in Publication Data
A catalogue record has been requested

ISBN 0–415–26904–0

Contents

Preface

This monograph is the third of a series devoted to endothelium-dependent hyperpolarizations. It consists of the Proceedings of the Third International Symposium devoted to this topic, which was held in Vaux de Cernay (France) from June 14 to 16, 2000. The first two meetings established the existence of endothelium-derived hyperpolarizing factor (EDHF) but also revealed the multiplicity of chemical factors potentially involved in endothelium-dependent hyperpolarizations. The third symposium continued to expand the worldwide interest in knowledge in the matter, but, in particular, highlighted the emerging role of gap junctional communication in the genesis of the phenomenon.

The first twelve chapters discuss the role of gap junctions in cardiovascular responses in general, and in endothelium-dependent hyperpolarizations in particular. The next set of fourteen chapters pursue the debate, that was so vivid in the previous symposium, as to the chemical identity of EDHF, focusing on the two surviving candidates: K^+ and EETs, with the timid appearance of another derivative of arachidonic acid in Chapter 27. The following three chapters conclude by ruling out NO as a major EDHF, at least in mice. The last part of the monograph deals with the impact of physiology, including hormonal modulation, and pathology (regenerated endothelium, hypertension, diabetes, oxidative stress, ischemia and radiation) on endothelium-dependent hyperpolarization. The last two experimental chapters describe the effects of converting enzyme inhibition on the deleterious effects of aging and hypertension on the phenomenon. As usual, the last chapter attempts to wrap it all up and to provide a reasonable summary of two days of most exciting science.

As always with multiauthored texts, the responsibility for the scientific content rests with the individual authors. Hence, all the statements made are not necessarily endorsed by the editor. His task has been mainly to select the authors, to streamline their texts, and to achieve as much uniformity of presentation as possible.

EDHF 2000 will be of interest not only to physiologists and pharmacologists puzzled by the complexity of the interactions between the endothelium and the underlying vascular smooth muscle cells, but also to clinical researchers and to the physicians who treat patients with cardiovascular diseases. Indeed, the understanding of the nature and role of EDHF already appears to be crucial in the quest for an improvement in the treatment of hypertension, diabetes, ischemia-reperfusion and other vascular disorders.

Acknowledgements

The participants of the Third International Symposium on Endothelium-Derived Hyperpolarizing Factor will not forget the charm and dedication of Mrs Denise Maggi, and Mrs Susan Bosio. This monograph would not have been possible without the total dedication of Mr Robert R. Lorenz who took responsibility for the illustrations. The administrative help of Ms Pascale Olivier was instrumental in compiling the unified reference list. The editor would like to thank most sincerely Dr Laurent Perret of the Institut de Recherches Internationales Servier, who supported the endeavor to try to make this monograph into a reasonably uniform text, despite the many contributors. He would also like to thank the authors most sincerely for their collaboration and understanding when faced with extensive editing of their manuscript. Last, but not least, the staff at the publishers should be complimented for their efficient handling of the manuscript.

Contributors

Abe, K.
Department of Anatomy
Graduate School of Medicine
Hokkaido University
Sapporo 060-8638
Japan

Abe, I.
Department of Medicine and Clinical
Science
Graduate School of Medical Sciences
Kyushu University
Fukuoka 812-8582
Japan

Adeagbo, A.S.O.
Department of Physiology and
Biophysics
University of Louisville
Louisville KY 40292
USA
Tel: 1 502 8 527 561
Fax: 1 502 8 526 239
e-mail: asadea01@gwise.louisville.edu

Akaishi, Y.
Department of Pharmacology
Graduate School of Medicine
Hokkaido University
Sapporo 060-8638
Japan

Angelini, G.D.
Division of Cardiac, Anaesthetic and
Radiologic Sciences
University of Bristol
Bristol Royal Infirmary
Bristol BS2 8HW
UK

Ayajiki, K.
Department of Pharmacology
Shiga University of Medical Science
Seta
Ohtsu 520-2192
Japan

Bartlett, I.S.
The John B. Pierce Laboratory
Yale University School of Medicine
290 Congress Avenue
New Haven CT 06519
USA

Bauersachs, J.
Medizinische Universitätsklinik
Würzburg
Josef Schneider-Straße 2
D-97080 Würzburg
Germany
Tel: 49 9312 015 301
Fax: 49 9312 015 302
e-mail: j.bauersachs@medizin.uni-
wuerzburg.de

Bény, J.-L.
Department of Zoology and Animal
Biology
University of Geneva
30 Quai Ernest-Ansermet
CH-1211 Geneva 4
Switzerland
Tel: 41 22 702 6766
Fax: 41 22 781 1747
e-mail: jean-louis.beny@zoo.unige.ch

Berg, G.A.
Department of Cardiothoracic Surgery
University of Glasgow
Western Infirmary
Glasgow G11 6NT
UK

Berman, R.S.
Department of Diagnostic Radiology
Wales Heart Research Institute
University of Wales College
of Medicine
Cardiff CF14 4XN
UK

Beyer, E.C.
Department of Pediatrics
University of Chicago
Chicago IL 60637
USA

Boyle, J.P.
Department of Cell Physiology and
Pharmacology
University of Leicester
Leicester LE1 9HN
UK

Brandes, R.P.
Institut für Kardiovaskuläre Physiologie
Klinikum der J.W. Goethe-Universität
Theodor-Stern-Kai 7
D-60590 Frankfurt am Main
Germany
Tel: 49 69 6301 6995
Fax: 49 69 6301 7668
e-mail: brandes@em.uni-frankfurt.de

Bredenkötter, D.
Institut für Kardiovaskuläre Physiologie
Klinikum der J.W. Goethe-Universität
Theodor-Stern-Kai 7
D-60590 Frankfurt am Main
Germany

Brink, P.R.
Department of Physiology and
Biophysics
SUNY at Stony Brook
Stony Brook NY 11794
USA
Tel: 1 631 4443 124
Fax: 1 631 4443 432
e-mail: peter@patch.pnb.sunysb.edu

Bryan Jr., R.M.
Department of Anesthesiology
Baylor College of Medicine
One Baylor Plaza
Houston TX 77030
USA

Buralli, S.
Department of Internal Medicine
University of Pisa
Via Roma, 67
56100 Pisa
Italy

Burnham, M.
School of Biological Sciences
University of Manchester
Oxford Road
Manchester M13 9PT
UK

Busse, R.
Institut für Kardiovaskuläre Physiologie
Klinikum der J.W. Goethe-Universität
Theodor-Stern-Kai 7
D-60590 Frankfurt am Main
Germany

Cambarrat, C.
Division Pathologies Cardiaques et
Vasculaires
Institut de Recherches Servier
11 rue des Moulineaux
92150 Suresnes
France

Campbell, W.B.
Cardiovascular Research Center
Medical College of Wisconsin
8701 Watertown Plank Road
Milwaukee WI 53226
USA

Capdevila, J.
Department of Medicine and
Biochemistry
Vanderbilt University Medical School
Nashville TN 37232
USA

Chataigneau, T.
UMR CNRS 7034
Faculté de Pharmacie
Université Louis Pasteur
de Strasbourg
BP24
67401 Illkirch cedex
France
Tel: 33 3 90 244127
Fax: 33 3 90 244313
e-mail: cthierry@aspirine.u-strasbg.fr

Chaytor, A.T.
Department of Diagnostic Radiology
Wales Heart Research Institute
University of Wales College of Medicine
Cardiff CF14 4XN
UK
Tel: 44 12920 742 912
Fax: 44 12920 744 726
e-mail: chaytor@cf.ac.uk

Childres, W.F.
Department of Anesthesiology
Baylor College of Medicine
One Baylor Plaza
Houston TX 77030
USA

Christ, G.J.
Department of Urology
Albert Einstein College of Medicine
Bronx NY 10461
USA

Christ, M.
Institut für Klinische Pharmakologie
Universitätsklinikum Mannheim
D-68167 Mannheim
Germany

Coats, P.
Department of Biomedical and
Biological Sciences
Glasgow Caledonian University
Cowcaddens Road
Glasgow G4 0BA
UK
Tel: 44 141 3313 209
Fax: 44 141 3313 208
e-mail: p.coats@gcal.ac.uk

Cocks, T.M.
Department of Pharmacology
University of Melbourne
Parkville
Victoria 3010
Australia
Tel: 61 383445678
Fax: 61 383448328
e-mail:
t.cocks@pharmacology.unimelb.edu.au

Coleman, H.A.
Department of Physiology
Monash University
Clayton, Melbourne
Victoria 3800
Australia
Tel: 61 3 9905 2520
Fax: 61 3 9905 2547
e-mail: h.coleman@med.monash.edu.au

Corriu, C.
UMR CNRS 7034
Faculté de Pharmacie
Université Louis Pasteur de Strasbourg
67401 Illkirch cedex
France

De Vriese, A.S.
Renal Unit
Ghent University Hospital
De Pintelaan 185
B-9000 Gent
Belgium
Tel: 32 9 240 5301
Fax: 32 9 240 4599
e-mail: an.devriese@rug.ac.be

Ding, H.
Smooth Muscle Research Group
Department of Pharmacology and
Therapeutics
University of Calgary Faculty of
Medicine
Calgary, Alberta T2N 4N1
Canada
Tel: 1 403 2208 402
Fax: 1 403 2702 211
e-mail: hding@ucalgary.ca

Dominiczak, A.F.
Department of Medicine and
Therapeutics
University of Glasgow
Western Infirmary
Glasgow G11 6NT
UK

Dora, K.A.
Department of Pharmacy and
Pharmacology
University of Bath
Bath BA2 7AY
UK

Doughty, J.M.
Department of Physiology
University of Bristol
University Walk
Bristol BS8 1TD
UK

Edwards, G.
School of Biological Sciences
University of Manchester
Oxford Road
Manchester M13 9PT
UK

Edwards, D.H.
Department of Diagnostic Radiology
Wales Heart Research Institute
University of Wales College of Medicine
Cardiff CF14 4XN
UK

Emerson, G.G.
The John B. Pierce Laboratory
Yale University School of Medicine
290 Congress Avenue
New Haven CT 06519
USA

Errington, R.J.
Department of Medical Biochemistry
University of Wales College of Medicine
Cardiff CF14 4XN
UK

Ertl, G.
Medizinische Universitätsklinik
Würzburg
Josef Schneider-Straße 2
D-97080 Würzburg
Germany

Falkner, K.C.
Department of Biochemistry and
Molecular Biology
University of Louisville
Louisville KY 40292
USA

Félétou, M.
Départment Diabéte et Maladies
Métaboliques
Institut de Recherches Servier
11 rue des Moulineaux
92150 Suresnes
France
Tel: 33 1 55 72 22 73
Fax: 33 1 55 72 24 40
e-mail: michel.feletou@fr.netgrs.com or
feletou@netgrs.com

Fisslthaler, B.
Institut für Kardiovaskuläre Physiologie
Klinikum der J.W. Goethe-Universität
Theodor-Stern-Kai 7
D-60590 Frankfurt am Main
Germany
Tel: 49 69 6301 6995
Fax: 49 69 6301 7668
e-mail: fisslthaler@em.uni-frankfurt.de

Fleming, I.
Institut für Kardiovaskuläre
Physiologie
Klinikum der J.W. Goethe-Universität
Theodor-Stern-Kai 7
D-60590 Frankfurt am Main
Germany

Fournet-Bourguignon, M.-P.
Division Pathologies Cardiaques
et Vasculaires
Institut de Recherches Servier
11 rue des Moulineaux
92150 Suresnes
France

Fujii, K.
Department of Medicine and Clinical
Science
Graduate School of Medical Sciences
Kyushu University
Fukuoka 812-8582
Japan
Tel: 81 92 642 5256
Fax: 81 92 642 5271
e-mail: fujii@intmed2.kyushu-u.ac.jp

Fujioka, H.
Department of Pharmacology
Shiga University of Medical Science
Seta
Ohtsu 520-2192
Japan

Fukao, M.
Department of Pharmacology
Graduate School of Medicine
Hokkaido University
Sapporo 060-8638
Japan
Tel: 81 11 706 6921
Fax: 81 11 706 78 24
e-mail: fukao@med.hokudai.ac.jp

Fukuta, H.
Department of Physiology
Nagoya City University Medical School
Mizuho-Ku
Nagoya 467-8601
Japan

Fulep, E.E.
Reproductive Sciences
Department of Obstetrics and
Gynecology
University of Texas Medical Branch
Galveston TX 77555-1062
USA

Funae, Y.
Department of Chemical Biology
Osaka City University Medical School
Osaka 545-8585
Japan

Gardener, M.J.
School of Biological Sciences
University of Manchester
Oxford Road
Manchester M13 9PT
UK
Tel: 44 1612 755 487
Fax: 44 1612 755 600
e-mail: matt.gardener@man.ac.uk

Garfield, R.E.
Reproductive Sciences
Department of Obstetrics and
Gynecology
University of Texas Medical Branch
Galveston TX 77555-1062
USA

Garland, C.J.
Department of Pharmacy and
Pharmacology
University of Bath
Bath BA2 7AY
UK
Tel: 44 1225 323 358
Fax: 44 1225 323 359
e-mail: c.j.garland@bath.ac.uk

Gauthier, K.M.
Department of Pharmacology and
Toxicology
Medical College of Wisconsin
8701 Watertown Plank Road
Milwaukee WI 53226
USA

Ghiadoni, L.
Department of Internal Medicine
University of Pisa
Via Roma, 67
56100 Pisa
Italy

Goddard-Finegold, J.
Department of Pediatrics
Baylor College of Medicine
One Baylor Plaza
Houston TX 77030
USA

Goto, K.
Department of Medicine and Clinical
Science
Graduate School of Medical Sciences
Kyushu University
Fukuoka 812-8582
Japan
Tel: 81 92 642 5256
Fax: 81 92 642 5271
e-mail: fujii@intmed2.kyushu-u.ac.jp

Griffith, T.M.
Department of Diagnostic
Radiology
Wales Heart Research Institute
University of Wales College
of Medicine
Cardiff CF14 4XN
UK
Tel: 44 029 207 431 070
Fax: 44 02 920 744 726
e-mail: griffith@cardiff.ac.uk

Gurney, A.M.
Department of Physiology and
Pharmacology
University of Strathclyde
27 Taylor Street
Glasgow G4 ONR
UK

Hamilton, C.A.
Department of Medicine and
Therapeutics
University of Glasgow
Western Infirmary
Glasgow G11 6NT
UK
Tel: 44 141 2112 042
Fax: 44 141 3392 800
e-mail: c.a.hamilton@clinmed.gla.ac.uk

Harder, D.R.
Cardiovascular Research Center
Medical College of Wisconsin
8701 Watertown Plank Road
Milwaukee WI 53226
USA
Tel: 1 414 4565 611
Fax: 1 414 4566 515
e-mail: dharder@mcw.edu

Harris, D.
School of Biomedical Sciences
University of Nottingham Medical
School
Queen's Medical Centre
Nottingham NG7 2UH
UK

Hashitani, H.
Department of Physiology
Nagoya City University Medical
School
Mizuho-Ku
Nagoya 467-8601
Japan

Hillier, C.
Department of Biomedical and
Biological Sciences
Glasgow Caledonian University
Cowcaddens Road
Glasgow G4 OBA
UK

Hirakawa, Y.
Department of Cardiovascular Medicine
Graduate School of Medical Sciences
Kyushu University
Fukuoka 812-8582
Japan

Hirano, K.
Department of Molecular Cardiology
Graduate School of Medical Sciences
Kyushu University
Fukuoka 812-8582
Japan

Hutcheson, I.R.
Department of Diagnostic Radiology
Wales Heart Research Institute
University of Wales College
of Medicine
Cardiff CF14 4XN
UK

Imaeda, K.
Department of Physiology
Nagoya City University Medical School
Mizuho-Ku
Nagoya 467-8601
Japan

Imaoka, S.
Department of Chemical Biology
Osaka City University Medical School
Osaka 545-8585
Japan

Isoda, T.
Division of Cardiology
John Hopkins University School
of Medicine
600 North Wolfe Street
Baltimore MD 21287
USA

Jarajapu, Y.P.
Department of Biomedical and
Biological Sciences
Glasgow Caledonian University
Cowcaddens Road
Glasgow G4 OBA
UK

Joshua, I.G.
Department of Physiology and
Biophysics
University of Louisville
Louisville KY 40292
USA

Kanaide, H.
Department of Molecular Cardiology
Graduate School of Medical Sciences
Kyushu University
Fukuoka 812-8582
Japan

Kanno, M.
Department of Pharmacology
Graduate School of Medicine
Hokkaido University
Sapporo 060-8638
Japan

Kass, D.A.
Division of Cardiology
John Hopkins University School
of Medicine
600 North Wolfe Street
Baltimore MD 21287
USA

Kendall, D.A.
School of Biomedical Sciences
University of Nottingham Medical
School
Queen's Medical Centre
Nottingham NG7 2UH
UK

Kitabatake, A.
Department of Cardiovascular
Medicine
Graduate School of Medicine
Hokkaido University
Sapporo 060-8638
Japan

Kleschyov, A.L.
UMR CNRS 7034
Faculté de Pharmacie
Université Louis Pasteur
de Strasbourg
67401 Illkirch cedex
France

Koslowski, M.
Department of Microbiology and
Pathology
University of Southampton
Southampton General Hospital
Southampton SO16 6YD
UK
Tel: 44 1703 794 827
Fax: 44 1703 796 869
e-mail:
matthiaskoslowski@hotmail.com

Kraemer, R.
Cardiovascular Research Center
Medical College of Wisconsin
8701 Watertown Plank Road
Milwaukee WI 53226
USA

Lameire, N.H.
Renal Unit
Ghent University Hospital
De Pintelaan 185
B-9000 Gent
Belgium

Langton, P.D.
Department of Physiology
University of Bristol
University Walk
Bristol BS8 1TD
UK
Tel: 44 1179 289 142
Fax: 44 1179 288 923
e-mail: phil.langton@bris.ac.uk

Lesage, L.
Division Pathologies Cardiaques
et Vasculaires
Institut de Recherches Servier
11 rue des Moulineaux
92150 Suresnes
France

Lindegger, N.
Department of Zoology and Animal
Biology
University of Geneva
Quai Ernest-Ansermet 30
CH-1211 Geneva 4
Switzerland

Liu, M.-Y.
Department of Pharmacology
Graduate School of Medicine
Hokkaido University
Sapporo 060-8638
Japan

Marrelli, S.P.
Department of Anesthesiology
Baylor College of Medicine
One Baylor Plaza
Houston TX 77030
USA
Tel: 1 713 7987 720
Fax: 1 713 7987 644
e-mail: marrelli@bcm.tmc.edu

Marsh, W.L.
Department of Diagnostic Radiology
Wales Heart Research Institute
University of Wales College of Medicine
Cardiff CF14 4XN
UK

Martin, P.E.M.
Department of Diagnostic Radiology
Wales Heart Research Institute
University of Wales College of Medicine
Cardiff CF14 4XN
UK
Tel: 441 2920 742 912
Fax: 441 2920 744 905
e-mail: martinpe@cardiff.ac.uk

Matoba, T.
Department of Cardiovascular Medicine
Graduate School of Medical Sciences
Kyushu University
Fukuoka 812-8582
Japan

Medhora, M.
Cardiovascular Research Center
Medical College of Wisconsin
8701 Watertown Plank Road
Milwaukee WI 53226
USA
Tel: 1 414 4565 612
Fax: 1 414 4566 515
e-mail: medhoram@mcw.edu

Michaelis, U.R.
Institut für Kardiovaskuläre
Physiologie
Klinikum der J.W. Goethe-Universität
Theodor-Stern-Kai 7
D-60590 Frankfurt am Main
Germany

Minamiyama, Y.
Department of Biochemistry
Osaka City University Medical School
Osaka 545-8585
Japan

Mosse, I.V.
Institute of Pharmacology and
Toxicology
Academy of Medical Sciences
14 Eugene Pottier Street
03057 Kiev
Ukraine

Mukai, Y.
Department of Cardiovascular
Medicine
Graduate School of Medical Sciences
Kyushu University
Fukuoka 812-8582
Japan

Muller, B.
UMR CNRS 7034
Faculté de Pharmacie
Université Louis Pasteur de Strasbourg
67401 Illkirch cedex
France
Tel: 33 3 88 67 69 67
Fax: 33 3 88 66 46 33
e-mail: bmuller@pharma.u-strasbg.fr

Nakashima, M.
Surgical Center
Saga Medical School
Saga 849-8501
Japan

Narayanan, J.
Cardiovascular Research Center
Medical College of Wisconsin
8701 Watertown Plank Road
Milwaukee WI 53226
USA

Nawate, S.
Department of Cardiovascular
Medicine
Graduate School of Medicine
Hokkaido University
Sapporo 060-8638
Japan

Newby, A.C.
Division of Cardiac, Anaesthetic and
Radiologic Sciences
University of Bristol
Bristol Royal Infirmary
Bristol BS2 8HW
UK

Niu, X.
Cardiovascular Research Center
Medical College of Wisconsin
8701 Watertown Plank Road
Milwaukee WI 53226
USA

O'Brien, R.C.
Department of Medicine
Monash University
Clayton, Melbourne
Victoria 3800
Australia

Okada, S.
Department of Pathology
Okayama University
Okayama 700-8558
Japan

Okamoto, H.
Cardiovascular Research Center
Medical College of Wisconsin
8701 Watertown Plank Road
Milwaukee WI 53226
USA

Okamura, T.
Department of Pharmacology
Shiga University of Medical Science
Seta
Ohtsu 520-2192
Japan
Tel: 81 77 548 2181
Fax: 81 77 548 2183
e-mail: okamura@belle.shiga-med.ac.jp

Osipenko, O.N.
Department of Physiology and
Pharmacology
University of Strathclyde
27 Taylor Street
Glasgow G4 ONR
UK

Oyekan, A.O.
Center for Cardiovascular Diseases
Texas Southern University
Houston TX 77004
USA

Pagliaro, P.
Department of Clinical and Biological
Sciences
University of Turin
Orbassano
10041 Turin
Italy

Paolocci, N.
Division of Cardiology
John Hopkins University School of Medicine
600 North Wolfe Street
Baltimore MD 21287
USA
Tel: 1 410 9557 153
Fax: 1 410 9550 852
e-mail: npaolocc@mail.jhmi.edu or
drass@bme.jhu.edu

Parkington, H.C.
Department of Physiology
Monash University
Clayton, Melbourne
Victoria 3800
Australia
Tel: 61 3 9905 2505
Fax: 61 3 9905 2547
e-mail: helena.parkington@med.
monash.edu.au

Parshikov, A.V.
Institute of Pharmacology and
Toxicology
Academy of Medical Sciences
14 Eugene Pottier Street
03057 Kiev
Ukraine

Pathi, V.
Department of Cardiothoracic Surgery
University of Glasgow
Western Infirmary
Glasgow G11 6NT
UK

Pfister, S.L.
Department of Pharmacology and
Toxicology
Medical College of Wisconsin
8701 Watertown Plank Road
Milwaukee WI 53226
USA
Tel: 14 144 568 285
Fax: 14 144 566 545
e-mail: spfister@mcw.edu

Pierce Jr., W.M.
Department of Pharmacology and
Toxicology
University of Louisville
Louisville KY 40292
USA

Prough, R.A.
Department of Biochemistry and
Molecular Biology
University of Louisville
Louisville KY 40292
USA

Quignard, J.F.
Départment Diabéte et Maladies
Métaboliques
Institut de Recherches Servier
11 rue des Moulineaux
92150 Suresnes
France

Randall, M.D.
School of Biomedical Sciences
University of Nottingham Medical
School
Queen's Medical Centre
Nottingham NG7 2UH
UK
Tel: 44 1159 709 484
Fax: 44 1159 709 259
e-mail: michael.randall@nottingham.
ac.uk

Reid, J.L.
Department of Medicine and
Therapeutics
University of Glasgow
Western Infirmary
Glasgow G11 6NT
UK

Reure, H.
Division Pathologies Cardiaques
et Vasculaires
Institut de Recherches Servier
11 rue des Moulineaux
92150 Suresnes
France

Roche, W.R.
Department of Microbiology and
Pathology
University of Southampton
Southampton General Hospital
Southampton SO16 6YD
UK

Roman, R.J.
Cardiovascular Research Center
Medical College of Wisconsin
8701 Watertown Plank Road
Milwaukee WI 53226
USA

Saade, G.R.
Reproductive Sciences
Department of Obstetrics and
Gynecology
University of Texas Medical Branch
Galveston TX 77555-1062
USA

Saavedra, W.F.
Division of Cardiology
John Hopkins University School
of Medicine
600 North Wolfe Street
Baltimore MD 21287
USA

Saboureau, D.
Division Pathologies Cardiaques
et Vasculaires
Institut de Recherches Servier
11 rue des Moulineaux
92150 Suresnes
France

Sakuma, I.
Department of Cardiovascular
Medicine
Graduate School of Medicine
Hokkaido University
Sapporo 060-8638
Japan

Salvetti, A.
Department of Internal Medicine
University of Pisa
Via Roma, 67
56100 Pisa
Italy

Sato, A.
Department of Pharmacology
Graduate School of Medicine
Hokkaido University
Sapporo 060-8638
Japan

Schiestel, D.
UMR CNRS 7034
Faculté de Pharmacie
Université Louis Pasteur
de Strasbourg
67401 Illkirch cedex
France

Schmitz-Winnenthal, F.-H.
Institut für Kardiovaskuläre
Physiologie
Klinikum der J.W. Goethe-Universität
Theodor-Stern-Kai 7
D-60590 Frankfurt am Main
Germany

Segal, S.S.
The John B. Pierce Laboratory
Yale University School of Medicine
290 Congress Avenue
New Haven CT 06519
USA
Tel: 1 203 5629 901 ext. 253
Fax: 1 203 6244 950
e-mail: sssegal@jbpierce.org

Selemidis, S.
Department of Pharmacology
University of Melbourne
Parkville
Victoria 3010
Australia

Shimokawa, H.
Department of Cardiovascular Medicine
Graduate School of Medical Sciences
Kyushu University
Fukuoka 812-8582
Japan
Tel: 81 92 642 5360
Fax: 81 92 642 5374
e-mail: shimo@cardiol.med.kyushu-
u.ac.jp

Sollini, M.
Department of Zoology and Animal
Biology
University of Geneva
Quai Ernest-Ansermet 30
CH-1211 Geneva 4
Switzerland

Soloviev, A.I.
Institute of Pharmacology and
Toxicology
Academy of Medical Sciences
14 Eugene Pottier Street
03057 Kiev
Ukraine
Tel: 38 044 446 02 88
Fax: 38 044 241 88 85
e-mail: s.a.pharm@naverex.kiev.ua

Spitzbarth, N.
Department of Pharmacology and
Toxicology
Medical College of Wisconsin
8701 Watertown Plank Road
Milwaukee WI 53226
USA

Stefanov, A.V.
Institute of Pharmacology and
Toxicology
Academy of Medical Sciences
14 Eugene Pottier Street
03057 Kiev
Ukraine

Stoclet, J.-C.
UMR CNRS 7034
Faculté de Pharmacie
Université Louis Pasteur
de Strasbourg
67401 Illkirch cedex
France

Stuart-Smith, K.
Division of Cardiac, Anaesthetic and
Radiologic
Sciences
University of Bristol
Bristol Royal Infirmary
Bristol BS2 8HW
UK

Suzuki, H.
Department of Physiology
Nagoya City University
Medical School
Mizuho-Ku
Nagoya 467-8601
Japan
Tel: 81 52 853 8129
Fax: 81 52 842 1538
e-mail: hisuzuki@med.nagoya-cu.ac.jp

Taddei, S.
Department of Internal Medicine
University of Pisa
Via Roma, 67
56100 Pisa
Italy
Tel: 390 50 551 110
Fax: 390 50 553 407
e-mail: s.taddei@int.medi.unipi.it

Taheri, M.R.
Cardiovascular Research Center
Medical College of Wisconsin
8701 Watertown Plank Road
Milwaukee WI 53226
USA

Takano, H.
Department of Anatomy
Graduate School of Medicine
Hokkaido University
Sapporo 060-8638
Japan

Takeshita, A.
Department of Cardiovascular
Medicine
Graduate School of Medical Sciences
Kyushu University
Fukuoka 812-8582
Japan

Tare, M.
Department of Physiology
Monash University
Clayton, Melbourne
Victoria 3800
Australia

Thollon, C.
Division Pathologies Cardiaques
et Vasculaires
Institut de Recherches Servier
11 rue des Moulineaux
92150 Suresnes
France

Tishkin, S.M.
Institute of Pharmacology and
Toxicology
Academy of Medical Sciences
14 Eugene Pottier Street
03057 Kiev
Ukraine

Toda, N.
Department of Pharmacology
Shiga University of
Medical Science
Seta
Ohtsu 520-2192
Japan

Triggle, C.
Smooth Muscle Research Group
Department of Pharmacology and
Therapeutics
University of Calgary Faculty of
Medicine
Calgary, Alberta T2N 4N1
Canada

Van de Voorde, J.
Department of Physiology and
Pathophysiology
University of Ghent
De Pintelaan 185
B-9000 Gent
Belgium
Tel: 32 9 240 33 42
Fax: 32 9 240 30 59
e-mail: johan.vandevoorde@rug.ac.be

Vanheel, B.
Department of Physiology and
Pathophysiology
University of Ghent
De Pintelaan 185
B-9000 Gent
Belgium
Tel: 32 9 240 3341
Fax: 32 9 240 3059
e-mail: bert.vanheel@rug.ac.be

Vanhoutte, P.M.
Institut de Recherches Internationales
Servier
6 place des Pléiades
92415 Courbevoie cedex
France

Vedernikov, Y.P.
Reproductive Sciences
Department of Obstetrics and Gynecology
University of Texas Medical Branch
Galveston TX 77555-1062
USA
Tel: 1 409 7470 488
Fax: 1 409 7722 261
e-mail: yvederni@utmb.edu

Vilaine, J.-P.
Division Pathologies Cardiaques
et Vasculaires
Institut de Recherches Servier
11 rue des Moulineaux
92150 Suresnes
France
Tel: 33 1 55 72 2304
Fax: 33 1 55 72 24 30
e-mail: jean.paul.vilaine@fr.netgrs.com

Virdis, A.
Department of Internal Medicine
University of Pisa
Via Roma, 67
56100 Pisa
Italy

Voskuil, C.E.
Cardiovascular Research Center
Medical College of Wisconsin
8701 Watertown Plank Road
Milwaukee WI 53226
USA

Walker, S.D.
Department of Pharmacy and
Pharmacology
University of Bath
Bath BA2 7AY
UK

Watanabe, S.
Department of Anatomy
Graduate School of Medicine
Hokkaido University
Sapporo 060-8638
Japan

Watanuki, S.
Department of Pharmacology
Graduate School of Medicine
Hokkaido University
Sapporo 060-8638
Japan

Weston, A.H.
School of Biological Sciences
University of Manchester
Oxford Road
Manchester M13 9PT
UK

Wigg, S.J.
Department of Medicine
Monash University
Clayton, Melbourne
Victoria 3800
Australia

Willecke, K.
Department of Molecular Genetics
University of Bonn
Römerstraße 164
D-53117 Bonn
Germany
Tel: 49 228 734 210
Fax: 49 228 734 263
e-mail: genetik@uni-bonn.de

Yamamoto, Y.
Department of Physiology
Nagoya City University
Medical School
Mizuho-Ku
Nagoya 467-8601
Japan

Zhang, C.C.
Cardiovascular Research Center
Medical College of Wisconsin
8701 Watertown Plank Road
Milwaukee WI 53226
USA

1　What do gap junctions do anyway?

P.R. Brink, E.C. Beyer and
G.J. Christ

Gap junction channels composed of connexins are the sites that allow the diffusion of small solutes from cell to cell exclusive of the extracellular space. To accomplish this each cell of two adjacent cells contributes half of the connexins required, in the form of a hemichannel, to form a gap junction channel. Three generic gap junction channel types are possible: (a) Channels composed of 12 identical connexins are homomeric/homotypic channels; (b) Heterotypic channels consist of two connexins, six of one type in one hemichannel and six of another in the other; (c) A heteromeric channel contains at least two or more connexins within one hemichannel. The connexins represent a multigene family with at least 15 identified mammalian connexins. The movement of charge through gap junctions necessary for the propagation of action potentials is well established in excitable cells but in non-excitable systems the role of gap junction mediated communication has been harder to illustrate and relate to physiological function. To understand the role gap junction channels might play in tissues such as the vascular wall of arteries and veins it is necessary to determine the various properties that gap junction channels possess. Voltage dependent gating, channel type, permselectivity, regulation/modulation of channel type, gating and permselectivity, and life cycle (connexin assembly/degradation) are all parameters which could potentially affect the transit of a solute from cell to cell and hence any syncytial (multicellular) response.

1. GENERAL PROPERTIES OF GAP JUNCTION CHANNELS

There are five general properties or processes that need to be considered when trying to understand the role of gap junctions in tissues. They are: channel type, gating properties; permselectivity; life cycle; and the regulation/modulation of these properties or processes.

1.1. Channel types

A Gap junction channel is composed of 12 connexin subunit proteins. There are three generic gap junction channel types. There are homotypic gap junctions composed of 12 identical connexin subunit proteins with each cell of an adjacent cell pair contributing two identical halves or hemichannels. A second type is the heterotypic gap junction channel consisting of two distinct connexins, six of one type in one hemichannel and six of another in the other. A third type is a heteromeric gap junction, where at least one of the two hemichannels contains more than one type of connexin. Homotypic channels have been characterized extensively in terms of their biophysical properties (Veenstra *et al.*, 1995, 1994). The majority of heterotypic forms possible using the oocyte system have been reviewed (White and Bruzzone, 1996). Other investigators have demonstrated heterotypic channel types in transfected mammalian cells (Bukauskas *et al.*, 1995; Brink *et al.*, 1997; Valiunas *et al.*, 2000) as well. A number of investigators have presented evidence for heteromeric channel types (Brink *et al.*, 1997; He *et al.*, 1999; Elenes and Moreno, 2000) although there is still some controversy with regard to the physiological significance of these findings.

1.2. Voltage dependent gating

Voltage dependent gating is a hallmark of gap junctions but the transjunctional voltage steps and the durations necessary to elicit reduction in junctional conductance are too large to be of importance under normal physiological conditions. Voltage steps of at least 25–30 mV, but more often 60 mV, with durations of many to hundreds of milliseconds are needed to elicit voltage dependent gating in gap junction channels (Veenstra *et al.*, 1994; Banach *et al.*, 2000; Ramanan *et al.*, 1999). Junctional currents can be recorded in response to voltage steps of different amplitude and sign from a primary culture of smooth muscle cells derived from saphenous vein using dual perforated patch clamp (Figure 1.1).

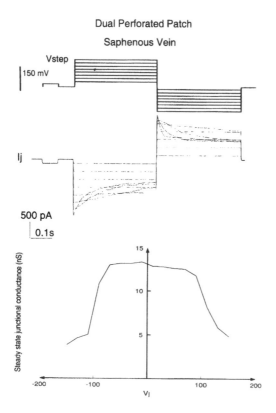

Figure 1.1 Dual perforated patch clamp of an isolated saphenous vein cell pair. The cells were a primary culture derived from an explant. The upper trace illustrates the voltage steps used. One cell of the pair was stepped while the other was held at a potential of Vm = 0 mV. The currents generated in that cell represent junctional current, which is shown as the middle tracing. The lower panel shows the steady state Vj–Gj relationship for the same data set.

In those experiments on saphenous vein smooth muscle the duration of the steps was 400 mS, which might not be sufficient to reach true steady state. Regardless, the reduction in junctional conductance typically observed with large transjunctional voltages is similar to that typically observed for Cx43 transfected into connexin-devoid cells and cardiac cells (Wang and Veenstra, 1997; Wang *et al.*, 1992). Multi-channel recordings are often obtained from cell pairs including vascular smooth muscle (Figure 1.2). In such an experiment one cell of a pair was stepped to 40 mV while the other was held at 0 mV using the dual whole cell recording mode with CsCl as the major salt in the pipettes, the traces are mirror images of each other. The channel behavior is identical to homotypic Cx43 recorded in transfected cells normally devoid of connexin expression. With data like this is possible to determine the mean open and closed times of gap junction channels (Brink *et al.*, 1996a). The average mean open time at ±40 mV was about 2 s and at ±60 mV it is about 1 s. The mean closed time at ±40 mV is about 0.6 s and 0.4 s at ±60 mV. The open probability at ±40 mV is 0.77, and 0.55 at ±60 mV. These values are consistent with the macroscopic data (see Figure 1.1).

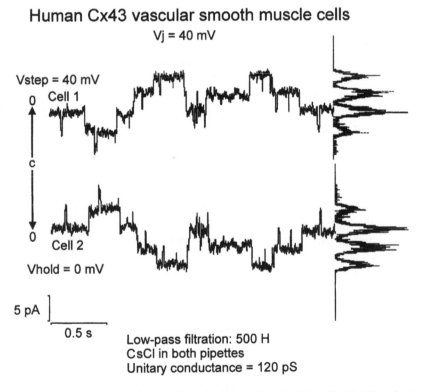

Human Cx43 vascular smooth muscle cells

Vj = 40 mV

Vstep = 40 mV

0   Cell 1

c

0   Cell 2

Vhold = 0 mV

5 pA

0.5 s

Low-pass filtration: 500 H
CsCl in both pipettes
Unitary conductance = 120 pS

Figure 1.2 Multichannel recordings from a cell pair. Vj = 40 mV. The pipette solutions contained CsCl, which reduced non-junctional currents. The recordings are identical in both cells. However, any activity observed in the stepped cell and not in the cell held at Vm = 0 results from the activity of non-junctional channels. The extreme right-hand side of the figure shows amplitude histograms for the two tracings. There are at least four active channels.

In many cases heterotypic Vj–Gj relationships show asymmetry (White and Bruzzone, 1996). This is thought to arise if the gating polarity of the two hemichannels is of opposite sign (Brink *et al.*, 1997; Valiunas *et al.*, 2000). The heteromeric Vj–Gj relationship is typically symmetric but often appears to display weaker voltage dependence than the homotypic counterparts (Beyer *et al.*, 2000; Brink *et al.*, 1997, 2000).

1.3. Permselectivity of gap junction channels

The connexin types present in smooth muscle are Cx40, Cx37, and most dominantly Cx43 (Beyer, 1993). Endothelial cells also contain the same connexins but Cx37 is most abundant *in situ*. These three connexins and all other connexins, which form gap junction channels regardless of type (homotypic, heterotypic or heteromeric (He *et al.*, 1999; Valiunas *et al.*, 2000; Brink *et al.*, 1997; White and Bruzzone, 1996)), display voltage dependent gating. A number of studies have illustrated the basic selectivity properties of Cx43, Cx40 and to a lesser degree Cx37 and Cx45 (Wang and Veenstra, 1997; Beblo and Veenstra, 1997; Veenstra *et al.*, 1994, 1995). Using variants of an established method (Kolodny, 1971) it has been shown that Cx43 allows the passage of ADP and ATP (Goldberg *et al.*, 1998). Transjunctional flux was not determined but rather the equilibrium time was estimated to be 20 minutes from cell to cell. CyclicAMP diffuses through Cx43 channels with a permeation rate 1/10 that of K^+ in ventricular myocytes, and furthermore, is able to affect contractility in recipient cardiac myocytes (Tsien and Weingart, 1976).

In tissues such as the vascular wall where more than one connexin is present, a number of additional questions must be addressed to better understand how gap junction permselectivity might play a role in physiological processes. Examples are whether or not the permselectivity properties are the same for homotypic Cx43, Cx37 and Cx40 or whether or not the properties of heterotypic and heteromeric channels differ significantly.

Conductance data has been collected in a number of studies for Cx43, Cx40 and Cx37 (Figure 1.3; Wang and Veenstra, 1997; Belbo and Veenstra, 1997; Veenstra *et al.*, 1994, 1995; Brink *et al.*, 2000). The approach has been to monitor single channel conductance using different cations while always using Cl^- as the anion, or alternatively, varying the anion and always using K^+ as the cation. The data reveal that there is little variation in cation permeablility among these three connexin types. That is, unitary conductance declines in all three connexin types as salt conductivity declines. The notable differences occur with regard to anions. Both Cx37 and Cx40 gap junction channel unitary conductance changes only slightly with varied anions indicating that these two channels are not very permeant to anions. In contrast, Cx43 shows poor discrimination with regard to cations or anions. As such, the permselectivity properties are different from connexin to connexin. How those properties will affect the transit of charged solutes such as second messengers is still unknown. Extrapolating from the Cx43 data it is clear that a number of second messenger molecules could be sufficiently permeable and have half-lives long enough to warrant consideration as potent cell-to-cell effectors.

For heterotypic and heteromeric channels the permselectivity properties have yet to be determined. Of particular interest are the heteromeric forms and the potential they provide for a varied number of channel types, each of which could possess unique selectivity properties (Elenes and Moreno, 2000; He *et al.*, 1999). Assuming that any

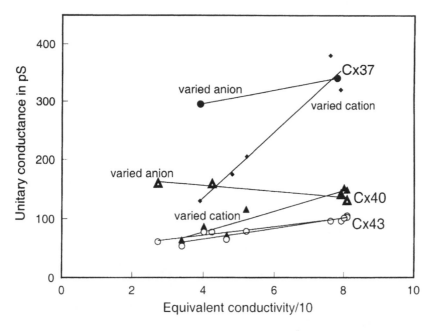

Figure 1.3 Unitary conductance in a particular salt is plotted against conductivity. Unitary conductance for Cx37, Cx40 and Cx43 homotypic channels was determined using different cations and anions. For the data on varied anions K^+ was the cation. For the data on varied cations Cl^- was the anion used. See text for further details. Triangles: Cx40; filled circles diamonds: Cx37; open circles: Cx43.

two connexins have equal affinity for each other and are present in equal amounts yields 192 possible heteromeric forms (Brink *et al.*, 1997).

The normally sparse innervation density in vascular smooth muscle, along with the lack of action potentials, point to gap junction channels as essential in effecting uniform membrane potential among coupled cells. In addition, gap junctions allow the transfer of second messengers such as cyclicAMP, inositolphosphate (IP_3) and calcium (Tsien and Weingart, 1976; Christ *et al.*, 1992; Sneyd *et al.*, 1995; Brink, 1998). Thus both electrotonic current spread and diffusion of signal molecules via gap junctions are potential candidates in coordinating a functional syncytium such as smooth muscle (Christ *et al.*, 1993, 1994, 1999; Christ and Barr, 2000).

1.4. Life cycle

Important factors, which have the potential to affect cell-to-cell coupling, are the synthesis, trafficking and degradation of connexins. Changes in any one of these parameters could result in alteration of the number of gap junction channels functioning to link two cell interiors. The half-life of Cx43 has been determined to be between 1.5 and 3.5 hours (Laird, 1996). Cx37 has similar turnover dynamics in stably transfected cells (Larson *et al.*, 1997). The turnover of Cx40 has not yet been determined. The rapid turnover of connexins implies an ability to modify cell-to-cell coupling over a time frame of hours. Interestingly, tissue modeling has implicated that

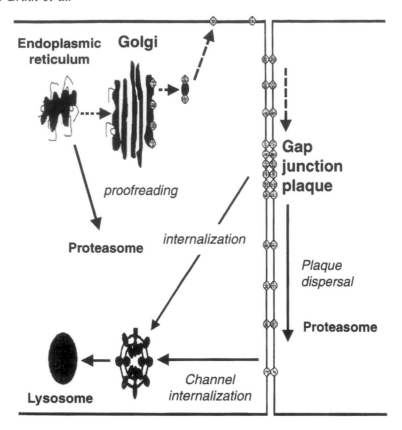

Figure 1.4 Gap junction lifecycle. The processes of biosynthesis, assembly, and degradation of subunit gap junction proteins are illustrated. Cytoplasmic organelles are indicated in bold. Biosynthetic steps are indicated by broken arrows. Proteolytic steps are indicated by solid arrows and italics. The connexin is a polytopic membrane protein which is initially synthesized by Endoplasmic reticulum-associated ribosomes. It is likely that mis-folded (or mis-assembled) connexins are targeted for degradation by the proteasome. Conflicting data suggest that connexins are assembled into hexameric hemichannels either in the endoplasmic reticulum or Golgi apparatus. Hemi-channels dock with counterparts from the adjacent cell, and then associate to form gap junction plaques containing many channels. Degradation of gap junctions involves both the proteasome and the lysosome. Some ultrastructural studies have suggested that gap junctions may be internalized (as "annular gap junctions"), while other studies have supported disruption of plaques. It is reasonable to assume that final digestion of gap junctions occurs in the lysosome. The proteasome may be involved in initial proteolysis of plaques/channels.

the most likely dynamic alteration in coupling associated with life cycle would be a reduction in channel number. Up regulation or increases in channel number are possible and probable but would do little to alter the efficiency of coupling in an already well-coupled system such as vascular smooth muscle (Christ *et al.*, 1994).

Most connexins are synthesized on ribosomes associated with the endoplasmic reticulum (ER) and inserted into the membrane of endoplasmic reticulum such that the loops connecting membrane-spanning regions, which are to become the extra-cellular loops, face its lumen. Hemichannels are formed in the trans-Golgi network (Musil and Goodenough, 1993) or in the endoplasmic reticulum (Falk *et al.*, 1994). The hemichannels are then trafficked to the membrane via vesicles. Such connexin-containing particles/vesicles (in the synthetic or degradative pathway) have been visualized by the expression of Cx43 linked to green fluorescent protein (Jordon *et al.*, 1999). Conversely, gap junction channel/connexin degradation may involve membrane internalization. Connexin proteolysis involves both lysosomal and proteasomal pathways, and it may be regulated by protein ubiquitination and/or phosphorylation (Laird, 1996; Laing and Beyer, 1995; Laing *et al.*, 1997). Various regulatory processes might affect many of the steps of synthesis, trafficking and degradation which in turn define the life cycle of the connexins (Figure 1.4).

1.5. Regulation/modulation of membrane processes: the role of kinases

1.5.1. Kinases affect K and calcium channel activity in vascular smooth muscle

Vascular smooth muscle cells utilize membrane potential as a major tool in determining the magnitude of vasoconstriction and dilatation (Jackson, 2000). The regulation of K channel activity is known to be an important component as action potential mediated excitation is not normally present. In general, hyperpolarization results in dilatation and depolarization results in constriction. Further, a number of studies have shown protein kinase A (PKA), protein kinase G (PKG) and protein kinase C (PKC) messenger systems are integral to vascular responsiveness. A number of vasodilators enhance K channel activity (K_{ATP}, ATP dependent potassium channels) via cyclicAMP linked to protein kinase A and Big potassium channels (BK_{Ca}) via cyclicGMP linked to protein kinase G, while vasoconstrictors, via protein kinase C, inhibit potassium channel activity (K_{ATP}, BK_{Ca} and K_v) (Standen and Qualyle, 1998; Carrier *et al.*, 1997; Fukao *et al.*, 1999). In addition, there is interdependence between calcium influx via L-type channels and ryanodine receptor mediated calcium flux resulting in "sparks". Sparks represent transient (ms) and highly localized elevations of intracellular calcium subjacent to the plasma membrane. Sparks are not sufficient to cause contraction. Thus the calcium flux affects the open probability of BKCa channels, which in turn affect resting potential and tone (Jagger *et al.*, 1998). The greater the spark frequency, the greater the BK_{Ca} activity, resulting in a tendency toward relaxation (Jagger *et al.*, 1998). In addition, L-type calcium channels are also sensitive to the activity of the protein kinases in vascular smooth cells (Obejero-Paz *et al.*, 1998; Belevich *et al.*, 1998). Clearly, the kinases are intimately involved in the modulation of calcium and K^+ channels, and thus their actions on these channels affects vascular tone. Is the same true for gap junction channels?

1.5.2. Are the kinases important to the physiology of gap junctions?

The majority of work devoted to kinase effects on junctional membranes has been in cardiac myocytes and vascular smooth muscle cells (Table 1.1). Most of the observations have been made using dual whole cell patch clamp with only a few observations using dual perforated patch. Application of carbachol or exposure to membrane permeant cyclic GMP resulted in a 30% reduction in junctional conductance, but when the dual perforated patch method was used no change in junctional conductance was observed (Takens-Kwak and Jongsma, 1992). The dose–response curve using heptanol as an uncoupler was the same for whole cell or perforated mode (Takens-Kwak *et al.*, 1992). Activation of protein kinase C via phorbol ester (TPA) in the same system resulted in a 15% increase in junctional conductance in dual whole cell mode while in dual perforated mode the increase was 46% (Kwak *et al.*, 1995c). Not surprisingly, an intact cytosolic environment is an important determinant of the effects of second messenger modulation.

In almost all cases where single channel events were recorded, shifts in the number of events at particular conductive levels were reported in response to activators or inhibitors of kinases. Halothane uncoupling was generally employed to reveal multi-channel activity. The shifts were often correlated with the phosphorylation state of one of the major connexins found in cardiac and vascular smooth muscle, in particular Cx43 (Moreno *et al.*, 1994). In a few studies, dye transfer was also monitored, in an attempt to determine changes in permselectivity. Application of phorbol ester in dual perforated mode or whole cell mode caused junctional conductance to increase but dye spread from cell to cell was reduced (Kwak *et al.*, 1995c). Event histograms of channel conductance versus the number of events in multichannel records revealed a downward shift (i.e. more transitions of lesser conductance). This correlated well with the notion of reduced dye transfer, but is hard to explain in terms of increased

Table 1.1 Messenger mediated kinase effects on macroscopic junctional conductance

	Whole cell	*Perforated cell*	*References*
Rat heart			
8br-cyclicGMP	reduced Gj 24–30%	no effect	TakensKwak and Jongsma, 92 Kwak *et al.*, 95b
Carbachol	reduced Gj ~30%	no effect	TakensKwak and Jongsma, 92
8br-cyclicAMP	no effect	not done	Kwak and Jongsma, 96
8br-cyclicAMP	increased Gj ~30%	not done	Burt and Spray, 88
Phorbol ester (TPA)	15% increase in Gj	46% increase in Gj	Kwak *et al.*, 95c
Isoproterenol	Increased Gj	not done	DeMello, 88
Rat vascular smooth muscle Corpra cavernosa			
8br-cyclicGMP	no effect	not done	Moreno *et al.*, 93
8br-cyclicAMP	no effect	not done	Moreno *et al.*, 93
Phenylephrine	no effect	not done	Moreno *et al.*, 93
Phorbol ester (TPA)	increased Gj 50%	not done	Moreno *et al.*, 93
Isoproterenol	decreased Gj 20%	not done	Moreno *et al.*, 93
A7r5 cells			
8br-cyclicAMP	decreased Gj 15%	not done	Moore *et al.*, 91
8br-cyclicGMP	no effect	not done	Moore *et al.*, 91

macroscopic junctional conductance. Increased open probability for Cx43, and most likely many other connexins, seems an unlikely explanation for the increased conductance as the open probability has been estimated to be near unity when transjunctional voltage is small (Brink *et al.*, 1996a). Further, the greater frequency of events reported in the halothane-induced uncoupling state is not necessarily an indicator of increased open probability (Christ and Brink, 1999). A greater number of events for a particular conductive state could translate into less mean open time and longer closed times. If so, then the data at hand imply recruitment (Kwak *et al.*, 1995c). Only one study has correlated event histograms and amplitude histograms of the same multichannel recording and illustrated that the frequency of events was inversely proportional to the weights of the amplitude histogram for human Cx43 gap junction channels (Christ and Brink, 1999).

2. IS GAP JUNCTION VOLTAGE DEPENDENCE AN IMPORTANT FACTOR IN A FUNCTIONAL SYNCYTIUM LIKE THE VASCULAR WALL?

To answer this question it is necessary to describe the basic function of a vascular syncytium. In this case one can focus on three channel types that play important roles in the maintenance of vascular tone. They are calcium, potassium and gap junction channels. All three of these channels have been implicated in hypertension, either in the form of altered activity, or altered expression (Martens and Gelband, 1998; Giulumian *et al.*, 1999; Arii *et al.*, 1999; Seiden *et al.*, 2000; Haefliger *et al.*, 1997; Moore *et al.*, 1991). Both K and calcium channels are essential in determining the resting potential of any single smooth muscle cell (Jackson, 2000), but it is the gap junction channel that has the potential to create functional (syncytial) groups within a tissue. These considerations beg the question: whether or not in well-coupled cells there is a circumstance where transjunctional voltage is large enough to trigger voltage dependent processes (Figure 1.1).

This is best answered by asking what the expected transjunctional voltage would be during an action potential where the membrane potential can vary over 100 mV. A good example derives from cardiac myocytes, which are excitable. In the heart, a typical ventricular myocyte is 80 μm long with a radius of 7–8 μm, and a myoplasmic resistance of 300–400 ohms-cm. The maximum rate of rise for the action potential is 100 V/s and conduction velocity is 50 cm/s. The predicted maximal transjunctional voltage is 3–4 mV using the relationship $Vc = [(V/s)/\theta]^*L$, where Vc is the voltage drop across the cell, V/s is the maximum rate of rise, θ is the conduction velocity, and L is the cell length. As such, about 0.3 to 0.4 pA passes through each channel assuming that there are about 10,000-gap junction channels/disk (an underestimate). Only when the total number of channels is 1000 or less does the transjunctional voltage from an action potential increase to a magnitude large enough to trigger voltage dependent gating (Brink *et al.*, 1996b). In cases where passive spread occurs, transjunctional voltages are even smaller; assuming that junctional conductance is approximately equal to, or less than, the input resistance of an isolated cell. Vascular smooth muscle and endothelial cells appear to be non-excitable, making transjunctional voltage to seem even less likely to be rate-limiting. While a number of studies have illustrated action potential-like wave forms utilizing non-physiological bath solutions for vascular smooth muscle cells (Geland and Hume, 1992; Yamazaki *et al.*, 1992; Cole *et al.*, 1996) none has provided direct evidence that these waveforms are propagated. Further, there has been no demonstration of conducted action potentials under normal physiological conditions. The small transjunctional voltages predicted to occur across gap junctions in response to electrical signals, whether passively or actively spread, indicate that voltage dependent gating of gap junctions is not important physiologically. In this light, it is questionable whether there is regulation or modulation of voltage-dependence, which might render it physiologically relevant. If so, the kinases are likely candidates to be involved in such a process, in terms of regulation, mainly because of the potential phosphorylation sites on C-terminus of the connexins (Lau *et al.*, 2000). The question then becomes: Is voltage dependence subject to regulation or modulation via kinases? The answer to this question is no. Indeed, activation of protein kinase A and C did not alter the kinetics or steady state voltage gating in human corpus cavernosum cells (Moreno *et al.*, 1993).

3. WHAT DO GAP JUNCTIONS DO IN VASCULAR SMOOTH MUSCLE?

Coordinated contraction or relaxation of vascular smooth muscle is not the result of propagated action potentials. A coordinated contractile response can be initiated by a neurotransmitter for example but the mechanism necessary to recruit cells in sparsely innervated tissue along with long diffusion distances, transmitter volatility, tortuosity factors, and neuronal and non-neuronal uptake processes argue against sufficient transmitter concentration to activate all the cells throughout the vascular wall (Bevan and Torok, 1970; Hirst and Neilds, 1978; Christ *et al.*, 1993; Ramanan *et al.*, 1998).

There is growing evidence for the role of gap junctions in coordinated contraction and relaxation in vascular smooth muscle (Christ *et al.*, 1993, 1994, 1999; Ramanan *et al.*, 1998). The following observations lend support to the notion that one or a few cells are activated by synaptic release of a transmitter on the basalar/adventitial border which results in the generation of messengers able to diffuse from cell to subsequent cell within the vascular wall resulting in each cell contracting. The observations are: (a) Contraction in response to phenylephrine is inhibited by heptanol (a known uncoupling agent); (b) Heptanol is ineffective in inhibiting KCl induced contractions; (c) Heptanol effectiveness in inhibiting phenylephrine contractions is dependent on the exposure-time. The longer the time of phenylephrine exposure (many minutes), the less effective heptanol is in reducing the amplitude of contraction (Figure 1.5); (d) Pre-exposure to heptanol always results in reduced contractile response upon exposure to phenylephrine but contractile force increases as the duration of exposure to alpha adrenergic agonists increases; and (e) The time course of cell shortening in freshly isolated cells for KCl or phenylephrine induced contraction is on the order of seconds.

Heptanol's ineffectiveness in blocking KCl contraction is consistent with diffusion of K^+ throughout the vascular wall. The time to half concentration for a $100\,\mu m$ wall thickness is 10 sec for K^+ where the extracellular diffusion coefficient (D_e) is $1.7 \times 10^{-5}\,cm^2/s$. D_e for K^+ in the rat aortic wall was estimated to be $3 \times 10^{-7}\,cm^2/s$ (Christ *et al.*, 1999) based on the rising phase (Tau of one to two minutes) of contraction in organ bath for a 100 μm thick wall. The approximately 50x suppression ($1.7 \times 10^{-5}/3 \times 10^{-7}$) is thought to be the due to tortousity factors. The slow one to two minute Tau for KCl induced contraction is consistent with the suppressed diffusion coefficient. There is no need for gap junctions in this case as all the cells are bathed in elevated K^+ within a few minutes and thus stimulated to contract.

How is it possible for heptanol to block the phenylephrine response? If heptanol is applied a few minutes after phenylephrine application it causes a reduction in contractile strength. If it is applied 25 minutes or longer after phenylephrine application then it is unable to cause a significant reduction in contraction (Christ et al., 1999). This observation is consistent with phenylephrine stimulating the cells at the advential/medial border (and perhaps the endothelial smooth muscle border?) to produce a message, which must diffuse to the subjacent layer via gap junctions. This assumes heptanol diffuses rapidly enough to penetrate a few cell layers deep to effect a blockade of junctional communication deeper into the vascular wall. With prolonged phenylephrine exposure, phenylephrine directly activates more cells, as it slowly diffuses deeper into the vascular wall. With longer exposure times, therefore, phenylephrine removes the need for gap junction-mediated signaling. An estimate of $D_e = 5 \times 10^{-8}$ cm²/s for phenylephrine in the vascular wall (100 μm thickness) has also been made on the basis of the time dependent heptanol blockade (Christ et al., 1999). Early estimates of the D_e for phenylephrine diffusion into the vascular wall were in the 10^{-7} cm²/s range (Bevan and Torok, 1970). An underlying assumption is that the diffusion of the intercellular signal (message) must be on the order of the K^+ diffusion rate through the extracellular space in the vascular wall.

The aforementioned discussion considers exclusively the role of intercellular communication among myocytes in the modulation of vascular tone. Heterocellular (extracellular or intercellular) communication between endothelial cells and myocytes is also critical to the control of vascular tone (Little et al., 1995; Xia et al., 1995; Dora et al., 1997; Bartlett and Segal, 2000; Emerson and Segal, 2000). Additional physiological and biophysical considerations come into play when evaluating intercellular communication between these very distinct vascular wall cell types. For example, differential cellular volumes and impedance mismatches must be overcome for physiologically relevant intercellular signal spread to occur. Another issue that warrants consideration is that the opportunity for heterocellular cell to cell contact is diminished by the presence of the internal elastic lamina. Both the former and the latter issues will be exacerbated in progressively larger vessels as the number of layers of myocytes increases. Finally, the opportunity for, and probability of, both heteromeric and heterotypic channels is greater, in light of the presence of the third connexin subtype in endothelial cell, that is, Cx37.

In free solution the diameter of K^+ unhydrated is 0.27 nm and D_e is 1.7×10^{-5} cm²/s. For phenylephrine whose size is 0.6 nm (unhydrated, between the size of glucose and lactose) the predicted D_e in free solution is 5×10^{-6} cm²/s. Thus the apparent suppression factor for phenylephrine (free solution versus vascular wall; $1.7 \times 10^{-5}/1 \times 10^{-7}-5 \times 10^{-8}$) is 50–100×, similar to K^+. Using the standard relationship ($x_{1/2} = 0.67\sqrt{D_e^* T}$) to estimate the distance ($x_{1/2}$) 50% of the molecules have traveled for some time T reveals that for K^+ 50% reach a distance of 90 μm with a D_e of 3×10^{-7} at 300 s. For phenylephrine 50% reach 90 μm with a D_e of 5×10^{-8} at $T = 1500$ s. Thus the difference in D_e for K^+ and phenylephrine in the vascular wall is consistent with the K^+ contraction insensitivity to heptanol and the sensitivity

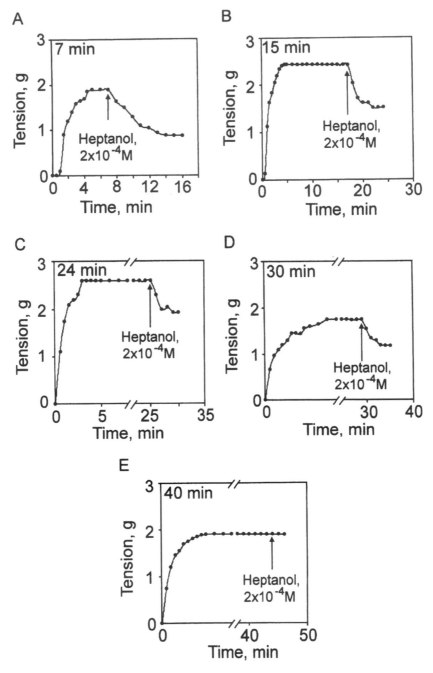

Figure 1.5 Addition of heptanol (2×10^{-4} M) resulted in a time-dependent relaxation of the phenylephrine-induced contraction. The magnitude of the observed heptanol-induced relaxation diminished with increased time after the addition of phenylephrine, in the continued presence of the agent. For these experiments, all tissues were equivalently pre-contracted to about 80% of their respective maxima. Reproduced from Christ *et al.*, 1999, with permission.

of the phenylephrine contraction to the latter. Taken together, these data and interpretation strongly suggest a physiological role for gap junctions in vascular smooth muscle.

4. CONCLUSIONS

With five distinct parameters to modulate gap junctions, spread out among the three distinct connexin types known to be present in the vascular wall, there are clearly many physiological scenarios available to regulate intercellular communication in the vasculature. One must further consider this incredible diversity/plasticity in junctional communication in light of the tremendous diversity in density and geometry of the perivascular innervation, as well as the structure and histology of different segments of the vascular network. When viewed in this context, it is clear that intercellular communication through gap junctions can play manifold roles in the initiation, maintenance and modulation of vascular tone in blood vessels throughout the vascular tree. Therefore, elucidating the precise role of intercellular communication in modulating tone in physiologically distinct vasculature will be critical to the improved understanding of vascular function, as well as the etiology and therapy of vascular disease.

2 Cardiovascular gap junctions: functional diversity, complementation and specialization of connexins

Klaus Willecke

This chapter reviews recent results related to the characterization of cardiovascular vascular gap junctions. The functions of connexin40, -43 and -45 have been studied using targeted mouse mutants of these genes. The following results are discussed: impaired myocardial conduction and vasodilatation along arterioles of connexin40 deficient mice; additive effects of connexin40 and -43 on ventricular conduction and cardiac morphogenesis; vascular maturation depending on connexin45 during embryonic development; and functional replacement of connexin43 by connexin32 or -40 and endothelium-specific ablation of connexin43 in transgenic mice.

Connexins are the protein subunits of vertebrate gap junctions, which are intercellular channels through which ions, metabolites and second messenger molecules below a molecular mass of about 1000 Daltons can diffuse. Gap junctions are organized in most tissues as plaques, which are aggregates consisting of few to many thousands of channels. Although these structures look similar when studied by electron microscopy, it was found that connexin proteins are encoded by a large gene family of at least 15 related genes in the mammalian genome (Simon and Goodenough, 1998; Manthey *et al.*, 1999). These genes are differentially expressed depending on the cell type. Some connexin genes are expressed in very few cell types, others are active in many but not all cell types. For unknown reasons, all types of cell appear to express more than one connexin. In ectopic expression systems, like Xenopus oocytes or transfected mammalian cells (Willecke and Haubrich, 1997), connexins can contribute to homotypic or heterotypic gap junction channels that are formed by docking of two hemichannels comprised of the same or different connexin isoforms, respectively. Some types of connexin hemichannels appear to be incompatible. In addition, at least some of the connexin proteins can be assembled to heteromeric hemichannels consisting of different subunits (Brink *et al.*, 1997).

The existence of the large connexin gene family in comparison with the relative uniform structure led researchers to question why so many different but related connexin genes have been generated and maintained during evolution. Most likely there must be functional differences between gap junctions in different organs or cell types. In order to verify this prediction, it is necessary to compare cells or whole animals deficient in one of the connexin genes with the wild type situation. The only mammal where mutations can be introduced at any targeted position in the genome is the laboratory mouse. Thus, several connexin-deficient mouse mutants have been generated and characterized.

Table 2.1 Expression of connexins in different regions of myocardium and blood vessel walls of the mouse

Myocardium	Blood vessel wall
Atria: Cx40, Cx45, Cx43 (low)	Endothelium: Cx37, Cx40, Cx43
Atrioventricular node: Cx40, Cx45	Smooth muscle cells: Cx40[2], Cx43[2], Cx45
His bundle: Cx40, Cx45	
Purkinje fibers: Cx40 (proximal parts)	
Cx40, Cx43 (distal parts)	
Ventricles: Cx43[1]	
(working myocardium)	

Notes
1 Besides high levels of Cx43, very low levels of Cx40 and Cx45 appear to be expressed in the ventricular wall.
2 The expression level of Cx40 and Cx43 differs in capillaries, arterioles, and arteries.

This chapter summarizes recent results from the author's laboratory, describing the function of cardiovascular gap junctions in the mouse. In the atrium of mouse myocardium, connexin(Cx)40, -43, and -45 are expressed. In conductive ventricular myocardium, Cx40 and -45 were found and the ventricular myocardium expressed mainly Cx43 and probably to a much lesser extent Cx40 and Cx45 (Table 2.1). It was postulated many years ago that the intercellular propagation of action potentials that leads to contraction of the heart is mediated by gap junction channels. Furthermore, the coordinated blood flow by adaptation of the arterial lumen to different physiological needs may at least partially depend on functional gap junction channels between smooth muscle cells and/or endothelial cells. The characterization of transgenic mouse mutants deficient in the mentioned connexin genes should – at least in principle – allow us to clarify the extent to which the postulated functions of cardiovascular gap junctions can be fulfilled by the different connexins expressed.

1. IMPAIRED MYOCARDIAL IMPULSE PROPAGATION AND VASODILATATION ALONG ARTERIES IN CONNEXIN40 DEFICIENT MICE

Cx40 deficient mice are viable and fertile (Kirchhoff *et al.*, 1998; Simon *et al.*, 1998). Thus, either the lack of Cx40 gap junction channels has no effect on development or it can be compensated by other connexins which may be expressed together with Cx40 in the same cells. Upregulation of another myocardial connexin was not found in hearts of adult Cx40 deficient mice. Since several of the electrocardiographic parameters were prolonged, it was concluded that Cx40 deficient mice exhibited lower atrial and ventricular conduction velocities compared to wild type mice (Kirchhoff *et al.*, 1998; Simon *et al.*, 1998). About 20% of Cx40 deficient mice showed atrium derived abnormalities in the cardiac rhythm but none of the wild type mice tested did (Kirchhoff *et al.*, 1998). In these experiments, avertin was used as anesthetic for transgenic mice and controls. No cardiac arrhythmias were observed in independently generated Cx40 deficient mice of similar genetic background (Simon *et al.*, 1998), studied with another anesthetic, sodium pentobarbital. Thus, the frequency of arrhythmias may be influenced by the narcotic agent. In order to solve this discrepancy, Cx40 deficient mice are currently being studied by means of telemetric measurements of the electrocardiogram in the conscious state. A more detailed study of the Cx40 deficient mice showed that the Cx40 deficiency affects sinusnode function and is associated with disturbances in sinoatrial and atrioventricular conduction. Furthermore, atrial tachyarrhythmias could be induced by atrial burst pacing using transesophageal stimulation in Cx40 deficient mice but not in heterozygous or wild type mice (Hagendorff *et al.*, 1999). This has also been found with epicardial electrodes in open chest mice under urethane anesthesia. Atrial conduction velocity was reduced by 30% in the Cx40 deficient heart but ventricular conduction was unaffected. This led to the conclusion that Cx40 channels are important determinants of conduction in the atrium and in the atrio-ventricular conduction system (Verheule *et al.*, 1999). Most recently, using an array of more than two hundred electrodes on the heart of open-chest mice, it was found that the Cx40 deficient mice suffer from a right bundle branch block in the myocardium (van Rijen *et al.*, 2000).

The conduction of vasomotor signals has also been studied along arterioles of the cremaster muscle of male Cx40 deficient mice (de Wit *et al.*, 2000). Short pulses of hyperpolarizing endothelium-derived vasodilators, depolarizing K^+ solutions or norepinephrine were locally applied and the amplitudes of vasodilatation along the arterioles were recorded. The spreading of vasodilatations, triggered by acetylcholine or bradykinin, was reduced markedly in Cx40 deficient mice, whereas vasoconstrictions, induced by K^+, decreased equally with distance in Cx43 deficient and wild type mice. The arterial blood pressure was about 25% higher in Cx40 deficient mice than in wild type mice. Future experiments have to decide whether this result was due to lack of Cx40 in the endothelium or perhaps due to the nerve activity-dependent regulation of blood flow (de Wit *et al.*, 2000). These results provide direct experimental proof that connexin activity can contribute to the regulation of blood flow and affect blood pressure. Whether or not other vascular connexins (Table 2.1) also contribute to impulse propagation in vascular walls and impair blood pressure is not yet known.

2. ADDITIVE EFFECTS OF CONNEXIN40 AND -43 ON VENTRICULAR CONDUCTION AND CARDIAC MORPHOGENESIS

Mice deficient in Cx43 died postnatally with a morphological abnormality of the heart (Reaume *et al.*, 1995). The right ventricular outflow tract was blocked so that blood could not be aerated in the lung. This is probably due to abnormal migration of neural crest cells which contribute to the morphogenesis of the right ventricular outflow tract (Huang *et al.*, 1998). Heterozygous Cx43(+/−) mice were viable and exhibited no severe defects in cardiac morphogenesis, although conflicting results on the conduction velocity in the myocardium of these mice have been published (Thomas *et al.*, 1998; Morley *et al.*, 1999). Cx40(−/−) mice showed reduced cardiac conduction but only mild morphological defects (Kirchhoff *et al.*, 1998). When investigating to what extent Cx40 and Cx43 can complement one another in cardiac morphogenesis and physiology, it appeared that all double mutants Cx40(−/−)/Cx43(+/−) showed cardiac malformations and died postnatally. In most of these animals common atrioventricular junctions with abnormal atrioventricular connection were found, much more severe than that seen occasionally in Cx40(−/−) mice. Furthermore, ventricular septal defects, premature closure of the ductus arteriosis and subcutaneous edemas were noted. The analysis of electrocardiograms of adult double heterozygous (Cx40(+/−)/Cx43(+/−) mice showed that both connexins had additive effects on ventricular, but not on atrial conduction. Cx40 and Cx43 proteins are coexpressed only in distal parts of ventricular conductive myocardium. Since Cx43 haploinsuffiency worsened the morphological phenotype of Cx40 deficiency, whereas Cx40 haploinsuffiency did not alter the phenotype of Cx43 deficiency, the functions of the Cx40 and Cx43 in cardiac morphogenesis are likely to be specific for each connexin isotype (Kirchhoff *et al.*, 2000). The molecular mechanisms which underlie the complementary, isotype specific effects of Cx40 and Cx43 in myocardium remain to be elucidated but the general effects of two connexins expressed in the same organ (i.e., additive and isotype specific functions) may also be valid for other organs.

3. CONNEXIN45 IS ESSENTIAL FOR VASCULAR MATURATION DURING EMBRYONIC DEVELOPMENT

In order to check the expression pattern of the Cx45 gene based on studies using Cx45 antibodies, a LacZ reporter gene was engineered in place of the Cx45 coding region in mouse embryonic stem cells. This generated Cx45 deficient mice (Krüger *et al.*, 2000). Using tissues from Cx45(+/−) heterozygous mice, the expression of the LacZ gene was analyzed by X-Gal staining which reflects the expression of Cx45 mRNA. Unexpectedly, X-Gal staining was found in all tissues where vascular or visceral smooth muscle cell layers had been cross-sectioned (Figure 2.1A). This finding was verified by isolation of the aorta and preparation of protein extracts which were used for immunoblotting with Cx45 antibodies. The general expression of Cx45 in smooth muscle cells has not been noticed before, presumably because the gap junction plaques in these cells are too small to be detected by immunofluorescence signals.

Cx45 deficient mouse embryos died between embryonic day 9.5 and 10.5. Abnormal maturation of blood vessels was observed in the yolk sac, placenta and embryo proper. In the Cx45 deficient yolk sac, initially formed blood vessels were not remodelled into a tree of appropriately sized, distinct vessels; instead a large endothelium-lined vascular lumen was present. In the labyrinthine part of the placenta, less branching of the embryonic vessels and invasion of maternal sinuses were found. In Cx45(−/−) embryos, the dorsal aortae were narrowed or absent, except for a normal or dilated part near the tail. The hearts of most Cx45 deficient embryos were dilated in the left ventricle, possibly because of overload due to the narrow embryonic vessels. Furthermore, the Cx45 deficient arteries failed to develop a smooth muscle cell layer. Taken together, these findings indicate that the Cx45(−/−) embryos die from malnutrition and shortage of aerated blood. The different effects of the lack of Cx45 in different parts of the embryonic vasculature imply the existence of different signaling pathways regulating intra- and extraembryonic vascular development. Furthermore, it is possible that some functions of Cx45 could be taken over by an(other) connexin(s) expressed in these cells of embryonic blood vessels.

The amount of transforming growth factor TGFβ1 in the epithelial layer of the yolk sac and in the myocardium was strongly decreased at embryonic day 9.5, relative to wild type embryos (Krüger *et al.*, 2000). Thus, Cx45 is required for the maintenance of TGF β1 expression in the yolk sac and heart. These findings led to the conclusion

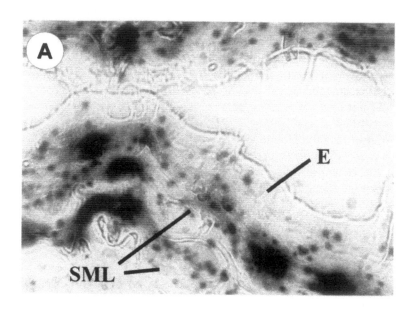

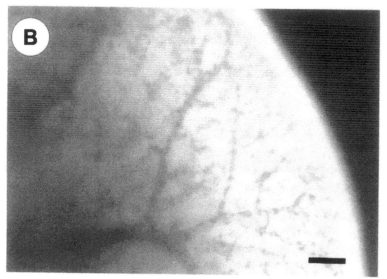

Figure 2.1 A. Transcriptional expression of the Cx45 gene in adult blood vessels of Cx45$^{+/-}$ mice, indicated by LacZ staining (Krüger *et al.*, 2000). The smooth muscle cell layer (SML) of the cross-sectioned mouse aorta is stained intensely blue. Only occasionally weak signals were observed in the endothelium (E). Thus, we conclude that the Cx45 gene is expressed in smooth muscle cells of the blood vessel wall. Scale bar: 15 μm. B. Transcriptional activity of the Cx43 gene in blood vessels of 11.5 dpc embryonic brain detected by LacZ staining of a Cx43$^{fl/+}$; TIE2-Cre-mouse. TIE2-Cre-mediated deletion of the floxed Cx43 allele led to expression of nuclear-localized β-galactosidase activity under control of transcriptional regulatory elements of the Cx43 gene. Based on colocalization of β-galactosidase activity with other markers we conclude that the deletion of the Cx43 gene has occurred in virtually all endothelial cells (Theis *et al.*, submitted for publication, 2000b). Scale bar: 150 μm.

that some of the cardiovascular defects might be due to failure of TGF β1 to trigger specific signaling pathways. It should be of interest to elucidate the molecular mechanism of vascular development in which Cx45 is involved.

Very recently Kumai *et al.* (2000) have also described the characterization of Cx45 deficient mice. These authors noticed that the cardiac walls of these mice displayed an endocardial cushion defect. Furthermore, the level of the Ca^{2+} dependent transcription factor NF-ATC1 was strongly decreased in Cx45 (−/−) endocardium. It remains to be investigated whether the vascular or the cardiac abnormalities occur first in Cx45 deficient mouse embryos.

4. CONNEXIN32 AND -43 CAN FUNCTIONALLY REPLACE CONNEXIN43 IN THE MYOCARDIUM BUT NOT DURING GAMETOGENESIS

In order to distinguish between general and specialized functions of connexin genes, we generated two connexin "knock-in" mice (Plum *et al.*, 2000). These are mouse mutants in which the coding region of Cx43 has been removed and the coding DNAs of Cx32 or Cx40 have been inserted instead (designated as Cx43KI32 or Cx43KI40 mice). Both experiments were carried out using the "double replacement" method of homologous recombination in embryonic stem cells (Theis *et al.*, 2000a). Heterozygous mice in which only one allele of Cx43 had been replaced by Cx32 or Cx40 (i.e., Cx43$^{43/32}$ or Cx43$^{43/40}$) were fertile and coexpressed the inserted connexin gene together with Cx43 in all tissues where Cx43 is normally expressed. Heterozygous mothers (Cx43$^{43/32}$) could not breast-feed normal size litters to weaning age. Since their breasts were full of milk, it is likely that the milk could not be ejected, possibly because the myoepithelial cells did not contract sufficiently (Plum *et al.*, 2000). Cx43 was expressed in myoepithelial cells in the alveolar periphery, while Cx32 (and Cx26) were expressed in mammary epithelium (Pozzi *et al.*, 1995). Perhaps aberrant gap junction communication in the epithelium and myoepithelium compartments in the breast of Cx43$^{43/32}$ mice could cause this effect. Heterozygous Cx43$^{43/40}$ mothers did not show this phenomenon.

Homozygous mouse mutants (Cx43KI32 and Cx43KI40) showed normal life expectancy but were infertile. The hearts of Cx43KI32 mice exhibited very mild morphological defects, whereas the hearts of Cx43KI40 mice appeared normal. Spontaneous ventricular arrhythmias were observed in most Cx43KI40 mice and rarely in Cx43KI32 mice but were not found in controls (Plum *et al.*, 2000). Thus, the inserted Cx32 or Cx40 can largely rescue the cardiac defect (block of the right ventricular outflow tract) seen in Cx43 deficient mice (Reaume *et al.*, 1995). Although Cx43 deficient mice die shortly after birth, embryos of both sexes show severe germ cell deficiency at embryonic day 11.5, before the onset of overt sexual dimorphism (Juneja *et al.*, 1999). This deficiency can be partially compensated by Cx32 or Cx40, since the ovaries of female Cx43KI32 or Cx43KI40 mice appear to be normal, although these animals show largely reduced fertility. The corresponding male mice are infertile. Secondary spermatogonia or further differentiated stages of spermatogenesis were never found in these animals. Therefore, Cx32 and Cx40 cannot rescue the defects in male spermatogenesis which apparently require the expression of Cx43. We do not know the exact cell type and mechanism for which the expression of Cx43 is essential during spermatogenesis. It should also be noted that Cx43KI32 and Cx43KI40 mice are considerably smaller than wild type controls of the same age. Thus, there is also a non-compensated effect on the body size. These results suggest that the diversity of connexin genes is due to functional specialization of gap junctional intercellular communication in certain cell types and tissues. Some functional requirements can be met more or less efficiently by other connexin isoforms.

5. ENDOTHELIUM SPECIFIC ABLATION OF CONNEXIN43

As mentioned, the deletion of Cx43 in the whole mouse genome led to postnatal lethality, thus precluding functional studies of the Cx43 gene in older mice. In order to circumvent this problem, the Cx43 coding region in transgenic mice was flanked by loxP sites, namely recognition sites of the cre recombinase. In addition, these mice carry a silent LacZ reporter gene that becomes transcriptionally activated after Cx43 deletion in those cells in which the Cx43 promoter is active. These mice were crossed with other transgenic mice that expressed the cre recombinase under control of TIE2 transcriptional elements specifically in endothelial cells. In the progeny of these crosses, specific LacZ expression was found in all endothelial cells (Theis *et al.*, 2000b) (Figure 2.1B). The results indicate widespread endothelial expression of Cx43 during embryonic development but in adult mice this expression was limited to capillaries and small vessels. When the floxed Cx43 mice were crossed with other mice that expressed the cre recombinase ubiquitously, similar endothelial levels of LacZ expression were found as observed after crossing with TIE2-cre mice. Thus, this experimental method allowed estimation that Cx43 was deleted from nearly all the endothelial cells in these mice. The Cx43 flox/-TIE2-cre mice were viable and developed normally. These mice did not have an altered arterial blood pressure (Theis *et al.*, 2000b), unlike mice deficient for Cx40 (that is also expressed in endothelial cells; Table 2.1) which exhibit an elevated arterial blood pressure compared to control mice (de Wit *et al.*, 2000). Thus, the functional roles of Cx43 and Cx40 in endothelial cells appear to be different, although it is possible that the elevation in arterial blood pressure may be a consequence of Cx40 lacking in other than endothelial cells. The specific ablation of Cx43 in the endothelium should provide a useful tool to clarify the role of this connexin in endothelial functions, such as regulation of vascular tone, wound healing and arteriosclerosis.

6. CONCLUSIONS

Different connexin subunits appear to contribute in an additive and complementary manner to cardiovascular gap junctions. In none of these cases, however, were the ions and/or metabolites identified which diffuse through these channels and cause the effects described. In order to fully understand the functional characteristics of connexin channels, it is necessary to identify these molecules and clarify how the different connexin channels are involved in intercellular signalling. The functional characterization of connexin mouse mutants can provide more and more detailed insights into the molecular physiology of gap junction channels. General "knock-out" mutants, in which most or all of the coding region of a connexin gene is lacking, can give hints to the general function of a given connexin gene. When the general "knock-out" mutation is lethal, as in the case of Cx43 and Cx45, it is necessary to bypass this lethality by generating inducible or cell type specific connexin mutants. Eventually, this increasingly refined approach should also provide an answer to the question: To what extent does the action of endothelium-derived hyperpolarizing factor(s) require gap junctions in the vascular wall?

ACKNOWLEDGMENTS

I would like to thank my coworkers for their enthusiasm and hard work in finishing the mentioned projects in our laboratory. The help of Olaf Krüger and Martin Theis with the preparation of Figure 2.1 and critical reading of this manuscript is gratefully acknowledged. Our investigations were supported by grants of the Deutsche For-schungsgemeinschaft (SFB 284, projects C1 and C6; SFB 400, project B3), by the Biomed program of the European Community and by the Fonds der Chemischen Industrie.

3 Endothelium and smooth muscle pathways for conduction along resistance microvessels

Steven S. Segal, Geoffrey G. Emerson and Iain S. Bartlett

Blood flow control involves the interplay of signaling between endothelial cells and smooth muscle cells in vascular resistance networks. The conduction of electrical signals along the blood vessel wall through gap junctions is highly effective at coordinating vasodilatation (through hyperpolarization) and vasoconstriction (through depolarization) via electromechanical coupling in smooth muscle. In the hamster cheek pouch, the signals for vasodilatation and vasoconstriction conduct along arterioles. In the cheek pouch retractor muscle, the signal for vasodilatation conducts along arterioles and feed arteries, while constriction spreads via perivascular sympathetic nerves. To define the roles of endothelium and smooth muscle as conduction pathways in resistance microvessels of these tissues, intracellular recording and selective light-dye damage to endothelial cells or to smooth muscle cells were performed. In cheek pouch arterioles, homologous coupling within endothelium and within smooth muscle provides parallel pathways for electrical signaling, with the specificity of the stimulus determining which cell layer is effective. Thus, depolarization (e.g., to phenylephrine) is conducted along the smooth muscle layer, independently of the endothelium. In turn, hyperpolarization (e.g., to acetylcholine) conducts along the endothelium (releasing EDHF) and also along the smooth muscle. For feed arteries of the retractor muscle, endothelial cells conduct hyperpolarization; although the smooth muscle cells are ineffective as a conduction pathway, they are electrically coupled to endothelial cells. Such differences in the nature of cell-to-cell coupling between vascular beds may reflect corresponding variations in the functional expression of gap junctions. Nevertheless, across tissues, conduction along the endothelium coordinates relaxation of smooth muscle within and among resistance microvessels, whether through EDHF release or through direct electrical coupling.

Peripheral vascular resistance begins with feed arteries, which control the volume of blood flowing into the tissue (Williams and Segal, 1993). Upon entering the tissue, feed arteries give rise to the arteriolar network, which controls the distribution and magnitude of blood flow throughout the tissue. Vasodilatation and vasoconstriction can be integrated and coordinated within resistance networks through the initiation of electrical signals which conduct through gap junctions between smooth muscle cells and endothelial cells in the vessel wall (Segal and Duling, 1986; Little *et al.*, 1995a; Xia *et al.*, 1995b; Welsh and Segal, 1998; Emerson and Segal, 2000a,b). Initial studies of the conduction of electrical signals in arterioles disregarded the endothelial cell layer and assumed that coupling between adjacent smooth muscle cells provided the signaling pathway (Hirst and Neild, 1978). However, both electrical and dye coupling between endothelial cells are prevalent in arterioles and feed arteries (Welsh and Segal, 1998; Emerson and Segal, 2000a). Whereas homologous coupling within respective cell layers has been confirmed in cheek pouch arterioles (Little *et al.*, 1995b; Welsh and Segal, 1998), the nature of coupling between smooth muscle cells and endothelial cells has remained controversial. In isolated arterioles and resistance arteries, heterologous 'myoendothelial' gap junctions and electrical coupling have appeared to be manifest (Little *et al.*, 1995b; Sandow and Hill, 2000; Emerson and Segal, 2000b). In contrast, for arterioles controlling blood flow in the cheek pouch, smooth muscle cell and endothelial cell layers have appeared to be electrically distinct (Welsh and Segal, 1998), with smooth muscle cell hyperpolarization and relaxation reflecting the release of EDHF (Welsh and Segal, 2000). Such differences between studies may reflect regional variation in the functional expression of gap junctions, in signal transduction pathways, as well as experimental conditions.

This brief review is concerned with defining the properties of conduction in resistance microvessels, with particular attention given as to how these properties can vary between tissues that differ in structure and function. It focuses on the hamster cheek pouch and its contiguous retractor muscle (Grasby *et al.*, 1999), as these preparations are used routinely to study microvascular flow control in epithelium and skeletal muscle, respectively, and have provided key insight into the nature of conducted vasomotor responses (Segal and Duling, 1986; Xia and Duling, 1995a; Xia *et al.*, 1995b; Welsh and Segal, 1998; Segal *et al.*, 1999; Bartlett and Segal, 2000; Emerson and Segal, 2000a,b). For both tissues, the microvessels studied (i.e., arterioles and feed arteries) typically contain a single, continuous layer of smooth muscle cells wrapped circumferentially around a monolayer of endothelial cell (Haas and Duling, 1997; Bartlett and Segal, 2000; Emerson and Segal, 2000a,b).

1. METHODS

Experiments were performed *in vivo* using the cheek pouch or retractor muscle of male hamsters anesthetized with sodium pentobarbital (65 mg/kg). The inability to perform intracellular recording from arterioles embedded within skeletal muscle fibers, or from feed arteries *in vivo* (which pulse with arterial pressure), led to *in vitro* experiments on intact, pressurized vessel segments (length, 3–5 mm). Thus, feed arteries were dissected, cannulated at both ends, secured in a vessel chamber, and pressurized to 75 mmHg (as measured *in vivo*). Exposed cheek pouch, retractor muscle, and isolated vessel preparations were superfused continuously with physiological saline solution maintained at body temperature. All procedures were approved by the Institutional Animal Care and Use Committee.

1.1. Vasoactive stimuli

Acetylcholine (1 M), norepinephrine or phenylephrine (5×10^{-1} M), KCl (1 M) and bradykinin (10^{-3} M) were dissolved in deionized H_2O and backfilled into glass micropipettes (tip diameter, 1–3 µm). The micropipette was positioned with its tip adjacent to the vessel wall. A brief stimulus (typically 500–1000 ms) was applied; acetylcholine, norepinephrine or phenylephrine were delivered using micro-iontophoresis, while KCl and bradykinin were delivered with pressure ejection (Welsh and Segal, 1998; Bartlett and Segal, 2000; Emerson and Segal, 2000a). A response was recorded at the 'local' site of release, the vessel was allowed to recover, and then the stimulus was repeated for each response recorded at defined distances along the vessel (typically 0.5 and 1 mm). These stimuli produce negligible tachyphylaxis, evoke maximal responses at the local site, and delivery is complete before the onset of the vasomotor response (typically a lag of about two seconds). Although conducted responses are bidirectional, upstream locations were observed for criterion measurements to preclude the possibility of stimulus convection in the bloodstream. Moving the pipette tip more than 100 μm from the vessel typically eliminated vascular responses, confirming the focal nature of stimulation.

To activate perivascular nerves, micropipettes were filled with isotonic saline and connected to a square-wave stimulator, positioned as above, and a five-second train was delivered at 32 Hz. A Ag/AgCl reference electrode secured to the edge of the preparation served as the reference electrode. Sodium nitroprusside (10^{-5} M) was added to the superfusion solution to evaluate maximum diameter and vasomotor tone.

1.2. Electrophysiology

Intracellular recordings were obtained in arterioles (diameter, 30–50 μm) or feed arteries (diameter, 50–70 μm) using glass microelectrodes (Welsh and Segal, 1998; Emerson and Segal, 2000a,b). In some experiments, both local and conducted responses were recorded from the same cell by moving the stimulus micropipette while maintaining the intracellular recording. Cell labeling with a fluorescent dye (e.g., Lucifer yellow or fluorescein-conjugated dextran) in the recording microelectrode enabled visualization of the specific cell(s) recorded from, such that smooth muscle cells encircle the vessel while endothelial cells align with the vessel axis (Welsh and Segal, 1998; Emerson and Segal, 2000a,b).

1.3. Light-dye damage

For *in vivo* experiments, fluorescein isothiocyanate conjugated to bovine serum albumin (molecular weight, 70 kDa) was delivered as a bolus intravenously (Bartlett and Segal, 2000). Conjugation of the dye to this plasma protein facilitated its retention within the vascular compartment, enabling endothelial cell damage to be produced from within the vessel lumen (Figure 3.1). To selectively disrupt smooth muscle cells, a micropipette filled with the dye solution was positioned abluminally to continuously perifuse a segment of the vessel. Complimentary experiments using fluorescein-conjugated dextran (70 kDa) confirmed that cell-layer selective light-dye damage with fluorescein does not depend upon the 'carrier' molecule (Emerson and Segal, 2000a). In the presence of either luminal or abluminal dye exposure, a central segment (about 250 μm long) of the vessel was illuminated to excite the dye and damage the membranes of adjacent cells (Figure 3.1). Between successive periods of dye illumination, responses to acetylcholine and phenylephrine released onto the illuminated segment were evaluated to ascertain the functional integrity of endothelial cells and smooth muscle cells, respectively (Bartlett and Segal, 2000; Emerson and Segal, 2000a). Upon completion of experiments, staining with propidium iodide (which labels dead or dying cells) or Hoechst 33342 (which labels all cells to which it has access) independently confirmed the specificity and location of cellular damage (Bartlett and Segal, 2000; Emerson and Segal, 2000a).

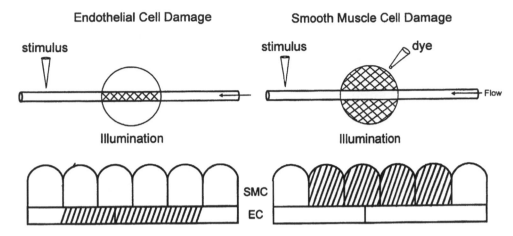

Figure 3.1 Illustration of light-dye technique to selectively damage endothelial cells (EC; left) or smooth muscle cells (SMC; right). The circle of illumination (about 250 µm) is determined by the field diaphragm in the light path. The effect of illumination upon a specific cell layer (EC or SMC) is determined by where the fluorochrome is present during illumination (intravascular for EC; abluminal perifusion with dye for SMC), indicated by the cross-hatch in each upper panel. Corresponding cell damage is indicated by hatching in lower panels; each represents one side of the vessel wall. A stimulus micropipette (e.g., containing acetylcholine or phenylephrine) is shown positioned to evaluate conduction through the illuminated segment; repositioning the micropipette to the illuminated segment is used to evaluate the (loss of) functional responses to a stimulus in the illuminated region. Flow arrow indicates direction of blood *in vivo* and superfusion *in vitro*.

2. RESULTS

2.1. Cheek pouch arterioles

All experiments using selective light dye damage in cheek pouch arterioles were performed *in vivo* (Bartlett and Segal, 2000). Following luminal light-dye treatment, acetylcholine applied to the illuminated central segment no longer evoked a response, though vasodilatation to sodium nitroprusside remained intact. Further, vasodilatation to bradykinin reversed to vasoconstriction, confirming that endothelial cell damage was not 'selective' for acetylcholine. When acetylcholine was delivered 500 µm downstream from the illuminated segment, vasodilatation conducted through the region containing damaged endothelial cells and into the proximal region of the arteriole (Figure 3.2). Thus, once initiated from a segment with intact endothelium, vasodilatation conducted along the smooth muscle layer despite disruption of the endothelial cell pathway. Phenylephrine released at the local site or at the illuminated site evoked vasoconstriction that conducted along the arteriole, confirming the integrity of the smooth muscle pathway.

Following abluminal light-dye treatment, responses to phenylephrine at the illuminated site were abolished. When phenylephrine was released 500 µm downstream, vasoconstriction conducted up to, but not beyond the region of smooth muscle cell damage (Figure 3.2). Nevertheless, acetylcholine released at the illuminated site readily evoked conducted responses, despite the lack of a vasomotor response from

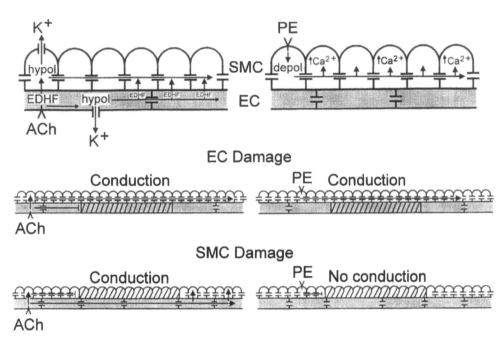

Figure 3.2 Proposed pathways for conduction along hamster cheek pouch arterioles. Cartoon
illustrates conclusions based upon findings in Welsh and Segal, 1998, 2000; Bartlett
and Segal, 2000. Phenylephrine (PE) evokes smooth muscle cell (SMC) depolarization
(depol) that conducts along the smooth muscle cell layer independent of the
endothelium, giving rise to vasoconstriction. Damage to the smooth muscle
conducting pathway blocks conducted vasoconstriction. Acetylcholine (ACh)
evokes endothelial cell (EC) hyperpolarization (hypol) by promoting K^+ efflux;
concomitant release of EDHF promotes K^+ efflux and hyperpolarization in adjacent
smooth muscle. Once initiated, hyperpolarization conducts along either (or both) cell
layer(s). Endothelial cell damage has no effect on conducted vasodilatation initiated
from a region with endothelial cells still intact. Smooth muscle cell damage is bypassed
by conduction along the intact endothelium, which promotes smooth muscle cell
hyperpolarization and vasodilatation beyond the region of damage. Parallel lines
between cells indicate gap junctions.

damaged smooth muscle cells. The latter finding confirmed the integrity of the
endothelial cell signaling pathway despite disruption of overlying smooth muscle cells.
Control experiments verified that, following either luminal or abluminal light-dye
damage, local (direct) responses to acetylcholine and phenylephrine delivered on either
side of the illuminated segment remained intact, confirming localization of cellular
damage to the illuminated segment. Further, illumination without dye did not effect
conduction (or cellular integrity), nor did the presence of dye without illumination.

2.2. Retractor muscle arterioles and feed arteries

For *in vivo* preparations, acetylcholine evoked vasodilatation that conducted with
little decrement along feed arteries, which are typically devoid of branches. In contrast, the conduction of vasodilatation in arteriolar networks decayed markedly with

distance, indicating that branching of the conduction pathway dissipated the conducted response (Segal and Neild, 1996). Norepinephrine or KCl evoked pronounced constriction of arterioles and of feed arteries. In sharp contrast to the conduction of vasoconstriction elicited by these stimuli in cheek pouch arterioles (Xia and Duling, 1995a; Welsh and Segal, 1998; Bartlett and Segal, 2000), vasoconstrictor responses of retractor vessels were constrained to the vicinity of the stimulus (Segal *et al.*, 1999). In turn, electrical stimulation with a microelectrode evoked constriction that spread rapidly along feed arteries and arterioles. The latter responses were inhibited with tetrodotoxin or blockade of α-adrenoceptors, confirming the release of norepinephrine along perivascular sympathetic nerves.

When studied *in vitro*, feed arteries readily conducted vasodilatation in response to acetylcholine (Emerson and Segal, 2000a,b). In contrast, vasoconstriction to norepinephrine, phenylephrine, or KCl did not conduct, while focal stimulation of sympathetic nerves constricted the entire vessel (Emerson and Segal, unpublished data). Thus, feed arteries displayed similar vasomotor properties both *in vivo* and *in vitro*. Intracellular recording with dye labeling revealed that acetylcholine evoked hyperpolarization along endothelial and smooth muscle layers. Following light-dye damage of endothelial cells (Figure 3.1), vasodilatation and hyperpolarization evoked

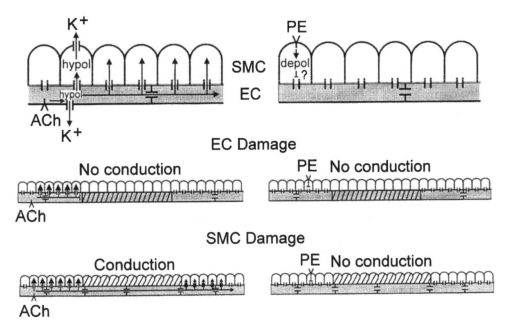

Figure 3.3 Proposed pathways for conduction along hamster retractor muscle feed arteries. Cartoon illustrates conclusions based upon findings in Segal *et al.* (1999), Emerson and Segal (2000a,b). Phenylephrine (PE) evokes smooth muscle cell (SMC) contraction that is constrained to the site of α-adrenoceptor activation; depolarization (depol) has not been confirmed. Damage to the smooth muscle layer is without effect, as it does not serve as a conduction pathway. Acetylcholine (ACh) evokes endothelial cell (EC) hyperpolarization (hypol) that is conducted along the endothelium. Hyperpolarization and relaxation of smooth muscle cells reflect direct electrical coupling through myoendothelial gap junctions along the vessel. Damage to the endothelial cell conduction pathway blocks conducted vasodilatation despite the integrity of the smooth muscle layer.

at the downstream end conducted up to, but not through, the segment containing damaged endothelial cells (Figure 3.3). This result is distinct from that described above for cheek pouch arterioles following endothelial cell damage, where smooth muscle cells served as an alternate conduction pathway. When smooth muscle cells were selectively damaged, vasodilatation initiated downstream conducted without impairment through (and could be initiated from) the treated segment, as found in cheek pouch arterioles.

3. DISCUSSION

The endothelium has been favored as a cellular pathway for conduction, attributable to the orientation of endothelial cells along the vessel axis, their pronounced dye coupling, and the location and extent of gap junctions between neighboring endothelial cells (Haas and Duling, 1997; Welsh and Segal, 1998). However, resolution of the endothelial cell conduction pathway, as well as the smooth muscle cell conduction pathway, has been ambiguous because both cell layers remained intact during previous studies. Refining the light-dye technique has enabled selective disruption of endothelium or smooth muscle, thereby facilitating the resolution of the role(s) of these respective cell layers in both the initiation and conduction of vasodilatation and vasoconstriction. Further, through applying this technique to comparable vessels from vascular beds supplying adjacent tissues that differ in structure and function, striking regional differences in signaling pathways have been revealed.

3.1. Light-dye treatment

Cellular damage with light-dye treatment relies on the production of free radicals when a fluorochrome is excited in the presence of oxygen. These highly reactive intermediates attack membrane components of nearby cells, leading to cell death (Rumbaut and Sial, 1999; Bartlett and Segal, 2000). The extent of cellular damage varies with the dye species used; fluorescein appears particularly effective (Rumbaut and Sial, 1999) and was used here. Earlier studies that have used light-dye to damage endothelial cells in microvessels have injected a bolus of sodium fluorescein into the peripheral circulation of rodents while intensely illuminating arterioles for a period of about 30 seconds (Rosenblum, 1986; Koller *et al.*, 1989). While this approach damages endothelial cells, the hydrophilic nature of the dye salt enables it to readily escape the vascular compartment, where it may concomitantly injure smooth muscle cells (Bartlett and Segal, 2000). To resolve this situation, 'impermeant' conjugates of fluorescein were presented intraluminally to damage endothelium or abluminally to damage smooth muscle (Figure 3.1). This has resulted in reproducible cell-type specific results using longer, controlled periods of illumination both *in vivo* (Bartlett and Segal, 2000) and *in vitro* (Emerson and Segal, 2000a).

3.2. Cellular pathways for conduction

As defined for the experiments described above, the conduction of vasomotor responses reflects changes in membrane potential that are conducted along the vessel wall. Whereas vascular smooth muscle is the 'final effector' of these vasomotor responses through electromechanical coupling, it is essential to define the signaling pathways that initiate and that conduct the electrical signals that give rise to smooth muscle contraction or relaxation. Neurotransmitters have been effective in probing the nature of these signaling events due to their selective effects on smooth muscle as well as endothelium. With smooth muscle cells, for example, norepinephrine and phenylephrine bind to α_1-adrenoceptors to activate an inward cation current (Wang *et al.*, 1993), promoting depolarization and the conduction of vasoconstriction (Xia and Duling, 1995a; Welsh and Segal, 1998). With endothelial cells, acetylcholine activates muscarinic receptors to stimulate Ca^{2+}-activated K^+ channels (Busse *et al.*, 1988) and thereby evoke hyperpolarization through K^+ efflux. Further, hyperpolarization of smooth muscle is often observed when endothelial cells are intact (Welsh and Segal, 1998; Campbell and Harder, 1999; Emerson and Segal, 2000a). Whereas smooth muscle hyperpolarization can reflect the spread of current from endothelial cells via myoendothelial gap junctions (Sandow and Hill, 2000; Emerson and Segal, 2000b), considerable evidence indicates that ACh-induced hyperpolarization of smooth muscle cells is indirect and depends upon the release of endothelium-derived hyperpolarizing factors (EDHFs) (Campbell and Harder, 1999; Félétou and Vanhoutte, 1999).

In cheek pouch arterioles, selective disruption along one cell layer revealed that either smooth muscle or endothelium can serve as a conduction pathway, with the nature of the stimulus determining which layer initiates and/or conducts the response (Figure 3.2). The elimination of conducted vasoconstriction with smooth muscle damage is consistent with intracellular recordings showing that phenylephrine (and norepinephrine) evoked depolarization of, and conduction along, the smooth muscle layer without altering the membrane potential of endothelial cells (Welsh and Segal, 1998). *In vitro* studies of cheek pouch arterioles have indicated the presence of myoendothelial coupling, as enabled by the presence of gap junctions between respective cell layers (Little *et al.*, 1995a,b). However, as observed *in vivo*, the elimination of conducted vasoconstriction with selective smooth muscle damage (Figure 3.2) is inconsistent with this interpretation, as myoendothelial coupling between cell layers on either side of damaged smooth muscle cells should enable the conducted response to bypass the region of cell damage.

A variety of signaling molecules that can regulate the conductance of gap junctions (e.g., cyclic nucleotides, Ca^{2+} and nitric oxide (Spray and Burt, 1990; Lu and McMahon, 1997)) are produced in response to blood pressure and flow. Thus, with the loss of transmural pressure and blood flow upon isolation for *in vitro* studies, the elimination of tangential wall stress and luminal shear stress may influence gap junctional coupling relative to *in vivo* conditions, as may penetration of a cell with a micropipette. Such variables may, in part, explain the controversy surrounding the nature of signaling between microvascular smooth muscle cells and endothelial cells for cheek pouch arterioles studied *in vitro* – where myoendothelial coupling has been implicated (Little *et al.*, 1995b; Xia *et al.*, 1995b; Dora *et al.*, 1997), and those studied *in vivo* – where myoendothelial coupling has not been apparent (Welsh and Segal, 1998; Bartlett and Segal, 2000).

The ability of cheek pouch arteriolar smooth muscle to serve as an 'alternative' pathway for conducted vasodilatation following endothelial cell damage is consistent with intracellular recordings showing that acetylcholine evokes hyperpolarization of (and conduction along) the smooth muscle as well as the endothelial cell layer (Welsh and Segal, 1998). Nevertheless, electrophysiological responses in smooth muscle cells were characteristically longer than from those recorded in adjacent endothelial cells (Welsh and Segal, 1998), suggesting a heterocellular signaling mechanism other than direct electrical coupling through myoendothelial gap junctions. In the presence of 17-octadecynoic acid (an antagonist of EDHF production by cytochrome P450 enzymes), conducted vasodilatation was inhibited by 50 to 70% (Welsh and Segal, 2000). Further, this antagonist inhibited hyperpolarization of smooth muscle in response to acetylcholine without altering that of endothelial cells, consistent with selective inhibition of an EDHF.

Findings from cheek pouch arterioles studied *in vivo* therefore suggest that activation of muscarinic receptors on endothelial cells can stimulate cytochrome P450 enzymes to produce metabolites of arachidonic acid that rapidly hyperpolarize and relax the surrounding smooth muscle cells. In such fashion, once smooth muscle cell hyperpolarization is initiated in a region containing intact endothelium, the smooth muscle layer readily conducts the signal along the arteriole, irrespective of the endothelial cell pathway (Figure 3.2). Alternatively, with selective regional damage to smooth muscle cells, the conduction of vasodilation through the region of damage implies that hyperpolarization conducted along the endothelium to promote relaxation of intact smooth muscle cells; e.g., through release of EDHF (Figure 3.2).

3.3. Regional differences in behavior

Tissue-specific differences are apparent in how vasoconstriction is transmitted along resistance microvessels of the retractor muscle compared to those of the cheek pouch. For example, whereas vasoconstriction conducted along the smooth muscle layer of arterioles in the cheek pouch (Welsh and Segal, 1998; Bartlett and Segal, 2000), it did not conduct in arterioles or feed arteries of the retractor muscle (Segal *et al.*, 1999). This difference also suggests that microvascular smooth muscle cells of the retractor muscle are not coupled to the extent shown for those of the cheek pouch in vessels of similar size and wall morphology. At the molecular level, this may in turn be attributed to regional heterogeneity in the distribution of connexin isoforms (Gabriels and Paul, 1998; Yeh *et al.*, 1999).

Arterioles and feed arteries of the retractor muscle are richly invested by sympathetic nerves (Grasby *et al.*, 1999); when stimulated, they release norepinephrine onto smooth muscle cells along the entire resistance network (Segal *et al.*, 1999). In contrast, arterioles studied in the cheek pouch are devoid of sympathetic innervation (Grasby *et al.*, 1999). The cheek pouch is an epithelial tissue with relatively low metabolic requirements and undergoes modest changes in blood flow. In contrast, blood flow to the retractor muscle undergoes more than a ten-fold increase from rest to intense activity (data not shown), while sympathetic innervation of skeletal muscle is central to the regulation of cardiovascular homeostasis during exercise (O'Leary *et al.*, 1991). Given the robust sympathetic innervation of the retractor muscle, and the lack of these nerves in the epithelial pouch (Grasby *et al.*, 1999) it is hypothesized that regional variations in perivascular innervation may influence the expression and coupling properties of gap junctions in microvascular smooth muscle and endothelium.

Multiple pathways exist for signals underlying vasodilatation and vasoconstriction to travel along the wall of resistance microvessels. Selective damage to smooth muscle and to endothelial cell layers has provided new insight into the role of each cell layer as a signaling pathway, as well as how such pathways may vary between vascular beds. Across preparations, endothelial cell integrity is required for initiating conducted vasodilatation with acetylcholine. Whereas the smooth muscle layer may provide an alternative pathway for conducting vasodilatation in cheek pouch arterioles, the integrity of the endothelium is required for conduction in feed arteries of the retractor muscle. Vasoconstriction is initiated with the release of phenylephrine or norepinephrine onto smooth muscle cells of resistance vessels of both tissues. While vasoconstriction conducts from smooth muscle cell to smooth muscle cell along cheek pouch arterioles, it does not conduct along feed arteries or arterioles of the retractor muscle studied under similar experimental conditions. Nevertheless, the entire resistance network of the retractor muscle is readily constricted through activation of perivascular sympathetic nerves. Such differences indicate that the biophysical determinants of conduction can vary between vascular beds that supply tissues that differ in structure and function.

ACKNOWLEDGMENTS

We thank Donald G. Welsh for substantive contributions to this work. This research was supported by grants RO1-HL41026 and RO1-HL56786 from the Heart, Lung, and Blood Institute of the National Institutes of Health, United States Public Health Service. G.G. Emerson was supported by Medical Scientist Training Program GM07205. I.S. Bartlett was supported by postdoctoral fellowship 9920265T from the Heritage Affiliate of the American Heart Association.

4 Membrane potential and calcium responses evoked by acetylcholine in submucosal arterioles of the guinea-pig small intestine

*Hiroyasu Fukuta, Kenro Imaeda,
Hikaru Hashitani, Yoshimichi
Yamamoto and Hikaru Suzuki*

In isolated submucosal arterioles of the guinea-pig small intestine, changes in membrane potential and intracellular Ca^{2+} evoked by acetylcholine were measured using intracellular microelectrodes and fura-2 fluorescence, respectively. In arterioles depolarized with Ba^{2+}, acetylcholine repolarized the membrane (hyperpolarization), with an associated decrease in membrane resistance. The hyperpolarization was inhibited by blocking K^+-channels with charybdotoxin and apamin or by inhibiting gap junctions with 18β-glycyrrhetinic acid. Acetylcholine increased the Ca^{2+} level in fresh arterioles (within two hours). The Ca^{2+}-responses decayed with time and finally disappeared in old arterioles (over three hours old). Ba^{2+} elevated Ca^{2+} level, and acetylcholine increased the level further in fresh arterioles and reduced it in old arterioles. The acetylcholine-induced reduction of Ca^{2+} level in old arterioles was attenuated in the presence of charybdotoxin. High-K^+ solution increased Ca^{2+} levels, and acetylcholine elevated the level further in fresh arterioles but produced no response in old arterioles. The acetylcholine-induced elevation of Ca^{2+} was observed only in fresh arterioles with intact endothelial cells, while Ba^{2+} elevated Ca^{2+} irrespective of the presence or absence of endothelial cells. In old arterioles, the Ca^{2+}-responses were inhibited by charybdotoxin, but not by apamin, 4-aminopyridine or glibenclamide. After inhibiting gap junctions with 18β-glycyrrhetinic acid, voltage-clamp experiments revealed that acetylcholine increases an outward K^+-current in endothelial cells but not in smooth muscle cells. The results indicate that acetylcholine increases endothelial Ca^{2+} and hyperpolarizes the cell membrane by activating Ca^{2+}-sensitive K^+-channels. The endothelial hyperpolarization may be propagated to smooth muscle cells through gap junctions.

Acetylcholine produces endothelium-dependent hyperpolarization in many types of vascular smooth muscles (Garland *et al.*, 1995), and the mediator may be an endothelium-derived hyperpolarizing factor (EDHF) (Chen *et al.*, 1988; Félétou and Vanhoutte, 1988). However, the nature of this factor is controversial. The involvement of humoral substances such as metabolites of arachidonic acid (Hecker *et al.*, 1994), cannabinoids (Randall *et al.*, 1996) or K^+ (Edwards *et al.*, 1998) has been considered. The hyperpolarization of smooth muscle could also be produced by an electrotonic spread of potentials from the endothelial cells (Marchenco and Sage, 1994, 1996; Yamamoto *et al.*, 1999). In fact, membrane potentials of both endothelial and smooth muscle cells show synchronized couplings (Von der Weid and Bény, 1993; Bény and Pacicca, 1994; Yamamoto *et al.*, 1998).

The acetylcholine-induced hyperpolarization may depend on the activation of K^+-channels, since the amplitude of the potential inversely relates to the concentration of potassium ions in the solution (Chen *et al.*, 1988; Chen and Suzuki, 1989). The inhibition of this hyperpolarization by charybdotoxin and apamin, but not by glibenclamide, Ba^{2+} or 4-aminopyridine, suggests that the main K^+-channels activated are of Ca^{2+}-sensitive type (Murphy and Brayden, 1995; Marchenco and Sage, 1996; Hashitani and Suzuki, 1997; Nishiyama *et al.*, 1998). Myo-endothelial gap junctions exist (Chaytor *et al.*, 1998), and functional communication between endothelial and smooth muscle cells has been confirmed using dyes transferable through gap junctions (Little *et al.*, 1995). Membrane potential changes occurring in endothelial cells can be propagated to smooth muscle cells through gap junctions (Bény and Pacicca, 1994), and the opposite is also the case (Yamamoto *et al.*, 1999). These observations suggest that the distribution of K^+-channels activated by acetylcholine is difficult to determine in experiments using conventional microelectrode techniques alone.

Attempts were made to localize the site of K^+-channels activated by acetylcholine in submucosal arterioles, using conventional microelectrode and patch clamp techniques. Changes in intracellular Ca^{2+} concentrations during stimulation with acetylcholine were also measured using fura-2 fluorescence. The detailed experimental methods have been reported elsewhere (Hashitani and Suzuki, 1997; Yamamoto *et al.*, 1998, 1999; Fukuta *et al.*, 1999). The results indicate that in this arteriole, acetylcholine increases Ca^{2+} only in endothelial cells and thus activates Ca^{2+}-sensitive K^+-channels to hyperpolarize the endothelial cell membrane. As the membrane potential changes in smooth muscle cells parallel those in the endothelial cells, a possible propagation of potentials from endothelium to smooth muscle must be considered.

1. MEMBRANE RESPONSES

Conventional microelectrode techniques were applied to submucosal arterioles prepared from the guinea-pig small intestine (Hirst, 1977), and electrical responses of the cell membrane produced by acetylcholine were measured. At rest, the membrane was quiescent, with the resting potential ranging between $-65\,mV$ and $-75\,mV$. Acetylcholine (up to $10^{-5}\,M$) produced negligible changes in the membrane potential. An inhibition of the inward rectifier K^+-channels with 5×10^{-5}–$5 \times 10^{-4}\,M$ Ba^{2+} (Edwards and Hirst, 1991) depolarized the membrane to -40 to $-50\,mV$ and initiated oscillatory changes in the membrane potential (10–$30\,mV$). In the presence of Ba^{2+}, acetylcholine (10^{-9}–$10^{-5}\,M$) hyperpolarized the membrane in a concentration-dependent manner, with the maximal amplitude being about $25\,mV$ at $10^{-6}\,M$ acetylcholine (Hashitani and Suzuki, 1997). The amplitude of electrotonic potentials produced by current injection was reduced during the acetylcholine-induced hyperpolarization, indicating that ionic conductance was increased. The acetylcholine-induced hyperpolarization was inhibited by $10^{-7}\,M$ charybdotoxin, and was abolished (Figure 4.1) or converted to depolarization response by the combination of charybdotoxin and apamin ($10^{-7}\,M$). Charybdotoxin and apamin inhibit intermediate and small conductance Ca^{2+}-sensitive K^+-channels, respectively (Adams, 1994; Nelson and Quayle, 1995), suggesting that these K^+-channels are involved in the acetylcholine-induced hyperpoarization.

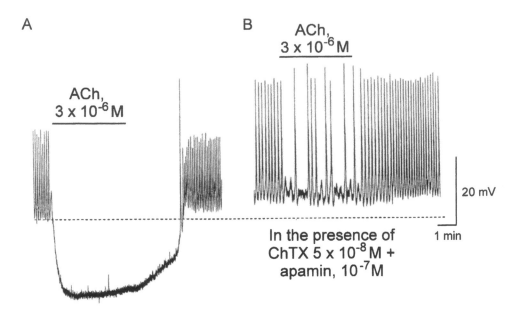

Figure 4.1 Acetylcholine-induced hyperpolarization and its inhibition by charybdotoxin and apamin. Acetylcholine (ACh, 3×10^{-6} M) was applied in the absence (A) and presence of 5×10^{-8} M charybdotoxin (CTX) and 10^{-7} M apamin (B). 5×10^{-4} M Ba^{2+} was present throughout. Both responses were recorded from the same cell in the submucosal arterioles of guinea-pig ileum. Dotted line indicates membrane potential levels produced by Ba^{2+} alone.

2. Ca^{2+}-RESPONSES

In fura-2 loaded arterioles, acetylcholine produced a sustained increase in Ca^{2+}, and the Ca^{2+}-response of similar amplitude was evoked by repetitive (three to five times at intervals 10–15 min) stimulation of the arteriole with acetylcholine. However, the amplitude of the Ca^{2+}-response decreased with time and finally disappeared at around three hours after fura-2 loading. Arterioles were divided into two groups based on the time after loading with fura-2, a fresh (within one to two hours) and old arteriole (over three to four hours). Acetylcholine produced an increase in Ca^{2+} in fresh arterioles but did not produce any obvious response in old preparations. Ba^{2+} (5×10^{-4} M) elevated Ca^{2+} levels in fresh and old arterioles to a similar extent, and acetylcholine further elevated the Ca^{2+} level in fresh arterioles, but reduced it in old arterioles (Figure 4.2). Attempts were made to observe the Ca^{2+}-responses produced by acetylcholine or Ba^{2+} in arterioles after the endothelial cells had been removed mechanically. In the absence of endothelial cells, acetylcholine did not but Ba^{2+} did elevate Ca^{2+} levels (Figure 4.3). These results indicate that acetylcholine elevates Ca^{2+} in endothelial cells while Ba^{2+} elevates Ca^{2+} in smooth muscle cells. High-K solution (38.8 mM$[K^+]_o$) elevated Ca^{2+} levels in both fresh and old arterioles, and acetylcholine increased the Ca^{2+} level further in fresh arterioles, but evoked no obvious response in old arterioles (Figure 4.4), suggesting that the acetylcholine-induced Ca^{2+} responses in smooth muscle cells are produced by hyperpolarization of the cell membrane.

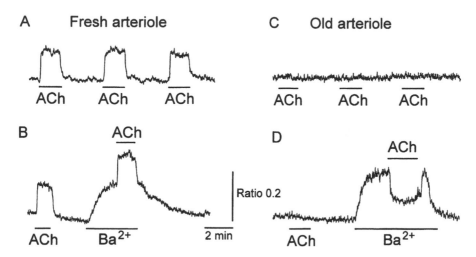

Figure 4.2 Ca^{2+}-responses produced by acetylcholine in fresh and old arterioles. Ca^{2+}-responses produced by acetylcholine (ACh, 10^{-6} M) in fresh (left) and old (right) submucosal arterioles loaded with fura-2. The arterioles were stimulated three times with acetylcholine in fresh (A) and old (C) arterioles. Acetylcholine was applied in the absence and presence of 5×10^{-4} M Ba^{2+} in fresh (B) and old (D) arterioles.

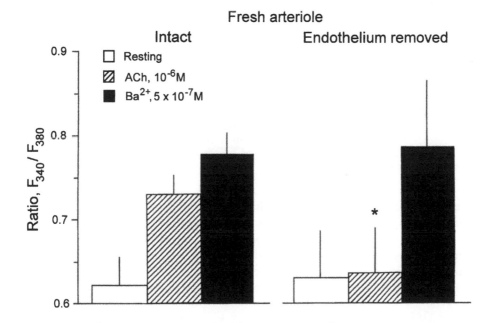

Figure 4.3 Ca^{2+}-responses produced by acetylcholine and Ba^{2+} in submucosal arterioles with or without endothelial cells. Fresh mesenteric arteries with and without endothelium were stimulated with 10^{-6} M acetylcholine (ACh) or 5×10^{-4} M Ba^{2+}, and peak amplitude of the Ca^{2+} responses was measured. Data show as means $\pm$ standard deviation ($n = 5-8$). The asterisk indicates a statistically significant reduction compared to intact arterioles ($p < .05$). (From Fukuta *et al.*, 1999, by permission.)

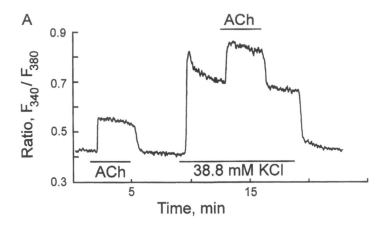

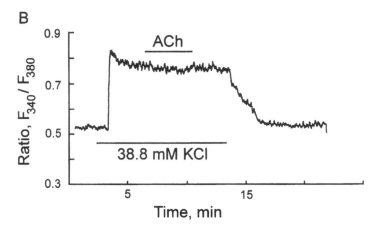

Figure 4.4 Effects of high-K solution on Ca^{2+}-responses. Ca^{2+}-responses produced by acetylcholine (ACh, 10^{-6} M) in the presence of $38.8\,mM[K^+]_o$ solution. A: fresh arteriole; B: old arteriole. In fresh arterioles, the acetylcholine-responses were similar in the absence and presence of high-K solution. (From Fukuta *et al.*, 1999, by permission.)

The effects of several types of K^+-channel inhibitors were tested on the acetylcholine-induced Ca^{2+} responses in fresh and old arterioles. In fresh arterioles, the Ca^{2+}-responses produced by acetylcholine were not altered by charybdotoxin, apamin, 4-aminopyridine or glibenclamide. In old arterioles, the inhibitory responses produced by acetylcholine in the presence of Ba^{2+} were attenuated by charybdotoxin but not by apamin, 4-aminopyridine or glibenclamide (Figure 4.5).

3. MEMBRANE ACTIVITIES OF FUNCTIONALLY ISOLATED SMOOTH MUSCLE AND ENDOTHELIAL CELLS

In isolated segments of the mesenteric arteriole, membrane currents evoked by acetylcholine were recorded from smooth muscle and endothelial cells using the patch-clamp

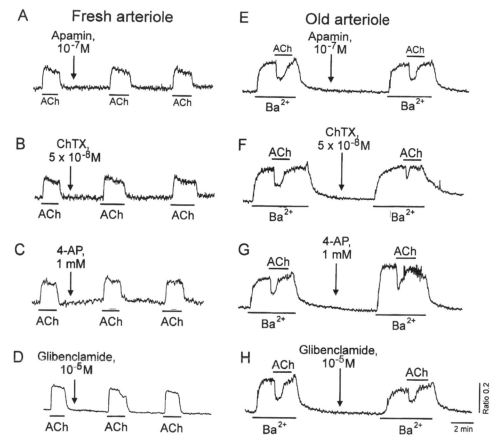

Figure 4.5 Effects of K-channel inhibitors on the Ca^{2+}-responses produced by acetylcholine in submucosal arterioles. Fura-2 loaded fresh (A–D) and old arterioles (E–H) were stimulated with 10^{-6} M acetylcholine (ACh), in the absence and presence of 10^{-7} M apamin (A), 5×10^{-8} M charybdotoxin (CTX, B), 10^{-3} M 4-amino-pyridine (4-AP, C) and 10^{-5} M glibenclamide (D). In old arterioles, 5×10^{-4} M Ba^{2+} was applied to elevate the Ca^{2+} level. Bar at the right-hand side indicates fluorescence ratio (F_{340}/F_{380}) of 0.2.

method in whole-cell configuration. These cells were electrically connected to each other through gap junctions to form a functional syncytium. Functional isolation of the patched cell from the surrounding cells was performed by inhibiting gap junctional communications using 18β-glycyrrhetinic acid (Yamamoto *et al.*, 1998). In the presence of 18β-glycyrrhetinic acid (2×10^{-5} M), the currents required to depolarize the membrane by 10 mV were reduced to a minimum, and acetylcholine did not produce any detectable currents in the smooth muscle (Figure 4.6). The current–voltage relationships produced by ramp pulse were of the outward rectifier type, and the relationship did not change in the presence of acetylcholine. After the gap junctional connections had been blocked by 18β-glycyrrhetinic acid, acetylcholine produced an outward current in endothelial cells (Figure 4.6). The subtraction of control currents from those obtained in the presence of acetylcholine indicated that the

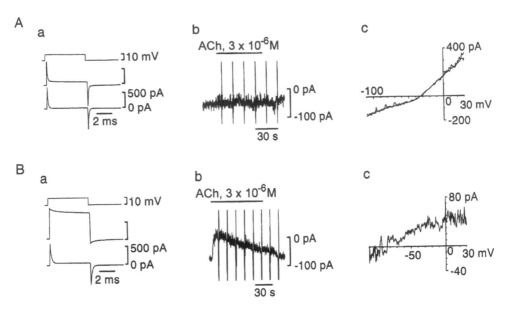

Figure 4.6 Acetylcholine-induced membrane currents in endothelial and smooth muscle cells. In the whole-cell voltage-clamp configuration, membrane currents required to depolarize the membrane by 10 mV in a smooth muscle (Aa) or an endothelial cell (Ba) were measured before (middle trace) and during application of 2×10^{-5} M 18β-glycyrrhetinic acid (bottom trace). Note the reduction of current required in the presence of 18β-glycyrrhetinic acid. Membrane currents evoked by 3×10^{-6} M acetylcholine (ACh) were measured from smooth muscle (Ab) and endothelial cells (Bb) of the mesenteric arteriole, in the presence of 2×10^{-5} M 18β-glycyrrhetinic acid. Acetylcholine affected the membrane currents only in the endothelial cell. Truncated vertical deflections are currents elicited by ramp pulses. The current–voltage relationships produced by ramp pulses in the absence and presence of acetylcholine were recorded from smooth muscle cells (Ac). The two relationships were nearly identical. The current produced by acetylcholine in the endothelial cell was extracted by subtracting the current–voltage relationships obtained in the absence of acetylcholine from those in the presence of acetylcholine (Bc). Acetylcholine activated an outward current with reversal potential around -90 mV.

acetylcholine-activated currents increased linearly by the membrane depolarization, with the reversal potential around -90 mV, suggesting that they were carried mainly by potassium ions. The acetylcholine-induced hyperpolarization recorded from smooth muscle cells using microelectrodes is also inhibited by 18β-glycyrrhetinic acid, in a reversible manner (Yamamoto *et al.*, 1999). These results indicate that acetylcholine activates endothelial K^+-channels and thus produces hyperpolarization only in endothelial cells, without altering ionic conductance in smooth muscle membrane.

4. DISCUSSION

In vascular tissues, many types of K^+-channels are present in smooth muscle (Nelson and Quayle, 1995) and endothelial cell membrane (Adams, 1994), as deduced from the actions of the inhibitors of K^+-channel subtypes. In submucosal arterioles of the guinea-pig small intestine, the acetylcholine-induced hyperpolarization was sensitive to charybdotoxin and apamin, suggesting the possible contribution of Ca^{2+}-sensitive K^+-channels (Nelson and Quayle, 1995). These results are in good agreement with those obtained in other arteries such as the rabbit mesenteric artery (Murphy and Brayden, 1995), the rat aorta (Marchenco and Sage, 1996), the rat mesenteric artery (Chen and Cheung, 1997) and the guinea-pig coronary artery (Nishiyama *et al.*, 1998). Possible involvement of inward rectifier type of K^+-channels in the acetylcholine-induced hyperpolarization is also reported in some arteries (Edwards *et al.*, 1998). Smooth muscle cells of the submucosal arterioles are endowed with this type of K^+-channels, which can be inhibited by Ba^{2+} (Edwards and Hirst, 1991). However, the contribution of inward rectifier K^+-channels in the acetylcholine-induced hyperpolarization must be minimal in the submucosal arteriole studied, since the present experiments are carried out in the presence of Ba^{2+}.

In some arteries, acetylcholine hyperpolarizes the cell membrane of vascular smooth muscle with fast and slow components. The latter component is inhibited by indomethacin or diclofenac, a known inhibitor of enzyme cyclooxygenase. These results indicate that endothelial prostanoids released by acetylcholine also hyperpolarize the membrane of arterial smooth muscle (Murphy and Brayden, 1995; Parkington *et al.*, 1993, 1996; Nishiyama *et al.*, 1998; Yajima *et al.*, 1999). The prostanoid-induced hyperpolarization is characterized by a slow onset and prolonged duration in response to acetylcholine, possibly because of the slow diffusion and/or action of the prostanoid (Zhang *et al.*, 1996; Yajima *et al.*, 1999). The prostanoid-induced component of the acetylcholine-induced hyperpolarization is inhibited by glibenclamide or 4-aminopyridine (Nishiyama *et al.*, 1998). Glibenclamide and 4-aminopyridine are inhibitors of ATP-sensitive K^+-channels and delayed rectifier K^+-channels, respectively (Nelson and Quayle, 1995). However, glibenclamide also inhibits prostaglandin receptors (Zhang *et al.*, 1991). These results suggest that the K^+-channels activated by endothelial prostanoids are of the delayed rectifier type (Nishiyama *et al.*, 1998). Thus, there are at least two types of K^+-channels activated during stimulation with acetylcholine. The hyperpolarization produced by EDHF is insensitive to inhibitors of EDRF and prostanoids (Chen *et al.*, 1988). In submucosal arterioles, the acetylcholine-induced hyperpolarization is not significantly altered by indomethacin or N^ω-nitro-L-arginine (Hashitani and Suzuki, 1997), suggesting that the main component of the hyperpolarization is produced by EDHF. This is also supported by the observation that the hyperpolarization is inhibited by charybdotoxin and apamin but not by 4-aminopyridine.

Ca^{2+}-sensitive K^+-channels may be activated by an increase in intracellular Ca^{2+} (Adams, 1994; Nelson and Quayle, 1995). Therefore, it is reasonable to speculate that the activation of these K^+-channels is accompanied by an increase in the intracellular Ca^{2+} concentration. The measurement of fura-2 fluorescence indicated that in submucosal arterioles, acetylcholine elevates Ca^{2+} only in endothelial cells, in agreement with other tissues (Schilling and Elliott, 1992). No positive Ca^{2+} response was evoked by acetylcholine in arterioles after removal of the endothelial cells. Thus, the K^+-channels activated during stimulation with acetylcholine may be distributed mainly in endothelial cells. This interpretation was confirmed by recording membrane potentials directly from endothelial cells after inhibiting gap junctional communications from surrounding cells. Acetylcholine indeed produces hyperpolarization of the membrane in endothelial cells by activation of K^+-channels, but does not hyperpolarize the cell membrane of vascular smooth muscle (Yamamoto *et al.*, 1999). Yet, this agonist produces hyperpolarization in the smooth muscle cells of intact arterioles (Hashitani and Suzuki, 1997; Yamamoto *et al.*, 1999). Thus, in submucosal arterioles, the hyperpolarization of smooth muscle cells presumably results from an electrotonic spread of hyperpolarization originating in the endothelial cells. Alternatively, acetylcholine produces a substance in endothelial cells (EDHF) which permeates through gap junctions but not the cell membrane, and this substance then stimulates K^+-channels of the smooth muscle membrane from the inside of cells.

In the porcine coronary artery, fura-2 is removed from endothelial cells much faster than from smooth muscle cells (Kuroiwa *et al.*, 1995), and this may also be the case in submucosal arterioles. That is, the acetylcholine-induced elevation of Ca^{2+} in fresh arterioles may represent the response of endothelial cells, while the absence of Ca^{2+}-response by acetylcholine in old arterioles may be due to the loss of fura-2 from these same cells. Ba^{2+} elevates Ca^{2+} levels in either fresh or old arterioles, to a similar extent, and the actions of Ba^{2+} are also observed in the absence of endothelial cells, indicating that Ba^{2+} acts primarily on the smooth muscle cells. Therefore, the reduction of the Ba^{2+}-elevated Ca^{2+} levels by acetylcholine observed in old arterioles may be the response of smooth muscle cells. Thus, fura-2 may be a useful tool to differentiate Ca^{2+} responses evoked by acetylcholine in smooth muscle and endothelial cells. The elevation of Ca^{2+} levels by high-K solution may be also the response of smooth muscles, since endothelial cells do not possess voltage-sensitive Ca^{2+}-channels in the cell membrane (Adams, 1994). The inhibition of the acetyl-choline-induced Ca^{2+}-responses by charybdotoxin in old arterioles, and also the absence of the Ca^{2+}-response in the presence of high-K solution suggest that the responses of arteriolar smooth muscle during stimulation with acetylcholine may be due to the hyperpolarization of the cell membrane.

5. CONCLUSION

Acetylcholine increases Ca^{2+} in endothelial cells and hyperpolarizes the membrane by activating Ca^{2+}-sensitive K^+-channels. This endothelial hyperpolarization probably is conducted to smooth muscle cells through gap junctions in an electrotonic manner. The resulting hyperpolarization of the cell membrane of vascular smooth muscle reduces intracellular Ca^{2+} and thus induces vasodilatation.

5 The effects of ouabain, 18α-glycyrrhetinic acid and connexin-mimetic peptides on intercellular communication in cells expressing a Cx43-GFP chimeric protein

Patricia E.M. Martin, R.J. Errington and Tudor M. Griffith

EDHF-type relaxations are attenuated by the steroidal compounds ouabain and 18α-glycyrrhetinic acid and connexin-mimetic peptides homologous to the Gap 26 and 27 domains of connexin43 (Cx43). In the present study the effects of these agents on the function and integrity of gap junctions were investigated in cultured cells. HeLa cells were transfected with cDNA encoding a chimeric Cx43 protein in which the carboxyl terminus on Cx43 was fused to the amino terminus of Green Fluorescent Protein (GFP), thus establishing functional gap junctions that can be directly visualized by GFP autofluorescence. Functionality was monitored by microinjection of Lucifer yellow into individual cells. Incubation with either ^{43}Gap 26 or ^{43}Gap 27 (5×10^{-4} M) resulted in about 50% reduction in dye transfer. Incubation with 18α-glycyrrhetinic acid (2.5×10^{-5} M) reduced functionality by about 90% as did ouabain at concentrations of 1×10^{-6} M $- 1 \times 10^{-4}$ M, but ouabain was without effect at 1×10^{-7} M. By contrast in A7r5 cells, ouabain concentrations of 3×10^{-4} M and above were necessary to attenuate the transfer of the dye. Visualization of Cx43-GFP by fluorescence microscopy showed that the peptides affected neither the number nor the distribution of gap junction plaques in the cell membrane. Time lapse microscopy of A7r5 cells expressing Cx43-GFP was used to analyse the effect of 18α-glycyrrhetinic acid and ouabain on gap junction stability and integrity. Disassembly and internalization of plaques was observed around 30 minutes after the addition of 2.5×10^{-5} M 18α-glycyrrhetinic acid to the cells. Gap junctions were not disrupted following treatment with 1 mM ouabain. The results suggest that connexin-mimetic peptides, 18α-glycyrrhetinic acid and ouabain block gap junctional communication by different mechanisms.

Gap junction intercellular communication channels form at the plasma membrane of adjacent cells providing a low resistance pathway for the exchange of regulatory ions and molecules smaller than 1 kDa between neighbouring cells (Goodenough *et al.*, 1996). The formation of a functional gap junction channel involves oligomerization of six connexin subunits to form a hexameric connexon or hemi-channel. This is trafficked through the cell to the plasma membrane where it aligns and docks with a hemi-channel from a neighbouring cell to form a gap junction. These channels aggregate into plaques at the plasma membrane (Evans *et al.*, 1999). At least twenty different isoforms of connexins have been identified in mammals, all of which share a common topology, with two extracellular loops, four transmembrane domains, one intracellular loop and amino and carboxyl termini located in the cytosol (Goodenough *et al.*, 1996). In the mammalian vascular wall Cx43, Cx40 and Cx37 (termed according to their molecular mass in kDa, determined from cDNA sequences) are the predominant isoforms expressed (Christ *et al.*, 1996). Gap junctions can be formed of one or more specific connexin isoform resulting in homomeric and heteromeric combinations with differing functional properties (He *et al.*, 1999; Beyer *et al.*, 2000; Brink *et al.*, 1997; Valiunas *et al.*, 2000).

Endothelium-derived hyperpolarizing factor (EDHF) mediates endothelium-dependent vascular relaxations that are independent of nitric oxide and prostanoid synthesis (Mombouli and Vanhoutte, 1997). Although the chemical nature of EDHF remains controversial, it is now accepted that such EDHF-type responses may involve diffusion of EDHF from the endothelium to the smooth muscle via myoendothelial gap junctions rather than the extracellular space (Chaytor *et al.*, 1998; Taylor *et al.*, 1998; Dora *et al.*, 1999; Fleming, 2000). Such responses are attenuated by peptides homologous to the first and second extracellular loops of Cx43, [43]Gap 26 and [43]Gap 27 respectively (Chaytor *et al.*, 1999; Dora *et al.*, 1999; Griffith *et al.*, this volume), and by the aglycone 18α-glycyrrhetinic acid (Taylor *et al.*, 1998; Chaytor *et al.*, 1999) and the glycoside ouabain (Feletou and Vanhoutte, 1988; Makino, 2000; Van de Voorde and Vanheel, 2000; Harris *et al.*, 2000), which have a similar steroidal structure.

The present work was undertaken to investigate the effects of these agents on the function and integrity gap junctions. The approach taken utilized a chimeric Cx43 protein in which the carboxyl terminus of Cx43 was fused to the amino terminus of Green Fluorescent Protein (GFP) (Paemeleire *et al.*, 2000). When transfected into the communication incompetent HeLa Ohio cell line this chimeric protein targets to the plasma membrane and establishes intercellular coupling in these cells as determined by the ability of cells intracytoplasmically injected with the fluorescent dye Lucifer yellow to transfer the dye to neighbouring cells (Paemeleire *et al.*, 2000). Immunolocalization studies using an antibody to Cx43 showed that the expression of Cx43 and Green Fluorescent Protein were coincident in transfected COS-7 and HeLa cells and Western blotting analysis confirmed that a protein of the predicted molecular mass (74 kDa) was expressed (Paemeleire *et al.*, 2000). Thus the direct effect of the peptides, 18α-glycyrrhetinic acid and ouabain on the functionality of Cx43-GFP gap junctions could be determined by quantifying changes in dye transfer. Furthermore, tagging connexins with GFP permits direct visualisation of connexin trafficking in live cells (Jordan *et al.*, 1999; Holm *et al.*, 1999; Paemeleire *et al.*, 2000) and enables time lapse microscopy to be used to determine directly the effect of ouabain and 18α-glycyrrhetinic acid on gap junction integrity and stability.

1. MATERIALS AND METHODS

1.1. Materials

All reagents were purchased from Sigma (Poole, UK) unless otherwise stated.

1.2. Chimeric connexin-GFP cDNA

Cx43 cDNA was fused inframe to the amino terminus of enhanced-GFP (eGFP) in the vector pe-GFP-N1 (Clontech). The open reading frame of wild type Cx43

(Beyer *et al.*, 1987) was amplified by the polymerase chain reaction from a plasmid containing the full length cDNA using appropriate oligonucleotide primers introducing *BglII* restriction enzyme sites at the 5′ and 3′ end of the cDNA respectively. This was ligated into the *BglII* site of peGFP-N1, transformed into DH5α cells and positive clones were selected by miniplasmid preparation and sequencing (Paemeleire *et al.*, 2000).

1.3. Cell culture

The smooth muscle cell line, A7r5 (ECACC, Wiltshire, UK), or HeLa Ohio cells, an epithelial cell line (ECACC, Wiltshire, UK) were maintained in Dulbecco's modified Eagles medium (DMEM), supplemented with 10% foetal calf serum, penicillin/streptomycin (100 µg/ml), amphotericin (100 µg/ml) and L-glutamine (2 mM) (GibcoBRL).

For immunocytochemical analysis and time lapse microscopy studies A7r5 cells were cultured in 24 mm^2 coverglass chambers (Labtek) and were transfected with 0.25 µg Cx43-GFP cDNA using Lipafectamine 2000 (Gibco BRL). The expression of Cx43 was confirmed by staining the cells with a monoclonal antibody against Cx43 (1:250 dilution, Chemicon). The secondary antibody was goat anti-mouse conjugated to Alexa 488 (1:700 dilution, Molecular Probes).

To establish stable HeLa cell populations expressing Cx43-GFP subconfluent monolayers of HeLa cells were transfected with Cx43-GFP cDNA. Forty-eight hours after transfection positive cells were selected with medium supplemented with Geneticin (G418-sulphate 4 mg/ml, Promega) and after three weeks cells positive for Green Fluorescent Protein were sorted by a fluorescence activated cell sorter using the fluorescein filter set. The selected cell populations were then maintained in the above medium supplemented with Geneticin (4 mg/ml) (Paemeleire *et al.*, 2000).

1.4. ^{43}Gap 26, ^{43}Gap 27, 18α-glycyrrhetinic acid and ouabain

The effects of ^{43}Gap 26 and ^{43}Gap 27, ouabain and 18α-glycyrrhetinic acid on direct cell to cell communication were assessed by studying transfer of Lucifer yellow CH (charge −2, MW 457 Da). HeLa cells stably transfected with Cx43-GFP cDNA were seeded at a density of 1×10^6 cells per 60 mm diameter tissue culture. Protein expression was enhanced by addition of 5×10^{-3} M sodium butyrate to the medium 18 hours prior to the experiments (George *et al.*, 1998b). Confluent monolayers were then incubated in Leibowitz L-15 medium (GibcoBRL) for 90 minutes at 37 °C. In some experiments, ^{43}Gap 26 or ^{43}Gap 27 peptide (5×10^{-4} M) were present during this incubation period. In other experiments the cells were preincubated with ouabain (1×10^{-7}–1×10^{-3} M) or 18α-glycyrrhetinic acid (2.5×10^{-5} M) for 60 and 30 minutes, respectively. Similarly the effect of ouabain and 18α-glycyrrhetinic acid were tested on A7r5 cells. Following intracytoplasmic microinjection of Lucifer yellow, cells were fixed in 4% paraformaldehyde, and the percentage of injections resulting in dye transfer to zero, one to four and more than five neighbouring cells (for HeLa cells) and zero to four, five to ten and more than ten neighbouring cells (for A7r5 cells) under each experimental condition assessed on an Axiovert fluorescence microscope (Zeiss, UK) linked up with a Hamamatsu ORCA digital camera and kinetic imaging software.

1.5. Time lapse microscopy and image analysis

Forty hours after transfection of A7r5 cells with Cx43-GFP, they were washed twice in phosphate buffered saline and the medium was replaced with 1 ml of a calcium-free solution of 1 mM Tris/10 mM Hepes at pH 7.5. The cells were viewed under a Zeiss Axiovert 100 microscope linked up with a BIORAD MRC 1024ES laser scanning system. Images were collected every 30 seconds in batches of 15 minutes for 60 minutes prior to treatment of the cells with 2.5×10^{-5} M 18α-glycyrrhetinic acid or 1×10^{-3} M ouabain. Following addition of the drug images were collected every 30 seconds in 15-minute batches for up to 90 minutes followed by image analysis using the BIORAD Lasersharp software. Time frames 1, 15 and 30 of each batch of images were assigned the colour channels red, green and blue, respectively, so that image superposition could provide information about the dynamics of Cx43-GFP trafficking in the cell. If there was limited movement of the connexins the merged image would be white as red, blue and green channels merged. The appearance of colour consequently reflects the directional movement of the Cx43-GFP protein.

2. RESULTS

2.1. Cellular localization of Cx43-GFP

Analysis by confocal microscopy showed that Cx43-GFP was targeted to the plasma membrane giving characteristic punctate staining of gap junction plaques in both HeLa and A7r5 cells (Figures 5.1 and 5.2). In A7r5 cells the chimeric protein was targeted to the plasma membrane giving a pattern of expression similar to endogenously expressed Cx43 (Figure 5.1).

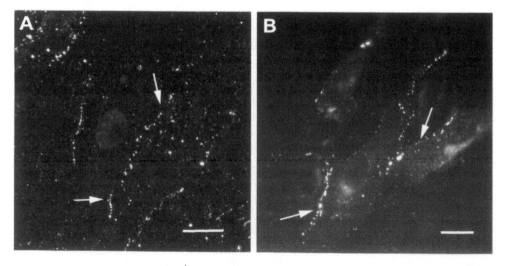

Figure 5.1 Expression of Cx43 and Cx43-GFP in A7r5 cells. A: Confluent monolayers of A7r5 cells were fixed and stained with a primary monoclonal antibody against Cx43 and secondary anti-mouse conjugated Alexa 488 secondary antibody. B: A7r5 cells were transfected with Cx43-GFP cDNA and viewed 24 hours after transfection for Cx43-GFP autofluorescence. Note the similar distribution of native Cx43 and Cx43-GFP in A and B. Arrows indicate gap junction staining. Bar = 10 μm. (*see Color Plate 1*)

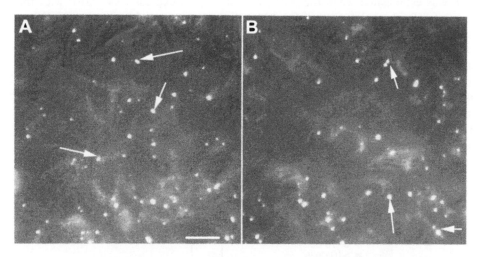

Figure 5.2 The effect of [43]Gap 27 on plaque distribution in HeLa cells expressing Cx43-GFP. Superimposed images of phase contrast and Cx43-GFP autofluorescence showing punctate gap junction locations at points of cell to cell contact in (A) non-treated cells and (B) cells treated with 5×10^{-4} M [43]Gap 27 peptide. Note similar distribution of staining. Arrows indicate typical Cx43-GFP gap junction plaques. Bar = 10 μm. (*see Color Plate 2*)

2.2. Functionality of gap junctions

2.2.1. HeLa cells expressing Cx43-GFP

Under non-transfected conditions, HeLa cells are poorly coupled and are generally unable to transfer dye to more than five neighbouring cells. Intercellular commu-

Table 5.1 The effect of gap peptides, ouabain and 18α-glycyrrhetinic acid on dye transfer in HeLa cells expressing Cx43-GFP

	% of cells transferring Dye ± SEM		
	0 Cells	*1–4 cells*	*>5 cells*
Native HeLa cells (negative control)	99 ± 1	1 ± 1	0
Cx43-GFP HeLa cells (positive control)	10 ± 8	18 ± 4	72 ± 12
5×10^{-4} M [43]Gap 26	40 ± 4	17 ± 3	$43 \pm 1^*$
5×10^{-4} M [43]Gap 27	43 ± 20	30 ± 4	$29 \pm 21^*$
1×10^{-7} M ouabain	8 ± 7	31 ± 4	62 ± 10
1×10^{-6} M ouabain	21 ± 3	65 ± 5	$13 \pm 4^*$
1×10^{-5} M ouabain	24 ± 23	72 ± 17	$4 \pm 5^*$
1×10^{-4} M ouabain	44 ± 12	53 ± 7	$3 \pm 4^*$
2.5×10^{-5} M 18α-GA	93 ± 9	7 ± 9	0^*

Notes
HeLa cells expressing Cx43-GFP were assessed for their ability to transfer Lucifer yellow before and after treatment of the cells with 5×10^{-4} M [43]Gap 26 or [43]Gap 27 for 90 minutes, 1×10^{-6}–1×10^{-4} M ouabain for 60 minutes or 2.5×10^{-4} M 18α-glycyrrhetinic acid (18α-GA) for 30 minutes. The results are expressed as the % of cells transferring dye to zero, one to four or more than five neighbouring cells. Data shown as means ± SEM. Experiments were performed in triplicate and are representative of 90 injections per set. The asterisks indicate a statistically significant effect compared to positive control cells ($p < .005$).

nication was established when the cells were selected to express Cx43-GFP with the majority of cells then able to transfer dye to five or more neighbouring cells. When the cells were treated with ^{43}Gap 26 or ^{43}Gap 27 (5×10^{-4} M) there was a reduction (about 50%) in the extent of dye transfer to five or more cells and an associated increase in the number of cells transferring dye to one to four cells (Table 5.1).

Treatment of the HeLa cells with 18α-glycyrrhetinic acid almost completely abolished dye transfer (Table 5.1). Exposure of the HeLa cells to ouabain at concentrations of 1×10^{-6} M, 1×10^{-5} M and 1×10^{-4} M resulted in marked attenuation ($\sim$90%) of dye transfer to more than five neighbouring cells and a corresponding increase in the number of cells transferring dye to one to four cells or in a nonfunctional status, whereas 1×10^{-7} M was without significant effect (Table 5.1).

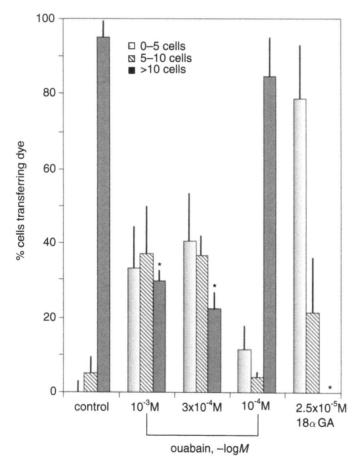

Figure 5.3 The effect of ouabain and 18α-glycyrrhetinic acid on intercellular coupling of A7r5 cells. The ability of confluent monolayers of A7r5 cells to transfer Lucifer yellow was assessed before (control) and after treatment of the cells with 1×10^{-4} M, 3×10^{-4} M and 1×10^{-3} M ouabain for 60 minutes or 2.5×10^{-5} M 18α-glycyrrhetinic acid (18α-GA) for 30 minutes. Experiments were performed in triplicate and are representative of 30 injections per set. Data are shown as means $\pm$ SEM. The asterisks indicate a statistically significant effect of the treatment ($p < .005$).

2.2.2. A7r5 cells

Experiments were also performed to investigate the effect of ouabain on the ability of A7r5 cells, which endogenously express Cx43 and Cx40, to transfer Lucifer yellow. Under normal conditions A7r5 cells exhibit a high degree of intercellular coupling with more than 80% of cells rapidly transferring dye to ten or more neighbouring cells. In these cells ouabain (1×10^{-4} M) was without effect, although incubation with 3×10^{-4} M and 1×10^{-3} M ouabain attenuated intercellular dye coupling by about 70%. Incubation of the cells with 2.5×10^{-5} M 18α-glycyrrhetinic acid for 30 minutes attenuated dye transfer by 80% (Figure 5.3).

2.3. Stability of gap junctions following drug treatment

2.3.1. HeLa cells

HeLa cell monolayers expressing Cx43-GFP were examined for Cx43-GFP plaque distribution before and after treatment of the cells with connexin-mimetic peptides by exploiting the autofluorescence of GFP. Direct microscopic visualization and counting of plaques at the plasma membrane showed that the connexin-mimetic peptides did not affect the number or distribution of the plaques with control cells having 34.4 ± 6.5 plaques per field of view and [43]Gap 27 treated monolayers with 36.5 ± 4.1 plaques per field of view (Figure 5.2). A similar lack of effect on plaque number and distribution was found with [43]Gap 26 (data not shown).

2.3.2. A7r5 cells

The effect of 18α-glycyrrhetinic acid and ouabain on gap junction stability and integrity was monitored by time lapse microscopy of A7r5 cells transfected with Cx43-GFP before and after drug treatment. Connexin trafficking events were analysed as described in section 1.5 giving a visual description of the vesicular movement over the time period. Under normal conditions Cx43-GFP gap junction plaques at the plasma membrane were stable as reflected by the high degree of white punctate staining (Figures 5.4A and B). There was often lateral movement along the plasma membrane and some evidence of intracellular movement of connexons to and from the plasma membrane, as reflected by the colour variations in the merged images (Figures 5.4A and B). Following exposure to 18α-glycyrrhetinic acid (2.5×10^{-5} M) there was a distinct change in the stability of the gap junction plaques (Figures 5.4C and D) with disruption and internalization occurring as early as 15–30 minutes after drug treatment. Exposure of the cells to 18α-glycyrrhetinic acid for 45–60 minutes resulted in further plaque disruption as they were removed from the plasma membrane and internalized. This is reflected by the spectrum of red, green and blue vesicles in the merged images (Figures 5.4D and E).

In contrast to 18α-glycyrrhetinic acid treatment, exposure of transfected A7r5 cells to ouabain did not disrupt gap junction plaques even at concentrations of 1×10^{-3} M (Figures 5.5A–D). Delivery of new connexons to the plasma membrane was still evident 30–45 minutes after exposure of the cells to ouabain (Figure 5.5C) and large plaques were still intact even 60 minutes after drug treatment (Figure 5.5D). However, a decrease in the overall rate of connexin trafficking was noted as observed by the

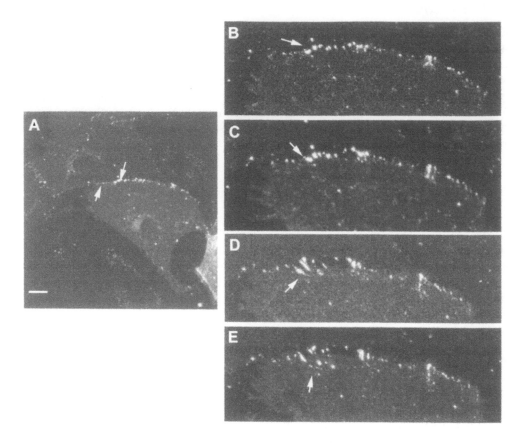

Figure 5.4 The effect of 18α-glycyrrhetinic acid on gap junction integrity in A7r5 cells. A7r5 cells were transfected with Cx43-GFP cDNA and 40 hours after transfection trafficking data was collected and analysed. A: Merged image of Cx43-GFP expression in A7r5 cells under normal conditions. B–D: Focus on the plasma membrane of the image in panel A. B: 15 to 30 minutes, C: 45 to 60 minutes before 18α-glycyrrhetinic acid treatment. At 65 minutes into the experiment 18α-glycyrrhetinic acid (2.5×10^{-5} M) was added. D and E show plaque disassembly occurring at 15–30 and 45–60 minutes after exposure to 18α-glycyrrhetinic acid. A–C: arrows indicate intact gap junctions; D and E: arrows indicate disassembled plaques. Bar = 10 μm. (*see Color Plate 3*)

progressive increase in the colocalization of the three image frames at 30–45 minutes and 60–75 minutes after exposure of the cells to ouabain (Figures 5.5C and D) compared to untreated conditions (Figure 5.5B).

3. DISCUSSION

In the present study mammalian cell expression systems have been used to study the effect of agents that attenuate EDHF-type relaxations on the functionality and integrity of gap junctions. Fusion of GFP to the carboxyl terminus of connexins permits the study of intracellular trafficking, biogenesis and functional properties of connexins

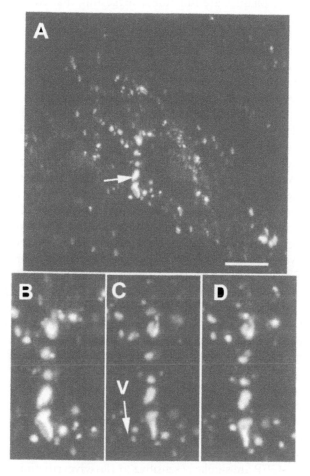

Figure 5.5 The effect of ouabain on the integrity of Cx43-GFP gap junctions. A7r5 cells were transfected with Cx43-GFP cDNA and 40 hours after transfection trafficking data was collected and analysed. A: merged image of 15–30 minutes under normal conditions. B–D focus on the plasma membrane of cells in panel A. B: 15 to 30 minutes under normal conditions. Ouabain (1×10^{-3} M) was added 30 minutes into the experiment. C: 30 to 45 minutes after exposure to ouabain: trafficking of connexons to the plasma membrane is evident as seen by movement of vesicle V (red → green → blue). D: 60 to 75 minutes after exposure to ouabain: reduced trafficking of connexons is evident as seen by the increased colocalisation of the three time points. Note that the plaques are still intact. Bar $= 10\,\mu$m. (*see Color Plate 4*)

(Jordan *et al.*, 1999; Holm *et al.*, 1999; Paemeleire *et al.*, 2000; Martin *et al.*, 2000). These chimeric proteins allow the dynamics of connexin trafficking events to be studied in live cells as they form channels that transfer fluorescent dyes such as Lucifer yellow with similar efficiency as their wild type counterparts (Jordan *et al.*, 1999; Paemeleire *et al.*, 2000; Martin *et al.*, 2000). Furthermore patch clamp techniques have shown that gap junctions composed of Cx43-GFP have similar electrical properties as wild type Cx43 except for a slightly reduced sensitivity to transjunctional voltage

(Bukauskas *et al.*, 2000). Only large plaques are functional suggesting that clustering may be important for opening of gap junction channels (Bukauskas *et al.*, 2000). The versatility of CxGFP chimerae in studying the physiological role of gap junctions is exemplified further by studies showing the direct involvement of gap junction plaques in Ca^{2+} wave propagation (Paemeleire *et al.*, 2000). The present study has further exploited the versatile nature of Cx43-GFP chimerae by studying the effect of peptides homologous to the first and second extracellular loops of Cx43, ouabain and 18α-glycyrrhetinic acid on gap junction functionality and integrity. Each of these agents has been reported to inhibit EDHF type relaxations (Chaytor *et al.*, 1999; Dora *et al.*, 1999; Taylor *et al.*, 1998; Félétou and Vanhoutte, 1988; Harris *et al.*, 2000).

[43]Gap 26 and [43]Gap 27 caused a reduction in the ability of HeLa cells expressing Cx43-GFP to transfer Lucifer yellow. These peptides attenuate EDHF-type relaxations and endothelium-dependent hyperpolarizations in rabbit mesenteric arteries (Chaytor *et al.*, 1999; Dora *et al.*, 1999). Both peptides reduced the number of cells transferring Lucifer yellow to more than five neighbouring cells with a corresponding three-fold increase in the number transferring the dye to less than four neighbours, and were therefore equi-effective in their ability to attenuate intercellular communication. Direct visualisation of gap junction plaques constructed from Cx43-GFP by fluorescence microscopy demonstrated that [43]Gap 26 and [43]Gap 27 affect neither their number nor distribution at points of cell to cell contact between HeLa cells, suggesting that the interaction of the peptides with the extracellular loops of Cx43 affects the permeability of already established connexons by inducing a subtle conformational change rather than affecting stability and docking of connexons so as to cause plaque disassembly. This lack of major structural disruption is consistent with the rapid and reversible nature of the inhibition of EDHF-mediated relaxations by [43]Gap 27 previously observed in the rabbit superior mesenteric artery (Chaytor *et al.*, 1998).

The aglycone 18α-glycyrrhetinic acid inhibits EDHF-type relaxations in rabbit vessels and it attenuates gap junctional coupling in a wide variety of cell types (Davidson and Baumgarten, 1988; Taylor *et al.*, 1998). The present results show that the gap junctions formed by Cx43-GFP are similarly sensitive to 18α-glycyrrhetinic acid and that it efficiently attenuates dye transfer in A7r5 cells. The mechanism of action of 18α-glycyrrhetinic acid varies at differing concentrations. Low concentrations (5 μM), result in a rapid and reversible inhibition of gap junctional intercellular coupling in alveolar epithelial cells (Guo *et al.*, 1999). At higher concentrations the aglycone causes reductions in phosphorylation of Cx43 and protein abundance, associated with a decrease in mRNA synthesis. Furthermore, the number of plaques at the plasma membrane is reduced (Guo *et al.*, 1999). The versatility of the Cx43-GFP chimeric protein allowed the study of the effect of 18α-glycyrrhetinic acid on gap junction plaques in transfected A7r5 cells in real time. The disassembly of plaques commenced 15–30 minutes after exposure of the cells to 18α-glycyrrhetinic acid. The lateral movement of connexons or small plaques along the plasma membrane was replaced by an unzipping effect of the gap junctions and internalization of the released vesicles. The exact pathway taken for internalization of these plaques is unknown but it is likely that this takes place via a proteosomal or lysosomal route (Laing and Beyer, 2000).

Ouabain attenuates EDHF-type relaxations in a number of arterial systems including rat mesenteric arteries and canine and porcine coronary arteries (Félétou and Vanhoutte 1988; Makino *et al.*, 2000; Van de Voorde and Vanheel, 2000; Harris *et al.*,

2000), although others have reported that ouabain has no direct effect on EDHF-type relaxations in rat hepatic and guinea-pig basilar arteries (Andersson *et al.*, 2000; Zygmunt *et al.*, 2000). The structural similarity of ouabain to 18α-glycyrrhetinic acid and the controversial reports on the efficacy of ouabain to inhibit EDHF-type responses led to an investigation of the action of ouabain on gap junctional intercellular communication and integrity. The results show that in HeLa cells expressing Cx43-GFP ouabain nearly abolished dye transfers at concentrations of $1 \times 10^{-6}-1 \times 10^{-3}$ M, but at 1×10^{-7} M was without effect. Similar results were also observed in COS-7 cells, which express low amounts of Cx43 (George *et al.*, 1998a Harris *et al.*, 2000). Ouabain also attenuated dye transfer in A7r5 cells, but was effective only at concentrations of 1×10^{-3} M and 3×10^{-4} M. These differences may be explained by the levels of connexins expressed by these cell types. The HeLa cells are relatively weakly coupled compared to the A7r5 cells which rapidly transfer dye to more than 20 neighbouring cells. Gap junctions in A7r5 cells can be formed from both Cx40 and Cx43 isoforms and the composition of the heteromeric gap junctions is expected to be very sensitive to the ratio of contributing connexins (He *et al.*, 1999; Brink *et al.*, 2000; Beyer *et al.*, 2000). The heteromeric channels formed may all have variable conductance, gating and permeability properties thus providing different mechanisms for controlling chemical and electrical communication (He *et al.*, 1999).

When the effect of ouabain on gap junction integrity was analysed by time lapse microscopy in A7r5 cells transfected with Cx43-GFP no disassembly of the gap junction plaques was observed, which generally remained intact 90 minutes after exposure to ouabain. However, there was an associated decrease in the overall movement of the Cx43-GFP protein. The effects of ouabain on functionality and trafficking may in part be explained by other actions such as blockade of the Na^+/K^+ ATPase pump, a consequence of which is an increase in levels of intracellular free Ca^{2+}. Increases in cytosolic Ca^{2+} levels trigger uncoupling of gap junction channels in a variety of cell types (reviewed by Delage and Deleze, 2000). However, the level of Ca^{2+} required to produce uncoupling is variable, for example, with Novikoff hepatoma cells (Lazrak and Peracchia, 1993), primary cultures of glial cells (Giaume and Venance, 1998) and osteoblast cells (Schirrmacher *et al.*, 1996) exhibiting high Ca^{2+} sensitivity. An increase in intracellular Ca^{2+} can be observed by monitoring levels of Fura red fluorescence following incubation of A7r5 cells transfected with Cx43-GFP with ouabain (unpublished observations). In osteoblast-like cells ouabain also cause increases Ca^{2+} concentrations which are associated with decreases in the spread of Lucifer yellow to neighbouring cells (Schirrmacher *et al.*, 1996). Furthermore, increased Ca^{2+} levels reduce the vesicular trafficking rates of Cx43-GFP in stable HeLa cell populations (unpublished observations). However, mammalian cardiomyocytes are more resistant to Ca^{2+} induced uncoupling (Burt *et al.*, 1982; Maurer *et al.*, 1987). Such variable susceptibility to inceases in Ca^{2+} may contribute to the differences observed in dye transfer between the different cell types in the present study.

4. CONCLUSION

Cx43-GFP chimerae provide a versatile tool for studying the dynamics of gap junction stability and integrity. The results show that connexin-mimetic peptides do not disrupt or destabilise gap junction plaques but attenuate intercellular communication. The present data confirm in real time that 18α-glycyrrhetinic acid causes plaque disassembly (Guo *et al.*, 1999). This disassembly of gap junction plaques helps explain the attenuation of EDHF-type relaxations observed in isolated arteries (Taylor *et al.*, 1998; Chaytor *et al.*, 1999). Ouabain, despite its structural similarity to 18α-glycyrrhetinic acid does not cause plaque disruption in smooth muscle cells, but an overall reduction in connexin trafficking rates. The attenuation of dye transfer may, in part be explained by increased levels of intracellular Ca^{2+} causing channel closure. The controversial results reported with ouabain in terms of EDHF-like response may be due to level of connexin expression and different connexin combinations being expressed in the various arteries studied leading to a differential susceptibility to increases in Ca^{2+} concentration.

ACKNOWLEDGEMENTS

This work was supported by the MRC. We acknowledge Prof. W.H. Evans in whose lab work on the Cx43-GFP chimerae was initiated.

6 Role of gap junctions in endothelium-dependent hyperpolarizations

M.J. Gardener, M. Burnham,
A.H. Weston and G. Edwards

In rat mesenteric and hepatic arteries the endothelium-dependent hyperpolarizations can be explained by the direct effects on smooth muscle of K^+ liberated from the endothelium. However, in other preparations in which there is a good EDHF-response, K^+ appears neither to hyperpolarize nor to relax the vascular smooth muscle. In these vessels, myoendothelial gap junctions might conduct endothelial cell hyperpolarization to the underlying smooth muscle or be the pathway through which any hyperpolarizing factor is transferred to these cells. In the present study, the effects of two gap junction inhibitors (Gap 27 and carbenoxolone) on the EDHF-responses in the guinea-pig internal carotid, the pig coronary and the rat hepatic and mesenteric arteries were investigated using microelectrode techniques. Using reverse transcriptase-polymerase chain reaction (RT-PCR) the presence of mRNA corresponding to all three vascular connexins, Cx37, Cx40 and Cx43 was detected in whole mesenteric and hepatic, pig coronary and guinea-pig internal carotid arteries. Gap junctions are formed from connexins and immunofluorescence staining of frozen sections of these blood vessels revealed the presence (and distribution) of Cx37, Cx40 and Cx43. Although the relative distribution of the connexins did not differ between preparations with the exception of the guinea-pig internal carotid artery, the data indicates that gap junctions have only a minor, if any, role in the EDHF-response of the rat hepatic and mesenteric arteries. However, these structures may be important in the guinea-pig internal carotid and pig coronary arteries.

In mesenteric and hepatic arteries of the rat endothelium-dependent hyperpolarizations can largely be explained by direct effects on smooth muscle of K^+ liberated from the endothelium via calcium-sensitive K^+-channels (Edwards *et al.*, 1998). However, in other preparations such as the guinea-pig internal carotid artery or the pig coronary artery, K^+ neither hyperpolarizes nor relaxes the vascular smooth muscle and thus cannot represent endothelium-derived hyperpolarizing factor (EDHF) (Edwards *et al.*, 1999; Quignard *et al.*, 1999). Thus, on the basis of the sensitivity of their smooth muscle to K^+, these four blood vessels can be grouped as K^+-sensitive (rat hepatic and mesenteric arteries) and K^+-insensitive (guinea-pig internal carotid and pig coronary arteries) preparations.

Gap junctions have been implicated in the response to 'endothelium-derived hyperpolarizing factor' in rabbit aorta and mesenteric artery and in the guinea-pig internal carotid artery (Chaytor *et al.*, 1998; Edwards *et al.*, 1999). However, gap junction inhibitors were found to have little, if any, effect on the endothelium-dependent hyperpolarizations in rat hepatic or mesenteric arteries (Edwards *et al.*, 1999). Thus, it may be that in K^+-sensitive preparations, gap junction coupling is not essential for the endothelium-dependent hyperpolarization (Edwards *et al.*, 1999) whereas these structures may have a more important role in K^+-insensitive vessels (Edwards *et al.*, 1999; Edwards *et al.*, 2000).

The basic building blocks of gap junctions are the connexins, of which three types (Cx37, Cx40 and Cx43) have been identified in endothelial and/or vascular smooth muscle cells (see Brink, 1998). Thus, the aim of this study was to compare the distribution of these connexins in guinea-pig carotid and pig coronary arteries (tissues which do not hyperpolarize to K^+) with that in rat mesenteric and hepatic arteries (in which K^+ hyperpolarizes the smooth muscle).

1. METHODS

1.1. Preparation of blood vessels

Hepatic and mesenteric arteries were obtained from male Sprague-Dawley rats (150–200 g body weight). Internal carotid arteries were dissected from Duncan-Hartley guinea-pigs (400–480 g body weight). Pig hearts were obtained from the local abattoir and transported to the laboratory in ice-cold Krebs solution (time from heart removal to vessel dissection approximately 45 min). The left anterior descending coronary artery was dissected free and cleaned of adherent fat and connective tissue.

All preparations were either used immediately after dissection or fixed for immuno-histochemistry.

1.2. Reverse transcriptase-polymerase chain reaction

1.2.1. Total RNA isolation

Whole blood vessels were dissected in ice-cold Krebs and either used immediately or stored in RNAlater (Ambion) for later processing. Total RNA was obtained using the Qiagen RNeasy mini kit for extraction from animal tissue. Briefly, the tissue was weighed. Thirty mg were placed in a 12 ml Falcon tube with 600 µl homogenization buffer containing guanidinium isothiocyanate and β-mecaptoethanol to inactivate RNases, and homogenized with a rotor homogenizer until a uniform solution was obtained. The lysate was then centrifuged at more than 10,000 rpm for 3 min, after which the supernatant was retained and the pelleted matter discarded. Three separate wash steps were performed using high salt and ethanol-containing buffers to remove contaminants. The total RNA was then eluted using RNase-free water.

1.2.2. Reverse transcription

Reverse transcription was carried out according to the protocol for Superscript II reverse transcriptase for all tissues used, except for total RNA from guinea-pig internal carotid artery which was reverse-transcribed using Sensiscript due to low total RNA yield.

1.2.3. PCR

PCR reactions were carried out using gene-specific primers (or homology-based for all guinea-pig connexins and pig connexin, Cx40), 0.6 µM final concentration, 0.25 mM deoxyribonucleoside5'-triphosphases (dNTPs), 1x Taq buffer (5 µl 10x buffer in 50 µl final reaction volume), 0.5 µl cDNA, 0.25 µl ExTaq (5 units/µl) and nuclease-free water to 50 µl. Reactions were subjected to a hot start (94 °C for 5 min after which ExTaq was added) to prevent non-specific annealing of primers.

After amplification, products were subjected to electrophoresis at 120 V on a 1% agrose gel containing 1.26×10^{-6} M ethidium bromide bathed in 0.5x TBE (44.5 mM Trizma base, 56 mM boric acid, 0.99 mM EDTA in milliQ purified water) containing 1.26×10^{-6} M ethidium bromide and visualized under UV light.

All products have been sequenced to confirm their identity.

1.3. Immunostaining

1.3.1. Fixing and sectioning of tissue and immunostaining

After dissection, arteries were fixed in 4% paraformaldehyde in phosphate-buffered saline (McLean and Nakane, 1974) for 30 min and then placed overnight in cryo-protectant (85% sucrose in phosphate-buffered saline (PBS) for porcine coronary artery, 30% sucrose for all others). Small artery segments were embedded in OCT® compound (Sakura), rapidly frozen and 4 µm cryostat sections were transferred to silanated slides.

For immuno-labelling, tissue sections were blocked with 1% w/v bovine serum albulmin (BSA) in PBS containing 5% v/v normal goat serum, incubated with primary antibodies overnight at 4 °C, and washed in phosphate-buffered saline. Slides were incubated with secondary antibodies conjugated to Texas red or Cy3 (Jackson ImmunoResearch, USA (via Stratech Scientific UK)) for 40 min, together with a blue nuclear label, 4',6-diamidino-2-phenylindole (DAPI). (Sigma, UK.)

1.3.2. Primary antibodies

Mouse monoclonal anti-Cx43 (Chemicon, USA) and rabbit polyclonal anti-mouse Cx37, Cx40 (ADI, USA), were employed as appropriate.

1.4. Solutions

The phosphate-buffered saline contained 8.4 mM Na_2HPO_4, 2.0 mM NaH_2PO_4, 145 mM. The Krebs solution contained 118 mM NaCl, 3.4 mM KCl, 2.5 mM $CaCl_2$, 1.2 mM KH_2PO_4, 1.2 mM $MgCl_2$, 11 mM glucose, 25 mM $NaHCO_3$.

1.5. Drugs, kits and enzymes

The following were used: agrose (molecular biology grade, Roche Diagnostics, Lewes, UK), boric acid (Sigma, Poole, UK), EDTA (Sigma, Poole, UK), ethidium bromide (Sigma, Poole, UK), ExTaq, 10x ExTaq buffer and 2.5 mM dNTP mixture (TaKaRa Biomedical via BioWhittaker Wokingham, UK), β-mecaptoethanol (Sigma, Poole, UK), paraformaldehyde (BDH, Lutterworth, UK), RNeasy mini kit (Qiagen, Crawley, UK), sucrose (BDH, Lutterworth, UK), Sensiscript reverse transcriptase (Qiagen, Crawley, UK), Superscript II (GibcoBRL, Paisley, UK), trizma base, (Sigma, Poole, UK), nuclease-free water (Promega, Southampton, UK).

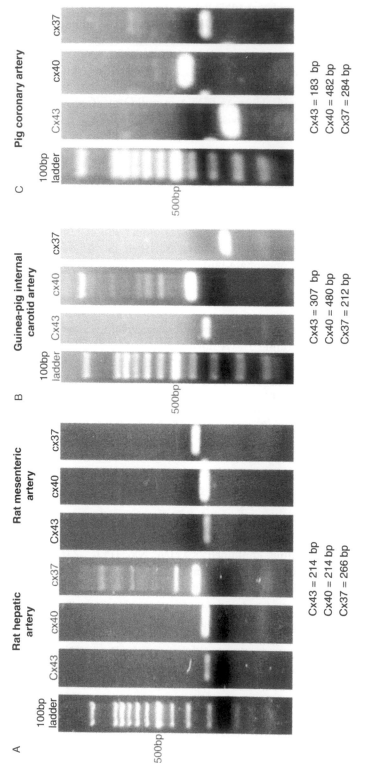

Figure 6.1 Results of RT-PCR experiments performed on whole blood vessels. The presence of the message for all three vascular connexins Cx37, Cx40 and Cx43 was detected in (A) rat hepatic and mesenteric arteries, (B) guinea-pig internal carotid and (C) porcine coronary arteries.

2. RESULTS

2.1. RT-PCR

The presence of mRNA encoding for Cx37, Cx40 and Cx43 was detected in total RNA samples obtained from whole rat mesenteric and hepatic as well as guinea-pig internal carotid and pig coronary artery (Figure 6.1).

2.2. Immunohistochemistry (Table 6.1)

2.2.1. Rat mesenteric and hepatic arteries

Staining with antibodies raised against Cx37, Cx40 and Cx43 showed that the distribution of these connexins and presumably the associated connexons and relevant gap junctions was mostly uniform throughout rat, pig and guinea-pig tissues studied. In the rat hepatic and mesenteric arteries, Cx37 was by far the most abundant with intense staining throughout the endothelial as well as the smooth muscle layer (Figure 6.2A(i and ii) respectively). The specificity of the Cx37 binding was confirmed by its complete inhibition in the presence of the antigenic peptide (not shown). Cx40 appeared to be uniformly distributed in the endothelium of both tissue types but was not evident in the smooth muscle (Figures 6.2B(i and ii)). Cx43 was the least abundant type with punctate distribution in endothelial cells and little evidence for its presence in the plasmalemma of myocytes (Figures 6.2C(i and ii)).

2.2.2. Guinea-pig internal carotid artery

Sections from the guinea-pig internal carotid artery were taken from the part of the blood vessel close to its exit from the carotid artery and from an area of the vessel distal to this where the blood vessel had greatly narrowed. These regions were termed the 'large' and the 'small' internal carotid arteries respectively. As in the rat preparations, Cx37 was again the most abundant in the guinea-pig internal carotid artery with staining throughout the vessel (Figure 6.3A). Cx40 was evenly distributed along the endothelium in the large and small internal carotid artery but was only present in the smooth muscle cells of the large sections (Figure 6.3B). In the small internal carotid artery, Cx43 was evident in the endothelium but was only sparsely distributed in the smooth muscle layer (Figure 6.3C left hand panel). In contrast, Cx43 was present in both the endothelium and smooth muscle of the large internal carotid artery sections and appeared to be expressed at levels similar to that of Cx37 (Figure 6.3C right hand panel).

Table 6.1 Comparison of connexin distribution

	Cx37		Cx40		Cx43	
	endo	*vsm*	*endo*	*vsm*	*endo*	*vsm*
Rat hepatic	+++	+++	++	(+)	+	(+)
Rat mesenteric	+++	+++	++	(+)	+	(+)
Guinea-pig (large) internal carotid	+++	+++	++	+	++	++
Pig coronary	+++	+++	++	(+)	+	(+)

A (i)　　　　　　　　(ii)

B (i)　　　　　　　　(ii)

C (i)　　　　　　　　(ii)

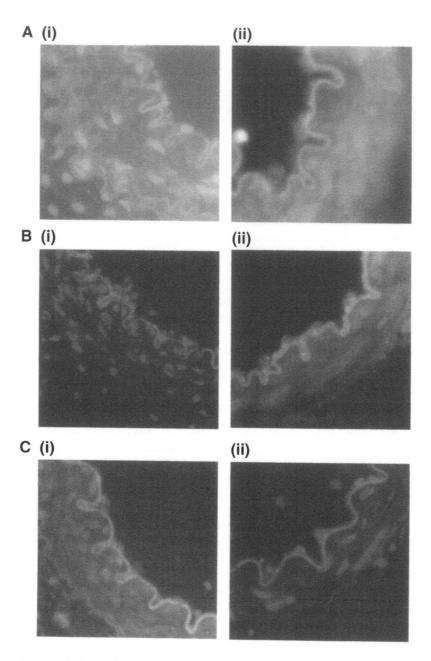

Figure 6.2 Connexin-specific immunostaining in rat hepatic and mesenteric arteries. Cx37 was abundant in both the endothelium and smooth muscle of the rat hepatic (A (i)) and mesenteric arteries (A (ii)), whereas Cx40 was restricted to the endothelium in both vessels (B (i) and (ii)). Cx43 was again evident in endothelium of both the hepatic and mesenteric arteries but also appeared at a low level in the media of these blood vessels (C (i) and (ii) respectively). (*see Color Plate 5*)

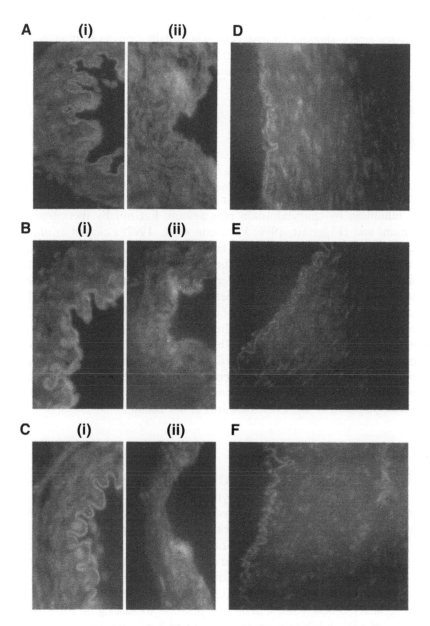

Figure 6.3 Connexin-specific immunostaining in the guinea-pig internal carotid artery and the porcine coronary artery. Cx37 staining was widespread in both the 'small' and 'large' internal carotid arteries (A (i) and (ii) respectively), and in the porcine coronary artery (D). Cx40 staining was restricted to the endothelium in the 'small' internal carotid artery (B (i)) but was evident in the media and endothelium in the 'large' internal carotid artery (B (ii)) as well as the porcine coronary artery (E). Cx43 expression was mainly endothelial in the 'small' internal carotid artery (C (i)) as was it in the porcine coronary artery (F) although there was some evidence for its expression in the smooth muscle. In the 'large' internal carotid artery, Cx43 was present in the endothelium but its expression was greatly increased in the smooth muscle (C (ii)). (*see Color Plate 6*)

2.2.3. Porcine coronary artery

The pig coronary artery showed similar connexin distribution to that in both rat hepatic and mesenteric arteries with Cx37 the most highly-expressed form (Figure 6.3D). Cx40 and Cx43 were more densely distributed in the endothelium than in the smooth muscle layer (Figures 6.3E and F).

3. DISCUSSION

3.1. EDHF and K$^+$

A unifying feature of the EDHF response in all preparations in which it has been studied is its inhibition by charybdotoxin plus apamin but not by iberiotoxin plus apamin (Zygmunt and Högestätt, 1996; Petersson et al., 1997; Eckman et al., 1998; Edwards et al., 1998; Yamanaka et al., 1998; Quignard et al., 1999). Almost certainly, the site of action of these toxins is on endothelial cell calcium-sensitive K$^+$ channels and these play a pivotal role in the EDHF pathway (Edwards et al., 1998, 2000). However, there are also notable differences between the EDHF responses in different preparations and this may be an indication of multiple 'hyperpolarizing factors' or of different mechanisms by which the endothelium influences the membrane potential of the underlying smooth muscle cells. Thus, a barium plus ouabain cocktail abolishes endothelium-dependent hyperpolarization in rat hepatic and mesenteric arteries (Edwards et al., 1998), whereas this combination of inhibitors has essentially no effect on the EDHF response in the guinea-pig carotid artery or the porcine coronary artery (Quignard et al., 1999; Edwards et al., 2000).

3.2. EDHF and gap junctions

Gap junctions have been implicated in the EDHF response, initially on the basis that known inhibitors also reduced the spasmolytic effect of EDHF (Kühberger et al., 1994; Chaytor et al., 1998) and later more directly by demonstration that gap junction inhibitors reduced the hyperpolarization (Dora et al., 1999; Edwards et al., 1999). One gap junction inhibitor which has been used for this demonstration is Gap 27, a peptide with a sequence identical to part of the second extracellular docking loop of Cx37 and Cx43. It has been assumed that the ability of this peptide to inhibit the EDHF reflects an action on the myo-endothelial junctions (Chaytor et al., 1998; Dora et al., 1999). However, using intact blood vessels, it is not possible to distinguish between the potential effects of such inhibitors on myo-endothelial gap junctions or on those between the smooth muscle layers. In the porcine coronary artery at least, there is emerging evidence that their site of action is predominantly on myocyte:myocyte junctions (Edwards et al., 2000). Nevertheless, irrespective of the site of action of the gap junction inhibitors, it is notable that Gap 27 has only a small inhibitory effect on the EDHF response in the rat mesenteric artery and it is essentially without effect on the response in the rat hepatic artery (Edwards et al., 1999). Thus, the primary aim of the present study was to determine whether *differential distribution* of connexins could explain the relative importance of gap junctions in the EDHF response in different tissues.

Whereas vascular endothelial cells express Cx37, Cx40 and Cx43, smooth muscle cells are thought to possess only Cx40 and Cx43 (see Brink, 1998). In the present study, Cx37 was the most abundantly-expressed connexin in both the smooth muscle and endothelial cells from all tissues investigated. Cx43 was the least expressed in these arteries with diffuse staining in the endothelium of all the vessels studied. The only blood vessel with Cx43 staining of any significance was the guinea-pig internal carotid artery. However, this was only seen in sections taken from near to its point of exit from the carotid artery. This is expected as Cx43 is up-regulated at sites of turbulence such as vessel bifurcations (Cowan *et al.*, 1998; Gabriels and Paul, 1998; van Kempen and Jongsma, 1999).

It seems likely that Cx37 represents the main potential target for inhibition of coupling by Gap 27. However the uniform expression of Cx37 in all the blood vessels studied suggests that the differences in the sensitivity of the EDHF response to inhibition by gap junction inhibitors cannot be explained by differential expression of connexins. The expression of Cx40 was confined to the endothelium in the arteries from the rat but could also be seen in smooth muscle cells from the guinea-pig internal carotid and pig coronary artery. Cx40 does not share homology with Cx43 and Cx37 at the region of the second extracellular loop, the locus Gap 27 was designed to mimic. It is therefore reasonable to assume that Gap 27 will not inhibit gap junctions containing solely Cx40 (homotypic gap junctions) and may only partially inhibit junctions comprising other connexins in addition to Cx40. This could well explain the inability of Gap 27 to inhibit EDHF in microelectrode recordings taken via the intima of the porcine coronary artery compared to the recordings from the adventitial side of the porcine coronary and guinea-pig internal carotid arteries (Edwards *et al.*, 2000). Over the distance from the endothelium to the electrode (approximately 20 cells in the porcine coronary artery) the coupling between these layers of cells can be reduced significantly by Gap 27 inhibiting some of the gap junctions present. However, coupling between the endothelium and first layer of smooth muscle cannot be inhibited because of the high levels of Cx40-containing gap junctions present in the endothelium and presumably in the myo-endothelial gap junctions. The differences seen between the rat hepatic and mesenteric arteries and guinea-pig internal carotid and porcine coronary arteries might be explained by the numbers of myo-endothelial gap junctions and their connexin make-up. Although speculative, the rat hepatic artery might represent a vessel with very poor myo-endothelial coupling while the porcine coronary and guinea-pig internal carotid arteries represent well-coupled vessels with the mesenteric artery occupying an intermediate position.

4. CONCLUSIONS

In the present study, the presence of Cx37, Cx40 and Cx43 was detected in all four blood vessels studied. However, there was no obvious correlation between connexin distribution and the possible role of gap junctions in the EDHF-responses of these vessels. Although it is tempting to speculate that myo-endothelial gap junctions are involved in those vessels which do not hyperpolarize when exposed to an increase in extracellular K^+, the resolution of the methodologies employed did not allow such junctions to be clearly visualized.

7 Heterogeneity of EDHF-type relaxations of rabbit and rat arteries analysed with peptides homologous to the extracellular loops of connexins 37, 40 and 43

Tudor M. Griffith, Andrew T. Chaytor, Rodney S. Berman and David H. Edwards

The contribution of gap junctional communication to acetylcholine-evoked relaxations in rabbit ear resistance arteries and rat hepatic and mesenteric arteries has been investigated with peptides homologous to the Gap 26 and 27 domains of the first and second extracellular loops of connexins (Cxs) 37, 40 and 43. These peptides were designated according to the nomenclature ^{37,40}Gap 26, ^{43}Gap 26, ^{37,43}Gap 27 and ^{40}Gap 27. N^G-nitro-L-arginine methyl ester (L-NAME, 3×10^{-4} M) attenuated maximal relaxations to acetylcholine by approximately 70% in the rabbit central ear artery (G_0), but only by 30% in its second branch generation (G_2). The residual responses, attributed to endothelium-derived hyperpolarizing factor (EDHF), were essentially abolished by ^{43}Gap 26 and ^{37,43}Gap 27 in both arteries. In the rat hepatic artery EDHF-type relaxations were unaffected by ^{37,40}Gap 26, ^{43}Gap 26, ^{37,43}Gap 27, ^{40}Gap 27, and combinations of peptide targeted to Cx40 (^{37,40}Gap 26 plus ^{40}Gap 27) or Cx43 (^{37,43}Gap 27 plus ^{43}Gap 26). By contrast, peptide combinations simultaneously targeting both Cxs40 and 43 (i.e., ^{37,40}Gap 26 plus ^{43}Gap 26, ^{37,43}Gap 27 plus ^{40}Gap 27, ^{37,40}Gap 26 plus ^{37,43}Gap 27 or ^{43}Gap 26 plus ^{40}Gap 26) decreased maximal relaxations by 30–90% in hepatic and mesenteric arteries. The findings provide evidence that the contribution of gap junctions to acetylcholine-induced responses in the rabbit ear vasculature increases with diminishing blood vessel size and is inversely related to functional NO activity. Whilst EDHF-type relaxations involve direct intercellular communication via Cx43 in the rabbit, intercellular coupling via both Cx40- and Cx43-containing gap junction channels is essential for the mediation of such responses in the rat.

Endothelium-dependent vascular relaxations observed in the presence of inhibitors of nitric oxide (NO) and prostanoid synthesis are widely attributed to an endothelium-derived hyperpolarizing factor (EDHF). Although the existence of EDHF has been demonstrated in cascade bioassay (Mombouli *et al.*, 1996), and in 'sandwich' strip preparations (Hutcheson *et al.*, 1999), in rabbit arteries and veins there is evidence that this factor normally transfers from endothelium to smooth muscle via myoendothelial gap junctions following stimulation by agonists such as acetylcholine, rather than the extracellular space (Chaytor *et al.*, 1998; Dora *et al.*, 1999; Yamamoto *et al.*, 1999; Griffith and Taylor, 1999). Gap junctions are formed by two interlocked hemi-channels or connexons, which are contributed by coupled cells, with each connexon constructed from six transmembrane protein subunits called connexins that cross the cell membrane four times with two loops exposed extracellularly (Kumar and Gilula, 1996). Interdigitation of these extracellular loops, followed by a 30° rotation, results in channel docking and the formation of an aqueous central pore (Perkins *et al.*, 1998). Clusters of up to several hundred individual gap junctions in plaque-like structures permit the direct intercellular transfer of ions and molecules smaller than 1 kDa in size at localized sites in the cell membrane (Bukauskas *et al.*, 2000). At least 20 connexin (Cx) subtypes have been identified in mammalian tissues and these are conventionally classified according to their molecular weight in kDa with endothelial and vascular smooth muscle cells variably expressing Cx37, Cx40 and Cx43 according to species and vessel type (Carter *et al.*, 1996; Brink, 1998; van Kempen and Jongsma, 1999). In theory, myoendothelial gap junctions could thus contain homotypic channels in which each contributing connexon is constructed from the same connexin subtype (e.g., Cx43/Cx43), heterotypic channels in which each connexon is constructed from a different subtype (e.g., Cx37/Cx43) and heteromeric channels in which each connexon contains a mixture of different connexin proteins.

In the rabbit mesenteric artery, whose smooth muscle cells express predominantly the Cx43 protein subtype, EDHF-type relaxations and hyperpolarizations evoked by acetylcholine are rapidly and reversibly abolished by a short synthetic undecapeptide that possesses sequence homology with the Gap 27 domain of the second extracellular loop of Cx43 (here denoted as [37,43]Gap 27 as the sequence is also common to Cx37, Table 7.1) (Chaytor *et al.*, 1998). [37,43]Gap 27 also inhibits EDHF-type relaxations in the rabbit jugular vein, thus demonstrating the generality of the gap junction mechanism (Griffith and Taylor, 1999). Changes in just three amino acids in the Gap 27 sequence leading into the fourth transmembrane Cx43 domain, so as to confer homology with Cx40 (here denoted as [40]Gap 27, Table 7.1), abolish its ability to inhibit EDHF-type relaxations in rabbit mesenteric arteries, confirming that its action is highly connexin-specific (Chaytor *et al.*, 1999). Indeed, in confluent COS-7 monolayers, a fibroblast cell line which expresses Cx43 as its only functional protein (George *et al.*, 1998), [37,43]Gap 27 attenuates intercellular diffusion of the fluorescent dye Lucifer yellow, whereas [40]Gap 27 is without effect (Chaytor *et al.*, 1999). [37,43]Gap 27 has also been shown to inhibit EDHF-type hyperpolarization in guinea-pig carotid and porcine coronary arteries (Edwards *et al.*, 1999, 2000), but is relatively inactive in rat mesenteric and hepatic arteries (Edwards *et al.*, 1999). Indeed, in rat arteries it has been suggested that K^+ ions released from the endothelium directly into the extracellular space serve as an EDHF by activating inwardly-rectifying smooth

Table 7.1 Amino acid sequences of the four peptides used in the study

	Gap 26	Gap 27
Cx37	VCYDQAFPISHIR	SRPTEKTIFII
Cx40	VCYDQAFPISHIR	SRPTEKNVFIV
Cx43	VCYDKSFPISHVR	SRPTEKTIFII

Notes
The Gap 26 and Gap 27 domains are conserved in man, rat and mouse and are located in the first and second extracellular connexin loops, respectively. Because of sequence overlap the peptides are designated as [37,40]Gap 26, [43]Gap 26, [37,43]Gap 27 and [40]Gap 27.

muscle K^+ channels and the Na^+/K^+ ATPase, thereby promoting hyperpolarization and relaxation (Edwards *et al.*, 1998). In contrast to the rabbit mesenteric artery, however, smooth muscle cells from some rat arteries express both Cx40 and Cx43 connexin subtypes, thus allowing the possibility that homotypic Cx40 channels, that should in theory be insensitive to inhibition by [37,43]Gap 27, could contribute to myoendothelial gap junctional communication in this species.

In arteries from the rat mesenteric bed, EDHF-type responses become progressively larger as vessel size decreases (Hwa *et al.*, 1994; Shimokawa *et al.*, 1996). In the rabbit ear, also, the mechanisms that underlie the vasodilator response to acetylcholine are spatially heterogeneous, being mediated predominantly by NO in the central ear artery but possessing the characteristics of an EDHF-type response in branch arteries with a diameter less than 100 µm (Berman and Griffith, 1997, 1998). The present study has attempted to define the role of gap junctions in the genesis of spatial heterogeneity in the mechanisms underlying acetylcholine-induced vasodilatation within the rabbit ear vascular network using peptides homologous to Cx43. Connexin-mimetic peptides designed to exploit similarities and differences in the amino acid sequences of the Gap 26 and 27 domains of Cxs 37, 40 and 43 (Table 7.1) were employed to determine whether the dual expression of Cxs 40 and 43 underlies the apparent species heterogeneity in the mechanisms underlying the EDHF phenomenon in the rabbit and the rat.

1. METHODS

1.1. Isolated ring preparations

Male New Zealand White rabbits (2.5–3.0 kg) were killed using intravenous sodium pentobarbitone (120 mg/kg) and male Wistar rats (200–250 g) were killed by a blow to the head followed by cervical dislocation. Rings (1–2 mm width) were obtained from the rabbit central ear artery (generation G_0) and rat hepatic artery and studied by a standard myograph technique in Holman's buffer (composition in mM: NaCl 120, KCl 5, $CaCl_2$ 2.5, NaH_2PO_4 1.3, $NaHCO_3$ 25, glucose 11, and sucrose 10) containing indomethacin (1×10^{-5} M) which was maintained at 37 °C and at pH 7.2–7.4 by oxygenation with 95% O_2/5% CO_2. Tension was initially set at 0.5 g in G_0 rings and 0.25 g in hepatic arteries. During an equilibrium period of 30–60 min the tissues were repeatedly washed with fresh buffer and tension readjusted as necessary following stress relaxation.

1.2. Cannulated arterial segments

Isolated second generation branch arteries (generation G_2) were perfused *in situ* in isolated intact ears from which a skin flap was dissected to expose a suitable territory. Having identified a G_2 vessel for study, a fine polypropylene cannula of appropriate diameter was inserted through a hole cut in the wall of the central ear artery close to the junction of the first generation (G_1) artery from which the G_2 artery originated. The cannula was then fed along this G_1 artery until its tip was immediately proximal to the origin of the G_2 artery selected for study and secured with suture. All flow was diverted into artery by a ligature placed on the parent vessel immediately distal to the tip of the cannula. The G_2 artery was severed 3–8 mm distal to its origin depending on local anatomy and the skin flap replaced to prevent drying and perfused with oxygenated Holman's buffer containing indomethacin (1×10^{-5} M) at 37 °C at a flow rate of 0.2 ml min^{-1} for an initial incubation period of 30 min. An air-filled compliance chamber connected via a T piece was used to damp pressure fluctuations to within 5% of the mean. Isolated rat mesenteric arteries (3rd order, *ca.* 10 mm length, 300–400 μm diameter) were cannulated and mounted in a Living Systems pressure myograph (LSI, Burlington, USA) containing gassed Holman's buffer at 37 °C. Intraluminal pressure was held constant at 40 mmHg under conditions of no flow and external vessel diameter monitored continuously by an automatic tracking system.

1.3. Experimental protocols

In rabbit G_0 and G_2 arteries concentration–response curves to acetylcholine were obtained following constriction with a combination of 5-hydroxytryptamine (1×10^{-6} M) and histamine (1×10^{-6} M). Depending on the protocol followed, these curves were constructed in the presence and absence of L-NAME (3×10^{-4} M), [37,40]Gap 26 (3×10^{-4} M or 5×10^{-4} M), [37,43]Gap 27 (3×10^{-4} M) or a combination of L-NAME with these peptides. Inhibitors were administered 30–60 min prior to inducing the constriction. Rat hepatic artery rings were incubated with L-NAME (3×10^{-4} M) and indomethacin (1×10^{-5} M) in all experiments and were preconstricted with (3×10^{-7} M) phenylephrine before cumulative concentration–response curves to acetylcholine were obtained. The effects of incubation with [37,40]Gap 26, [43]Gap 26, [37,43]Gap 27 or [40]Gap 27 (each at 6×10^{-4} M) and all possible combinations of these peptides in pairs (3×10^{-4} M for each individual peptide) were also studied. In rat mesenteric segments, the effects of extraluminal administration of [37,40]Gap 26 plus [43]Gap 27 and [43]Gap 26 plus [40]Gap 27 (each peptide at 3×10^{-4} M) on EDHF-type responses evoked by acetylcholine were also examined following constriction by phenylephrine (1×10^{-6} M).

2. STATISTICAL ANALYSIS

Data are given as mean $\pm$ SEM, where *n* denotes the number of animals studied for each data point. Concentration–response curves were assessed by one-way analysis of variance (ANOVA) followed by a multiple comparisons test. Changes in the concentration of acetylcholine causing half-maximal relaxation (EC$_{50}$) and maximal relaxation (expressed as % reversal of agonist-induced constriction, R_{max}) were evaluated by a Student's *t*-test and considered significant when *p* was less than .05.

3. DRUGS

Acetylcholine chloride, histamine dihydrochloride, 5-hydroxytryptamine (as creatinine sulphate complex), phenylephrine, indomethacin, and N^G-nitro-L-arginine methyl ester were obtained from Sigma, Poole, UK. Gap peptides were synthesized by Severn Biotech or SigmaGenosys, UK. Purity was greater than 95%.

4. RESULTS

4.1. Connexin-mimetic peptides and relaxations to acetylcholine in rabbit ear arteries

In G_0 rings constricted by 5-hydroxytryptamine (1×10^{-6} M) and histamine (1×10^{-6} M), relaxations to acetylcholine were reduced compared to control and concentration–response curves shifted to the right following a 30 min incubation with either ^{43}Gap 26 or ^{37,43}Gap 27 at concentrations of 3×10^{-4} M (Figure 7.1). Each peptide reduced maximal relaxations to acetylcholine by about 20% with an associated two to three fold rightward shift in EC_{50} (Table 7.2), but did not significantly affect force development in response to the combination of 5-hydroxytryptamine and histamine (data not shown). Time-matched control responses to acetylcholine were also obtained and showed no significant attenuation of relaxation over time, thereby confirming the viability of the endothelium during the experimental protocols (Figure 7.1). Experiments were also performed with ^{43}Gap 26 at a concentration of 5×10^{-4} M, to determine if the inhibitory effects of the peptide were maximal at 3×10^{-4} M. The EC_{50} obtained for acetylcholine-induced relaxation at the higher concentration was $3.0 \pm 1.0 \times 10^{-6}$ M with a maximal relaxation of $72 \pm 6.0\%$ ($n = 4$) and these values did not differ significantly from those obtained with the lower concentration of ^{43}Gap 26 (Table 7.2).

L-NAME (3×10^{-4} M) substantially attenuated the relaxations evoked by acetylcholine in preconstricted G_0 rings, reducing the maximal response by about 70%

Table 7.2 Effects of connexin-mimetic peptides and N^G-nitro-L-arginine methyl ester (L-NAME) on responses to acetylcholine in isolated rabbit ear G_0 arterial rings and perfused G_2 arteries

	n	$R_{max}(\%)$	$EC_{50}(\mu M)$
G_0			
Control	21	89 ± 2	1.3 ± 0.4
L-NAME	9	$21 \pm 4^*$	$3.2 \pm 0.9^*$
^{43}Gap 26	6	$72 \pm 7^*$	$3.3 \pm 0.9^*$
L-NAME + ^{43}Gap 26	4	$2 \pm 2^{*,\dagger}$	–
^{37,43}Gap 27	6	$68 \pm 10^*$	$4.3 \pm 0.9^*$
L-NAME + ^{37,43}Gap 27	5	$9 \pm 5^{*,\dagger}$	–
G_2			
Control	16	89 ± 4	1.2 ± 0.5
L-NAME	8	$59 \pm 11^*$	4.3 ± 1.8
^{43}Gap 26	3	$43 \pm 9^*$	4.6 ± 3.3
L-NAME + ^{43}Gap 26	4	$5 \pm 2^{*,\dagger}$	–
^{37,43}Gap 27	5	$35 \pm 17^*$	$9.7 \pm 5.5^*$
L-NAME + ^{37,43}Gap 27	4	$1 \pm 1^{*,\dagger}$	–

Notes
Tone was induced by the combination of 5-hydroxytryptamine (1×10^{-6} M) and histamine (1×10^{-6} M). L-NAME and connexin-mimetic peptides were each administered at a concentration of 3×10^{-4} M. Data are shown as means $\pm$ SEM. The asterisks and the daggers indicate statistically significant differences versus control and the presence of L-NAME only, respectively ($p < .05$).

(Figure 7.1). In the additional presence of [43]Gap 26 or [37,43]Gap 27 (3×10^{-4} M), responses to acetylcholine were virtually abolished (Figure 7.1). Force development was slightly increased by L-NAME, but not further affected by incubation with either [43]Gap 26 or [37,43]Gap 27 (data not shown).

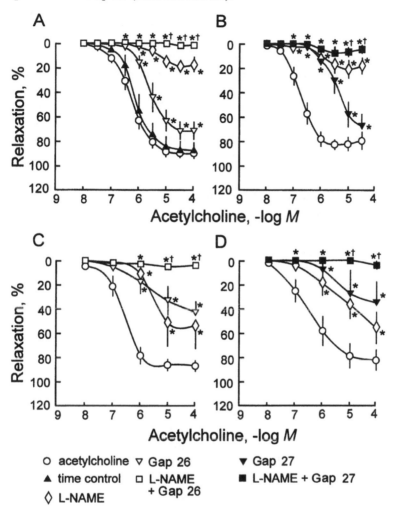

Figure 7.1 Effects of connexin-mimetic peptides on concentration–relaxation curves to acetylcholine in isolated rabbit G_0 arterial rings and isolated perfused G_2 arteries constricted with the combination of 5-hydroxytryptamine (1×10^{-6} M) and histamine (1×10^{-6} M). (A,B) In G_0 rings, responses were attenuated to an approximately equivalent extent by 3×10^{-4} M [43]Gap 26 and [37,43]Gap 27, whereas 3×10^{-4} M N^G-nitro-L-arginine methyl ester (L-NAME) caused substantially greater inhibition. The combination of L-NAME with either [43]Gap 26 or [37,43]Gap 27 essentially abolished relaxation. In (A) time-matched controls are shown for comparison. (C,D). In perfused G_2 arteries, [43]Gap 26 and [37,43]Gap 27 both inhibited the control depressor response to a greater extent than L-NAME, although the combination of L-NAME and either peptide again almost abolished relaxation. Data are shown as means ± SEM; n values are given in Table 7.1. Asterisks and daggers indicate statistically significant differences versus control and the presence of L-NAME only, respectively ($p < .05$).

In the presence of either [43]Gap 26 or [37,43]Gap 27 (3×10^{-4} M), maximal relaxations to acetylcholine in perfused segments of G_2 arteries in which pressure was elevated by the combination of 5-hydroxytryptamine (1×10^{-6} M) and histamine (1×10^{-6} M) were reduced by about 50% (Figure 7.1), with a four- to eight-fold rightward shift in EC_{50} (Table 7.2). Neither peptide exerted significant effects on pressure development in response to the combination of 5-hydroxytryptamine and histamine (data not shown).

The maximal depressor response induced by acetylcholine in G_2 segments, following pressure elevation with 5-hydroxytryptamine (1×10^{-6} M) and histamine (1×10^{-6} M), was significantly reduced by about 30% following incubation with L-NAME (3×10^{-4} M) (Figure 7.1). Incubation with L-NAME plus either [43]Gap 26 or [37,43]Gap 27 (3×10^{-4} M) virtually abolished responses (Figure 7.1). The perfusion pressure was elevated significantly by L-NAME but not affected further by either [43]Gap 26 or [37,43]Gap 27 (data not shown).

4.2. Connexin-mimetic peptides and relaxations to acetylcholine in the rat hepatic artery

Rings of hepatic artery were constricted by phenylephrine (3×10^{-7} M) in the presence of L-NAME (3×10^{-4} M) and indomethacin (1×10^{-5} M). EDHF-type relaxations were maximal at a concentration of 1×10^{-5} M acetylcholine with a maximal response of about 80% of the phenylephrine-induced tone. Incubation with [37,40]Gap 26, [43]Gap 26, [37,43]Gap 27 or [40]Gap 27 (each at 6×10^{-4} M) did not significantly alter maximal relaxations or the EC_{50} for acetylcholine compared to control (Figure 7.2).

4.3. Paired peptide combinations in the rat hepatic artery

Incubation with [37,40]Gap 26 plus [40]Gap 27 or [43]Gap 26 plus [37,43]Gap 27 (3×10^{-4} M for each component) did not alter EDHF-type relaxations evoked by acetylcholine when compared to control (Figure 7.3). Following incubation with [37,40]Gap 26 plus [43]Gap 26 or [37,43]Gap 27 plus [40]Gap 27 (3×10^{-4} M for each component) maximal EDHF-type relaxations to acetylcholine were reduced significantly (Figure 7.4, Table 7.3). EC_{50} values were not altered significantly following incubation with [37,40]Gap 26 plus [43]Gap 26, whereas there was a significant rightward shift following incubation with [43]Gap 26 plus [40]Gap 27 (Table 7.3). Incubation with [37,40]Gap 26 plus [37,43]Gap 27 (3×10^{-4} M for both) inhibited maximal EDHF-type relaxations (Figure 7.4, Table 7.3) with a significant shift in EC_{50} values (Table 7.3). [43]Gap 26 plus [40]Gap 27 peptide similarly inhibited the maximal response to acetylcholine (Figure 7.4, Table 7.3) with an associated shift in EC_{50} values (Table 7.3).

4.4. Paired peptide combinations in the rat mesenteric artery

In segments of mesenteric artery constricted by phenylephrine (1×10^{-6} M) in the presence of L-NAME (3×10^{-4} M) and indomethacin (1×10^{-5} M), EDHF-type relaxations were maximal at a concentration of 1×10^{-6} M acetylcholine with a maximal response of about 50% of the phenylephrine-induced tone. Following pre-incubation with [37,40]Gap 26 plus [43]Gap 26 or [37,43]Gap 27 plus [40]Gap 27 (3×10^{-4} M

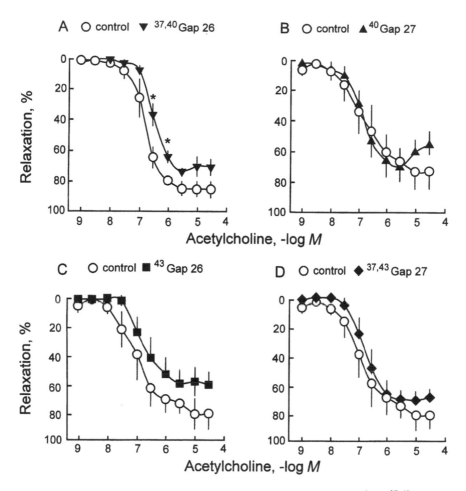

Figure 7.2 Concentration–response curves showing that 6×10^{-4} M ^{37,40}Gap 26 (A), ^{40}Gap 27 (B), ^{43}Gap 26 (C) or ^{37,43}Gap 27 (D) were substantially without effect on EDHF-type relaxations to acetylcholine in rat hepatic artery rings. Data are shown as means ± SEM; $n = 5$ in each case. Asterisks indicate statistically significant differences versus control ($p < .05$).

for each component) maximal relaxations to acetylcholine were reduced by about 90% (Figure 7.5).

5. DISCUSSION

The present study has provided evidence that connexin-mimetic peptides homologous to specific domains of the first and second extracellular loops of the connexins found in the vascular wall can be used to analyse the role of gap junctional communication in the EDHF response to acetylcholine in arteries of rabbit and rat. In the rabbit, peptides homologous to the Gap 26 or 27 domains of Cx43 effectively abolished EDHF-type relaxations to acetylcholine in ear arteries of different sizes, although the

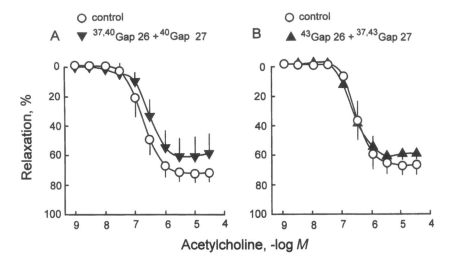

Figure 7.3 Concentration–response curves showing that peptide combinations targeted to either (A) Cx40: [37,40]Gap 26 plus [40]Gap 27 (3×10^{-4} M for each, $n = 5$) or (B) Cx43: [43]Gap 26 plus [37,43]Gap 27 (3×10^{-4} M for each, $n = 4$) did not significantly affect EDHF-type relaxations to acetylcholine in rat hepatic artery rings. Data are shown as means ± SEM.

Table 7.3 Effects of combinations of connexin-mimetic peptides on EDHF-type relaxations to acetylcholine in rat hepatic arteries

	n	$R_{max}(\%)$	EC_{50} (nM)
Control	4	80 ± 8	66 ± 10
[37,40]Gap 26 + [43]Gap 26	4	56 ± 5*	130 ± 40
Control	6	75 ± 6	36 ± 4
[37,43]Gap 27 + [40]Gap 27	6	50 ± 7*	171 ± 80*
Control	5	81 ± 9	91 ± 8
[37,40]Gap 26 + [37,43]Gap 27	5	48 ± 5*	141 ± 40*
Control	5	67 ± 3	314 ± 50
[43]Gap 26 + [40]Gap 27	5	29 ± 4*	730 ± 60*

Notes
Tone was induced by phenylephrine (3×10^{-7} M). L-NAME and each component peptide were administered at a concentration of 3×10^{-4} M. Data are shown as means ± SEM. The asterisks indicate statistically significant differences versus control ($p < .05$).

relative contribution of this mechanism was greater in distal arteries from this bed. By contrast, in rat hepatic and mesenteric arteries, the simultaneous administration of peptides that targeted Cxs40 and 43 was found necessary to attenuate the response to acetylcholine, suggesting that EDHF-type relaxations in this species require the participation of gap junctions constructed from both connexin subtypes. The findings highlight major regional differences in the mechanisms that contribute to endothelium-dependent relaxations within the same vascular network, and suggest that the reported apparent interspecies differences in the involvement of gap junctions in the EDHF phenomenon in rabbit and rat arteries may not reflect differences in fundamental mechanisms of relaxation.

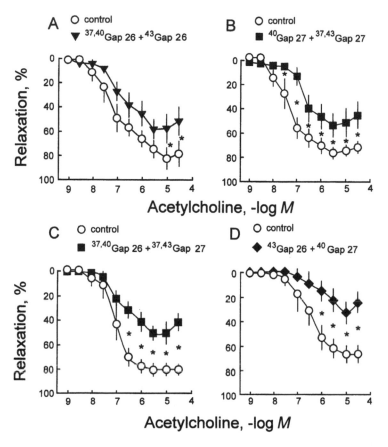

Figure 7.4 Concentration–response curves showing significant inhibition of EDHF-type relaxations to acetylcholine in rat hepatic artery rings by the peptide combinations [37,40]Gap 26 plus [43]Gap 26 (A), [40]Gap 27 plus [37,43]Gap 27 (B), [37,40]Gap 26 plus [37,43]Gap 27 (C) and [43]Gap 26 plus [40]Gap 27 (D). Each peptide component was administered at 3×10^{-4} M. Data are shown as means $\pm$ SEM; *n* values are given in Table 7.3. Asterisks indicate statistically significant differences versus control ($p < .05$).

5.1. Rabbit ear resistance arteries

The magnitude of the maximal response to acetylcholine and its potency as an endothelium-dependent agonist were similar in rings of rabbit central ear artery (G_0, ~800 μm diameter) and perfused segments of its second branch generation (G_2, ~100 μm diameter). However, [43]Gap 26 and [37,43]Gap 27 caused similar reductions (about 20%) in the maximal relaxation evoked by acetylcholine in G_0, whereas the maximal depressor response evoked by acetylcholine was reduced by nearly 55% in G_2. The inhibitory effects of these peptides were also associated with approximately equivalent rightward shifts in acetylcholine concentration–response curves, there being a two to three fold decrease in the potency of this agonist in G_0 rings, and a larger four to eight fold decrease in G_2 segments. By contrast, NO was demonstrated to play a greater functional role than gap junctions in G_0, with L-NAME reducing the

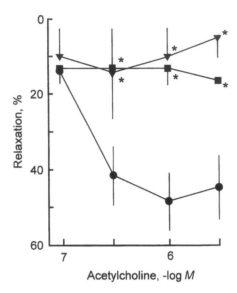

Figure 7.5 Concentration–response curves showing attenuation of EDHF-type relaxations to acetylcholine in rat mesenteric artery segments in the presence of [37,40]Gap 26 plus [37,43]Gap 27 (A) or [43]Gap 26 plus [40]Gap 27 (B). Each peptide component was administered at 3×10^{-4} M. Data are shown as means ± SEM ($n = 3$–12). Asterisks indicate statistically significant differences versus control ($p < .05$).

maximal response to acetylcholine by about 70%, but only by about 30% in G_2. These residual EDHF-type responses were critically dependent on gap junctional communication and effectively abolished by [43]Gap 26 and [37,43]Gap 27 in both G_0 rings and G_2 segments. The findings therefore provide a mechanistic explanation for previous X-ray microangiographic observations in the perfused intact rabbit ear in which the contribution of NO to acetylcholine-induced dilatation was found to decrease with diminishing vessel size (Berman and Griffith, 1998).

The variable role played by EDHF in arteries of different sizes is likely to be multifactorial. Observations that myoendothelial gap junctions are approximately twice as numerous in third order arteries (diameter about 350 μm) than first order arteries (diameter about 500 μm) from the rat mesentery, suggest that regional differences in anatomy could lead to an apparent "upregulation" of EDHF-type relaxations in the most distal arteries (Sandow and Hill, 2000). Regional variations in the pathways that mobilize Ca^{2+} to maintain contraction could also generate spatial heterogeneity as EDHF-mediated hyperpolarizations are associated with a decrease in the influx of Ca^{2+} via L-type voltage-operated channels (Bolz *et al.*, 1999). In the rat aorta, for example, contraction is largely independent of Ca^{2+} influx and the EDHF component of relaxation weak, whereas in small rat mesenteric vessels contraction is more dependent on Ca^{2+} influx and agonists stimulate large EDHF-type responses (Hwa *et al.*, 1994; Shimokawa *et al.*, 1996; Tomioka *et al.*, 1999). NO may inhibit the synthesis of EDHF through a cGMP-dependent pathway (Olmos *et al.*, 1995; Kessler *et al.*, 1999). In theory this could explain the reciprocal relationship between the contribution of NO and EDHF to relaxation in the G_0 and G_2 arteries observed in the present study as well as an inverse correlation between the magnitudes of NO- and EDHF-type relaxations in individual rings of rabbit superior mesenteric artery (Hutcheson *et al.*, 1999).

5.2. Rat hepatic and mesenteric arteries

Maximal relaxations evoked by acetylcholine in the presence of L-NAME and indomethacin were of the order of 65–85% of phenylephrine-induced tone in rings of rat hepatic artery. A spectrum of peptides was used to define the contribution of gap junctional communication to these EDHF-type responses, namely [37,40]Gap 26, [43]Gap 26, [37,43]Gap 27 and [40]Gap 27. However, at concentrations of 6×10^{-4} M, none of these peptides modulated relaxation in isolation, and in experiments in which two peptides were employed at concentrations of 3×10^{-4} M each, combinations targeted to Cx40 ([37,40]Gap 26 plus [40]Gap 27) or to Cx43 ([37,43]Gap 27 plus [43]Gap 26) were also devoid of inhibitory activity. In marked contrast, peptide combinations targeted specifically to the Gap 26 or Gap 27 domains (i.e., [37,40]Gap 26 plus [43]Gap 26 or [37,43]Gap 27 plus [40]Gap 27) resulted in about 30% inhibition of the maximal relaxation. The most effective combinations, however, targeted the Gap 26 and 27 domains of Cxs40 and 43 simultaneously (i.e., [37,40]Gap 26 plus [37,43]Gap 27 and [43]Gap 26 plus [40]Gap 27), and decreased the maximal relaxations by 40% to 50%. As inhibition of EDHF-type relaxation in the rat hepatic artery was incomplete, it cannot be discounted that other mechanisms, such as hyperpolarization caused by K^+ efflux from the endothelium (Edwards *et al.*, 1999), play a contributory role in this blood vessel. However, in parallel experiments employing isolated segments of rat mesenteric artery studied under isobaric conditions, the [37,40]Gap 26 plus [37,43]Gap 27 and [43]Gap 26 plus [40]Gap 27 combinations both almost abolished EDHF-type relaxations evoked by acetylcholine. It remains to be established if regional variations in the connexin expression of hepatic and mesenteric arteries contribute to these apparent differences in response.

5.3. Mechanism of action of connexin-mimetic peptides

Immunohistological studies indicate that gap junctions cluster in plaques at points of intercellular contact in which there may often be co-localization of different connexin subtypes. For example, co-localization of Cx40 and Cx43 has been reported in the wall of both rat arteries and hamster arterioles (Little *et al.*, 1995; Hong and Hill, 1998). However, the precise connexin composition of myoendothelial gap junctions remains to be established, and it is likely that this differs between vessel types as there are substantial variations between the relative expression of Cx37, Cx40 and Cx43 by the endothelium and the smooth muscle of elastic and muscular arteries, and even within the same organ (Hong and Hill, 1998; van Kempen and Jongsma, 1999; Hwan Seul and Beyer, 2000). It is also unknown if co-localization of Cxs40 and 43 has functional consequences in the context of the EDHF phenomenon as these connexins form not only heterotypic Cx40/Cx43 channels but also heteromeric channels that possess unique gating properties conferred by interactions between different hetero-domains of the two connexin proteins (Gu *et al.*, 2000).

In cultured HeLa cells transfected to express a chimeric Cx43-GFP protein that forms functional gap junctions which render these cells communication competent, direct visualization of the fluorescent protein has demonstrated that neither [37,43]Gap 27 nor [43]Gap 26 affect the number and distribution of plaques at points of cell to cell contact (Martin *et al.*, this volume). This suggests that connexin-mimetic peptides decrease the permeability of already established gap junctions by interacting with their extracellular connexin loops to induce either a subtle misalignment in connexon–connexon docking or a conformational change in connexin protein structure that modulates channel gating, rather than causing gross plaque disassembly. This lack of plaque disruption is consistent with the rapid and reversible nature of the inhibition of EDHF-mediated relaxations by [37,43]Gap 27 (Chaytor *et al.*, 1998). By contrast, other established inhibitors of gap junctional communication such as the 18α-isoform of glycyrrhetinic acid, which similarly inhibit EDHF-type relaxations in rabbit arteries and veins (Taylor *et al.*, 1998; Griffith and Taylor, 1999), may cause irreversible disassembly and internalization of gap junction plaques after relatively short exposure times (Martin *et al.*, this volume).

Although the transfer of an EDHF from endothelium to smooth muscle via myoendothelial gap junctions appears essential for the existence of EDHF-type relaxations evoked by acetylcholine in rabbit arteries (Chaytor *et al.*, 1998), a diffus-ible mediator would subsequently be expected to spread to deeper layers of smooth muscle cells within the vessel wall via gap junctions, thereby enhancing the overall hyperpolarizing response. Connexin-mimetic peptides cannot, however, be used to define the relative importance of such homocellular and heterocellular communication pathways as they inhibit direct communication between vascular smooth muscle cells at concentrations similar to those that abolish EDHF-type relaxations (Chaytor *et al.*, 1997). Whether the electrotonic spread of hyperpolarization from the endothelium to smooth muscle, and subsequently between smooth muscle cells in successive layers of the vessel wall, contributes to EDHF-type relaxations remains to be established. However, in porcine arteries electrotonic conduction of endothelial hyperpolarization extends only as far as the immediately subjacent smooth muscle, suggesting that the endothelium is unable to serve as a major source of electrical current (Bény *et al.*, 1997). Since electrical continuity between adjacent cells is dependent on gap junctional communication (Xia *et al.*, 1995; Brink, 1998), this mechanism should also theoret-ically be attenuated by connexin-mimetic peptides.

6. CONCLUSIONS

In the rabbit ear, NO/prostanoid independent relaxations to acetylcholine are dom-inated by a gap junction-dependent mechanism in blood vessels with a diameter less than 100 μm, suggesting that heterocellular gap junctional communication may be of particular importance in the regulation of microcirculatory perfusion. Gap junctional communication also underpins EDHF-type relaxations in rat arteries but in this species Cx40 and Cx43 channels are both essential for the mediation of NO/prosta-noid independent relaxations.

8 Myoendothelial and circumferential spread of endothelium-dependent hyperpolarization in coronary arteries

Stavros Selemidis and
Thomas M. Cocks

Endothelium-dependent vasodilatation in response to developing microthrombi provides an important feedback mechanism to increase flow and wash away. This 'reflex' mechanism, termed here the *Vanhoutte effect*, is proposed to protect vessels such as epicardial coronary arteries from thrombotic occlusion. However, it is difficult to envisage how focal endothelial stimulation in response to platelet activation evokes uniform segmental vasodilatation, necessary to increase vessel diameter and blood flow. Endothelium-derived NO and prosacyclin are likely to act only as local vasodilators and antiplatelet factors, which leaves the other endothelium-derived hyperpolarizing factor (endothelium-dependent hyperpolarization) as the possible coordinator of the *Vanhoutte effect*. Therefore, the aim of the present study was to determine whether focal stimulation of endothelium mediates hyperpolarization and relaxation of remote endothelium-denuded regions of the same annulus of the vessel. The main findings indicate that endothelium-dependent hyperpolarization of the smooth muscle in porcine and bovine epicardial coronary arteries spreads electrotonically around the circumference of the vessel to initiate a wave of relaxation. Both hyperpolarization and relaxation are not due to NO or prostacyclin, but depend on endothelial cell K_{Ca} channels, myoendothelial gap junctions and L-type voltage-operated Ca^{2+} channels. Therefore, these findings combined with the longitudinal spread of endothelial cell hyperpolarization and the well recognized antiplatelet effects of NO and prostacyclin indicate that coronary arteries have a remarkable capacity to avoid occlusive thrombosis.

Endothelium-dependent vasodilatation occurs in response to a variety of stimuli, all of which activate endothelial cells to release vasoactive substances such as NO and endothelium-dependent hyperpolarization. For instance, shear stress and pulsatile changes in pressure (Popp *et al.*, 1998) are two physiologically relevant stimuli for endothelium-dependent vasodilatation. Also, bradykinin which can be generated *in vitro* and *in vivo* by cleavage of endothelial-bound kininogen (van Iwaarden *et al.*, 1988; Hasan *et al.*, 1995) by plasma kallikrien (Nishikawa *et al.*, 1992), acts on B_2 kinin receptors to cause endothelium-dependent relaxation. Platelet aggregation is another physiological stimulus for endothelium-dependent relaxation (Cohen *et al.*, 1983). However, whilst shear stress, pulsatile changes in pressure and kininogen-derived bradykinin most likely activate the entire endothelial cell layer within an arterial segment to release endothelium-derived relaxing factors (EDRFs), adenosine diphosphate (ADP) and 5-hydroxytryptamine released by aggregating platelets at sites of vascular damage are likely to only act as local activators. This raises the question whether or not local endothelial cell activation by platelet aggregation and the subsequent release of EDRFs at this activation site, can be a sufficient stimulus for dilatation of the entire arterial annulus. An affirmative answer to this important question could be given if the activated endothelium was able to send an electrical signal to local underlying smooth muscle cells which could then travel around the circumference of the vessel via electrotonic coupling. Therefore, the aim of the present study was to determine whether locally released EDRFs in response to bradykinin, ADP and 5-hydroxytryptamine evoke circumferental spread of hyperpolarization to endothelium-denuded regions of the artery to relax the entire vessel.

1. METHODS

1.1. Dual chamber organ bath

3 mm (internal diameter) rings of pig right coronary artery and bovine left anterior descending coronary artery were cut open in a manner such that the circular smooth muscle ran in parallel with the length of the strip (Figure 8.1). The endothelium was removed from half of the strip by gentle abrasion with a Krebs-moistened cotton tipped applicator. The strip was then anchored to a horizontal organ bath chamber with one row of pins at the boundary between the regions of the artery with and without endothelium. A second row of pins was placed approximately 1.5 mm from the first row of pins into the region of the strip without endothelium. This endo-thelium-free region between the two rows of pins was termed the 'conduction zone'. Such an arrangement allowed independent recordings of changes in force from both ends of the strip, when each end was connected to a separate force transducer. A plastic partition was then placed between the rows of pins to isolate the two regions of the strip into separate leak-proof chambers perfused (4 ml/min) with warm (37 °C) Krebs solution. The lack of leak between the chambers was verified at the end of each experiment by perfusing one chamber with Evans blue (10 mg/ml) and then analysing the effluent of the other chamber spectrophotometrically. A 'leak-free' dual chamber organ bath allowed for region-specific application of endothelium-dependent vaso-dilators and of antagonists. Changes in membrane potential using standard intra-cellular microelectrode techniques (Selemidis *et al.*, 1998) were recorded from smooth muscle cells either approximately 1 mm beyond the conduction zone border of the region of artery without endothelium (i.e., approxiamtely 2.5 mm from the border of the region with endothelium) or from smooth muscle cells in the region of ar-tery with endothelium. Indomethacin (3×10^{-6} M) was present for all experiments on bovine rings, but was not necessary for those in pig coronary arteries since prostanoids do not contribute to endothelium-dependent relaxations in this tissue (Kilpatrick and Cocks, 1994).

1.2. Experimental protocol

After an equilibration period of 30 min, both the regions of artery (i.e., with and without endothelium) were stretched to a passive force level of 1 g and allowed a 30 min recovery period after which they were stretched a second time to 1 g passive force. Following a further 30 min equilibration period, strips were maximally contracted (F_{max}) with an isotonic high K^+ (125 mM K^+) depolarising solution. Once

Dual chamber bath

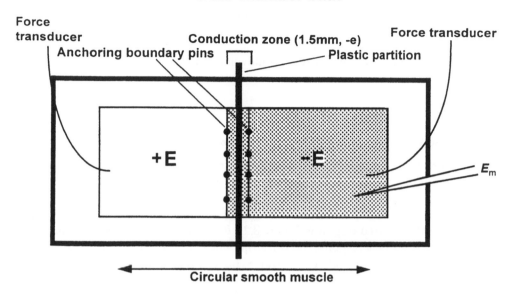

Figure 8.1 Schematic diagram showing a top view of the dual chamber organ bath. A ring of
coronary artery with a diameter of approximately 3 mm is cut open in a manner
such that the circular muscle runs parallel to the length of the preparation. This
strip of artery (approximately 9 mm in length) is then anchored with a row of pins
to the base of a sylgard-coated horizontal organ chamber. Half the strip on one side
of the row of pins is rubbed mechanically with a Krebs moistened cotton tip to
denude the endothelium. A second row of pins is placed approximately 1.5 mm from
the first row into region of the strip without endothelium ($-E$). This arrangement
allows force to be measured from the region of artery with endothelium
($+E$) independently of that without endothelium, as well as changes in membrane
potential using standard intracellular microelectrode techniques. A plastic partition
is then placed between the row of pins to isolate the two regions of the artery strip
into two separate leak-proof chambers with each chamber separately perfused with
Krebs solution. The above described partitioned, dual chamber organ bath allows
for region-specific application of endothelium-dependent vasodilators and antagonists
to the strip of artery.

a steady maximum contraction was achieved, the strips of artery were then incubated
in normal Krebs and strips were allowed to recover to their resting levels of passive
force. After 30 min, both regions of the strip were contracted to $\sim$40% F_{max} by
titrating the concentration of U46619 (10^{-8}–10^{-7} M) and once the level of active
force evoked by U46619 reached a stable plateau, the region with endothelium and
in some cases the region without endothelium were selectively exposed to single
applications of either bradykinin (5×10^{-6} M), substance P (5×10^{-8} M), ADP
(10^{-4} M), 5-hydroxytryptamine (10^{-5} M; in the presence of 3×10^{-6} M ketanserin to
inhibit any direct contractile response to 5-hydroxytryptamine; Cocks and Angus,
1983), thrombin (1 U/ml), sodium nitroprusside (10^{-5} M) or cromakalim (10^{-5} M).
Antagonists were added to either region of the partitioned chamber for 30 min
prior to contraction with U46619 and remained present for the duration of the
experiment.

1.3. Data presentation and statistical analysis

Relaxation was expressed as a percentage of the initial contraction to U46619 and calculated as means ± SEM. Differences in responses between treatment groups were compared statistically using Students' t-test for unpaired observations with significance accepted when p was less than .05. Peak hyperpolarizations from resting membrane potentials were measured in millivolts (mV).

2. RESULTS

2.1. Transferred relaxations and hyperpolarizations

In a dual chamber organ bath, when both the strips of pig coronary artery with and without endothelium were contracted with U46619, addition of bradykinin $(5 \times 10^{-7}$ M) to the strip with endothelium caused a relaxation in that region (local response) which always preceeded a similar but smaller relaxation in strip without endothelium (transferred response; Figure 8.2). Both substance P and bradykinin (not shown) failed to cause a response in both strips when applied only to the strip without endothelium confirming effective removal of the endothelium in that region (Figure 8.2). However, subsequent application of substance P to the strip with endothelium caused a similar pattern of local and transferred relaxations as bradykinin (Figure 8.2). Both local and transferred relaxations to bradykinin and substance P were unaffected by tetrodotoxin (3×10^{-7} M) (data not shown) and capsaicin (10^{-5} M) (data not shown).

A similar pattern of local and transferred responses to those obtained with bradykinin and substance P, also occurred with ADP (10^{-4} M; local, $56.2 \pm 7.3\%$, transferred, $50.6 \pm 5.8\%$, $n = 8$), 5-hydroxytryptamine (10^{-5} M; local, $69.6 \pm 8.6\%$, transferred, $24.3 \pm 10.2\%$, $n = 4$) and thrombin (1 U/ml; local, $69.8 \pm 1.1\%$, transferred, $56.0 \pm 4\%$, $n = 4$) when added either alone or in triple combination (local, $82.4 \pm 3.6\%$, transferred, $62.9 \pm 9.5\%$) to the region of artery with endothelium.

Application of bradykinin or substance P to the region of a pig coronary artery strip with endothelium caused local hyperpolarizations (bradykinin; 21.2 ± 2.5 mV, substance P; 23.0 ± 2.5 mV, $n = 6$) and transferred hyperpolarizations (bradykinin, 11.2 ± 1.3 mV; substance P, 11.8 ± 1.1 mV) to the region without endothelium (resting membrane potential; -44.6 ± 1.1 mV; $n = 30$). When the conduction zone of the strip of artery was severed mechanically, local endothelium-dependent relaxations and hyperpolarizations to bradykinin and substance P were unaffected but there was no transfer of relaxations or hyperpolarizations to the region of the strip without endothelium (data not shown).

N^{G}-nitro-L-arginine (L-NOARG, 10^{-4} M) significantly inhibited the local relaxations to bradykinin and substance P but had no effect on the transferred and hyperpolarizations (Figure 8.3). In addition, the local contraction to L-NOARG of 0.2 ± 0.01 g ($n = 6$) did not transfer to the endothelium-denuded region as either contraction or depolarisation (control resting membrane potential; -44.6 ± 1.1 mV; L-NOARG; 42.1 ± 1.1 mV, $n = 7$) and sodium nitroprusside (10^{-5} M), which caused maximum local responses, elicited neither hyperpolarization nor transfer of relaxation (Figure 8.4). Similar transfer of non-NO/non-prostanoid-dependent hyperpolarizations and relaxations to bradykinin occurred in strips of bovine coronary artery (data not shown).

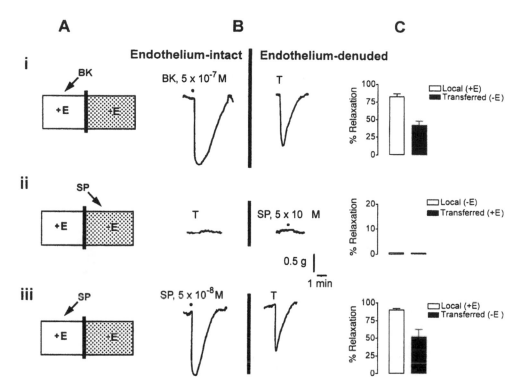

Figure 8.2 Demonstration of circumferential transfer of endothelium-dependent relaxations to bradykinin (BK) and substance P (SP) in the pig coronary artery. Each of the three schematic diagrams (i–iii) in column (A) of the dual chamber organ illustrate a single application of bradykinin and substance P that is region-specific (i.e., +E, with endothelium; −E, without endothelium). Exposure of a single strip of artery to the endothelium-dependent agonists occurred in the sequence illustrated in rows i–iii. Column (B) shows digitized original chart recordings of local relaxations and the resultant transfer (T) of effects in the same strip corresponding to the sequential application of bradykinin or substance P. Vertical (force; g) and horizontal (time; min) scale bars in column (B), apply for all traces. Column (C) shows group data as histograms from experiments described in rows i–iii. Relaxation is expressed as a % reversal of the U46619-induced contraction. Histograms represent the means ± SEM from ten experiments. In row i, selective application of bradykinin to the +E-region of the artery strip caused a local relaxation in that region and a transferred relaxation to the −E-region of the strip. The subsequent application of SP to the −E-region (row ii) resulted in a lack of response in both −E- and +E-regions of the strip, confirming the effective removal of the endothelium. Finally, row iii illustrates that exposure of the +E-region to substance P caused a local relaxation followed by transfer of relaxation to the −E-region, in a manner similar to that observed with bradykinin (row i).

2.2. Endothelium-dependent hyperpolarization mediates transferred relaxations and hyperpolarizations

When the endothelium-intact region of the strip of pig coronary artery was treated with the dual combination of apamin and charybdotoxin the transferred relaxations

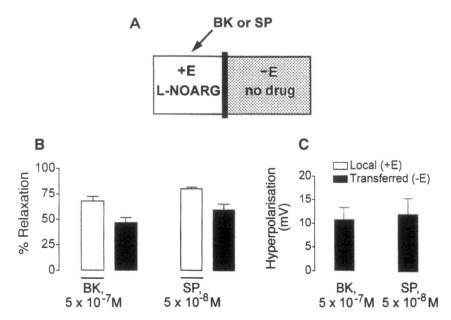

Figure 8.3 Evidence that the circumferential transfer of endothelium-dependent relaxations and hyperpolarizations to bradykinin (BK) and substance P (SP) in
the pig coronary artery are not due to NO. The schematic diagram of the dual
chamber organ bath in (A) illustrates a single application of either bradykinin
or substance P to the region of the artery strip with endothelium (+E), which
was treated for 30 min with the NO synthase inhibitor, L-NOARG (10^{-4} M).
(B) and (C) show group data as histograms of local and transferred
relaxations and transferred hyperpolarizations corresponding to application
of bradykinin and substance P. Relaxation is expressed as a % reversal of
the U46619-induced contraction and hyperpolarization as millivolts (mV).
Histograms represent the means $\pm$ SEM ($n = 5$–10).

and hyperpolarizations to bradykinin (Figure 8.5) were abolished, whereas the local
relaxations in the region of the strip with endothelium were not affected significantly.
Subsequent application of L-NOARG (10^{-4} M) to apamin and charybdotoxin-treated
preparations abolished the local relaxation to bradykinin (data not shown, $n = 2$). The
L-type voltage-operated Ca^{2+} channel inhibitor, nifedipine (3×10^{-7} M) inhibited the
transferred relaxation ($24.1 \pm 9.0\%$, $n = 6$) to bradykinin when applied to the region
of the strip with endothelium.

An inhibitor of cytochrome P450 2C, sulphaphenazole (10^{-5} M), had no effect on
both local and transferred relaxations to bradykinin (Figure 8.5).

The gap junction uncoupling agent, 18-β-glycyrrhetinic acid (5×10^{-5} M) inhibited
transfer of both relaxation (Figure 8.6) and hyperpolarization (data not shown) to
bradykinin without affecting the local relaxation when applied to the region of the
strip with endothelium but not when applied to the region without endothelium
(Figure 8.6).

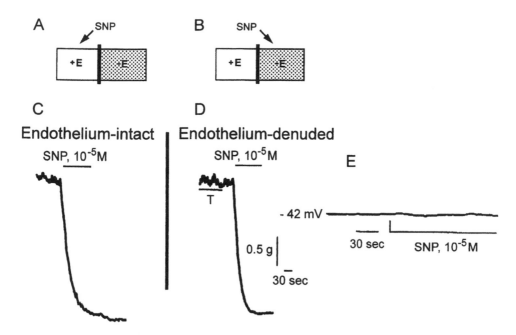

Figure 8.4 Demonstration that the NO donor, sodium nitroprusside (SNP; 10^{-5} M) does not cause circumferential transfer of relaxation and hyperpolarization in pig coronary artery. Schematic diagrams in (A) and (B) of a dual chamber organ bath illustrate sequential, region-specific (+E, with endothelium; −E, without endothelium) application of a single concentration of sodium nitroprusside in the same strip of artery. (C) and (D) Digitized original chart recordings of tension show local relaxation in the +E-region to sodium nitroprusside but no transfer (T) of this response to the −E-region of the artery, which then relaxed maximally to direct application of sodium nitroprusside Vertical (force; g) and horizontal (time; s) scale bars apply to both traces. (E) Lack of effect of sodium nitroprusside on membrane potential. Force traces in columns (A) and (B) and membrane potential recording in (E) are representative of five experiments.

3. DISCUSSION

The findings of the present study demonstrate for the first time that endothelium-dependent hyperpolarization acts as a remote inhibitory signalling mechanism in coronary arteries. That is, activation of endothelial cells at a discrete point of an annulus of artery causes hyperpolarization and relaxation of the smooth muscle at the activation site, which then spreads around the circumference of the vessel to cause relaxation in remote regions of the entire annulus. This circumferential transfer of relaxation is not due to NO, which is a local mediator, and it does not involve cytochrome-P450-derived metabolites of arachidonic acid. It does, however, appear to depend on myoendothelial gap junctions, endothelial cell K_{Ca} and L-type voltage-operated Ca^{2+} channels. Thus, endothelium-dependent hyperpolarization of smooth muscle is most likely not mediated by a factor *per se* in coronary arteries, but rather is due to spread of electrical current from the endothelium to the smooth muscle via myoendothelial gap junctions.

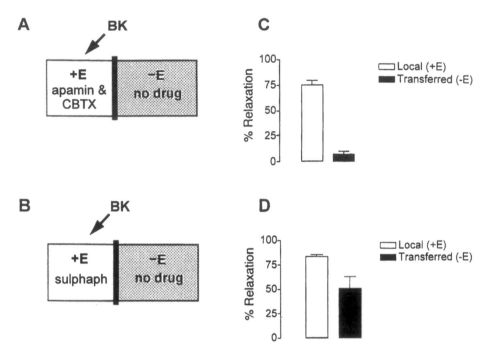

Figure 8.5 Evidence that the circumferential transfer of endothelium-dependent relaxations to bradykinin (BK) in pig coronary artery are due to K_{Ca} but not cytochrome P450 2C-dependent pathways of arachidonic acid metabolism. Both schematic diagrams (A and B) of the dual chamber organ bath illustrate application of bradykinin to the region of the artery strip with endothelium (+E) which was treated with either (A), a combination of apamin (10^{-7} M) and charybdotoxin (CBTX; 10^{-7} M) or (B) sulphaphenazole (sulphaph, 10^{-5} M). (A) and (B) represent different pig arteries. (C) and (D) show group data as histograms of local relaxations in the +E region and the resultant transferred relaxations in the −E-region to bradykinin. Relaxation is expressed as a % reversal of the U46619-induced contraction. Histograms represent means ± SEM ($n = 6$).

A novel technique (the dual chamber organ bath) was established to examine mechanisms of endothelium-dependent relaxation in large epicardial coronary arteries. In contrast to experiments conducted in isolated rings of coronary artery in classic organ chambers, where endothelium-dependent vasodilators activate all of the endothelium, this new dual chamber system enabled one region of the ring of the artery to be stimulated independently of the other. Thus, with this technique the hypothesis could be tested that endothelium-dependent hyperpolarization and relaxation of smooth muscle generated by a local source of endothelium can be conducted to remote distant smooth muscle could be tested. The results presented here demonstrate clear differences in the mechanisms by which the two main endothelium-dependent relaxing mechanisms in coronary arteries, NO and endothelium-dependent hyperpolarization, evoke relaxation of smooth muscle in large coronary arteries. NO is a local mediator, evoking relaxation only of smooth muscle underlying the site of endothelial cell activation, whereas endothelium-dependent hyperpolarization not only acts

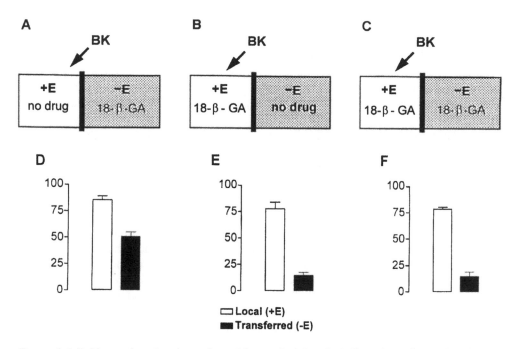

Figure 8.6 Evidence that the circumferential transfer of endothelium-dependent relaxation to bradykinin (BK) in pig coronary artery depends on myoendothelial gap junctions. The three schematic diagrams of the dual chamber organ bath in (A–C) illustrate application of bradykinin to the region of the artery strip with endothelium (+E). The schematic diagrams also illustrate region-specific application of the gap junction uncoupler 18-β-glycyrrhetinic acid (18-β-GA; 5×10^{-5} M). (D) and (F) show corresponding group data as histograms of local and transferred relaxations to bradykinin expressed as a % reversal of the U46619-induced contraction. Histograms represent means ± SEM ($n = 6$). In (D), despite selective treatment of the region of the strip without endothelium (−E) with 18-β-glycyrrhetinic acid, the selective application of bradykinin to the +E-region of the strip was still able to cause a local and transferred relaxation to the −E-region which was not significantly different to the control response (see Figure 8.2). By contrast, (E) and (F) show that application of 18-β-glycyrrhetinic acid to either the +E-region or to both regions of the artery strip had no significant effect on the local relaxation but nearly abolished the transferred relaxation to bradykinin.

locally, but also travels to remote smooth muscle by electrotonic coupling between endothelial and smooth muscle cells, as well as, between smooth muscle cells.

Several different mechanisms can be envisaged by which hyperpolarization can spread intercellularly between smooth muscle cells. First, it can be carried by diffusion of an intracellular messenger such as Ca^{2+}, inositol trisphospahate (IP_3) or cyclic adenosine monophosphate (cyclic AMP). Although diffusion of Ca^{2+} and small molecules like cAMP can influence cells over distances of millimeters, these processes are rather slow (at approximately 10 µm/s; i.e., approximately 150 s to travel over 1.5 mm) and as such are unlikely to account for spread of hyperpolarization observed in the pig coronary artery. Another mechanism by which hyperpolarization can spread between cells in the artery wall is a regenerative process, such as one that might involve a Ca^{2+}-induced Ca^{2+} release (i.e., a Ca^{2+} wave) (Young *et al.*, 1996). However, the speed of the Ca^{2+} wave would be expected to be governed by intracellular Ca^{2+} diffusion kinetics and even though it can theoretically travel over infinite distances it would most likely be too slow to account for the transferred responses observed in the present studies. An involvement of inhibitory nerves is unlikely as tetrodotoxin and capsaicin failed to affect the spread of hyperpolarization and relaxation. The finding that the endothelium-dependent transferred hyperpolarizations decayed by about 50% over a distance of 2.5 mm supports the possibility that the hyperpolarization spreads by an electrotonic, non-regenerative process. A similar decay has been demonstrated in the spread of electrical current applied by direct injection of hyperpolarization into pig coronary arterial smooth muscle cells (Bény, 1997). Thus, hyperpolarization decayed in an exponential manner but from a point source it could travel up to 5 mm with only approximately 50% decay (Bény, 1997). Further evidence in support of electrotonic movement of hyperpolarization along the smooth muscle layer in this artery was the additional finding (unpublished observations), that the transfer but not the initiation of the K_{ATP}-induced hyperpolarization of smooth muscle to cromakalim occurred in the presence of the K_{ATP} channel inhibitor, glibenclamide. This eliminates a possible regenerative action of K_{ATP} channels in the conduction of the transferred hyperpolarization to cromakalim but supports electrotonic movement of current through the smooth muscle media.

The finding that gap junction uncoupling agents, like 18-β-glycyrrhetinic acid abolished the non-NO hyperpolarization and transferred relaxations to bradykinin supports the idea that myoendothelial gap junctions are involved in the transmission of endothelium-dependent hyperpolarization to smooth muscle (Chatyor *et al.*, 1998; Sandow and Hill, 2000). However, block of gap junctions between smooth muscle cells by 18-β-glycyrrhetinic acid and thus the transmission of hyperpolarization along the smooth muscle media, might be an equally possible explanation for an alternative inhibitory action of these compounds on endothelium-dependent responses. One of the strengths of the dual chamber organ chamber is that it is possible to selectively apply antagonists to one region of the arterial strip. Thus, when 18-β-glycyrrhetinic acid was applied only to the region of the strip without endothelium it had no effect on either the transferred relaxations or smooth muscle tone induced by U46619. By contrast, when it was applied to the both regions of the strip, the transferred hyperpolarization and relaxation to bradykinin was abolished. These findings indicate that while 18-β-glycyrrhetinic acid does not inhibit homologous gap junctions between smooth muscle cells it might act as a selective inhibitor of myoendothelial gap junctions.

Given the likely scenario that myoendothelial gap junctions are involved in non-NO, hyperpolarization-dependent relaxations and that endothelial cells hyperpolarize in response to endothelium-dependent vasodilators, it seems logical to suggest that in coronary arteries electrotonic spread of hyperpolarization from the endothelium to the smooth muscle accounts for endothelium-dependent hyperpolarization and not a transferable factor. However, while electrotonic spread of current may explain the transfer of hyperpolarization around the circumference of the artery, via the smooth muscle media, a similar spread of hyperpolarization from the endothelium to the smooth muscle is not possible in large blood vessels like the pig coronary artery due to different biophysical characteristics of the two cell types (Bény and Paccica, 1994). Because the input resistance of the large smooth muscle media in pig coronary artery is low compared to the flat monolayer of endothelial cells, electrotonic movement of current from the endothelium to the smooth muscle would be insufficient to change the membrane potential in the smooth muscle layer (Bény and Paccica, 1994). This claim was based on the finding that the gap junction uncoupling agent halothane, had no effect on the endothelium-dependent hyperpolarization of smooth muscle to brady-kinin. The flow of current in the reverse direction however, which was possible and probably due to rectified gap junctions was inhibited by halothane. Therefore, it was concluded that a phenomenon other than passive electrical coupling between the two cell types, such as a paracrine endothelium-dependent hyperpolarization is required to be released by the endothelium to explain the regenerated hyperpolarization of the smooth muscle (Bény and Paccica, 1994). Since halothane might be selective for specific connexin subtypes (He and Burt, 2000) and therefore may show selectivity for specific gap junctions, halothane may fail to uncouple the myoendothelial gap junctions which transfer electrical signals in the direction of endothelium to the smooth muscle. An alternative possibility that incorporates a role for both a diffusible messenger with smooth muscle hyperpolarizing capabilities and myoendothelial gap junctions is that endothelium-dependent hyperpolarization is an ion, such as Ca^{2+} or even a small diffusible molecule like cyclic AMP or inositol triphosphate, which can spread via myoendothelial gap junctions from the endothelium to the smooth muscle.

3.1. Endothelium-dependent hyperpolarization protects against thrombosis: The Vanhoutte effect

Given the finding in large coronary arteries that focal stimulation of endothelium by 5-hydroxytryptamine, ADP and thrombin endothelium-dependent hyperpolarization-dependent circumferential spread of relaxation may be the main vasodilator mechanism derived from the endothelium in response to local stimuli like platelets. Thus, endothelium-dependent hyperpolarization may offer protection against thrombosis in diseased atherosclerotic coronary arteries.

The etiology of thrombosis is unknown, however, the primary influences that predispose blood vessels to thrombosis are endothelial cell injury and abnormal blood flow, both of which contribute to inappropriate platelet activation (For reviews see Falk, 1991; Wu and Thiagarajan, 1996; Lijnen and Collen, 1997). In diseased arteries, clots tend to develop when aggregating platelets adhere around the reactive 'shoulder' of eccentric lesions at sites of endothelial cell damage and high turbulent flow (Falk, 1991); the latter of which is accentuated by inappropriate release of potential spasmogens, thromboxane A_2 and 5-hydroxytryptamine and loss of local protective effects of NO and prostacyclin. The turbulent flow can cause further damage to the endothelium because such countercurrent blood flow increases the likelihood of platelet aggregation and clotting.

Whilst platelets play a central role in the progression of thrombogenesis, in particular in causing the initial obstruction to flow (Falk, 1991), their release of 5-hydroxytryptamine and ADP as they begin to clot in arteries like coronary arteries may be beneficial if these mediators are able to activate intact functional endothelial cells to evoke vasodilatation of the segment of blood vessel in which the clot is forming. Such 'reflex' vasodilatation can be advantageous for at least two reasons. First, the increase in blood flow associated with vasodilatation of the vessel increases the shearing forces at the endothelial cell monolayer. These forces can reduce the adhesion of incoming platelets to von Willebrand's factor and dislodge an early platelet thrombus (Lew *et al.*, 1985) by 'washing away' excess platelets before the clot is finally sealed by fibrin. Secondly, vasodilatation can promote fibrinolysis by diluting unwanted clotting factors and permitting an influx of fresh clotting factor inhibitors (Lijnen and Collen, 1995). Therefore, 5-hydroxytryptamine and ADP released from platelets and the endothelium-dependent vasodilatation they can mediate have the potential to restrict progression of a clot to the immediate site of injury.

The problem with this proposal, however, is that ADP and 5-hydroxytryptamine released from activated platelets at the site of endothelial cell injury will only, at best, activate other viable endothelial cells within the immediate region of the developed clot whereas dilatation of the entire vessel segment is necessary to change blood flow. The findings in the present study that focal stimulation of intact endothelium by ADP, 5-hydroxytryptamine and thrombin all evoked endothelium-dependent hyperpolarization-dependent circumferential spread of relaxation support the idea that such uniform segmental dilatation can be achieved by locally activated platelets.

A potential pitfall of our model of focal stimulation and thus, our intepretation of our data that endothelium-dependent hyperpolarization-dependent uniform segmental dilatation occurs to platelet aggregation, is, whether stimulation of half the strip of artery with perhaps an estimated 10,000 endothelial cells is representative of focal stimulation by platelets at a local site of injury *in vivo*. At the smallest level this would involve activation of a single endothelial cell. However, application of hyperpolarising current into a single endothelial cell in the hamster feed artery preparation *in vivo*, caused local vasodilatation and also a conducted hyperpolarization which travelled electrotonically via gap junctions up to 0.5 mm along the longitudinal length of the artery to evoke vasodilatation at that site (Emerson and Segal, 2000). Thus, it seems feasible that platelet activation of even a single endothelial cell may be a sufficient stimulus to evoke vasodilatation. If the mechanism of endothelium-dependent hyperpolarization-dependent uniform segmental dilatation operates simultaneously with the longitudinal spread of endothelial cell hyperpolarization between endothelial cells via homocellular gap junctions (Emerson and Segal, 2000), then it could be possible that focal stimulation of endothelial cells by platelet-derived vasodilators has the potential to dilate not only the immediate zone of activation, but the ascending and descending spread of hyperpolarization along the length of the artery suggests a much wider annulus of artery. Therefore, it is proposed that endothelium-dependent hyperpolarization-dependent uniform segmental dilatation, when activated by platelet-derived vasodilators, explains the initial hypothesis proposed by Vanhoutte in 1988; that 5-hydroxytryptamine and ADP released from platelets and the reflex vasodilatation they mediate disperses unwanted developing clots.

4. CONCLUSION

An important physiological role for endothelium-dependent hyperpolarization in coronary arteries is to preserve vasodilator function under pro-thrombotic conditions, especially when local vasoactive factors such as NO and prostacyclin cannot diffuse through atheromatous plaques (Bassenge and Heusch, 1990; Chester *et al.*, 1990). As such coronary arteries have a remarkable intrinsic capacity to avoid occlusive thrombosis and vasospasm.

9   Direct myoendothelial contacts in human pulmonary microvessels

*M. Koslowski, A.C. Newby, W.R. Roche,
G.D. Angelini and K. Stuart-Smith*

Endothelium-derived Hyperpolarizing Factor (EDHF) is important for the regulation of the vasomotor tone of small blood vessels and thus for the regulation of vascular resistance. Direct cell-to-cell contact in the form of gap junctions appears to be important for the signal transduction of EDHF. Although there is functional evidence for myoendothelial gap junctions, there is little direct morphological evidence for their existence in the systemic vasculature and there are no published studies about their existence in distal pulmonary blood vessels. The present study uses transmission electron microscopy to demonstrate direct myoendothelial contact in human pulmonary microvessels formed by membrane projections of contractile cells. In all likelyhood, they represent gap junctions and provide a pathway for signal transduction of EDHF.

Different endothelium-derived factors are involved in the regulation of the vasomotor tone, but Endothelium-derived Hyperpolarizing Factor (EDHF) is particulary implicated in the relaxation of the smooth muscle of distal arteries of small diameter (Shimokawa *et al.*, 1996; Griffith *et al.*, 1998). The phenomenon known as EDHF appears to consist of agonist-mediated hyperpolarization of the endothelial cell, followed by hyperpolarization of the underlying smooth muscle cell (Edwards *et al.*, 1999; Yamamoto *et al.*, 1999). This process probably requires close contact between the endothelial and smooth muscle cell layer, thus accounting for the prominence of EDHF in the thinner-walled microvasculature. For this reason, attention has focused on the possible role of myoendothelial gap junctions as the means whereby the EDHF 'signal' is transmitted from one cell to another. Blockade of hyperpolarization of smooth muscle cells by using gap junction inhibitors (Taylor *et al.*, 1998; Yamamoto *et al.*, 1999) highlights the potential importance of gap junctions for transmission of EDHF between endothelial and smooth muscle cells. Two hypotheses have been proposed about the nature of EDHF. Either EDHF is electrotonically transferred hyperpolarization via gap junctions from endothelial to smooth muscle cells (Yamamoto *et al.*, 1999), or a chemical factor represents EDHF and the gap junctions provide a pathway for the movement of this chemical factor from endothelial to smooth muscle cells (Campell *et al.*, 1996; Randall and Kendall, 1998). Indeed, gap junctions provide a pathway for direct movement of low-molecular-weight substances between adjacent cells and thereby activate signal transduction (Gabriels and Paul, 1998). Endothelial cell-to-endothelial cell and smooth muscle cell-to-smooth muscle cell junctions are well documented in systemic blood vessels and in the main stem of the pulmonary artery in a variety of species (van Kempen and Jongsma, 1999; Nakamura *et al.*, 1999). Although there is functional evidence for myoendothelial junctions in large systemic blood vessels (Little *et al.*, 1995; Bény and Conat, 1992), ultrastructural evidence of myoendothelial junctions in the microvasculature is rare (Svendsen *et al.*, 1990; Sandow and Hill, 2000). Myoendothelial junctions have not yet been described in pulmonary microvessels, the site of the pulmonary vascular resistance.

The aim of the present study was to determine morphologically whether or not myoendothelial cell coupling in microvessels of the human lung occurs.

1. MATERIAL AND METHODS

Segments of surgically removed human lungs, which were not involved by tumor or other nonneoplastic lung disease were chosen. These segments were perfusion-fixed in primary fixative (3% gluteraldehyde, 4% formaldehyde in 0.1 M Piperazine-N,N'-bis-2-ethanesulphonic acid buffer, pH 7.2) for five minutes. Small pieces were dissected out, immersed in the primary fixative for one hour, fixed in 1% buffered osmium tetroxide for one hour, dehydrated and embedded in Spurr resin. Silver sections were cut, stained with uranyl acetate and lead citrate and viewed on a Hitachi H7000 transmission electron microscope. One single section per cell was analysed in 100 endothelial cells. The average diameter of the analysed vessels was less than 400 μm.

2. RESULTS

The media of the pulmonary microvessels contained three to four smooth muscle layers (Figure 9.1). Membrane projections of contractile cells through fenestrae of the internal elastic lamina were found forming close cellular contacts with endothelial cells. In some sections these junctions are broad appositions (Figure 9.1), in other sections short and slender appositions (Figure 9.2). The outer layers of the two cell membranes appear to fuse focally within these appositions giving the appearance of short gap junctions (Figures 9.3 and 9.4). Broad membrane appositions ($n = 9$) occured with a frequency of 9% of sections and were commoner than shorter membrane projections ($n = 2$) with a frequency of 2% of sections. Myoendothelial junctions were smaller in area than areas of contact between endothelial cells (Figure 9.5).

All detected membrane projections forming myoendothelial junctions originated from contractile cells. No projections of endothelial cells through the internal elastic lamina were seen.

3. DISCUSSION

The present study demonstrates that human pulmonary microvessels contain anatomical structures that suggest the presence of myoendothelial gap junctions. Two morphological variants of myoendothelial junctions in form of broad membrane appositions and small, slender membrane projections were found. Similar structural observations have been made in the human saphenous vein (Svendsen *et al.*, 1990).

In the current experiments, transmission electron microscopy was carried out to investigate myoendothelial cell coupling in human pulmonary microvessels. This method is useful to identify cell-to-cell communications and detects possible gap

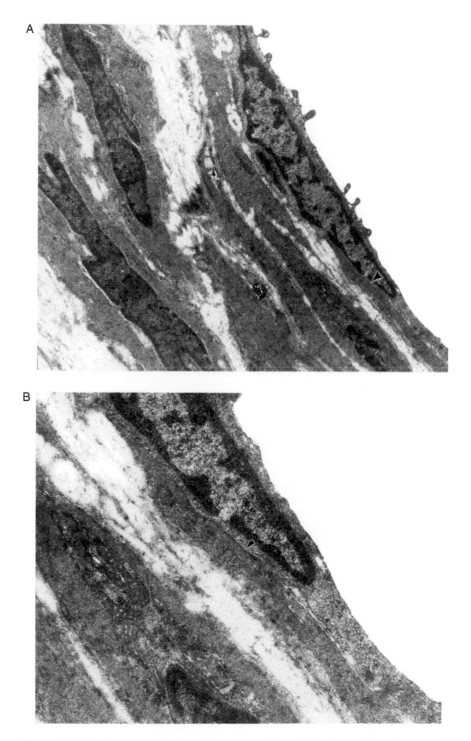

Figure 9.1 Membrane projection of a contractile cell forming a broad myoendothelial junction (arrows) (A: ×5000; B: ×20000). Three layers of smooth muscle cells are visible in Figure 9.1A.

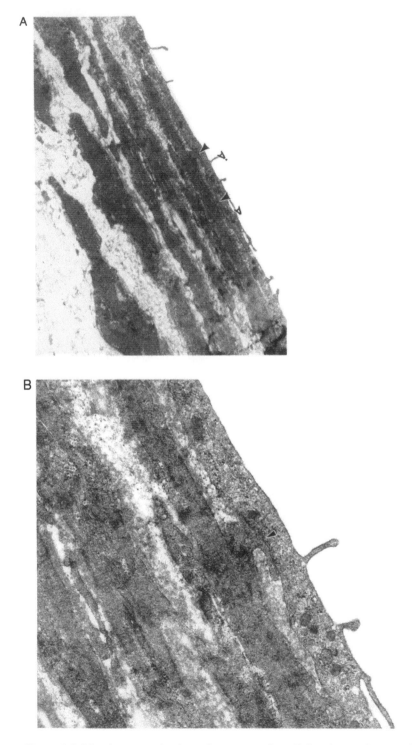

Figure 9.2 Membrane projection of a contractile cell forming a short and slender myo-endothelial junction (arrows) (A: ×5000; B: ×20000).

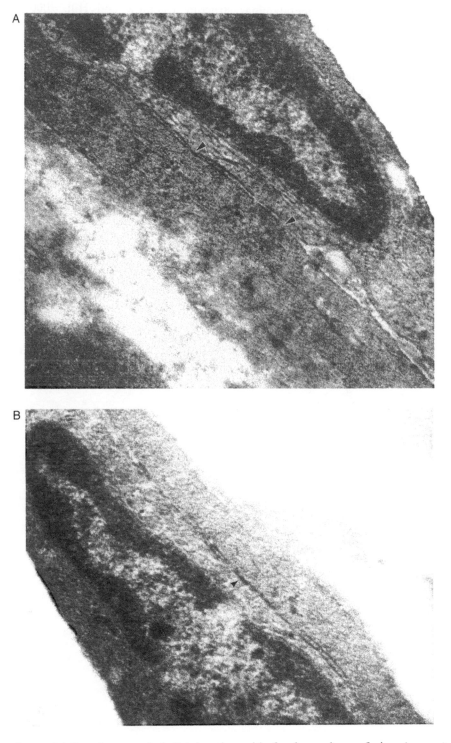

Figure 9.3 Broad myoendothelial junction with focal membrane fusion (arrows) resembling short gap junctions (×50000).

junctions by their typical pentalaminar structure (Sandow and Hill, 2000). The small size of myoendothelial junctions compared with interendothelial junctions may explain why direct anatomical evidence for endothelium-to-smooth muscle cell contact is rare (Spagnoli *et al.*, 1982; Sandow and Hill, 2000).

Myoendothelial junctions were found in 11 of 100 endothelial cells on single sections. Providing approximately 200 ultrathin serial sections could be made from one

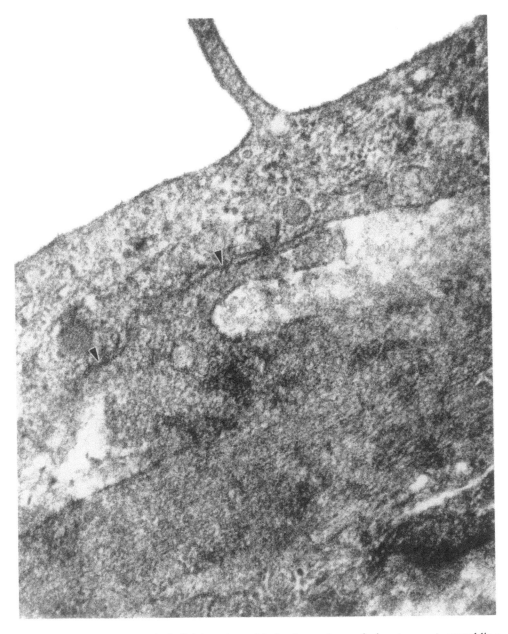

Figure 9.4 Slender myoendothelial junction with focal membrane fusion (arrows) resembling short gap junctions (×50000).

endothelial cell of 10–20 μm (Svendsen *et al.*, 1990), the present results suggest that approximately 20 myoendothelial junctions exist per endothelial cell in human pulmonary microvessels. The same number of myoendothelial junctions per endothelial cell were found in the distal mesenteric artery of the rat (Sandow and Hill, 2000). The number of myoendothelial junctions per endothelial cell is smaller in large arteries (Svendsen *et al.*, 1990; Sandow and Hill, 2000). This is readily explained by the thick internal elastic lamina which forms a considerable barrier between endothelial and smooth muscle cells in large conduit vessels (Svendsen *et al.*, 1990). Although one myoendothelial junction per endothelial cell appears sufficient to produce significant electrical changes in the smooth muscle layer (Sandow and Hill, 2000), smooth muscle cells in the layers closer to the adventitia of large vessels will be remote from any endothelial signal.

Myoendothelial gap junctions formed by membrane projections from endothelial cells through the internal elastic lamina to the smooth muscle (Svendsen *et al.*, 1990; Sandow and Hill, 2000) were not found in the present study. By contrast, membrane projections through the internal elastic lamina originating from contractile cells were easily identified. Either endothelial projections are not present in the pulmonary microvessels of the human lung, or they are much smaller in number than membrane projections arising from contractile cells and therefore they were not detected by single section electron microscopy.

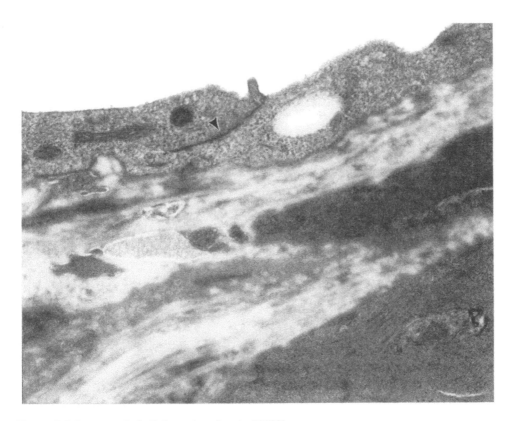

Figure 9.5 Large endothelial gap junction (×20000).

4. CONCLUSION

The present study shows that myoendothelial junctions are present in human pulmonary microvessels. It is likely that these membrane appositions contain gap junctions, the structure considered by many to be necessary for the cell-to-cell transmission of EDHF. They are small in size and more numerous than in large conduit vessels.

ACKNOWLEDGEMENT

This project is supported by the Division of Cardiac, Anaesthetic and Radiologic Sciences, University of Bristol.

10 Role of gap junctional communication in EDHF-mediated responses and mechanisms of K^+-induced dilatations

David Harris, Patricia E.M. Martin,
David A. Kendall, Tudor M. Griffith
and Michael D. Randall

The role of gap junctions in EDHF-mediated responses and the mechanisms of K^+-induced relaxation have been investigated in the rat isolated mesenteric arterial bed. Endothelium-derived hyperpolarizing factor (EDHF)-mediated responses to carbachol (in the presence of indomethacin and N^G-nitro-L-arginine methyl ester (L-NAME) were substantially reduced in the presence the gap junction inhibitors, 18α-glycyrrhetinic acid, SR141716A and palmitoleic acid, and also ouabain and clotrimazole. K^+ caused dilatations of preparations perfused with K^+ free buffer, which were sensitive to both ouabain and 18α-glycyrrhetinic acid but not to SR141716A, palmitoleic acid or clotrimazole. The relaxations to K^+ were reduced following inhibition of cycloxygenase and were abolished by removal of the endothelium. It is concluded that gap junctional communication plays a major role in endothelium-dependent relaxations mediated by EDHF and that K^+ causes dilatation in an endothelium-dependent manner, which is in part mediated via prostanoids.

EDHF-type relaxations involve myoendothelial gap junctions (Chaytor *et al.*, 1998). However, EDHF-type relaxations can also be explained by efflux of K^+ (Edwards *et al.*, 1998) from the endothelium (Gordon and Martin, 1983) through apamin plus charybdotoxin sensitive K^+ channels (Doughty *et al.*, 1999). The relaxation is thought to be due to activation of Na^+/K^+ATPases and opening of inward rectifier K^+ channels (Edwards *et al.*, 1998).

Activation of the Na^+/K^+ATPase by K^+, leading to relaxation, has been suggested on the basis of the inhibitory effects of ouabain (Hendrickx and Casteels, 1974). In the context of EDHF, the sensitivity of responses to ouabain has been controversial, with reports that ouabain inhibits endothelium-dependent hyperpolarization (but not relaxation) in canine coronary vascular smooth muscle (Feletou and Vanhoutte, 1988). In the rat hepatic artery ouabain also did not affect endothelium-dependent relaxations (Zygmunt and Högestätt, 1996). However, in the latter preparation high concentrations of ouabain in the presence of Ba^{2+} abolished EDHF and K^+ induced hyperpolarization but only modestly affected the relaxation responses (Edwards *et al.*, 1998).

In view of the proposal that K^+ might represent an EDHF, the aim of the present study was to investigate the comparative pharmacology of K^+-induced relaxations and EDHF-mediated responses. Given that heterocellular endothelial-smooth muscle gap junctional communication may play a critical role in EDHF-mediated responses the effects of the gap junction inhibitors, 18α-glycyrrhetinic acid (Davidson *et al.*, 1986; Chaytor *et al.*, 1999), palmitoleic acid (Domenighetti *et al.*, 1998) and

SR141716A (Chaytor *et al.*, 1999), have been investigated against both EDHF-mediated responses to carbachol and relaxations to K^+. In addition removal of the endothelium abolishes responses to K^+ thereby suggesting that K^+ may be acting on the endothelium to release autacoids (Okazaki *et al.*, 1998). Therefore, the effects of endothelial denudation on responses to carbachol and K^+ have also been examined.

1. METHODS

1.1. Isolated, perfused superior mesenteric arterial bed of the rat

Male Wistar rats were anaesthetized with sodium pentobarbital (60 mg/kg, intra-peritoneally) and killed by exsanguination. Following laporotomy, the superior mesenteric artery was cannulated and the arterial vasculature was dissected away from the guts, placed in a jacketed organ chamber (McCulloch *et al.*, 1997) and perfused at 5 ml/min with oxygenated Krebs–Henseleit solution (composition, $\times 10^{-3}$ M; NaCl 118, KCl 4.7, $MgSO_4$ 1.2, KH_2PO_4 1.2, $NaHCO_3$ 25, $CaCl_2$ 2, D-glucose 10; 37 °C). Indomethacin (10^{-5} M) and N^G-nitro-L-arginine methyl ester (L-NAME; 3×10^{-4} M) were added to the Krebs–Henseleit buffer in experiments involving carbachol in order to define EDHF as the mediator of NO- and prostanoid-independent relaxations to the endothelium-dependent dilator, carbachol (McCulloch *et al.*, 1997). In most experiments involving K^+-induced relaxations, a K^+-free Krebs–Henseleit solution was prepared by substituting KCl and KH_2PO_4 for equimolar concentrations of NaCl and Na_2HPO_4, respectively, to optimize the responses to K^+. Additional K^+ experiments were carried out in the presence of normal K^+-containing Krebs–Henseleit buffer.

1.2. Experimental protocol

Following equilibration (30 minutes), methoxamine (1.2×10^{-6} M) was added to the buffer to increase perfusion pressure by approximately 100 mmHg. The dilator effects of carbachol (acting via EDHF) or KCl were then assessed. The doses of KCl (1×10^{-6}–2.5×10^{-5} mol) were from stock concentrations of 1×10^{-3}–2.5×10^{-2} M, and the rapid injection of 1 ml boluses of stock solutions would have transiently resulted in concentrations in this range (1×10^{-3}–2.5×10^{-2} M).

In preparations receiving indomethacin (10^{-5} M), L-NAME (3×10^{-4} M), flurbi-profen (10^{-5} M), clotrimazole (a cytochrome P450 and widely accepted EDHF inhib-itor, 10^{-5} M), barium chloride ($BaCl_2$, 3×10^{-5} M) or ouabain (10^{-3} M) the agents were added to the buffer to achieve the desired concentration and allowed to equili-brate (30 minutes) prior to addition of dilators. 18α-glycyrrhetinic acid (10^{-4} M), palmitoleic acid (5×10^{-5} M) and SR141716A (10^{-5} M) were allowed to equilibrate for one hour. In some preparations, the endothelium was removed by perfusion of distilled water for three minutes (Wagner *et al.*, 1999).

1.3. Data and statistical analysis

The dose–response curves were fitted to a logistic equation (McCulloch *et al.*, 1997); the $-\log ED_{50}$ (pD_2) and maximal relaxation (R_{max}) values obtained were compared by ANOVA with Bonferroni's *post-hoc* test. In experiments measuring K^+ responses,

Student's *t*-tests for unpaired observations were performed at each dose and the response at the concentration of 2.5×10^{-2} M was taken as the maximum. *p* values less than .05 were considered to be statistically significant.

1.4. Drugs and reagents

Barium chloride was supplied by Aldrich Chem. Co. (Milwaukee, USA) and dissolved in saline. SR141716A was supplied by Sanofi (Montpellier, France) and dissolved in ethanol. All other drugs were supplied by Sigma Chemical Co. (Poole, UK) and dissolved in saline, except 18α-glycyrrhetinic acid, indomethacin, flurbiprofen and clotrimazole (dissolved in ethanol).

2. RESULTS

2.1. Carbachol

Carbachol, in the presence of indomethacin (10^{-5} M) and L-NAME (3×10^{-4} M), caused dose-dependent dilatations ($ED_{50} = (3.61 \pm 1.86) \times 10^{-9}$ mol; $R_{max} = 85.3 \pm 4.0\%$; Figure 10.1). Addition of ouabain (10^{-3} M), in the presence of indomethacin and L-NAME, essentially abolished these responses (Figure 10.1). Ba^{2+} (3×10^{-5} M) alone produced a modest inhibition of dilatation to carbachol (Figure 10.1). The combination of ouabain and Ba^{2+} also opposed the responses to carbachol (Figure 10.1).

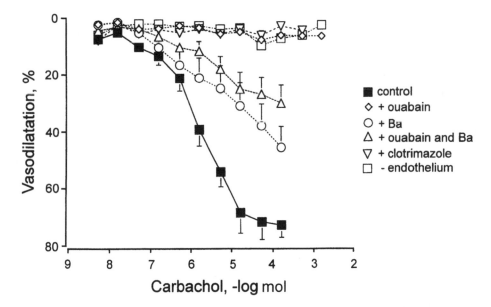

Figure 10.1 Dilatation to carbachol in the rat isolated mesenteric arterial bed in the presence of indomethacin (10^{-5} M) and N^G-nitro-L-arginine methyl ester (L-NAME; 3×10^{-4} M) (control; $n = 8$) and either ouabain (1×10^{-3} M; $n = 6$), $BaCl_2$ (Ba; 3×10^{-5} M; $n = 6$), the combination of $BaCl_2$ and ouabain, or clotrimazole (10^{-5} M; $n = 5$) and following removal of the endothelium ($n = 5$). Values are shown as mean $\pm$ SEM.

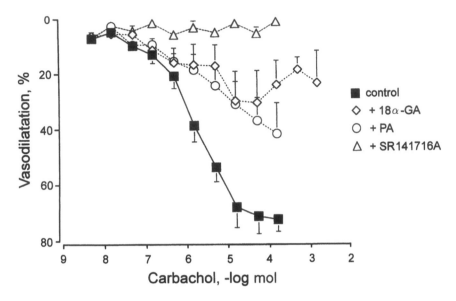

Figure 10.2 Dilatation to carbachol in the rat isolated mesenteric arterial bed in the presence of indomethacin (10^{-5} M) and N^G-nitro-L-arginine methyl ester (L-NAME; 3×10^{-4} M) (control; $n = 8$) and either 18α-glycyrrhetinic acid (18α-GA; 10^{-4} M; $n = 6$), palmitoleic acid (PA; 5×10^{-5} M; $n = 6$), or SR141716A (10^{-5} M; $n = 4$). Values are shown as mean ± SEM.

The addition of clotrimazole (10^{-5} M) or removal of the endothelium almost abolished relaxations to carbachol (Figure 10.1). The gap junction inhibitors, 18α-glycyrrhetinic acid (10^{-4} M), palmitoleic acid (5×10^{-5} M) and SR141716A (10^{-5} M) all significantly inhibited vasorelaxations to carbachol in the presence of indomethacin and L-NAME (Figure 10.2).

2.2. K^+

In normal buffer, potassium chloride (KCl, 10^{-3}–2.5×1^{-2} M) caused dilatations ($R_{max} = 46.6 \pm 8.5\%$; Figure 10.3). In K^+-free Krebs–Henseleit buffer, the dilatations were significantly greater ($R_{max} = 71.9 \pm 2.1\%$; Figure 10.3). Addition of indomethacin (10^{-5} M) significantly inhibited these relaxations ($R_{max} = 56.4 \pm 6.2\%$ at 2.5×10^{-2} M; Figure 10.3). The cycloxygenase inhibitor, flurbiprofen (10^{-5} M), also significantly inhibited K^+-evoked dilatations ($R_{max} = 64.7 \pm 1.5\%$; Figure 10.3). K^+ relaxations were significantly affected in the presence of L-NAME alone ($R_{max} = 63.2 \pm 3.1\%$; Figure 10.3). In the presence of 10^{-3} M ouabain, relaxation to K^+ was essentially abolished (Figure 10.4). Ba^{2+} (3×10^{-5} M significantly inhibited K^+ responses (Figure 10.4) and the combination of ouabain plus Ba^{2+} further attenuated these responses (Figure 10.4). Removal of the endothelium almost abolished K^+-induced relaxation ($R_{max} = 11.9 \pm 2.6\%$; Figure 10.3). However, clotrimazole (10^{-5} M), had no effect on dilatation to K^+ (Figure 10.4). 18α-glycyrrhetinic acid (10^{-4} M) significantly inhibited dilatation to K^+ (Figure 10.4) while SR141716A (10^{-5} M) and palmitoleic acid (5×10^{-5} M) had no significant effects on K^+-induced dilatations (Figure 10.4).

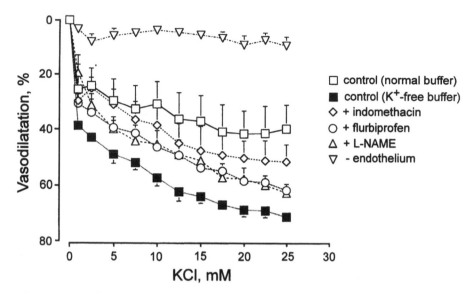

Figure 10.3 Dilatation to KCl in the rat isolated mesenteric arterial bed in the presence of either indomethacin (10^{-5} M; $n = 6$), flurbiprofen (10^{-5} M; $n = 5$), N^G-nitro-L-arginine methyl ester (L-NAME; 3×10^{-4} M; $n = 5$), normal buffer ($n = 4$) or K^+-free buffer ($n = 7$) and following endothelial denudation ($n = 6$). Values are shown as mean ± SEM.

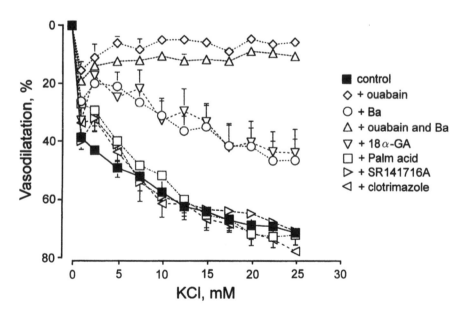

Figure 10.4 Dilatation to KCl in the rat isolated mesenteric arterial bed perfused with K^+-free buffer (control; $n = 7$) in the presence of either ouabain (10^{-3} M; $n = 6$), BaCl$_2$ (Ba; 3×10^{-5} M; $n = 6$), the combination of BaCl$_2$ plus ouabain ($n = 6$) 18α-glycyrrhetinic acid (18α-GA; 10^{-4} M; $n = 6$), palmitoleic acid (Palm Acid; 5×10^{-5} M; $n = 6$) or SR141716A (10^{-5} M; $n = 4$), clotrimazole (10^{-5} M; $n = 5$). Values are shown as mean ± SEM.

3. DISCUSSION

The present study demonstrates that EDHF-mediated and K^+-induced dilatations show different characteristics. The effects of the inhibitors on the relaxations to carbachol emphasise the role of gap junctional communication in EDHF-mediated vasorelaxation. By contrast, the dilatation to K^+ was found to be endothelium-dependent and in part mediated via prostanoids.

The inhibition of EDHF-type relaxations by the gap junction inhibitors 18α-glycyrrhetinic acid, SR141716A and palmitoleic acid is consistent with these responses being mediated via myoendothelial gap junctions (Chaytor *et al.*, 1998). In addition, clotrimazole has also been identified as a potent inhibitor of gap junctional communication (Harris *et al.*, 2000). Taken together, these findings add further weight to the proposal that EDHF-type relaxations involve direct endothelial-smooth muscle coupling via gap junctions (Chaytor *et al.*, 1998).

The K^+-evoked dilatation was less prominent in the presence of physiological concentrations of K^+, and in the rat aorta, K^+ induces relaxation only in K^+-free buffer and not in normal Krebs–Henseleit solution (Oh *et al.*, 2000). The K^+-evoked relaxations were also attenuated by 18α-glycyrrhetinic acid. However, neither SR141716A, palmitoleic acid nor clotrimazole affected these responses, leading to the conclusion that gap junctional communication does not contribute to K^+-evoked relaxations. These observations highlight fundamental differences between EDHF-mediated and K^+-induced dilatation, and also suggest that the action of 18α-glycyrrhetinic acid against K^+ involves pharmacological effects which are distinct from blockade of gap junctions, such as an ability to inhibit the Na^+/K^+ATPase (Terasawa *et al.*, 1992).

The strictly endothelium-dependent nature of the responses to K^+ observed in the present study does not support the hypothesis that K^+ ions released from the endothelium function as an EDHF (Edwards *et al.*, 1998). Furthermore, relaxations evoked by carbachol or by K^+ were abolished by ouabain, which mimicked the effects of endothelial denudation, thus excluding a major role for inwardly-rectifying K^+ channels. Ouabain blocks intercellular coupling in non-vascular cell types (Schirrmacher *et al.*, 1996) and also significantly inhibited the intercellular spread of Lucifer yellow via gap junctions in a model system (Harris *et al.*, 2000). This suggests that its inhibitory action against carbachol-evoked relaxations may, at least in part, be explained by effects on gap junctions. It is possible that similarities in the pharmacological profiles of ouabain and 18α-glycyrrhetinic acid, including the ability to block gap junctions, reflect their common basic steroidal structure. Indeed, 18α-glycyrrhetinic acid itself inhibits the Na^+/K^+ATPase in the canine kidney, albeit with a substantially greater IC_{50} ($\sim70\,\mu M$) than ouabain ($0.5\,\mu M$) (Terasawa *et al.*, 1992). Likewise the mechanism through which ouabain decreases gap junctional permeability in osteoblasts is secondary to the elevations in intracellular Ca^{2+} that are an expected consequence of Na^+ pump inhibition (Schirrmacher *et al.*, 1996).

The mechanisms underlying the effects of K^+ ions in the rat mesenteric bed are likely to involve stimulation of the endothelial Na^+/K^+ATPase and/or activation of inwardly-rectifying endothelial K^+ channels (Daut *et al.*, 1988; Laskey *et al.*, 1990). Both actions would be expected to promote hyperpolarization of the cell membrane to increase the electrochemical gradient for Ca^{2+} entry and promote Ca^{2+}-dependent synthesis of endothelial autacoids. This mechanism should in theory be susceptible to inhibition by 18α-glycyrrhetinic acid, as well as ouabain, thus explaining the ability of both compounds to attenuate or abolish, respectively, endothelium-dependent relaxations to K^+.

In the present study, clotrimazole abolished EDHF-type relaxations but was without effect on the relaxations evoked by K^+, further highlighting differences in the pathways activated by the two stimuli. The lack of effect of clotrimazole against K^+-induced relaxations would appear to exclude K^+ acting via EDHF release. The inhibitors of cycloxygenase indomethacin and flurbiprofen did, however, partly attenuate the responses to K^+ but not carbachol (McCulloch *et al.*, 1997), indicating that endothelium-derived prostanoids contribute towards K^+-induced relaxations.

4. CONCLUSION

The present investigation has shown that the mechanism of dilatation to K^+ is strictly endothelium-dependent and is, in part, mediated via prostanoids. Experiments with 18α-glycyrrhetinic acid, SR141716A, palmitoleic acid and clotrimazole have identified an important role for direct endothelium-smooth muscle coupling via gap junctions in the relaxations mediated via EDHF but not K^+. Therefore, differences in the pharmacology of EDHF and K^+ suggest that K^+ is unlikely to be an EDHF in the rat mesenteric arterial bed.

ACKNOWLEDGEMENTS

MDR thanks the British Heart Foundation for financial support. DH holds an MRC Studentship.

11 Comparison of α and β isoforms of glycyrrhetinic acid and carbenoxolone as inhibitors of EDHF-type relaxation

Andrew T. Chaytor, Wendy L. Marsh,
Iain R. Hutcheson and Tudor M. Griffith

The vascular actions of the lipophilic gap junction inhibitors 18α-glycyrrhetinic acid, 18β-glycyrrhetinic acid and the water-soluble hemisuccinate derivative of 18β-glycyrrhetinic acid, carbenoxolone, were investigated in constricted rings of rabbit superior mesenteric artery. EDHF-type relaxations to acetylcholine, observed in the presence of N^G-nitro-L-arginine methyl ester (L-NAME) and indomethacin, were attenuated by incubation with 18α-glycyrrhetinic acid, 18β-glycyrrhetinic acid or carbenoxolone in a concentration-dependent fashion. By contrast, none of these agents affected responses to sodium nitroprusside, an exogenous source of NO, and relaxations evoked by acetylcholine in the absence of L-NAME were attenuated by approximately 20%. 18α-glycyrrhetinic acid exerted no direct effect on vessel tone, whereas 18β-glycyrrhetinic acid and carbenoxolone caused relaxations. Relaxations to carbenoxolone were attenuated by endothelial denudation and by incubation with L-NAME, whereas those to 18β-glycyrrhetinic acid were unaffected. In conclusion, all three agents inhibit EDHF-type relaxations evoked by acetylcholine. Unlike 18α-glycyrrhetinic acid, carbenoxolone and 18β-glycyrrhetinic acid possess intrinsic relaxing properties which in the case of carbenoxolone involves functional enhancement of NO activity in addition to direct effects on vascular smooth muscle.

Endothelium-dependent relaxations to agonists such as acetylcholine may be mediated by nitric oxide (NO), prostanoids and an endothelium-derived hyperpolarizing factor (EDHF) (see Garland *et al.*, 1995; Mombouli and Vanhoutte, 1997 for reviews). The NO- and prostanoid-independent component of endothelium-dependent responses which arc attributable to the actions of an EDHF depend on gap junctional intercellular communication (Chaytor *et al.*, 1998; Hutcheson *et al.*, 1999; Griffith and Taylor, 1999). Gap junctions are membrane bound channels which are formed by the docking of two connexon hemichannels contributed by apposing cells. Each hemichannel is constructed from six connexin (Cx) protein subunits which oligomerize around a central aqueous pore that permits passage of electrical current and molecules smaller than 1 kDa in size. This allows direct intercellular communication between the cytoplasmic compartments of physically adjacent cells (Yeager and Nicholson, 1996). At least 20 connexin subtypes, classified according to molecular size, have been described in mammalian tissues with endothelial and vascular smooth muscle cells variably expressing Cxs 37, 40 and 43 (Carter *et al.*, 1996; Chaytor *et al.*, 1997; Li and Simard, 1999). Myoendothelial gap junctions have been demonstrated in rabbit carotid artery and could in theory consist of homotypic (e.g. Cx43/Cx43) and heterotypic (e.g. Cx37/Cx43) channels as well as heteromeric channels in which the contributing connexons are constructed from more than one connexin protein (Spagnoli *et al.*, 1982; Elfgang *et al.*, 1995; He *et al.*, 1999; Van Kempen and Jongsma, 1999).

Intercellular communication via gap junctions may be inhibited by glycyrrhetinic acid, a lipophilic steroidal aglycone derived from glycyrrhizic acid, which is found in the liquorice root, *Glycyrrhizia glabra* (Davidson *et al.*, 1986; Davidson and Baumgarten, 1988). Glycyrrhetinic acid exists in α and β isoforms, and studies have shown that both compounds are active in the blood vessel wall. 18α-glycyrrhetinic acid inhibits NO- and prostanoid-independent relaxations in rabbit iliac arteries at concentrations that do not directly affect vascular tone (Taylor *et al.*, 1998). Analogously, 18β-glycyrrhetinic acid inhibits endothelium-dependent hyperpolarizations of vascular smooth muscle (Yamamoto *et al.*, 1999), but exerts additional endothelium-independent effects that depress vascular smooth muscle tone (Taylor *et al.*, 1998). The disodium salt of the hemisuccinate derivative of 18β-glycyrrhetinic acid, carbenoxolone, is also an effective inhibitor of homocellular gap junctional communication in human fibroblasts (Davidson *et al.*, 1986; Davidson and Baumgarten, 1988), but its ability to modulate vascular tone through effects on the permeability of gap junctions has not previously been characterized. Furthermore, there is evidence that carbenoxolone promotes endothelium-dependent relaxations that are mediated via the NO pathway (Dembinska-Kiec *et al.*, 1991). In view of such apparent pharmacological differences between 18α-glycyrrhetinic acid, 18β-glycyrrhetinic acid and carbenoxolone, in the present study we have evaluated the relative merits and disadvantages of these agents as putative inhibitors of EDHF-type relaxations.

1. METHODS

1.1. Isolated ring preparations

Superior mesenteric arteries were removed from male New Zealand white rabbits (2.5 kg) which had been killed by injection of sodium pentobarbitone (120 mg/kg; i.v.) and transferred to cold Holman's solution of the following composition (mM): 120 NaCl; 5 KCl; 2.5 $CaCl_2$; 1.3 NaH_2PO_4; 25 $NaHCO_3$; 11 glucose; and 10 sucrose. Rings (2–3 mm wide) were cut and suspended in 3 ml organ baths containing gassed (95% O_2; 5% CO_2; pH 7.4) Holman's solution at 37 °C. Changes in isometric force were monitored using Dynamometer UFI force transducers (Lectromed, UK) connected to a Maclab 4e system (ADInstruments, UK). Tension was initially set at 0.5 g and during an equilibrium period of 1 hour the tissues were washed with fresh Holman's solution every 10–15 min with tension readjusted as necessary following stress relaxation. Rings without endothelium were prepared by gentle abrasion of the intimal surface of the blood vessel. All rings were initially tested for the presence or absence of endothelium by constriction of the tissue with 1×10^{-5} M phenylephrine and subsequent addition of 1×10^{-6} M acetylcholine.

1.2. Experimental protocols

Rings of superior mesenteric arteries with intact endothelium were contraced with phenylephrine (1×10^{-5} M) and cumulative concentration–response curves to acetylcholine obtained before and after a 45 min incubation with the inhibitor of NO synthase, N^G-nitro-L-arginine methyl ester (L-NAME, 3×10^{-4} M) in combination with the inhibitor of cyclooxygenase, indomethacin (1×10^{-5} M). To evaluate the effects of the glycyrrhetinic acid derivatives on the NO/prostanoid-independent component of the relaxations induced by acetylcholine, cumulative concentration–response curves to this agonist were obtained following a 1 hour incubation with 18α-glycyrrhetinic acid (to 3×10^{-4} M), 18β-glycyrrhetinic acid (to 1×10^{-3} M) or carbenoxolone (to 3×10^{-4} M). In some rings acetylcholine-induced relaxations were also assessed after incubation with these compounds for 1 hour in the absence of L-NAME and indomethacin. The effects of the vehicles used to dissolve 18α-glycyrrhetinic acid (DMSO) and 18β-glycyrrhetinic acid (ethanol) on vascular tone were investigated in control studies.

Possible direct effects of the glycyrrhetinic acid derivatives on vascular tone were compared in preparations with and without endothelium. Rings were constricted with phenylephrine (1×10^{-5} M) and cumulative concentration–response curves to 18α-glycyrrhetinic acid, 18β-glycyrrhetinic acid and carbenoxolone obtained. In some studies on rings with endothelium the blood vessels were incubated for 45 min with L-NAME (3×10^{-4} M). The effects of 18α-glycyrrhetinic acid (1×10^{-4} M), 18β-glycyrrhetinic acid (1×10^{-5} M) and carbenoxolone (3×10^{-4} M) on relaxations evoked by sodium nitroprusside were also examined in preconstricted endothelium-denuded rings following an initial 1 hour preincubation period. All drugs were supplied by Sigma, UK.

1.3. Statistical analysis

Data are given as mean $\pm$ SEM, where n denotes the number of animals studied for each data point. Concentration–response curves were assessed by one-way analysis of variance (ANOVA) followed by the Bonferroni multiple comparisons test. EC_{50} values and maximal relaxations (expressed as % reversal of phenylephrine-induced constriction) were compared by the Student's t-test for unpaired data. Differences were considered to be statistically significant when p was less than .05.

2. RESULTS

2.1. Control solution

Acetylcholine caused large relaxations of rings with endothelium with an EC_{50} of 0.12 ± 0.06 1×10^{-6} M (Figure 11.1). Maximal relaxations to acetylcholine were reduced significantly by $25 \pm 4\%$, $18 \pm 3\%$ and $17 \pm 3\%$ following incubation with 18α-glycyrrhetinic acid (1×10^{-4} M), 18β-glycyrrhetinic acid (1×10^{-5} M) and carbenoxolone (3×10^{-4} M), respectively, without significant effects on the EC_{50} value for relaxation.

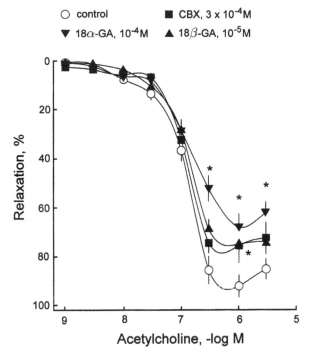

Figure 11.1 Effects of 1×10^{-4} M 18α-glycyrrhetinic aid, 1×10^{-5} M 18β-glycyrrhetinic acid or 3×10^{-4} M carbenoxolone (CBX) on acetylcholine-induced relaxations of rings with endothelium of rabbit superior mesenteric arteries under control conditions during contractions with phenylephrine (10^{-5} M) in the absence of L-NAME and indomethacin. Each gap junction inhibitor significantly attenuated the maximal response to acetylcholine ($n = 4$ for each). The asterisks indicate statistically significant differences ($p < .05$).

2.2. Presence of L-NAME plus indomethacin

2.2.1. 18α-Glycyrrhetinic acid

Acetylcholine evoked relaxations of rings with endothelium in the presence of L-NAME (3×10^{-4} M) and indomethacin (1×10^5 M), with an EC$_{50}$ of $0.37 \pm 0.01 \times 10^{-6}$ M (Figure 11.2a). The relaxations were attenuated in a concentration-dependent fashion following incubation with 18α-glycyrrhetinic acid over the range $10-100 \times 10^{-6}$ M, with maximal responses being attenuated by $93 \pm 2\%$ in the presence of 1×10^{-4} M 18α-glycyrrhetinic acid (Figure 11.2A). There was no change in EC$_{50}$ following incubation with 18α-glycyrrhetinic acid at concentrations up to 3×10^{-5} M. Concentrations up to 0.2% v/v of DMSO had no significant effect on EDHF-type responses.

2.2.2. 18β-Glycyrrhetinic acid

Acetylcholine evoked relaxations of rings with endothelium in the presence of L-NAME (3×10^{-4} M) and indomethacin (1×10^5 M), with an EC$_{50}$ of $0.22 \pm 0.05 \times 10^{-6}$ M (Figure 11.2B). In the presence of 18β-glycyrrhetinic acid there was again

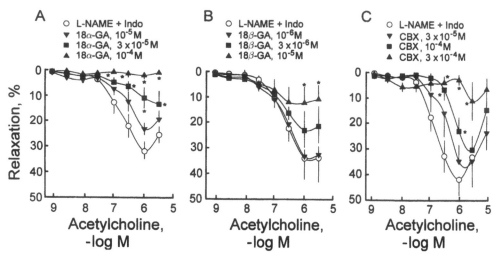

Figure 11.2 Effects of (A) 18α-glycyrrhetinic acid ($n = 5$), (B) 18β-glycyrrhetinic acid ($n = 4$) or (C) carbenoxolone ($n = 5$; CBX) on acetylcholine-induced relaxations of rings with endothelium of rabbit superior mesenteric arteries in the presence of L-NAME (3×10^{-4} M) and indomethacin (1×10^{-5} M). Each compound attenuated the EDHF-type relaxation to acetylcholine in a concentration-related manner. The asterisks indicate statistically significant differences versus L-NAME plus indomethacin ($p < .05$).

a concentration-dependent attenuation of relaxation, with maximal responses being reduced by $64 \pm 4\%$ in the presence of 18β-glycyrrhetinic acid 1×10^5 M (Figure 11.2B). The EC_{50} values were unaffected by 18β-glycyrrhetinic acid at any of the concentrations used. Ethanol, (up to 0.1% v/v) exerted no significant effect on EDHF-type responses.

2.2.3. Carbenoxolone

In the presence of L-NAME (3×10^{-4} M) and indomethacin (1×10^{-5} M), acetylcholine evoked EDHF-type relaxations with an EC_{50} of $0.21 \pm 0.07 \times 10^{-6}$ M (Figure 11.2C). Incubation with carbenoxolone (3×10^{-5} M) had no significant effect on the responses either in terms of EC_{50} ($0.40 \pm 0.01 \times 10^{-6}$ M) or maximum (Figure 11.2C). However, in the presence of 1×10^{-4} M carbenoxolone there was a significant increase in the EC_{50} to $0.79 \pm 0.03 \times 10^{-6}$ M and a small but significant reduction in the maximal response by $28 \pm 3\%$ (Figure 11.2C). At 3×10^{-4} M, carbenoxolone significantly inhibited maximal relaxation by $73 \pm 5\%$ (Figure 11.2C), although EC_{50} values did not differ significantly.

2.2.4. Reversibility

Submaximal inhibitory concentrations of 18α-glycyrrhetinic acid, 18β-glycyrrhetinic acid and carbenoxolone were employed to determine if their effects on EDHF-type relaxations were reversible. Following incubation with 3×10^{-5} M 18α-glycyrrhetinic

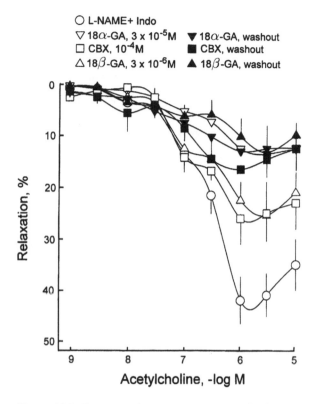

Figure 11.3 Concentration–response curves for EDHF-type relaxations to acetylcholine (ACh) in rings with endothelium of rabbit superior mesenteric arteries obtained in the presence of 3×10^{-5} M 18α-glycyrrhetinic acid ($n = 3$), 3×10^{-6} M 18β-glycyrrhetinic acid ($n = 3$) or 1×10^{-4} M carbenoxolone ($n = 3$; CBX), before (open symbols) and after (closed symbols) repeated washout of all drugs for 1 hour. No reversibility was observed with 18α-glycyrrhetinic acid, and progressive inhibition was observed with 18β-glycyrrhetinic acid and carbenoxolone. Indices of significance have been omitted for clarity of presentation.

acid, the exposure to increasing concentrations of acetylcholine after repeated washout of all drugs at 5-minute intervals for 1 hour revealed no restoration of the relaxation (Figure 11.3). Repeat concentration–response curves to acetylcholine obtained after washout of 3×10^{-6} M 18β-glycyrrhetinic acid or 1×10^{-4} M carbenoxolone demonstrated a progressive depression even after 1 hour washout (Figure 11.3).

2.3. Phenylephrine

Incubation with 18α-glycyrrhetinic acid at the highest concentration permitted by its limited solubility in vehicle (final bath concentrations: 18α-GA, 3×10^{-4} M; DMSO, 0.6% v/v) caused a small relaxation within 5 min which was subsequently sustained over 1 hour. Administration of either the 18α-glycyrrhetinic acid stock solution or DMSO caused similar reductions in phenylephrine-induced tone (18α-glycyrrhetinic acid: $16 \pm 4\%$, $n = 4$; DMSO: $17 \pm 5\%$, $n = 9$). By contrast, 0.2% DMSO or

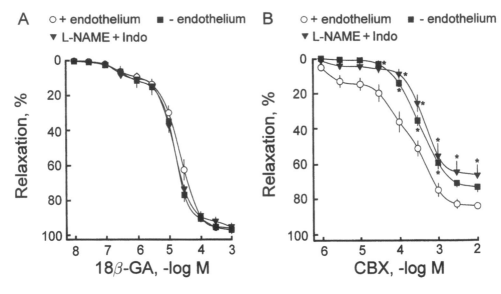

Figure 11.4 Effects of (A) 18β-glycyrrhetinic acid and (B) carbenoxolone (CBX) on the constrictor response to 1×10^{-5} M phenylephrine in rabbit superior mesenteric artery rings with endothelium in the presence ($n = 7$ and $n = 9$, respectively) and absence ($n = 7$ and $n = 6$, respectively) of L-NAME (3×10^{-4} M) and indomethacin (1×10^{-5} M) and in rings without endothelium ($n = 5$ and $n = 10$, respectively). The asterisks indicate statistically significant differences ($p < .05$).

1×10^{-4} M 18α-glycyrrhetinic acid, which resulted in the same final bath concentration of DMSO, did not affect arterial tone (data not shown).

18β-glycyrrhetinic acid induced concentration-dependent relaxations of rings with endothelium which were maximal at a concentration of approximately 1×10^{-3} M. These relaxations were unaffected either by incubation with L-NAME (3×10^{-4} M) or endothelial denudation (Figure 11.4A). The responses were attributable to a direct action of 18β-glycyrrhetinic acid as equivalent concentrations of the ethanol vehicle were without effect on tone.

Carbenoxolone evoked concentration-dependent relaxations of rings with endothelium which were maximal at a concentration approximately 1×10^{-2} M. Treatment with L-NAME (3×10^{-4} M) and indomethacin (1×10^{5} M) significantly attenuated the relaxation, causing an increase in EC_{50} and a significant reduction in maximal response (Figure 11.4B). Endothelial denudation caused a similar reduction in carbenoxolone-induced relaxation which was reflected by a significant increase in EC_{50} value and a significant reduction in maximal response (Figure 11.4B).

2.4. Sodium nitroprusside

In preparations without endothelium sodium nitroprusside induced concentration-dependent relaxations with an EC_{50} of $0.32 \pm 0.07 \times 10^{-6}$ M (Figure 11.5). Incubation with 18α-glycyrrhetinic acid (1×10^{-4} M), 18β-glycyrrhetinic acid (1×10^{-5} M) or carbenoxolone (3×10^{-4} M) did not significantly affect the EC_{50} value or the maximal

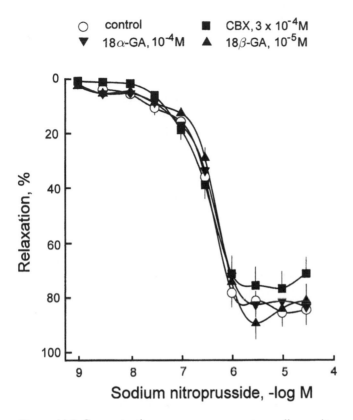

Figure 11.5 Concentration–response curves to sodium nitroprusside in rings without endothelium of rabbit superior mesenteric arteries showing that 18α-glycyrrhetinic acid (1×10^{-4} M), 18β-glycyrrhetinic acid (1×10^{-5} M) and carbenoxolone (3×10^{-4} M; CBX) ($n = 4$ in each case) did not significantly affect relaxation.

relaxation. The phenylephrine-induced contraction averaged 3.10 ± 0.40 g in the control situation, and 3.00 ± 0.20 g, 2.60 ± 0.20 g and 2.50 ± 0.30 g in the presence of 18α-glycyrrhetinic acid, 18β-glycyrrhetinic acid and carbenoxolone, respectively. Although 18β-glycyrrhetinic acid and carbenoxolone both caused small reductions in tone, this trend did not achieve statistical significance at the concentrations employed.

3. DISCUSSION

The present experiments demonstrate that the three structurally-related gap junction inhibitors, 18α-glycyrrhetinic acid, 18β-glycyrrhetinic acid and carbenoxolone, inhibit acetylcholine evoked NO- and prostanoid-independent relaxations in the rabbit superior mesenteric artery. Rank potencies against EDHF-type relaxations were 18β-glycyrrhetinic acid $> 18\alpha$-glycyrrhetinic acid $>$ carbenoxolone, with 10–30 fold higher concentrations of carbenoxolone being required to produce inhibitory effects equivalent to those of the parent 18β-glycyrrhetinic acid compound. The differential potencies of the three agents in the rabbit superior mesenteric artery contrast with early studies showing that they are equi-effective gap junction inhibitors in confluent human fibroblast monolayers in which direct cell–cell communication is reduced by 95% at concentrations around 1×10^{-5} M (Davidson *et al.*, 1986; Davidson and Baumgarten, 1988). Gap junctions allowing communication between cells in such monolayers are located superficially and it is possible that the apparently lower biological potency of carbenoxolone in the arterial wall reflects the presence of the hemisuccinate group, which decreases lipophilicity compared to 18β-glycyrrhetinic acid and may in some way reduce access to myoendothelial gap junctions.

Consistent with an action distal to the occupation of muscarinic receptors, 18α-glycyrrhetinic acid and 18β-glycyrrhetinic acid did not significantly affect the EC_{50} value for EDHF-type relaxations to acetylcholine, which remained in the sub-micromolar range until such responses were nearly abolished. This is consistent with the previous demonstration that 18α-glycyrrhetinic acid abolishes EDHF-type relaxations induced by cyclopiazonic acid, an agent which activates the endothelial cell through receptor-independent mechanisms by depleting Ca^{2+} stores and promoting capacitative Ca^{2+} influx (Taylor *et al.*, 1998). In the present study, non-specific effects of 18α-glycyrrhetinic acid, 18β-glycyrrhetinic acid and carbenoxolone on endothelial function were excluded by observations that relaxations to acetylcholine evoked in the absence of L-NAME were attenuated by only about 20% following an initial 1 hour incubation with these agents. As shown in experiments with connexin-mimetic peptides, this is likely to reflect the contribution of EDHF to the full response to acetylcholine observed in this blood vessel in the presence of NO synthesis (Chaytor *et al.*, 1998). Relaxations to sodium nitroprusside were unaffected by 18α-glycyrrhetinic acid, 18β-glycyrrhetinic acid or carbenoxolone indicating that these agents do not interfere with the ability of NO to cause relaxation of smooth muscle.

In cultured monolayers expressing Cx43, the interruption of intercellular communication by 18α-glycyrrhetinic acid, 18β-glycyrrhetinic acid and carbenoxolone is rapid (within 15–30 min), initially reversible, and is not associated with changes in the integrity of gap junction plaques (aggregates of gap junctions at points of cell–cell contact) or changes in the phosphorylation status of their connexin proteins (Guan *et al.*, 1996; Guo *et al.*, 1999). With longer incubations, however, there is time- and concentration-dependent dephosphorylation of Cx43, plaque disassembly, and progressive reductions in both Cx43 mRNA and protein expression as exposure times are extended from 30 min to 4 hours (Guan *et al.*, 1996; Guo *et al.*, 1999). In the present study the inhibitors were present in the organ chamber for 1 hour before concentration–relaxation curves to acetylcholine were obtained and their effects were found to be irreversible. Thus, EDHF-type relaxations to acetylcholine were not restored to their control value after washout of 18α-glycyrrhetinic acid for 1 hour, and in the case of 18β-glycyrrhetinic acid and carbenoxolone a progressive decrease in the EDHF-type response to acetylcholine became apparent even after the removal of the inhibitors from the buffer. Although there is some evidence that glycyrrhetinic acid and its derivatives bind to a specific membrane protein that possesses low affinity for mineralocorticoids, glucocorticoids and other steroids (Negishi *et al.*, 1991), the mechanism(s) through which they attenuate intercellular communication remain incompletely understood. Inhibition is unlikely to be specifically related to the steroidal structure of such compounds (Davidson *et al.*, 1986), and a direct causal link between connexin deposphorylation and plaque stability remains to be established.

Indeed, 18α-GA reportedly causes plaque disaggregation without affecting the phosphorylation status of Cx43 in C6 glioma cells (Goldberg *et al.*, 1996), and also attenuates Lucifer yellow dye transfer in HeLa cells transfected to express functional gap junctions constructed from connexin26 (Cx26), a connexin subtype that is not thought to be regulated by phosphorylation (George *et al.*, 1998).

It is possible that the apparently progressive inhibition of EDHF-type relaxations observed with 18β-glycyrrhetinic acid and carbenoxolone in the present study reflects non-specific toxic effects of glycyrrhetinic acid and its derivatives, which are generally most pronounced with compounds that possess the β configuration and after incubation times of several hours. In human fibroblasts, for example, 18β-glycyrrhetinic acid exerts toxic effects at relatively low concentrations, whereas toxicity is not apparent with 1×10^{-4} M 18α-glycyrrhetinic acid after 2 hours incubation and cell viability is reduced only after prolonged (20 hours) exposure at concentrations over 3×10^{-5} M (Davidson *et al.*, 1986; Davidson and Baumgarten, 1988). Carbenoxolone is also thought to exert greater cellular toxicity than 18α-glycyrrhetinic acid in fibroblasts (Davidson *et al.*, 1986). Toxicity may nevertheless also be a function of cell type. In C6 glioma cells, high concentrations of 18α-glycyrrhetinic acid (7.5×10^{-5} M) abolish dye transfer without affecting protein synthesis or cell viability (Goldberg *et al.*, 1995), whereas in pulmonary epithelial cells prolonged incubation with similar concentrations of 18α-glycyrrhetinic acid reduces protein expression and impairs their viability (Guo *et al.*, 1999).

The ability of 1×10^{-4} M 18α-glycyrrhetinic acid to abolish EDHF-type relaxations without affecting smooth muscle tone thus appears to make this compound particularly suitable as a pharmacological tool for studying the role of gap junctions in the regulation of vascular tone. By contrast, 18β-glycyrrhetinic acid and carbenoxolone both exerted concentration-dependent relaxing effects which at millimolar concentrations reversed phenylephrine-induced constriction by more than 70%. In this respect, relaxations evoked by 18β-glycyrrhetinic acid were evident at 10–30 fold lower concentrations than carbenoxolone, thus paralleling its greater potency as an inhibitor of EDHF-type relaxations, and resulted exclusively from a direct smooth muscle action. By contrast, relaxations to carbenoxolone were attenuated by removal of the endothelium or treatment with the NO synthase inhibitor L-NAME, implicating the additional participation of the NO pathway. Consistent with these findings, endothelium-independent relaxations to 18β-glycyrrhetinic acid have been documented in the rabbit iliac artery (Taylor *et al.*, 1998), and carbenoxolone promotes endothelium-dependent relaxations of the rat aorta through a mechanism that involves NO synthesis (Dembinska-Kiec *et al.*, 1991). Although additional direct effects of carbenoxolone on smooth muscle were not reported by these latter workers, responses were investigated only at concentrations up to 3×10^{-4} M, which in the present study caused relaxations equal to or less than 30%.

The present experiments with 18α-glycyrrhetinic acid and previous studies with gap junction peptides (Chaytor *et al.*, 1997) indicate that homocellular gap junctional communication between smooth muscle cells is not a determinant of the ambient smooth muscle force development induced by phenylephrine in the rabbit superior mesenteric artery. Effects on gap junctional communication are therefore unlikely to underlie the direct action of 18β-glycyrrhetinic acid and carbenoxolone against contraction. Indeed, carbenoxolone is thought to possess inhibitory activity against phosphodiesterases that inactivate adenosine $3':5'$ cyclic monophosphate (cyclic

AMP) and guanosine $3':5'$ cyclic monophosphate (cyclic GMP) (Amer *et al.*, 1974; Vapaatalo *et al.*, 1978). Since increased levels of cyclic AMP promote relaxation of smooth muscle, this mechanism could in theory contribute to the direct relaxing effects of carbenoxolone in the rabbit superior mesenteric artery, although it remains to be demonstrated experimentally that 18β-glycyrrhetinic acid indeed affects cyclic AMP phosphodiesterase. The NO-dependent component of carbenoxolone-induced relaxations is most likely to reflect inhibition of cyclic GMP phosphodiesterase, rather than increased NO synthesis, as carbenoxolone does not stimulate NO synthesis by pulmonary artery and aortic endothelial cells (Ullian *et al.*, 1996). Increased biological NO activity may also result from decreased inactivation by superoxide anions (Rubanyi and Vanhoutte, 1986; Gryglewski *et al.*, 1986). While it has been suggested that steroidal compounds may scavenge superoxide radicals (Hall *et al.*, 1987), this mechanism seems unlikely to be a major contributor to the endothelium-dependent action of carbenoxolone, as neither of the chemically-related 18α-glycyrrhetinic acid and 18β-glycyrrhetinic acid compounds enhanced functional NO activity. It is unknown whether or not carbenoxolone suppresses the generation of superoxide anions by endothelial cells, as reported for macrophages at concentrations within the micromolar range (Suzuki *et al.*, 1983).

4. CONCLUSION

18α-glycyrrhetinic acid, 18β-glycyrrhetinic acid and carbenoxolone inhibit NO- and prostanoid-independent relaxations evoked by acetylcholine in rings of the rabbit superior mesenteric artery with endothelium, consistent with the view that gap junctions are involved in EDHF-type relaxations in this blood vessel. However, at concentrations that exert significant inhibitory effects on EDHF-type responses, 18β-glycyrrhetinic acid and carbenoxolone both cause substantial reductions in constrictor tone through a direct action on smooth muscle, and in the case of carbenoxolone, an additional NO-dependent mechanism. 18β-glycyrrhetinic acid and carbenoxolone thus appear less specific than 18α-glycyrrhetinic acid as pharmacological probes for assessing the contribution of gap junctional communication to endothelium-dependent responses.

12 Inhibitory effect of 18-β-glycyrrhetinic acid on the relaxation induced by acetylcholine in the rat aorta

Bernard Muller, Deborah Schiestel,
Jean-Claude Stoclet and
Andrei L. Kleschyov

The purpose of the present study was to examine the potential effects of the isomers of glycyrrhetinic acid on the endothelium-dependent relaxation mediated by nitric oxide. In rat aortic rings, acetylcholine and the calcium ionophore A23187 produced an endothelium-dependent relaxing effect, which was abolished by the inhibitor of nitric oxide synthase, N^{ω}-nitro-L-arginine methyl ester. The relaxation evoked by acetylcholine was reduced by 18-β-glycyrrhetinic acid, but not by the 18-α-isomer. However, neither 18-α- nor 18-β-glycyrrhetinic acid affected the relaxation produced by A23187. In preparations without endothelium, neither 18-β-glycyrrhetinic acid nor 18-α-glycyrrhetinic acid modified the relaxation elicited by S-nitroso-N-acetylpenicillamine. These data suggest that 18-β-glycyrrhetinic acid inhibits the nitric oxide-dependent relaxing effect of acetylcholine in the rat aorta, by a mechanism distinct from inhibition of either nitric oxide synthase, gap junctions or the direct effect of nitric oxide in smooth muscle. The 18-β-isomer of glycyrrhetinic acid most likely interfered with the transduction pathways which led to the activation of endothelial nitric oxide synthase upon receptor stimulation. These data demonstrate that the inhibitory effects of 18-β-glycyrrhetinic acid are not limited to relaxation mediated by EDHF.

In isolated blood vessels, the respective contribution of nitric oxide, prostacyclin and EDHF to endothelium-dependent relaxation is usually addressed by drugs which may affect the synthesis, release and/or effects of these factors. Inhibitors of nitric oxide synthase or cycloxygenase are used to evaluate the role of nitric oxide and prostacyclin, respectively, and endothelium-dependent relaxations which are resistant to inhibition of these pathways are attributed to EDHF (Félétou and Vanhoutte, 1999). In some arteries, EDHF-like responses are inhibited by 18-β or 18-α-glycyrrhetinic acid (Taylor *et al.*, 1998; Fujimoto *et al.*, 1999; Fukuta *et al.*, 1999; Kagota *et al.*, 1999; Yamamoto *et al.*, 1999). As these lipophilic aglycones inhibit gap junctionnal communications (Davidson *et al.*, 1986; Davidson and Baumgarten, 1988; Guan *et al.*, 1996), hyperpolarization of vascular smooth muscle cells in some blood vessels may result from the electrical transfer and/or from the transfer of diffusible factors via gap junctions (Félétou and Vanhoutte, 1999).

Little information is available on the specificity of the isomers of glycyrrhetinic acid on EDHF-mediated responses. Especially, the potential effect of glycyrrhetinic acid on other endothelium-derived relaxing factors such as nitric oxide is not documented. The purpose of the present study was to determine whether or not the isomers of glycyrrhetinic acid affect the relaxation mediated by nitric oxide, either produced by endothelial nitric oxide synthase or delivered by a donor of nitric oxide. The rat aorta was chosen as model since in this large conduit artery, EDHF does not contribute to endothelium-dependent relaxations, and nitric oxide is the major if not the unique relaxing factor released by the endothelial cells (Rees *et al.*, 1990; Nagao *et al.*, 1992; Shimokawa *et al.*, 1996).

1. METHODS

1.1. Relaxation studies

The thoracic aorta (from male Wistar rats, 10–12 weeks old) was removed, cleaned of fat and connective tissues and cut into rings (2–3 mm long). In some cases, the endothelium was removed by rubbing the intimal surface of the rings with a curved forceps. Aortic rings were suspended (2 g of passive tension) in an organ chamber filled with Krebs solution (kept at 37 °C and bubbled with 95% O_2/5% CO_2). Tension was measured with an isometric force transducer. After an equilibration period of 60 min, the rings were contracted with norepinephrine (10^{-6} M) and acetylcholine (10^{-6} M) was applied to assess the presence or absence of functional endothelium. Endothelium was considered to be present when acetylcholine produced at least 30% relaxation. Rings were considered without endothelium when acetylcholine failed to produce relaxation. After a one hour washout-period (during which time the Krebs solution was replaced every 15 min), 18-α- or 18-β-glycyrrhetinic acid (3×10^{-5} M) or its vehicle (dimethylsulfoxide, 0.3%) was added. Forty-five minutes later, rings were contracted with norepinephrine (10^{-7} M in the case of rings without endothelium, 3×10^{-7} M for rings with endothelium). Once the contraction reached a steady state, acetylcholine, A23187 or S-nitroso-N-acetylpenicillamine was added in a cumulative manner. In the case of acetylcholine, preliminary experiments demonstrated that reproducible responses could be obtained with time on the same ring, in the absence of 18-α- or 18-β-glycyrrhetinic acid. Thus, the effect of glycyrrhetinic acid on the relaxation elicited by acetylcholine was investigated on the same ring. When N^ω-nitro-L-arginine methyl ester was used, it was added at the concentration of 3×10^{-4} M, 15 min before norepinephrine.

1.2. Chemicals

Acetylcholine, A23187, 18-α-glycyrrhetinic acid, 18-β-glycyrrhetinic acid, N^ω-nitro-L-arginine methyl ester, norepinephrine (from Sigma Chemical Co, France), S-nitroso-N-acetylpenicillamine (from ICN Biomedicals, France).

1.3. Expression of results and statistical analysis

Results are expressed as mean ± SEM of *n* experiments. Relaxing effects are expressed in percentage of the contraction obtained prior to addition of relaxing agents. Concentration that produced 50% relaxation (EC_{50} values) were determined by log-logit regression. Statistical comparisons were performed by one-way or multi analysis of variance. *p* values less than .05 were considered to be statistically significant.

2. RESULTS

In rat aortic rings with endothelium constricted with norepinephrine (3×10^{-7} M), acetylcholine and the calcium ionophore A23187 produced endothelium-dependent relaxation which were abolished in the presence of N^{ω}-nitro-L-arginine methyl ester (3×10^{-4} M, not shown). The relaxing effect of acetylcholine was reduced by 18-β-glycyrrhetinic acid (3×10^{-5} M) but not by the 18-α isomer (Figure 12.1). The percentages of relaxation induced by 10^{-6} M of acetylcholine (a concentration that produced a maximal relaxing effect) were 55.2 ± 4.9 ($n = 13$), 17.3 ± 3.2 ($n = 9$) and 53.0 ± 10.2 ($n = 4$) in the absence and in the presence of 3×10^{-5} M of 18-β- and 18-α-glycyrrhetinic acid, respectively. The effect of 18-β-glycyrrhetinic acid was statistically significant. By contrast, the relaxation produced by the calcium ionophore A23187 (10^{-6} M, a concentration that produced a maximal relaxation) in rings with endothelium was not affected by the two isomers of glycyrrhetinic acid (Figure 12.2). In preparations without endothelium constricted with norepinephrine, the relaxing effect produced by S-nitroso-N-acetylpenicillamine was not modified by the isomers of glycyrrhetinic acid (Figure 12.3). The EC_{50} values of S-nitroso-N-acetylpenicillamine were 163 ± 63 nM ($n = 12$), 166 ± 60 nM ($n = 8$) and 117 ± 50 nM ($n = 5$) in the absence and in the presence of 3×10^{-5} M of 18-β- and 18-α-glycyrrhetinic acid, respectively.

3. DISCUSSION

The main result of the present study is that 18-β-glycyrrhetinic acid inhibited the nitric-oxide-dependent relaxing effect of acetylcholine in the rat aorta. This effect of glycyrrhetinic acid is stereoselective, since the 18-α-isomer did not inhibit the relaxation elicited by acetylcholine.

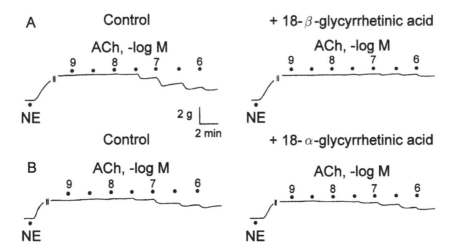

Figure 12.1 Representative traces (out of four to nine experiments) showing the relaxing effect of acetylcholine (Ach) in rat aortic rings with endothelium constricted with norepinephrine (NE, 3×10^{-7} M), before (control, in the presence of 0.3% dimethylsulfoxide) and after addition of 3×10^{-5} M of 18-β-glycyrrhetinic acid (A) or 18-α-glycyrrhetinic acid (B).

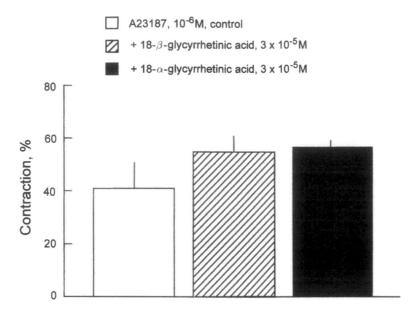

Figure 12.2 Effect of 18-β-glycyrrhetinic acid and 18-α-glycyrrhetinic acid (3×10^{-5} M) on relaxations to the calcium ionophore A23187 (10^{-6} M) in rat aortic rings with endothelium constricted with norepinephrine (3×10^{-7} M).

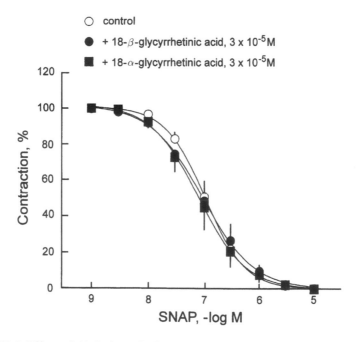

Figure 12.3 Effect of 18-β-glycyrrhetinic acid and 18-α-glycyrrhetinic acid (3×10^{-5} M) on relaxations to S-nitroso-N-acetylpenicillamine (SNAP) in rat aortic rings without endothelium constricted with norepinephrine (10^{-7} M).

The production of nitric oxide by the endothelium was stimulated using acetylcholine or the calcium ionophore A23187. Both drugs induce endothelium-dependent vasorelaxation which is abrogated by N^{ω}-nitro-L-arginine methyl ester, an inhibitor of nitric oxide synthase. This is consistent with the idea that in the rat aorta, nitric oxide is the major if not the only relaxing factor released by the endothelial cells (Rees *et al.*, 1990; Nagao *et al.*, 1992; Shimokawa *et al.*, 1996).

The 18-α-isomer of glycyrrhetinic acid affected neither the relaxation produced by S-nitroso-N-acetylpenicillamine, a donor of nitric oxide, nor the relaxing effect of the endothelium-dependent vasodilators, acetylcholine or A23187. By contrast, 18-β-glycyrrhetinic acid inhibited the relaxant effect of acetylcholine. It is unlikely that the inhibitory effect of 18-β-glycyrrhetinic acid on acetylcholine-induced relaxation was due to an impairement of the effect of nitric oxide at the level of smooth muscle. Indeed, 18-β-glycyrrhetinic acid did not modify the relaxant effect elicited by S-nitroso-N-acetylpenicillamine in preparations without endothelium. Therefore 18-β-glycyrrhetinic acid affected the relaxing effect of acetylcholine at a step upstream to the activation of soluble guanylyl-cyclase by nitric oxide in vascular smooth muscle cells.

In the rat aorta, the vasodilatation induced by nitric oxide may rely on gap junctional communications (Javid *et al.*, 1996). This interpretation was suggested by experiments showing that the vasodilator effect of acetylcholine is reduced by octanol and heptanol, two inhibitors of gap junctions. In the present study, the 18-α-isomer of glycyrrhetinic acid, which is a more selective inhibitor of gap junctions (Taylor *et al.*, 1998), did not affect the relaxation evoked by acetylcholine. Therefore, it seems unlikely that blockade of gap junction accounted for the inhibitory effect of 18-β-glycyrrhetinic acid on acetylcholine-induced relaxation. This is further supported by the lack of effect of 18-β-glycyrrhetinic acid on the relaxation elicited by the calcium ionophore A23187. This latter observation also excludes the possibility that 18-β-glycyrrhetinic acid inhibited the calcium/calmodulin-dependent activation of endothelial nitric oxide synthase. An antagonist effect of 18-β-glycyrrhetinic acid on endothelial muscarinic receptors appears unlikely, since in some arterial preparations, the response to acetylcholine is not affected by 18-β-glycyrrhetinic acid (Murai *et al.*, 1999). Taken together, the data of the present study suggest that 18-β-glycyrrhetinic acid may interfere with endothelium and nitric oxide-dependent relaxation by affecting a step of the transduction pathways which led to the activation of endothelial nitric oxide synthase upon receptor stimulation. These data also demonstrate that the inhibitory effects of 18-β-glycyrrhetinic acid are not limited to relaxations mediated by EDHF.

ACKNOWLEDGEMENTS

The authors thank Dr Catherine Corriu (UMR CNRS 7034) for critical reading of the manuscript.

13 A central role for endothelial cell potassium channels in EDHF-mediated responses

Kim A. Dora, Simon D. Walker and Christopher J. Garland

Of crucial importance to understanding endothelium-dependent hyperpolarization has been the demonstration that hyperpolarization within the endothelium can be blocked using a combination of apamin and charybdotoxin. As a consequence, these toxins together completely block the hyperpolarization and relaxation of smooth muscle which represents the end point of the endothelium-dependent hyperpolarizing factor (EDHF) pathway. This chapter discusses the concept that the potassium ions whose efflux causes the hyperpolarization of endothelial cells act as an EDHF, together with the passive spread of that hyperpolarization through myoendothelial gap junctions. The relative importance of each branch of the pathway varies in different arteries, but together they can explain the EDHF phenomenon.

The identity of endothelium-dependent hyperpolarizing factor (EDHF) still remains the subject of considerable controversy. In addition to a diffusible factor, electrical coupling between the endothelium and the smooth muscle cells could contribute to the EDHF response to a variable extent in different arteries. However, in spite of an increasingly complex picture, there are aspects of the pathway which are both clear and apparently universal. Probably the most significant of these is the fact that activation can be blocked in the combined presence of the potassium channel toxins apamin and charybdotoxin (Waldron and Garland, 1994; Corriu *et al.*, 1996). Other related facts are that an essential early step in the activation of all endothelium-dependent dilator pathways is an increase in the endothelial cell calcium concentration, and that this increase in calcium is associated with a hyperpolarization of the endothelial cell membrane (Busse *et al.*, 1989; Chen and Suzuki, 1990; Plane *et al.*, 1998).

Taken together, these points may in fact provide a comprehensive mechanistic explanation for endothelium-dependent hyperpolarizations, with no need to evoke the concept of an additional directly acting EDHF. Thus, stimulation of endothelial cells, for example following muscarinic receptor activation, will lead to an elevation in cytoplasmic calcium concentration which in turn will activate calcium-sensitive potassium channels and cause hyperpolarization. The hyperpolarization will result from efflux of potassium ions out of the cells, and these potassium ions may then act as an EDHF on the adjacent smooth muscle cells. In addition, if functional myo-endothelial gap junctions are present, the endothelial cell hyperpolarization may passively hyperpolarize the adjacent smooth muscle. In both cases, hyperpolarization of the smooth muscle will lead to relaxation if tone is present.

1. DOES THE SENSITIVITY TO APAMIN AND CHARYBDOTOXIN RESIDE WITHIN THE ENDOTHELIUM?

A range of potassium channel blocking agents has been used to attempt to block the EDHF pathway. However, in the rat mesenteric artery, the only totally effective approach was the use of a combination of inhibitors for calcium-activated potassium channels, apamin and charybdotoxin (Waldron and Garland, 1994) (Figure 13.1). Individually, each of these toxins only partially depressed the EDHF-mediated hyperpolarization and relaxation. This suggested that two separate and parallel pathways each mediated by a different type of potassium channel may underlie these effects. Subsequently, a number of groups using a variety of different arterial preparations have demonstrated the effectiveness of this toxin combination against EDHF responses, to the extent that block with apamin and charybdotoxin but not apamin and iberiotoxin is now an accepted defining characteristic of the EDHF response (e.g., Corriu *et al.*, 1996; Plane and Garland, 1996; Zygmunt and Hogestatt, 1996). Both toxins block calcium-activated potassium channels, but whereas apamin selectively blocks the small conductance calcium activated potassium

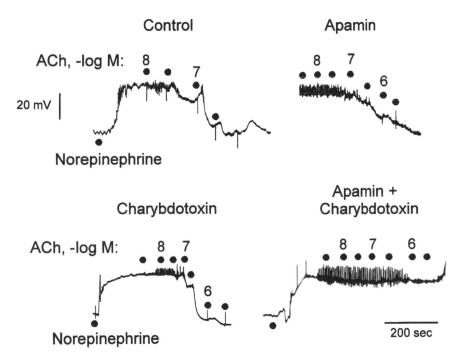

Figure 13.1 Hyperpolarization of smooth muscle to acetylcholine is sensitive to the combined application of apamin and charybdotoxin. Sharp microelectrode recording in a rat small mesenteric artery mounted in a wire myograph. Norepinephrine (5×10^{-7}–10^{-6} M) evoked depolarization which was reversed by increasing concentrations of acetylcholine (Control). Apamin (5×10^{-7} M) and charybdotoxin (3×10^{-8} M) each shifted the concentration–response curve, but only their combined presence abolished the EDHF-mediated response evoked by acetylcholine. Data from Waldron and Garland (1994).

channel (SK$_{Ca}$), charybdotoxin blocks both the large (BK$_{Ca}$) and intermediate conductance (IK$_{Ca}$) subtypes, and in addition, the voltage-sensitive delayed rectifier channel (K$_V$) (Ishii *et al.*, 1997; Lazdunski *et al.*, 1985; Zygmunt *et al.*, 1997). In contrast, iberiotoxin is selective against BK$_{Ca}$ channels, so its inability to substitute for charybdotoxin infers a role for IK$_{Ca}$ together with apamin-sensitive SK$_{Ca}$ in the EDHF pathway.

The fact that apamin reduced the EDHF response was at first sight surprising, as patch clamp studies had shown that while vascular smooth muscle cells exhibit clear BK$_{Ca}$ currents in a variety of arteries, it had not been generally possible to reveal any evidence for SK$_{Ca}$ currents. The blood vessels studied in this regard included the small mesenteric artery, which has been widely employed in studies on the EDHF pathway (Mistry and Garland, 1998). This suggested the possibility that the SK$_{Ca}$ channels, and thus apamin sensitivity, may in fact reside with the endothelium rather than the smooth muscle layers. In the isolated rat aorta, outward currents sensitive to block with apamin had been reported with a mean conductance consistent with current flow through SK$_{Ca}$ channels. Interestingly, two distinct conductances were recorded in the aorta, the larger of the two (6.7 pS) was resistant to the blocking action of apamin but sensitive to charybdotoxin (Marchenko and Sage, 1994, 1996).

The possibility that a similar profile existed in the endothelium of small resistance arteries, where the action of EDHF is known to be more predominant, was studied directly in hepatic and mesenteric arteries. In hepatic arteries, acetylcholine which only acts on the endothelium, evoked a hyperpolarization in the endothelial cells which was abolished with apamin and charybdotoxin and thus consistent with a location on the endothelium (Edwards *et al.*, 1998) (Figure 13.2). Endothelial cell hyperpolarization was also stimulated with an activator of IK$_{Ca}$ channels, 1-ethyl-2-benzimidazolinone (1-EBIO). This action was blocked with charybdotoxin but not

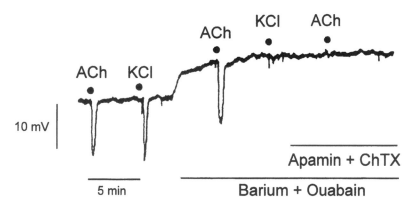

Figure 13.2 Endothelial cell hyperpolarization to acetylcholine is sensitive to the combined presence of apamin and charybdotoxin. Intracellular microelectrode recording in a pinned-out rat small hepatic artery. The endothelial cell hyperpolarized to bolus application of acetylcholine (ACh, 10^{-5} M) and raised extracellular potassium ion (K$^+$, 10 mM). The hyperpolarization to acetylcholine was not due to an efflux of K$^+$ through inwardly rectifying K$^+$ channels nor the Na$^+$/K$^+$ ATPase, but rather through apamin and charybdotoxin-sensitive K-channels. This shows directly that these K-channels are present in the endothelium. Modified from Edwards *et al.* (1998).

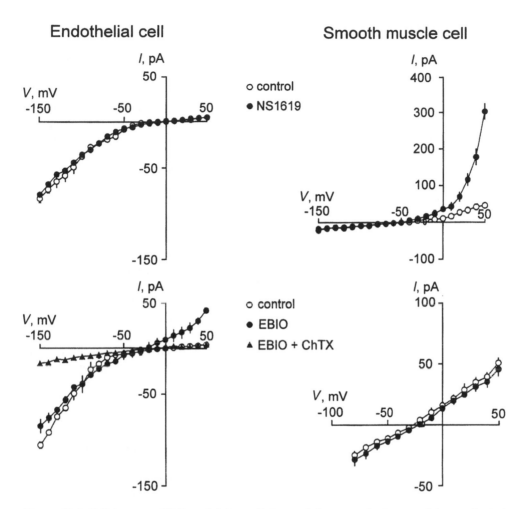

Figure 13.3 Cell-type specificity of intermediate- and large-conductance calcium-activated K-channels. Endothelial and smooth muscle cells were freshly isolated from rat small mesenteric artery and current (I)–voltage (V) relationships generated for K-currents using the whole-cell configuration of the patch-clamp technique. The activator of IK_{Ca}, 1-ethyl-2-benzimidazolinone (1-EBIO, 6×10^{-4} M), induced an outward K-current in the endothelial cells, which was reversed by charybdotoxin (ChTX, 2.5×10^{-7} M). 1-EBIO had no effect in smooth muscle cells. In contrast, the activator of BK_{Ca}, NS 1619 (3.3×10^{-5} M), induced an iberiotoxin-sensitive K-current in smooth muscle but not in endothelial cells. Each point represents the mean $\pm$ SEM ($n = 4$).

iberiotoxin (Edwards *et al.*, 2000). Patch clamp recordings from either smooth muscle or endothelial cells freshly isolated from rat small mesenteric arteries revealed outward current evoked in the former with the BK_{Ca} activator, NS 1619 and in the latter with 1-EBIO to activate IK_{Ca} (Walker *et al.*, 2000; Figure 13.3). Together, these data indicate that both IK_{Ca} and SK_{Ca} channels are present in the endothelium of resistance arteries and that they can be activated by endothelium-dependent agonists and blocked with apamin and charybdotoxin.

2. DOES POTASSIUM RELEASED FROM THE ENDOTHELIUM SERVE AS AN EDHF?

The possibility that potassium passing out of endothelial cells through SK_{Ca} and IK_{Ca} channels can act as an EDHF was suggested on the basis of similarities between acetylcholine and exogenous potassium, their respective pharmacological profiles and the direct measurement of apamin and charybdotoxin sensitive potassium release from the endothelium (Edwards *et al.*, 1998). Central to this suggestion, was the finding that increases in extracellular potassium concentration up to around 15 mM (from 4.8 mM) evoked smooth muscle hyperpolarization and relaxation in rat mesenteric and hepatic arteries. Both of these effects were depressed significantly in the presence of barium to block inwardly rectifying potassium channels (K_{ir}) and ouabain to block Na^+/K^+ ATPase. The equivalent EDHF responses evoked with acetylcholine were inhibited to a similar extent. The inhibitory action of barium and ouabain was more marked in the hepatic artery, suggesting that an additional mechanism operates in the mesenteric artery explaining the residual EDHF-mediated relaxation. Increases in potassium concentration also stimulated hyperpolarization in the endothelial cells. However, unlike the hyperpolarization of the endothelial cells to acetylcholine, this effect of potassium ion was not blocked with apamin and charybdotoxin. This was consistent with a role for potassium release *through* these channels and then acting as an EDHF on the smooth muscle cells.

The membrane potential and tension measurements reported by Edwards *et al.* (1998) were carried out in separate experiments. The former measurements were made at or close to the resting membrane potential, while the latter were recorded in the presence of contraction to enable relaxation to be measured. In the presence of prior depolarization and contraction evoked with the α_1-adrenergic agonist phenylephrine, increasing the potassium concentration evoked a robust, sustained and correlated hyperpolarization and associated relaxation in the mesenteric artery (Figure 13.4). Both of these effects were sensitive to the extent of the stimulation, being markedly depressed if the membrane depolarized beyond -38 mV and cells contracted in excess of 10 mN (Figure 13.4). The EDHF-mediated response to acetylcholine was not depressed in a similar way. However, whereas an additional mechanism may explain this discrepancy, it may in part reflect the extracellular potassium ion concentration. Although hyperpolarization and relaxation to 10.8 mM K^+ was blocked, increasing the concentration to 13.8 mM was able to stimulate hyperpolarization and relaxation (data not shown). A failure to take any account of the level of stimulation presumably underlies the recent inability to record impressive and reproducible relaxation to potassium in the mesenteric artery. In this study, only transient relaxation could be recorded to the addition of 5.5 mM potassium in 30–40% of the vessels studied (Lacy *et al.*, 2000). This crucial influence of prior stimulation also may help to explain the failure in this recent study to record any relaxation in endothelium-denuded vessels. Indeed, removal of the endothelium in our hands shifts the concentration–response curve to potassium to the right but does not depress the overall ability of the ion to evoke relaxation (Figure 13.4).

The fact that the level of membrane potential and tension in the smooth muscle can influence the response to potassium of course raises the question: does potassium contribute significantly to the EDHF pathway *in vivo*? This question remains to be answered directly, but the evidence available suggests that it may well contribute.

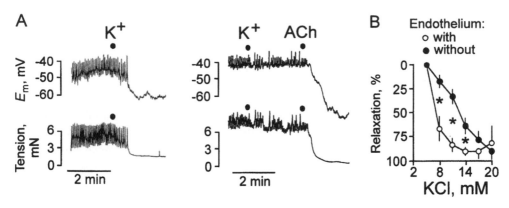

Figure 13.4 Relaxation and hyperpolarization to potassium ion is dependent on the level of stimulation and the presence of the endothelium. Rat small mesenteric arteries were mounted in a wire myograph. (A) Simultaneous recordings of tension and hyperpolarization to potassium ion (K^+, 10.8 mM) and acetylcholine (ACh, 10^{-6} M) demonstrate a lack of response to this concentration of potassium ion during high levels of stimulation, whereas the response to acetylcholine remains unchanged. At low levels of stimulation (below approximately -40 mV and 8 mN), potassium ion always evoked hyperpolarization and relaxation (data not shown). (B) The ability of potassium ion to evoke relaxation was partially dependent on hyperpolarization of the endothelial cells, in addition to a direct action on smooth muscle cells. Data are means $\pm$ SEM ($n = 10-14$ experiments) and were analyzed non-parametrically with the Mann-Whitney Test. The asterisks indicate statistically significant differences between treatments ($p < .05$).

In the isolated perfused mesenteric vascular bed, increasing potassium concentrations evoked an endothelium-independent vasodilatation, which was abolished in the presence of barium and ouabain. These blockers also significantly depressed the endothelium-dependent vasodilatation to acetylcholine obtained in the presence of inhibitors of NO synthase and cycloxygenase (Makino *et al.*, 2000). Although a high concentration of methoxamine was used as a stimulant in these experiments (the perfusion pressure was around 100 mmHg), potassium was still able to evoke dilatation. In isolated, pressurised mesenteric arteries, even when the pressure is as high as 120 mmHg, the resting membrane potential of the smooth muscle is still around -50 mV and under isobaric conditions wall tension actually decreases (Schubert *et al.*, 1996; Wesselman *et al.*, 1997). Furthermore, the action of potassium is not restricted to the mesenteric vasculature, as in pressurized cerebral and coronary arteries raising external potassium from 6 to 16 mM evoked a pronounced endothelium-independent vasodilatation (Knot *et al.*, 1996). In the light of all these observations it is surprising that in a recent study on isolated pressurized mesenteric arteries dilatation to potassium only occurred in 30% of the blood vessels, although acetylcholine had an effect in all cases (Doughty *et al.*, 2000). Whatever the explanation for the variability in response to exogenous potassium, the EDHF vasodilatation evoked with acetylcholine was sensitive to block with either barium and ouabain or gap junction inhibitors. This supports the suggestion that potassium ion and the spread of hyperpolarization from the endothelium together explain the EDHF response in the small mesenteric artery (Edwards *et al.*, 1998). So a considerable amount of evidence favours some role for potassium as an EDHF.

3. DO MYOENDOTHELIAL GAP JUNCTIONS CONTRIBUTE TO THE EDHF RESPONSE?

Gap junctions between endothelial and smooth muscle cells are potential sites where current may spread passively between the different cell types. Although there have been numerous reports in recent years showing close appositions between endothelial and smooth muscle cells, convincing anatomical evidence for true myoendothelial connections in blood vessels is extremely limited. The requirement is to show penta-laminar membrane associations between these cells with electron microscopy. Such connections have been observed within the mesenteric bed of the rat (Sandow and Hill, 2000). The incidence of these connections appears to relate inversely to the size of mesenteric vessel. So in mesenteric arteries, structures exist which could potentially allow hyperpolarization to spread from the endothelium to the smooth muscle and contribute to the EDHF-mediated response, perhaps explaining the component of the hyperpolarization which is resistant to block with barium and ouabain. The fact that the incidence of myoendothelial gap junctions appears to increase as the artery size decreases could then help to explain the increasing importance of the EDHF-mediated response in the smaller vessels.

The real difficulty in defining a possible role for current spread in the EDHF response has been the lack of selective agents to block gap junctions. The recent availability of novel gap peptides, designed to interact with the extracellular loop of the connexin proteins which form gap junctions and the use of glycyrrhetinic acid derivatives, have provided inhibitory agents with more specificity than those previously available, such as heptanol and halothane. However, these agents are also not devoid of other actions and there is no evidence to suggest that they act selectively against the myoendothelial gap junctions, as opposed to the homocellular connections within both the endothelium and smooth muscle layers. Nonetheless, Gap27 inhibits the EDHF induced smooth muscle hyperpolarization in the rabbit mesenteric artery (Dora *et al.*, 1999), and the water soluble glycyrrhetinic-acid derivative carbenoxolone inhibits EDHF evoked smooth muscle hyperpolarization in the mesenteric but not hepatic artery (Edwards *et al.*, 1999; Yamamoto *et al.*, 1999). These data together suggest that a significant component of the EDHF response in the mesenteric artery results from a spread of hyperpolarization from the endothelium to the smooth muscle cells.

4. DO OTHER FACTORS FUNCTION AS AN EDHF?

A large number of arterial preparations have been used to study the EDHF pathway. This chapter has concentrated on the rat mesenteric and hepatic arteries because these have been among the most extensively utilized vessels in this regard. However, two other preparations that have received considerable attention are the guinea-pig carotid and the porcine coronary arteries. In the both of these arteries, exogenous potassium does not appear to evoke any hyperpolarization in the smooth muscle, arguing strongly against any role as EDHF in these blood vessels (Quignard *et al.*, 1999). However, hyperpolarization of the smooth muscle in the carotid artery could be evoked after hyperpolarizing the endothelial cells with either EBIO or acetylcholine. The hyperpolarization of the smooth muscle, but not the endothelial cells, evoked by these agents was blocked with either carbenoxolone or Gap27. This indicates that in this artery the EDHF response can be explained simply by the spread of endothelial cell hyperpolarization (Edwards *et al.*, 1999). In the porcine coronary artery, 11,12-epoxyeicosatrienoic acid (11,12-EET) has been suggested to act as an EDHF (Fisslthaler *et al.*, 1999). However, both 11,12-EET and substance P hyperpolarized endothelial cells in this artery, an effect which was abolished by apamin and charybdotoxin. Although 11,12-EET caused direct hyperpolarization of the smooth muscle, this action was blocked with iberiotoxin. As the EDHF evoked hyperpolarization to substance P in this artery was unaffected by iberiotoxin, 11,12-EET cannot be acting directly as an EDHF in this blood vessel (Edwards *et al.*, 2000). However, it remains possible that it may serve as an intracellular modulator within the EDHF pathway. Although Gap27 reduced the endothelium-dependent smooth muscle hyperpolarization to substance P recorded with sharp microelectrodes passed through the adventitia, it did not reduce hyperpolarization in the sub-intimal smooth muscle cells. This suggests that Gap27 is ineffective against the myoendothelial spread of hyperpolarization in this artery, but that it does reduce an amplifying spread of hyperpolarization through the smooth muscle cell layers.

5. CONCLUSION

The two most important advances in the understanding of the EDHF phenomenon have been that the pathway can be completely inhibited by the combined application of apamin and charybdotoxin, and that this effect is due to a block of hyperpolarization *within* the endothelium. The potassium ions which leave the endothelial cell and cause that hyperpolarization can then act to evoke hyperpolarization of the smooth muscle in their own right. In addition, the hyperpolarization can spread passively through myoendothelial gap junctions. The relative importance of each of these routes will then vary in specific blood vessels depending on the responsiveness of the smooth muscle cells to potassium and the extent of heterocellular coupling. But hyperpolarization of the endothelial cells is the key step in the initiation of both branches of the EDHF pathway, and as this hyperpolarization and the EDHF pathway are blocked by apamin and charybdotoxin, there is no need to suggest that any other factors act as an EDHF.

14 Could the EDHF be K^+ in porcine coronary arteries?

Jean-Louis Bény, Monica Sollini and Nicolas Lindegger

The goal of the present study was to examine whether K^+ could be the endothelium-derived hyperpolarizing factor (EDHF) induced by substance P and bradykinin in porcine coronary arteries. A candidate EDHF molecule must be released by the endothelial cells upon stimulation by the kinins. Both peptides evoked a large outward K^+ current in cultured endothelial cells of porcine coronary arteries. A K^+ selective electrode recorded an increase in K^+ concentration in the extracellular medium in the media of the coronary artery upon stimulation with kinins. The scavenging of the candidate EDHF molecule must abolish the EDHF effect. In coronary strips, the scavenging of K^+ with cryptate 2.2.2 abolished the endothelium-dependent relaxations produced by substance P and bradykinin which are resistant to nitro-L-arginine and indomethacin. Application of the exogenous candidate EDHF molecule must mimic the effect of EDHF on smooth muscle cells. The perifusion of a medium supplemented with K^+ depolarized and contracted strips of coronary artery. However, the short application of exogenous K^+ ions hyperpolarized the smooth muscle cells. A mechanism of action that explains the effect of EDHF must be identified. Ouabain, an inhibitor of the Na^+-K^+ ATPase, abolished the endothelium-dependent relaxations resistant to nitro-L-arginine and indomethacin without inhibiting the relaxation to endothelium-derived nitric oxide. These results are compatible with the concept that, in the porcine coronary artery, K^+ ions released by the endothelial cells are EDHF and that these ions hyperpolarize and hence relax the smooth muscle exclusively by activating the Na^+-K^+ ATPase.

In porcine coronary arteries, the two kinins substance P and bradykinin relax the smooth muscles in an endothelium-dependent manner by releasing nitric oxide from the endothelium and by triggering the phenomenon known as EDHF (Bény and Brunet 1988; Pacicca *et al.*, 1992). During the endothelium-dependent relaxations caused by kinins, the membrane potential of endothelial cells and of underlying smooth muscle cells simultaneously hyperpolarizes in the same manner (Brunet and Bény, 1989). Two different hypotheses concerning the nature of EDHF could explain the synchrony of these two electrical events. EDHF could be either the resultant of an electrotonic conduction of the endothelial cells hyperpolarization to the neighbouring smooth muscle cells or K^+ ions released by the endothelial cells during their hyperpolarization (Chaytor *et al.*, 1998; Edwards *et al.*, 1998; Yamamoto *et al.*, 1999). The first hypothesis was tested using halothane as an uncoupler. Halothane uncoupled the electrotonic spread of a hyperpolarization of the smooth muscle cells to the endothelial cells, but did not inhibit the EDHF-mediated response (Bény and Pacicca, 1994). This observation made the "electrotonic hypothesis" rather unlikely. Therefore, experiments were designed to test whether EDHF can be K^+ ions in porcine coronary arteries.

To be EDHF, K^+ firstly should be released in sufficient amount by the endothelial cells upon stimulation by substance P and bradykinin. Secondly, endogenous released

K^+ should hyperpolarize the smooth muscle cells by an identifiable mechanism. Finally, exogenous K^+ should be able to mimic the effects of EDHF on the smooth muscle cells. In the present chapter, the evidences in favour and against these different events will be reviewed.

1. METHODS

1.1. Preparation of the tissues

Anterior descending branches of coronary arteries from domestic pig (*Sus scrofa*) were obtained at the slaughterhouse. The coronary lumen was rinsed by injection of cold, oxygenated (95% O_2, 5% CO_2) Krebs solution (mM: NaCl 118.7, KCl 4.7, $CaCl_2$ 2.5, KH_2PO_4 1.2, $NaHCO_3$ 24.8, $MgSO_4$ 1.2, glucose 10.1, pH 7.3–7.4). Adherent tissue was removed from sections of the coronary artery. Rings of about 2 mm width obtained from these sections were cut longitudinally to give strips of about 5 mm in length parallel to the circular smooth muscles. For some experiments, the endothelium was removed by gently rubbing the internal surface of the strip with a cotton tip. To check that the endothelium had been removed by this procedure, the response of the strip to substance P was tested (Pacicca *et al.*, 1992).

1.2. Pharmacological experiments

When mechanical tension was measured to obtain concentration–response curves, ligatures were attached to both ends of the strips, and these were suspended with a resting isometric tension of about 5 mN in a 85 µl tissue chamber (Pacicca *et al.*, 1992). To establish the concentration–response curves for substance P and bradykinin, U-46619 (3×10^{-7} M) was added to the perfusion fluid throughout the experiment to obtain a reproducible state of initial tension in the strip. The tension stabilized to about 5 mN. The strips were superfused with Krebs solution containing each concentration of the peptide in an ascending, non-cumulative manner for a sufficient time to allow full relaxation. A 10–20 min washout period was allowed between successive application. Peptides were administered to the preparations by diluting them directly in the plastic beaker that contained the perfusion solution. To reveal the EDHF-mediated response, nitro-L-arginine (L-NA, 10^{-4} M, an inhibitor of nitric oxide synthase) and indomethacin (10^{-5} M, an inhibitor of prostacyclin synthesis) were administered to the strips in the perfusion fluid for at least 25 min before the first application of the kinins.

When testing the effect of the K^+ chelator cryptate 2.2.2, only one concentration, causing 50% relaxation, of each peptide was used (Pacicca *et al.*, 1992). Preliminary experiments demonstrated tachyphylaxis in the presence of the chelator. Since tachyphylaxis would hide the peptide-induced relaxation shown in a typical concentration–response curve, it was necessary to test only one concentration of each kinin.

1.3. Primary culture of endothelial cells

Left anterior descending branches of pig coronary arteries were obtained at the slaughterhouse. The endothelial cells were collected by gentle rubbing of the internal face of the vessel with a scalpel. The cells were suspended in culture medium (M199) and plated on collagen coated glass coverslips in culture Petri dishes. Cells were used after two to five days of primary culture (Baron *et al.*, 1996).

1.4. Whole cell patch clamp recording

To measure the currents activated by the kinins, the whole cell patch clamp technique was used. (Hamill *et al.*, 1981). Recordings were performed on single cells, or small islets never exceeding four cells, to avoid space clamp problems. To determine the current–potential relationship, repetitive 300 ms voltage pulses were applied throughout the recording, usually reaching 30, 50 and 80 mV above the holding potential (varying between −60 and −20 mV). To normalize the results, the current conductance was expressed in density (pS/pF). Thus, membrane capacitance was measured before each experiment by applying a 10 mV voltage step. Experiments were performed at room temperature (20–22 °C) (Baron *et al.*, 1996).

1.5. Extracellular K^+ electrode

Two channels borosilicate glass capillaries were used (Clark Electromedical Instruments, Edenbridge, UK; theta style; OD: 2 mm). One channel was dedicated to be the reference channel in order to measure the potentials and the other one was the potassium sensor. Double-barreled capillaries were used to be sure to measure the potential in the same place where K^+ concentration was measured. After pulling the electrode, one of the two channels must be broken at the opposite side of the tip. This channel becomes the active channel where the K^+ ligand will be placed. To avoid its silanization, the intact channel was closed by melting the glass. The open channel was silanized with *N,N*-dimethyltrimethylsilylamine. Silane is vaporized at 250 °C in vacuum for 15 seconds into the future active channel. The silane binds hydroxyl groups of glass and provides its hydrophobicity. The electrodes were then beveled. The tip of the future active channel was filled over night in vacuum with valinomycin, a potassium-ion exchanger. After filling the tip with ligand, the melted side of the reference channel was opened and filled with 3 M NaCl. Krebs solution was injected into the active channel. A silver–silver chloride wire was inserted in each channel. The opposite end of the tip was then sealed with wax. Changes in the difference of potential between the active and the reference channels were measured using a high impedance differential amplifier. The calibration was performed before and after the measurement in the coronary strip. Immediately after calibration, the electrodes were used to record in the coronary strips. After crossing the endothelium and the internal elastic lamina the electrode was left in the same position for 20–25 min to allow extracellular K^+ to stabilize before the application of peptides (Coles and Tsacopoulos, 1977; Coles and Tsacopoulos, 1979; Munoz *et al.*, 1983).

1.6. Electrophysiological experiments

Strips were incubated in a 100 µl Perspex chamber, continuously perfused with oxygenated Krebs solution at 36 °C by means of a peristaltic pump (1.250 µl min^{-1}). An extremity of the strip was pinned on a silicon rubber surface with the intimal side facing up. The other extremity was fixed horizontally to a force transducer. Throughout the experiment U-46619 (3×10^{-7} M) was added to the perfusion fluid to obtain a reproducible state of initial tension in the strip. The membrane potential was measured using a conventional glass microelectrode (60–80 MΩ) filled with 3 M KCl. KCl (0.5–3 M in Krebs solution) was injected in 2–10 µl aliquots during 0.5 second directly into the perifusion fluid with a micro pipette. The tip of the pipette was applied to the surface of the incubation medium at different positions between the inlet and the outlet (aspiration tubing) of the chamber. These different positions changed the transit time of the "cloud" of KCl from about two to five seconds. The purpose of such applications of exogenous KCl was to mimic a transient release of this ion from the endothelial cells in localized areas, such as the myoendothelial bridges (Pacicca *et al.*, 1992).

1.7. Preparation of peptides and chemicals

The peptides bradykinin and substance P were each prepared at a concentration of 1 mg ml^{-1} in 0.25% acetic acid, acetylcholine at a concentration of 1 mg ml^{-1} in 0.9% NaCl. These solutions were stored as aliquots of 100 or 50 µl at $-20\,°$C until use. U-46619 was prepared at a concentration of 1 mg ml^{-1} in 75% ethanol. The inhibitors were prepared at a concentration of 10 mg ml^{-1} in 0.02% HCl for L-NA and at a concentration of 2 mg ml^{-1} in more than 99.8% ethanol for indomethacin. U-46619, the peptides and the inhibitors were diluted subsequently to the desired concentrations in Krebs solution. The other molecules were prepared directly in Krebs solution.

1.8. Drugs

The following agents were used: acetylcholine (Sigma, St. Louis, MO, USA), apamin (Alomone Labs, Jerusalem, Israel), 1,2-bis(2-aminophenoxy)ethane-*N*,*N*,*N'*,*N'*-tetra-acetic acid (BAPTA Sigma, St. Louis, MO, USA), bradykinin (Bachem Feinchemikalien, AG, Budendorf, Switzerland), charibdotoxin (Alomone Labs, Jerusalem, Israel), cryptate 2.2.2 (Kryptofix 2.2.2, Fluka, Buchs, Switzerland), *N*,*N*-dimethyltrimethyl-silylamine (silane, Fluka, Buchs, Switzerland), ethylene glycol-bis(β-aminoethyl ether) *N*,*N*,*N'*,*N'*-tetraacetic acid (EGTA, Sigma, St. Louis, MO, USA), iberiotoxin (Alomone Labs, Jerusalem, Israel), indomethacin (Sigma, St. Louis, MO, USA), nitroglycerin 0.2 mg ml^{-1} ethanol (G. Pohl-Boskamp Gmbh and Co., Hohenlockstedt, Germany), nitro-L-arginine (Aldrich, Steinheim, Germany), 17-octadecynoid acid (17-ODYA; Sigma, St. Louis, MO, USA), ouabain (Sigma, St. Louis, MO, USA), prostagladin F$_{2\alpha}$ (Sigma, St. Louis, MO, USA), substance P (Bachem Feinchemikalien, AG, Budendorf, Switzerland), U46619 (Cayman Chemical, Ann Arbor, USA), valinomycine (Fluka, Buchs, Switzerland).

1.9. Statistical analysis

Data were calculated as the mean ± standard error of the mean (SEM). Student's test for unpaired observations was used to compare results. A *p* value less than .05 was taken as significant; *n* refers to the number of observation.

2. RESULTS

2.1. Substance P and bradykinin activate a K$^+$ current

The stimulation of the cultured endothelial cells with substance P (10^{-7} M) and bradykinin (10^{-7} M) induced an outward current that developed rapidly and then gradually decreased. The slope conductance of the activated currents measured on different cells was expressed as a function of the cell capacitance to normalize the results. The membrane capacitance was 25.8 ± 1.6 pF ($n = 30$) for one cell, 43.9 ± 2.3 pF ($n = 19$) and 84.0 ± 3.4 pF ($n = 22$) for two and three coupled cells (Frieden *et al.*, 1999).

The maximal slope conductance induced by the effect of kinins were 258.7 ± 17.7 pS/pF ($n = 40$) for substance P, and 268.5 ± 18.7 pS/pF ($n = 46$) for bradykinin. These two values were not significantly different. With 5.6 mM extracellular K$^+$, the current reversal potentials were close to the K$^+$ equilibrium potential of -80 mV: for substance P -72.9 ± 0.8 mV ($n = 40$), and -73.7 ± 1.0 mV ($n = 46$) for bradykinin. With 40 mM K$^+$, the current reversal potentials were -25.8 ± 0.7 mV ($n = 5$) for substance P, and -27.2 ± 1 mV ($n = 5$) for bradykinin, for a calculated K$^+$ equilibrium potential of -30 mV (Frieden *et al.*, 1999).

Without intra- and extracellular Ca^{2+} (2×10^{-3} M EGTA in the bath and 5×10^{-3} M BAPTA in the patch pipette), no currents were elicited by the two kinins.

2.2. Apamin and iberiotoxin

To identify the different K$_{Ca}$ channels activated by the kinins, different K$_{Ca}$ channel inhibitors were tested. Apamin (10^{-6} M), a blocker of small conductance SK$_{Ca}$ channels (Latorre *et al.*, 1989), significantly reduced the slope conductance of the substance P-evoked current by 65% (92.8 ± 37.5 pS/pF, $n = 5$). Iberiotoxin (5×10^{-8} M), a blocker of large conductance BK$_{Ca}$ channels (Galvez *et al.*, 1990), did not significantly alter the substance P response (249.4 ± 34.4 pS/pF, $n = 11$). The addition of apamin plus iberiotoxin caused the same inhibition as apamin alone on the substance P-evoked current (100.1 ± 42.3 pS/pF, $n = 5$) (Frieden *et al.*, 1999).

On the contrary, the bradykinin induced response was not significantly affected by apamin. The current slope conductance averaged 280.0 ± 63.6 pS/pF ($n = 5$). Iberiotoxin significantly reduced (by about 40%) the K$^+$ current activated by bradykinin (164.1 ± 24.2 pS/pF, $n = 6$). Together, apamin plus iberiotoxin did not produce a higher inhibition than iberiotoxin alone: 154.2 ± 35.7 pS/pF ($n = 7$). The two toxins did not shift the current reversal potential of the currents activated by substance P or bradykinin (Frieden *et al.*, 1999).

2.3. Cytochrome P450 epoxygenase

The involvement of cytochrome P450 derived compounds was tested. Concentration–response curves were obtained on coronary strips with intact endothelium contracted with prostaglandin F$_{2\alpha}$, (10^{-5} M) in the presence of indomethacin (10^{-5} M) and L-NA (10^{-4} M), to reveal EDHF mediated relaxations. At 3×10^{-6} M, 17-ODYA, a suicide substrate of cytochrome P450 enzyme, did not change the concentration–response curve to substance P: The EC_{50} to the peptides was 0.27 ± 0.04 nM ($n = 11$) under control conditions and 0.32 ± 0.04 nM ($n = 8$) in the presence of the inhibitor. On the contrary, 17-ODYA caused a significant rightward shift of the concentration–response curve to bradykinin, with an EC_{50} of 15.1 ± 6.1 nM ($n = 7$) compared to 3.1 ± 0.6 nM ($n = 9$) under control conditions. It decreased the maximal relaxation to bradykinin by about 20%.

2.4. Epoxyeicosatrienoic acids and gating of endothelial cell K_{Ca} channels

Epoxyeicosatrienoic acids enhance the open state probability of a 285 pS KCa channel which is activated by bradykinin in endothelial cells of the pig coronary artery (Baron *et al.*, 1997). Therefore, the effect of 17-ODYA (3×10^{-6} M) was tested on the bradykinin-induced K^+ current. In the presence of the inhibitor, the maximal current slope conductance due to bradykinin was significantly inhibited by 35% (178.9 ± 36.8 pS/pF, $n = 11$). On the contrary, the response to substance P was not affected by 17-ODYA (248.7 ± 63.7 pS/pF, $n = 7$) (Frieden *et al.*, 1999).

2.5. K^+ concentration in the arterial wall

When the potassium selective electrode penetrated the tissue, an increase of K^+ concentration was recorded. The damage of the cells that were crossed by the electrode caused this transient increase. After about 20 minutes the extracellular K^+ concentration stabilized. When bradykinin or substance P were applied to the coronary strips the K^+ concentration increased to 141 ± 80 µM ($n = 4$) for substance P and 200 ± 106 µM ($n = 4$) for bradykinin. The time course of K^+ concentration increase was comparable to that of the hyperpolarization of the smooth muscle cells (Figure 14.1).

2.6. Exogenous K^+ ions relaxations

Strips without endothelium were tonically contracted with U-46619 (3×10^{-7} M). A solution of K^+ added to the Krebs solution that already contains 5.9 mM K^+ did not relax these strips but instead, increased the isometric force. On the contrary, when the strips were contracted by U-46619 (3×10^{-7} M) in the absence of K^+ in the incubation medium, the addition of 1.2×10^{-3} M K^+ relaxed the strip by $3 \pm 1\%$ ($n = 4$) and that to 5.9×10^{-3} M K^+ by $30 \pm 7\%$ ($n = 4$). These relaxations were abolished by ouabain (10^{-3} M; $n = 4$) (Bény and Schaad, 2000).

2.7. Exogenous K^+ ions and cell membrane potential

In these experiments, the coronary strips had an intact endothelium and were contracted with U-46619 (3×10^{-7} M). The membrane potential of the smooth muscle cells was -44 ± 2 mV ($n = 8$). This value was not significantly different from that recorded in the absence of U-46619. In this case, when 10 µl of K^+ (3 M) were injected into the incubation chamber close to the superfusion inlet, it depolarized the smooth muscle cells by 23 ± 1 mV ($n = 4$). On the other hand, when 5 µl of KCl (0.5 M) were

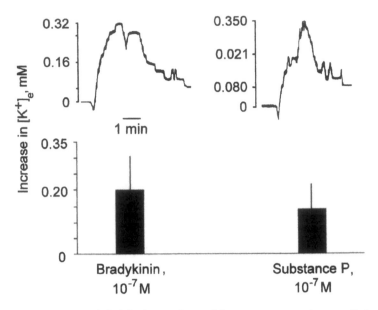

Figure 14.1 Upper panel: Original recordings of the measurement of extracellular $[K^+]$ in the media of a porcine coronary artery obtained with a double-barreled selective K^+ sensitive electrode. Effect of bradykinin (10^{-7} M; left) and substance P (10^{-7} M; right). Lower panel: aggregated results. Data shown as mean $\pm$ SEM.

injected close to the outlet, this caused a small, transient depolarization of 3 ± 1 mV ($n = 4$) followed by a hyperpolarization of 15 ± 1 mV ($n = 4$)(Bény and Schaad, 2000).

2.8. Source of endogenous K^+ ions

Apamin (10^{-7} M) plus charibdotoxin (10^{-4} M) reduced the relaxation to substance P (10^{-8} M) to $22 \pm 8\%$ and that of bradykinin (3×10^{-7} M) to $3 \pm 1.5\%$ compared to the relaxations observed in the absence of the toxins. Thus, when toxins inhibited the K^+ release, the EDHF mediated effect of substance P and bradykinin was reduced by about 72% and 96%, respectively (Bény and Schaad, 2000).

2.9. Role of endogenous K^+ ions

To chelate K^+ ions, a diazapolyoxa macrobicyclic complex, cryptate 2.2.2 (Kryptofix 2.2.2) was used. The effect of Kryptofix was tested on the EDHF mediated effect of substance P (10^{-8} M) and of bradykinin (3×10^{-7} M). In Krebs solution containing indomethacin and nitro-L-arginine, strips contracted with U-46619 (3×10^{-4} M) relaxed by $76 \pm 10\%$ to substance P and by $70 \pm 11\%$ to bradykinin. A concentration of 2×10^{-3} M Kryptofix 2.2.2 abolished these relaxations. The cryptate did not affect the membrane potential of the endothelial and smooth muscle cells, or the hyperpolarizing effect of the kinins on the latter. The effect Kryptofix 2.2.2 was reversible (data not shown). Since Kryptofix 2.2.2 is not totally specific, the same experiments were done in a solution without monovalent cations. The strips were contracted by U-46619. Substance P and bradykinin relaxed these strips by $53 \pm 13\%$ and $29 \pm 14\%$ respectively, in the presence of NO-synthase and cycloxygenase inhibitors. These relaxations were reduced by Kryptofix 2.2.2 (2×10^{-3} M) to $1 \pm 1\%$ for bradykinin and to $7 \pm 2\%$ for substance P. When the synthesis of nitric oxide and prostacylin was not inhibited, in the presence of cryptate, substance P and bradykinin relaxed the strip by 30% (Bény and Schaad, 2000).

2.10. Na$^+$-K$^+$ ATPase

Ouabain (5×10^{-7} M) abolished the endothelium-dependent relaxations produced by substance P and bradykinin resistant to indomethacin and nitro-L-arginine ($n = 4$). On the contrary, ouabain (5×10^{-7} M) did not abolish the relaxation caused by substance P (10^{-8} M; $13 \pm 7\%$; $n = 4$) and bradykinin (3×10^{-7} M; $7 \pm 4\%$; $n = 4$) in the absence of indomethacin and nitro-L-arginine (Bény and Schaad, 2000).

3. DISCUSSION

The molecule that is supposed to be the EDHF in porcine coronary arteries should be released by the endothelial cells upon stimulation by kinins. Many observations converge to confirm that indeed this is the case for K$^+$. This ion is responsible of the current that hyperpolarizes the endothelial cells. The main channels responsible for its release have been identified at the single channel level. When bradykinin stimulates endothelial cells, iberiotoxin-sensitive large conductance potassium channels are activated by cytosolic calcium. These channels are activated by physiological range of calcium because the epoxyeicosatrienoic acids stimulated by the kinin increase their sensitivity to this ion. These results are confirmed by manipulations of the synthesis of epoxyeicosatrienoic acids. Inhibition or activation of cytochrome P450 epoxygenase is reflected on the EDHF mediated response to bradykinin but not that to substance P (Fisslthaler *et al.*, 1999). Indeed, the latter does not stimulate the production of epoxyeicosatrienoic acids (Frieden *et al.*, 1999). In addition, the use of a selective K$^+$ electrode confirms the increase in extracellular concentration of K$^+$ upon stimulation with the kinins. Therefore K$^+$, without any doubt, fulfills the first criterium to be released from the endothelial cells in response to bradykinin and substance P.

The scavenging of endogenously released K$^+$ should abolish the EDHF relaxation. This experiment presents a major technical difficulty since K$^+$ is already present in the extracellular medium. Thus, to work at low K$^+$ concentration constitutes in itself a dramatic change in the experimental conditions. In addition, an ionic chelator is never perfectly specific. This implicates that this approach in any way will modify the incubation medium. Another problem results from the utilization as scavenger of a molecule like Kryptofix 2.2.2 which is not characterized pharmacologically. Nevertheless the results presented here steer onto the confirmation of the idea that endogenous K$^+$ is the EDHF. However, these results cannot be considered, because of the mentioned problems, as a final demonstration.

Exogenous K$^+$ should mimic the effect of EDHF on the smooth muscle cells. This is a necessary condition that must be fulfilled by the candidate EDHF molecule. This is the point that constitutes the major difficulty of the present study. Indeed, the application of exogenous K$^+$ to smooth muscle cells depolarizes and contracts them. This is at the opposite of expectations for a putative EDHF. However, circumstantial observations show that depending on how K^+ is applied to a coronary strip, the ion can repetitively hyperpolarize the smooth muscle cell. Therefore K^+ can be a hyperpolarizing factor. Two interpretations are envisaged. At first, in an intact tissue the concentration of extracellular K^+ is lower than in the incubation medium as a result of a continuous active pumping. In that case, as demonstrated in the present study, an increase in K^+, always hyperpolarizes and relaxes the smooth muscle cells. Unfortunately, a regional low extracellular K^+ concentration would be difficult to

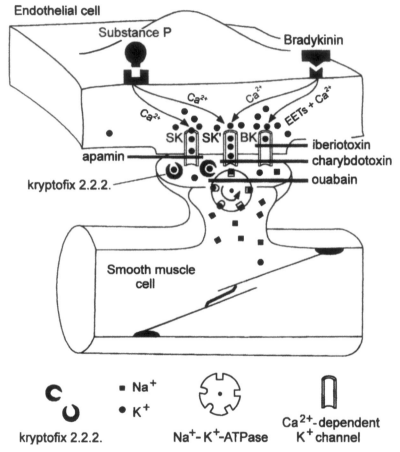

Figure 14.2 Sites of action of pharmacological tools used. In the endothelial cells of porcine coronary arteries, bradykinin and substance P induce the increase of cytosolic free calcium concentration via the inositol phosphate pathway. By that way bradykinin gates apamin-insensitive (charybdotoxin-sensitive) small conductance calcium-dependent potassium channels. Iberiotoxin-sensitive large conductance potassium channel are also gated because bradykinin activates the production of epoxyeicosatrienoic acids (EETs) and these molecules render the channels sensitive to calcium. Substance P gates apamin-sensitive and -insensitive (charibdotoxin sensitive) small conductance calcium-dependent potassium channels. For both peptides, the consequence is the release of potassium. This ion can be scavenged by Kryptofix 2.2.2. Extracellular potassium hyperpolarizes the smooth muscle cells by activating the electrogenic Na^+-K^+ ATPase which can be inhibited by ouabain.

measure with a K^+ sensitive electrode that is best suited to measure concentration-changes rather than absolute value. In addition, during tissue penetration with the electrode, the extracellular K^+ concentration increases because many cells are injured. Second, in an intact tissue, likely at the myoendothelial junctions, specialized areas may exist where the K^+ channels are concentrated close to regions of the smooth muscle cells rich in Na^+-K^+ ATPase (the K^+ receptors). This would constitute, in some way, a potassium "synapse". As a matter of fact, rubbing a coronary strip to remove the endothelium would damage such a structure. However, these two working hypotheses are purely speculative and no evidence exist now in favor or against them. Nevertheless, the present results demonstrated that K^+ can be the EDHF in the coronary artery although it should be remembered that this is the weakest point of the present demonstration.

The molecule that is supposed to be the EDHF should have a mechanism of action compatible with the knowledge on EDHF mediated responses. Thus, the inhibition of a component of this mechanism should abolish the EDHF phenomenon. The observation that a low concentration of ouabain abolishes the EDHF mediated response induced by the kinins fulfills this criterium.

With the two weak points mentioned above, K^+ ions appear to be the best candidate as EDHF in the porcine coronary artery (Figure 14.2). This conclusion seems in contradiction with that of Fisslthaler et al. (1999) who identified as epoxyeicosatrienoic acids EDHF in the porcine coronary artery. Epoxyeicosatrienoic acids, produced by cytochrome P450 epoxygenase, are synthesized upon stimulation of endothelial cells (Harder et al., 1995). In addition, the epoxyeicosatrienoic acids activate K_{Ca} channels on smooth muscle cells (Hu and Kim, 1993; Li and Campbell, 1997). Thus, epoxyeicosatrienoic acids relax and hyperpolarize smooth muscles, which suggests that they are EDHF (Hecker et al., 1994; Fisslthaler et al., 1999). Transfection of coronary arteries with cytochrome oxidase antisense oligonucleotides attenuate EDHF-mediated response (Fisslthaler et al., 1999). Unfortunately for technical reasons, these experiments were done on strips after 48 hour of incubation *in vitro*. In this situation the control strip exhibits in response to bradykinin a residual hyperpolarization which characterizes this organotypic cultured tissue. This hyperpolarization is different in time course and in intensity from the EDHF-mediated hyperpolarization of smooth muscle cells observed in fresh tissues. One interpretation is that this particular and residual hyperpolarization develops during the incubation of the strips *in vitro*. It is caused by epoxyeicosatrienoic acids and is different from the hyperpolarization attributed to EDHF. Our present results and conclusions are in agreement with the proposal that EDHF depends on the activity of cytochrome P450 (Fisslthaler et al., 1999). However, these manipulations have a strong influence on K_{Ca} channels gating and not on the EDHF synthesis (Baron et al. 1997).

4. CONCLUSION

K^+ fulfills, satisfactorily, most of the criteria required for being EDHF in porcine coronary arteries.

15 Nitro-L-arginine/indomethacin-resistant relaxations to acetylcholine in small gastric arteries of the rat: Effect of ouabain plus Ba^{2+} and relation to potassium ions

Johan Van de Voorde and Bert Vanheel

In several blood vessels, endothelium-dependent relaxations are in part mediated by an endothelium-derived hyperpolarizing factor (EDHF), the nature of which is unknown. Experiments were performed to investigate the hypothesis that in small gastric arteries of the rat EDHF might be identified as potassium ions, released by activation of endothelial K_{Ca}-channels and inducing relaxation by stimulation of Na^+/K^+-pump and the inward rectifier K^+ conductance. EDHF-induced relaxations (assessed as the nitro-L-arginine/indomethacin resistant component of acetylcholine-induced relaxations of preparations contracted with norepinephrine), but not sodium nitroprusside-induced relaxations are inhibited in the presence of ouabain plus Ba^{2+}. Ouabain is responsible for the greater part of the inhibition. This inhibition is reversible. Application of increasing concentrations of K^+ elicits in some preparations transient relaxations, but in a greater part of the preparations, there are no or only small relaxations. The K_{Ca}-channel opener NS 1619 elicits relaxation effects that are not diminished after removal of the endothelium and are not inhibited by ouabain plus Ba^{2+}. Similar results are obtained with 1-EBIO, a K_{Ca}-channel opener acting more selectively on endothelial cells. Thus, EDHF-mediated relaxation is sensitive to inhibition by ouabain plus Ba^{2+}, but the relation of this inhibitory influence to an action of K^+ as EDHF is unlikely.

Endothelial cells modulate tone of the underlying vascular smooth muscle cells by releasing endothelium-derived relaxing factors (EDRFs) under basal conditions and in response to agents such as acetylcholine. Among those relaxing factors, in contrast to nitric oxide (NO) and in some blood vessels also prostacyclin, the identity of endothelium-derived hyperpolarizing factor (EDHF) is not univocally established (Vanhoutte and Félétou, 1999).

Controversial evidence suggests that EDHF might be anandamide (Randall *et al.*, 1996; Chataigneau *et al.*, 1998) or an epoxyeicosatrienoic acid formed through a cytochrome P450-dependent mechanism (Hecker *et al.*, 1994; Campbell *et al.*, 1996; Corriu *et al.*, 1996; Van de Voorde and Vanheel, 1997; Vanheel and Van de Voorde, 1997; Drummond *et al.*, 2000). In certain blood vessels EDHF may be K^+-ions (Edwards *et al.*, 1998). Indeed, observations on rat hepatic and mesenteric arteries suggested that the increase in cytosolic calcium, seen after stimulation of endothelial cells with acetylcholine, activates endothelial K_{Ca}-channels leading to the efflux of K^+ into the myoendothelial space. This increase in K^+ would then hyperpolarize and relax the adjacent smooth muscle cells by activating the Na$^+$/K$^+$ pump and the inwardly rectifying K$^+$ channels (Edwards *et al.*, 1998).

The present study aimed to find out whether or not in small gastric arteries of the rat EDHF can be identified as the potassium ion. Therefore it was investigated: (a) whether or not EDHF-mediated relaxation is blocked after inhibition of the Na$^+$/K$^+$-pump and the inward rectifying K$^+$-channel with ouabain and Ba^{2+} respectively; (b) what is the influence of exogenous K$^+$; and (c) whether or not relaxations elicited by the K$_{Ca}$-channels openers NS 1619 and 1-EBIO (the latter acting more selectively on endothelial K$_{Ca}$-channels (Adeagbo, 1999; Edwards *et al.*, 1999b)), would be inhibited by removal of the endothelium or incubation with ouabain plus Ba^{2+}.

1. METHODS

1.1. Experimental procedure

Experiments (approved by the ethical committee on animal research of Ghent University) were performed on small gastric arteries (normalized diameter ranging from 180 to 504 µm) from young female Wistar rats (200–260 g). The animals were sacrificed by cervical dislocation. The arteries were dissected free and mounted in an automated dual small vessel myograph (model 500 A; J.P. Trading, Aarhus, Denmark). After isolation, the preparations were transferred to an organ chamber filled with 10 ml of Krebs–Ringer bicarbonate solution. Two stainless steel wires (40 µm diameter) were guided through the lumen of segments, having a length of 1.5–2 mm. One wire was fixed to a force-displacement transducer, and the other was connected to a micrometer. The preparations were allowed to equilibrate for 30 min in the Krebs–Ringer bicarbonate solution bubbled with 95% O$_2$ and 5% CO$_2$ at 37 °C. The arteries were then normalized to obtain optimal conditions for active force development (Mulvany and Halpern, 1977). In brief, the passive wall tension-internal circumference characteristics were determined. On the basis of this relation, the circumference was set to a normalized internal circumference (from which normalized diameter can be calculated) corresponding to 90% of the internal circumference that the vessels would have under a passive transmural pressure of 100 mmHg. After normalization, the preparations were allowed to equilibrate for at least 30 min. Thereafter the preparations were challenged three times with a mixture of K$^+$ 120 mM and norepinephrine 10^{-5} M. When reproducible contractions were obtained, cumulative concentration–relaxation curves to agonists were made during contractions to norepinephrine 10^{-5} M (eliciting 98% of the maximal contraction). All experiments were performed in the presence of the NO-synthase inhibitor nitro-L-arginine (L-NA, 10^{-4} M) and the cyclooxygenase inhibitor indomethacin (5 × 10^{-5} M) to exclude the potential involvement of NO and prostanoids in the observations.

1.2. Drugs

The experiments were performed using a Krebs–Ringer bicarbonate solution of the following composition (in mM): NaCl 135, KCl 5, NaHCO$_3$ 20, glucose 10, CaCl$_2$ 2.5, MgSO$_4$·7H$_2$0 1.3, KH$_2$PO$_4$ 1.2, and EDTA 0.026. High-K$^+$ (120 mM) solution was prepared by equimolar replacement of NaCl with KCl. Acetylcholine chloride, indomethacin, nitro-L-arginine, norepinephrine bitartrate and ouabain were obtained from Sigma (St. Louis, MO, USA). Barium chloride and sodium nitroprusside were obained from Merck (Darmstadt, Germany), NS 1619 from RBI (Natick, MA, USA) and 1-ethyl-2-benzimidazolinone (1-EBIO) from Tocris (Bristol, UK).

All concentrations are expressed as final molar concentrations in the organ chamber. Concentration–response curves were obtained by cumulative additions of small volumes (maximal 1%) into the experimental chamber. All solutions were prepared freshly by dilution from appropriate stock solutions. Stock solutions were made in water except for 1-EBIO and NS 1619 (dissolved in dimethylsulfoxide), acetylcholine (dissolved in phthalate buffer pH 4.0) and indomethacin (dissolved in ethanol).

1.3. Statistics

The data are shown as means $\pm$ SEM; n indicates the number of preparations tested. Statistical significance was evaluated using Student's t-test for paired observations. Differences were considered to be statistically significant when p was less than .05.

2. RESULTS

2.1. Ba^{2+} and ouabain

The simultaneous addition of Ba^{2+} (3×10^{-5} M) and ouabain (5×10^{-4} M) elicited no effect on basal tone in most preparations (16/26). In the remaining arteries a transient contraction was observed (2.39 ± 0.39 mN; $n = 10$). The contraction elicited with norepinephrine (10^{-5} M) was not significantly affected (12.98 ± 0.85 mN in the absence versus 12.49 ± 0.84 mN in the presence of Ba^{2+} plus ouabain; $n = 26$). In the combined presence of Ba^{2+} (3×10^{-5} M) and ouabain (5×10^{-4} M), added 15 min before the contraction of the preparations, EDHF-mediated relaxations were significantly impaired. Under the same experimental conditions, the combined presence of Ba^{2+} and ouabain had no influence on relaxations induced by sodium nitroprusside (Figure 15.1). In the presence of Ba^{2+} (3×10^{-5} M) alone, the L-NA/indomethacin-resistant relaxations to acetylcholine was not significantly shifted to the right, while the response was significantly impaired in the presence of ouabain (5×10^{-4} M) alone (Figure 15.1). Addition of Ba^{2+} as such had no influence on basal tone and on the contraction elicited by norepinephrine (15.45 ± 2.1 and 15.46 ± 1.9 mN in the absence and presence of Ba^{2+}, respectively; $n = 4$).

In another series of experiments the influence of different concentrations (5×10^{-4}, 5×10^{-5} and 5×10^{-6} M) of ouabain was investigated. In these experiments ouabain was added after contraction of the preparations with norepinephrine (10^{-5} M), 10 min before the addition of acetylcholine. In the experiments with 5×10^{-4} M ouabain, an additional concentration–response curve with acetylcholine was obtained 30 min after washout of the glycoside. At all concentrations used, ouabain caused a transient contraction followed by a more slowly developing relaxation. The responses to acetylcholine were still inhibited in the presence of 5×10^{-5} M, but not in the presence of 5×10^{-6} M of ouabain. The inhibitory effect of ouabain 5×10^{-4} M was reversible (Figure 15.2).

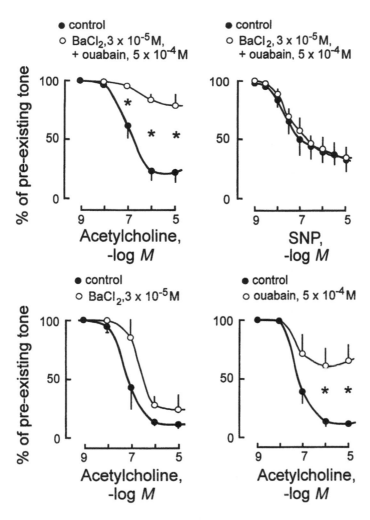

Figure 15.1 Relaxations (in percentage of the contraction to norepinephrine (10^{-5} M)) of increasing molar concentrations of acetylcholine and sodium nitroprusside (SNP) under control conditions and in the combined presence of Ba^{2+}(3×10^{-5} M) and ouabain (5×10^{-4} M) or in the presence of Ba^{2+} (3×10^{-5} M) or ouabain (5×10^{-4} M) alone. All experiments were performed in the presence of indomethacin and nitro-L-arginine. Data shown as means ± SEM ($n = 4$–9). The asterisks indicate statistically significant differences ($p < .05$) (reproduced with permission from Van de Voorde and Vanheel, 2000).

2.2. Potassium

The influence of increasing extracellular concentrations of K$^+$ was tested by cumulative additions of KCl, 1–15 mM, in preparations showing substantial L-NA/indomethacin-resistant relaxations in response to acetylcholine. In some arteries (14/29) transient relaxations (more than 10% of tone) were observed with the lower concentrations of K$^+$ (Figure 15.3). In the remaining segments no or minimal relaxations (less than 10% of

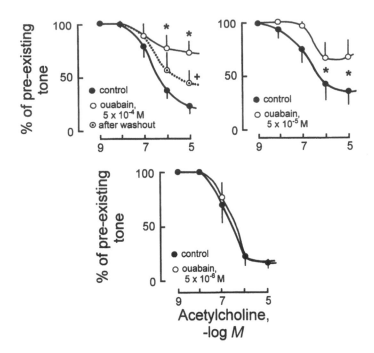

Figure 15.2 Relaxations (in percentage of the contraction to norepinephrine (10^{-5} M)) of increasing molar concentrations of acetylcholine under control conditions and in the presence of increasing concentrations (5×10^{-6}, 5×10^{-5} and 5×10^{-4} M) of ouabain. The pointed line represents the effect of acetylcholine after washing out 5×10^{-4} M ouabain for 30 min. All experiments were performed in the presence of indomethacin and nitro-L-arginine. Data shown as means ± SEM ($n = 4$–5). The asterisks and crosses indicate statistically significant difference ($p < .05$) with control and with ouabain 5×10^{-4} M, respectively (reproduced with permission from Van de Voorde and Vanheel, 2000).

tone) or even contractions were observed in response to K$^+$ (Figure 15.3) despite strong relaxing responses to additions of acetylcholine (Figure 15.4).

2.3. NS 1619 and 1-EBIO

After removal of the endothelium, resulting in a complete loss of the response to acetylcholine, the relaxations to NS 1619 ($n = 4$) and 1-EBIO ($n = 6$) were not significantly diminished (Figure 15.5). The responses to NS 1619 and 1-EBIO were not significantly altered by the administration of ouabain (5×10^{-4} M) plus Ba^{2+} (3×10^{-5} M) (Figure 15.5).

3. DISCUSSION

The experiments described were performed to determine whether or not K$^+$ is EDHF (Edwards *et al.*, 1998) in small gastric arteries of the rat. In this preparation, L-NA/indomethacin-resistant relaxations to acetylcholine are mediated by EDHF

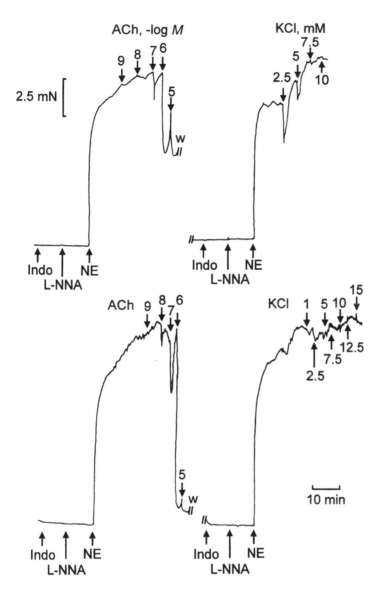

Figure 15.3 Original recordings of two experiments showing the effects of increasing concentrations of acetylcholine (−log molar) and of increasing millimolar concentrations of K$^+$ on isolated small gastric arteries of the rat. The preparations were contracted with norepinephrine (10^{-5} M) in the presence of indomethacin and nitro-L-arginine (reproduced with permission from Van de Voorde and Vanheel, 2000).

since the response completely disappears after removal of the endothelium and in the presence of high concentrations of K$^+$ (unpublished observations).

The observations with ouabain and Ba^{2+} confirm results obtained in hepatic and mesenteric arteries (Edwards *et al.*, 1998). The inhibitory influence of these substances relies mainly on blockade of the Na$^+$/K$^+$-pump since the inhibitory influence of

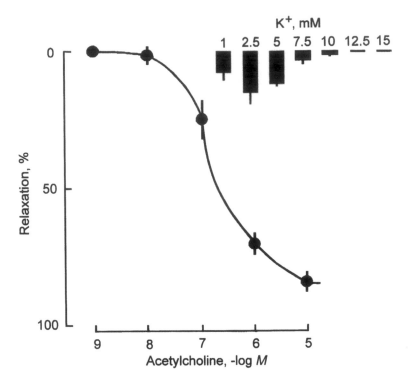

Figure 15.4 Relaxations (in percentage of the contraction to norepinephrine (10^{-5} M)) caused by increasing molar concentrations of acetylcholine and millimolar concentrations of K^+ in the same preparations. All experiments were performed in the presence of indomethacin and nitro-L-arginine. Data shown as means $\pm$ SEM ($n = 14–29$) (reproduced with permission from Van de Voorde and Vanheel, 2000).

ouabain is more pronounced than that of Ba^{2+}. The inhibitory influence of ouabain is reversible and specific since the non-EDHF-mediated relaxations elicited by sodium nitroprusside are not influenced by Ba^{2+} plus ouabain.

In the gastric artery, the high concentration of ouabain (10^{-3} M) originally used in hepatic artery (Edwards *et al.*, 1998) is not required for inhibition of EDHF-mediated relaxations. Indeed, lower concentrations are also active. At 5×10^{-6} M, no inhibition of the relaxation to acetylcholine is observed, although a transient contraction is still elicited in contracted preparations, illustrating that this concentration of ouabain is active. Various isoforms of Na/K-ATPase exist, with different sensitivities to ouabain. For the $\alpha_1\beta_1$ Na/K-ATPase isoenzyme in the rat, the inhibition constant (K_i) is in the order of $4 \times 10^{-5}–10^{-4}$ M, while the other isoenzymes are more sensitive to ouabain (K_i in the order of $3 \times 10^{-8}–2 \times 10^{-7}$ M) (Blanco and Mercer, 1998). The present data thus suggest the potential involvement of the $\alpha_1\beta_1$ Na/K-ATPase isoenzyme in the inhibitory influence of ouabain on EDHF-mediated relaxation, for as far as no aspecific effects of ouabain are involved. Also in the rat hepatic artery the endothelium-dependent smooth muscle hyperpolarization to acetylcholine is sensitive to lower concentrations of ouabain ($1–5 \times 10^{-7}$ M) (Edwards *et al.*, 1999b).

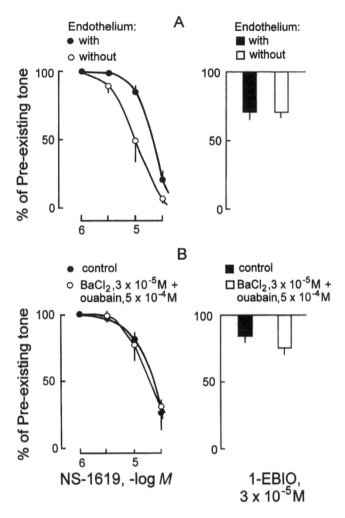

Figure 15.5 Relaxations (in percentage of the contraction to norepinephrine (10^{-5} M)) of increasing molar concentrations of NS 1619 and 1-EBIO (3×10^{-5} M) in preparations with and without endothelium (A) and in preparations in the absence and presence of Ba^{2+} (3×10^{-5} M) plus ouabain (5×10^{-4} M) (B). All experiments performed in the presence of indomethacin and nitro-L-arginine. Data shown as means $\pm$ SEM ($n = 4-5$) (reproduced with permission from Van de Voorde and Vanheel, 2000).

While the observations with Ba^{2+} and ouabain are in agreement with the suggestion of K^+ being EDHF, the results obtained with the addition of exogenous K^+ are not. Some of the preparations relaxed in a transient way in response to additions of small concentrations of the ion. However, most preparations showed no or only small relaxations, despite the fact that these blood vessels exhibited a strong EDHF-mediated response. If endogenous K^+-ions were EDHF, one would expect that addition of exogenous K^+ induces relaxation in all EDHF-sensitive preparations. Similar inconsistent and transient relaxations to additions of low concentrations of K^+ are observed in small mesenteric (Lacy *et al.*, 2000) and hepatic (Andersson *et al.*, 2000) arteries of the rat. The transient relaxations seen in part of the preparations in response to K^+ might be the consequence of the release of relaxing substances by perivascular nerves, as is the case in guinea-pig basilar artery (Zygmunt *et al.*, 2000).

In a further attempt to find out whether or not EDHF can be identified as K^+, experiments were performed using the K_{Ca}-channel opener NS 1619 (Olesen *et al.*, 1994; Holland *et al.*, 1996). If K^+ is released as EDHF by endothelial cells through activation of K_{Ca}-channels, direct activation of these channels should elicit a relaxation which is at least in part endothelium-dependent. However, preparations without endothelium (as evidenced by the lack of relaxation to acetylcholine) showed no diminished response to NS 1619 compared to preparations with endothelium.

That the response to NS 1619 is not diminished in preparations without endothelium might be due to an overwhelming influence of the K_{Ca}-channel openers on K_{Ca}-channels on the smooth muscle. Whatsoever, opening of K_{Ca}-channels in either smooth muscle or endothelial cells is expected to increase the K^+-concentration in the intercellular fluid surrounding the smooth muscle cells. According to the K^+-hypothesis (Edwards *et al.*, 1998) this increase in intercellular K^+ should activate the Na^+/K^+ pump and the inward rectifier. Therefore one could speculate that the response to NS 1619 is at least in part inhibited by ouabain plus Ba^{2+}. However, the present results clearly demonstrate the absence of an inhibitory effect of the combination on the relaxation induced by the K^+-channel opener.

It is unknown whether or not NS 1619 indeed activates endothelial K_{Ca}-channels. However, 1-EBIO acts more specifically on these channels (Adeagbo, 1999; Edwards *et al.*, 1999b). At least in rat hepatic arteries, 1-EBIO mimics the effects of EDHF, since it induces a hyperpolarization of the smooth muscle that is completely dependent on the endothelium and that is abolished by Ba^{2+} and ouabain (Edwards *et al.*, 1999b). The present experiments however do not support this view since the relaxation of rat gastric arteries to 1-EBIO is not dependent on the presence of endothelial cells and is not inhibited by Ba^{2+} plus ouabain. The present findings with the K_{Ca}-channel openers thus are not in line with the hypothesis of K^+ as the mediator of the relaxations attributed to EDHF in the rat gastric arteries. Other mechanisms than the opening of K_{Ca}-channels may contribute to the relaxant effect of NS 1619 (Edwards *et al.*, 1994) and possibly also of 1-EBIO. That EDHF in rat small gastric arteries is unlikely to be K^+ is supported also by membrane potential measurements (Vanheel and Van de Voorde, chapter 16, this volume).

The present study contributes to the evidence suggesting that K^+ is certainly not the universal EDHF. A similar conclusion has been reached in guinea-pig carotid and porcine coronary arteries (Quignard *et al.*, 1999), human subcutaneous arteries (Buus *et al.*, 2000), bovine coronary artery (Drummond *et al.*, 2000) and guinea-pig basilar artery (Zygmunt *et al.*, 2000). Even in the rat mesenteric (Vanheel and Van de Voorde, 1999; Lacy *et al.*, 2000) and rat hepatic (Andersson *et al.*, 2000) arteries, the evidence is not consistently in favor of K^+ as EDHF.

If K^+ is not EDHF, the inhibitory influence of ouabain plus Ba^{2+} on EDHF-mediated relaxation remains to be explained. Blocking the Na^+/K^+-pump with ouabain may lower the concentration gradient for K^+ across the membrane of the smooth muscle cell and diminish the driving force for K^+-efflux from these cells in response to EDHF. The latter often has been associated with opening of K^+-channels on the smooth muscle cells (Cohen and Vanhoutte, 1995; Garland *et al.*, 1995). At the level of the endothelial cells, the inhibition of the Na^+/K^+-pump and of the inward rectifier, which are also present in endothelial cells (Nilius *et al.*, 1997), may depolarize these cells and diminish the driving force on Ca^{2+}-influx, an essential step for triggering EDHF-mediated responses. Ouabain also can block gap junctional communication (Spray and Bennet, 1985; Watsky *et al.*, 1990). This action of ouabain needs to be considered in relation to EDHF-mediated effects since heterocellular gap junctional communications may be involved in EDHF-mediated relaxations and hyperpolarizations (Chaytor *et al.*, 1998; Taylor *et al.*, 1998; Edwards *et al.*, 1999a). Blockade of these gap junctions by ouabain could explain the inhibitory influence on EDHF-mediated relaxations observed in the present study.

ACKNOWLEDGMENTS

With thanks to E. Tack for the expert technical assistance.

16 Effects of barium, ouabain and K^+ on the resting membrane potential and endothelium-dependent responses in rat arteries

Bert Vanheel and Johan Van de Voorde

The possibility that extracellular K^+ ions represent EDHF was explored in main and small mesenteric and in small gastric arteries of the rat. The membrane potential of the smooth muscle cells was measured with conventional microelectrodes in the continuous presence of N^G-nitro-L-arginine and indomethacin. In the main mesenteric artery, inhibition of the inward rectifier with low concentrations of barium, which slightly depolarized the smooth muscle cells, did not affect the peak endothelium-dependent hyperpolarization induced by superfusion with acetylcholine. In small mesenteric arteries, in which barium depolarized the smooth muscle cells to a larger extent, the endothelium-dependent hyperpolarization to acetylcholine was increased. The additional application of a high concentration of ouabain further depolarized the smooth muscle cells of both arteries. In the combined presence of barium plus ouabain, the hyperpolarization elicited by acetylcholine was not abolished but decreased to 64% of the control response in the main arteries, and not significantly affected in small mesenteric arteries. Measurements with K^+ ion-selective microelectrodes did not reveal a rise in subendothelial K^+ activity in main mesenteric arteries during stimulation with acetylcholine. Increasing the K^+ concentration in the superfusate depolarized the smooth muscle cells of main and small mesenteric and of small gastric arteries. These findings argue against a role of smooth muscle inward rectifier K^+ channels and Na/K pumping in the acetylcholine-induced endothelium-dependent hyperpolarization in the studied blood vessels.

In most arteries, the chemical nature of EDHF is unclear, although several studies suggest that a non-prostanoid metabolite of arachidonic acid is involved (Adeagbo and Henzel, 1998; Cohen and Vanhoutte, 1995). Since the original proposal that EDHF is a cytochrome P450 monoxygenase generated metabolite of arachidonic acid (Rubanyi and Vanhoutte, 1987; Hecker *et al.*, 1994; Bauersachs, *et al.*, 1994), strong evidence suggests that the EDHF liberated by bradykinin in bovine and porcine coronary arteries is an epoxyeicosatrienoic acid or a mixture of such compounds (Campbell *et al.*, 1996; Popp *et al.*, 1996; Gebremedhin *et al.*, 1998; Fisslthaler *et al.*, 1999). This does not seem to be the case, however, for the EDHF liberated by acetyl-choline in blood vessels such as the carotid artery of the guinea-pig (Corriu *et al.*, 1996) and the hepatic (Zygmunt *et al.*, 1996) and main mesenteric (Vanheel and Van de Voorde, 1997) arteries of the rat.

In hepatic and small mesenteric arteries of the rat, a transient rise of the K^+ concentration in the myoendothelial space, due to the agonist-induced rise in intracellular calcium and subsequent increase in K^+ efflux from the endothelial cells, may hyperpolarize the adjacent smooth muscle through activation of the Na/K pump and the inward rectifying K$^+$ conductance (Edwards *et al.*, 1998). This proposal was substantiated by the demonstration of the inhibitory effect of ouabain and barium on both the endothelium-dependent hyperpolarizations of the smooth muscle cells induced by acetylcholine and on the hyperpolarizations induced by raising the K$^+$ concentration (Edwards *et al.*, 1998). Moreover, measurements with ion-selective microelectrodes showed transient increases in extracellular K$^+$ activity in the subendothelial space of the rat hepatic artery during stimulation of the endothelial cells with acetylcholine (Edwards *et al.*, 1998). In coronary arteries of the guinea-pig and the pig, however, exposure to ouabain plus barium did not affect endothelium-dependent hyperpolarizations (Quignard *et al.*, 1999). Moreover, raising extracellular K$^+$ concentration usually depolarized the vascular smooth muscle cells, indicating that K$^+$ does not represent EDHF in these blood vessels (Quignard *et al.*, 1999).

The present experiments were designed to investigate the influence of increases in extracellular K$^+$ concentration on the resting membrane potential of main mesenteric and small mesenteric and gastric arteries of the rat. In addition, the effect of barium and ouabain was investigated on endothelium-dependent hyperpolarizations induced by acetylcholine.

1. MATERIALS AND METHODS

1.1. Preparations

The mesentery or the stomach of 12–14 weeks old female Wistar rats, anaesthetized with an intraperitoneal injection of a lethal dose (200 mg/kg) of pentobarbitone, was excised and placed in cold normal Krebs–Ringer solution with composition (in mM): NaCl 135, KCl 5, NaHCO$_3$ 20, CaCl$_2$ 2.5, MgSO$_4$·7H$_2$O 1.3, KH$_2$PO$_4$ 1.2, EDTA 0.026, and glucose 10. This solution was continuously gassed with a 95% O$_2$–5% CO$_2$ gas mixture. A segment of the main mesenteric artery or of a small mesenteric or gastric artery was dissected free of adherent connective tissue. Rings (4–6 mm) of the main mesenteric artery were slit along their longitudinal axis and the vascular strip was pinned down, intimal side upwards, to the bottom of a small recording chamber kept at 35 °C. Segments (3–4 mm) of small mesenteric or gastric arteries were pinned out in the experimental chamber to penetrate from the adventitial side. After mounting of the small arteries they were opened by incision proximally and distally to the site of microelectrode impalement. The preparations were allowed to equilibrate for at least 60 min before starting the microelectrode impalements while being continuously superfused (3 bathvolumes/min) with control solution. This solution was supplemented with N$^\omega$-nitro-L-arginine (10^{-4} M) and indomethacin (5×10^{-5} M) to exclude interference from NO and prostanoids, respectively, and was oxygenated continuously (95% O$_2$–5% CO$_2$, pH 7.4).

1.2. Electrophysiological measurements

Transmembrane potentials were measured with conventional microelectrode techniques (Vanheel *et al.*, 1994). Microelectrodes were pulled with a vertical pipette puller (David Kopf, model 750, Tujunga, CA, USA) from filamented glass tubing (1 mm outer diameter; Hilgenberg, Germany). The microelectrodes were filled with 1 M KCl. Their electrical resistance, measured in the normal Krebs–Ringer solution, ranged from 40 to 80 MΩ. The measured potential was followed on an oscilloscope and traced with a pen recorder at low speed. Absolute values of membrane potential were taken as the difference of the stabilized potential after cell impalement and the zero potential upon withdrawal of the microelectrode from the cell. Changes in membrane potential produced by applications of acetylcholine or K$^+$ under control conditions and after experimental interventions (barium, ouabain) were usually measured in the same cell during continuous recordings. Barium was added to the superfusate for at least 10 min before challenging the preparations with acetylcholine. In the experiments in which ouabain was applied additionally, pre-exposure to this drug was limited to 10 min to allow full expression of its acute depolarizing effect (due to the loss of electrogenic pump activity) without extensive alteration of intracellular ion (especially K$^+$) concentrations. Exposures to acetylcholine or increased K$^+$ concentration were made by addition of these substances from the appropriate stock solutions to the superfusion solution. Both the influence of more prolonged exposures (4–6 min of superfusion with solution containing acetylcholine or increased K$^+$ concentrations) and of transient exposures were tested. The latter were applied by bolus addition of aliquots of appropriate stock solutions (made in the control fluid immediately before administration) to the inlet of the continuously perfused experimental chamber.

Measurements of the extracellular potassium activity were performed using liquid ion exchanger K$^+$-selective microelectrodes, constructed and calibrated as described previously (Vanheel *et al.*, 1990; Vanheel and de Hemptinne, 1992). Briefly, unfilamented glass tubings (1.5 mm outer diameter) were pulled to micropipettes. The pipettes were silanized by heating for about two hours at 180 °C, subsequent exposure (for 5 min) to vapours of tri-*n*-butylchlorosilane (Fluka, Switzerland), and further baking for at least three hours at 180 °C. Under microscopic control, the extreme tip of the silanized micropipettes was broken down to 1–2 μm to prevent involuntary cell impalement and to increase the response time of the microelectrodes. Silanized pipettes were then filled with a short column of valinomycin-based K$^+$ resin (Cocktail B, Fluka, Switzerland) and backfilled with 150 mM KCl. The ion-selective microelectrodes were connected with a driven shield to a high input impedance preamplifier (Analog Devices 311J), and the extracellular K$^+$ signal was referred to the virtual ground potential to which the experimental chamber was clamped. The slope of the K$^+$-selective microelectrodes was 59.3 ± 0.5 mV for a tenfold change in [K$^+$]. An extracellular K$^+$ activity coefficient of 0.75 was assumed.

1.3. Drugs

Indomethacin, N$^\omega$-nitro-L-arginine, acetylcholine chloride, ouabain and barium chloride were obtained from Sigma Chemical Co. All concentrations are expressed as final molar concentrations in the superfusion chamber. Ouabain was added as a solid directly to the warmed superfusate. Stock solutions of N$^\omega$-nitro-L-arginine and BaCl$_2$ were made in water, indomethacin was dissolved in anhydrous ethanol. Acetylcholine was dissolved in 50 mM potassium hydrogen phthalate buffer, pH 4.0, as a 10^{-2} M solution. Further dilutions (1:10 or 1:100) of the agonist were made in the control fluid immediately before addition to the superfusate.

1.4. Statistics

Results are expressed as means ± SEM. *n* indicates the number of preparations, each obtained from a different rat. Statistical significance was evaluated using Student's *t*-test for paired or unpaired observations, as appropriate, a *p*-value less than .05 indicating a statistically significant difference.

2. RESULTS

2.1. Control responses

During superfusion with the control solution containing N^ω-nitro-L-arginine (10^{-4} M) and indomethacin (5×10^{-5} M), the resting membrane potential of the smooth muscle cells of the main mesenteric artery was stable and averaged -52.5 ± 1.1 mV ($n = 20$). Exposure of the blood vessels to acetylcholine (3×10^{-7} M) for about 5 min induced a transient peak hyperpolarization of 9.7 ± 0.6 mV ($n = 12$). In the presence of the vasodilator, the membrane potential recovered towards its control level, recovery which was accelerated by washout of the substance (Figure 16.1). When allowing for 20–30 min washout periods between successive applications of acetylcholine, the

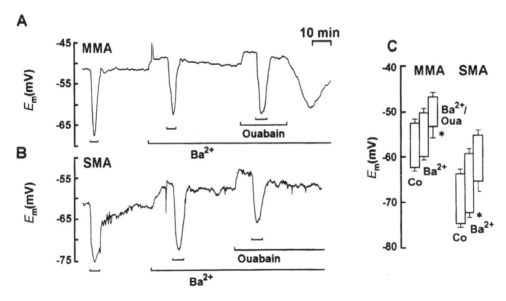

Figure 16.1 (A,B) Original recordings of the membrane potential (E_m) of smooth muscle cells of a main mesenteric artery (MMA), impaled from intimal side (A) and a small mesenteric artery (SMA), impaled from the adventitial side (B). The response to superfusion with a solution containing acetylcholine (3×10^{-7} M) (as indicated by the horizontal lines) is monitored under control conditions, in the presence of barium (Ba^{2+}, 3×10^{-5} M), and in the combined presence of barium and ouabain (5×10^{-4} M). Shortly after addition of barium in (A), the microelectrode was dislodged and re-impaled. (C) Mean change of the membrane potential of smooth muscle cells of the main (MMA) and small mesenteric artery (SMA) induced by acetylcholine under control conditions (Co), after exposure to barium and after additional application of ouabain (Ba^{2+}/ouab).

obtained responses were reproducible up to 90–100% of the original magnitude (Vanheel and Van de Voorde, 1997). In smooth muscle cells of small mesenteric arteries, the resting membrane potential was -65.0 ± 2.1 mV ($n = 9$) in the control fluid. Acetylcholine (3×10^{-7} M) reproducibly hyperpolarized the membrane by 11.2 ± 1.0 mV ($n = 8$) under control conditions (Figure 16.1).

2.2. Barium

Superfusion of main mesenteric artery strips with barium (3×10^{-5} M) containing fluid caused a steady depolarization of the resting membrane potential of the smooth muscle cells by 2.3 ± 0.2 mV ($n = 11$). In the presence of barium, the magnitude of the endothelium-dependent hyperpolarization elicited by acetylcholine was not decreased

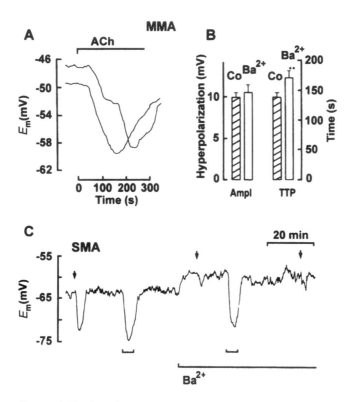

Figure 16.2 (A) Time course of the change in membrane potential (E_m) of a smooth muscle cell of the main mesenteric artery (MMA) in response to acetylcholine (ACh) in the absence (lower trace) and presence (upper trace, depolarized resting potential) of barium (3×10^{-5} M). (B) Amplitude of peak hyperpolarization (Ampl) and time taken to reach this peak (TTP) under control condition (Co, hatched columns) and after exposure to barium (Ba^{2+}, open bars). Values are means $\pm$ SEM ($n = 15$). Asterisks denote statistically significant difference ($p < .02$). (C) Original recording of the change in membrane potential (E_m) in response to transient (arrows) and more prolonged (horizontal bars) applications of acetylcholine in a smooth muscle cell of a small mesenteric artery (SMA) under control conditions and after exposure to barium (Ba^{2+}, 3×10^{-5} M).

(Figure 16.1). Conversely, in four of the eleven experiments an increase in hyperpolarization was noted while in the others a small decrease was apparent, the latter not discernable from the normal rundown of this response when the tissue was repeatedly challenged with acetylcholine. The peak hyperpolarization after exposure to barium averaged 9.6 ± 1.0 mV, which was not significantly different from the control hyperpolarization (Figure 16.1). In small mesenteric arteries, exposure to barium depolarized the smooth muscle cells by 4.5 ± 0.6 mV ($n = 4$). In the presence of barium, the acetylcholine-induced hyperpolarization was significantly increased to 13.1 ± 1.0 mV (Figure 16.1).

A consistent observation with barium was that, although the magnitude of the acetylcholine-induced peak hyperpolarization was not significantly decreased, it took longer to reach it, both in main and in small mesenteric arteries. Moreover, in eight of the experiments (pooled data from both types of vessel, $n = 15$), the hyperpolarization occurred in two distinct phases (Figure 16.2). The mean time from entrance of acetylcholine in the experimental chamber to the maximal membrane potential response was significantly increased from 139 ± 7 to 171 ± 11 sec (Figure 16.2).

In four small mesenteric arteries, the effect of barium on the transient application of acetylcholine was investigated. In these experiments, acetylcholine was added as a few drops from a diluted stock solution to the inlet of the experimental chamber. The transient stimulation of the endothelial cells with acetylcholine resulted with some delay in hyperpolarization of the membrane potential of the recorded smooth muscle cell. The peak of this membrane potential change occurred when acetylcholine was already washed out of the continuously perfused experimental chamber. After exposure to barium, responses to transient acetylcholine applications were greatly depressed. Conversely, superfusion with acetylcholine containing fluid under these conditions elicited an increased response (Figure 16.2).

2.3. Barium plus ouabain

The additional application of ouabain (5×10^{-4} M) to the vascular strips or segments further depolarized the smooth muscle cells on average by 3.5 ± 0.4 ($n = 7$, main arteries) and 4.0 ± 0.8 mV ($n = 4$, small arteries), respectively. After exposing the tissues for about 10 min to the Na/K pump inhibitor, the acetylcholine-induced hyperpolarization never was inhibited completely. In smooth muscle cells of the main artery, the acetylcholine-induced hyperpolarization averaged 6.2 ± 2.7 mV (significantly smaller than the control hyperpolarization), while the membrane potential change in smooth muscle cells of the small mesenteric arteries was not significantly different from control (10.0 ± 2.3 mV). Effective inhibition of the Na/K pump by ouabain was demonstrated by the transient hyperpolarization of the smooth muscle cells after washout of the drug (Figure 16.1).

2.4. Increases in K^+-concentration

In main mesenteric, small mesenteric and small gastric arteries, raising $[K^+]_o$ from 6.2 mM in the superfusion solution by 2, 4, 5 or 8 mM consistently depolarized the smooth muscle cells (Figure 16.3). Transient increases in extracellular K^+ concentration, effected by bolus injections to the flowing control fluid, also depolarized the smooth muscle cells of small mesenteric arteries (data not shown).

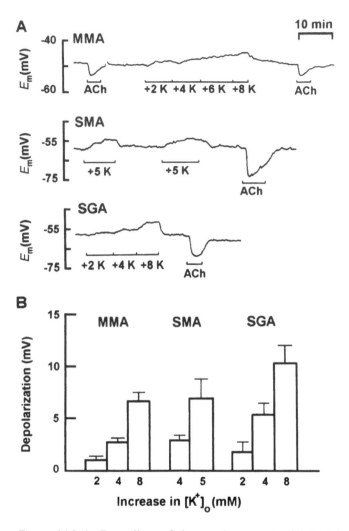

Figure 16.3 A. Recordings of the membrane potential (E_m) in a smooth muscle cell of the main mesenteric artery (MMA), small mesenteric artery (SMA) and small gastric artery (SGA) during superfusion with solution containing acetylcholine (ACh) or increasing millimolar concentrations of K^+ (K). B. Depolarization of the smooth muscle cell membrane potential by increases in extracellular K^+ concentration ($[K^+]_o$). Values are means ± SEM for four main mesenteric arteries (MMA), four small mesenteric arteries (SMA) and five small gastric arteries (SGA), respectively.

2.5. Extracellular K^+ activity

After insertion of the tip of a K^+-selective microelectrode through the endothelial layer of superfused main mesenteric arteries, the K^+ activity in the subendothelial space averaged 4.2 ± 0.1 mM, a value significantly lower than that in the superfusate (4.65 mM, Figure 16.4). Stimulation of the endothelial cells with up to 5×10^{-6} M

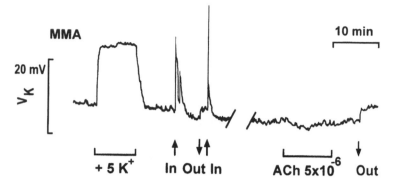

Figure 16.4 Recording of the output of a K$^+$-selective microelectrode (V_K) during a switch to a superfusate containing a higher K$^+$ concentration (+5 K$^+$) and during superfusion with acetylcholine (ACh, 5×10^{-6} M) containing solution after insertion in the subendothelial space (In) of a main mesenteric artery (MMA). During the break in the record the preparation was superfused for 23 min with control solution.

acetylcholine did not cause a rise in interstitial K$^+$ activity. The apparent mean K$^+$ activity changed to 4.0 ± 0.1 mM ($n = 4$).

3. DISCUSSION

Low concentrations of barium specifically block the inward rectifier K$^+$ current in vascular tissue (Nelson and Quale, 1995). The inward rectifier potassium channels in native rat arterial smooth muscle cells, including those of the mesenteric artery, consist of subunits of the K$_{ir}$ 2.1 isoform (Bradley *et al.*, 1999). One of the characteristics of this subfamily is that they display a high sensitivity to blockade by barium ($K_d = 3.5 \times 10^{-6}$ M at -60 mV; Bradley *et al.*, 1999). In the present experiments, 3×10^{-5} M barium was used. It was found that barium depolarized the smooth muscle cells of the main mesenteric artery by 2.3 mV, and those of the small arteries by 4.5 mV. This indicates that, in both arteries, the inward rectifier contributes to the setting of the membrane potential at rest. The fact that the barium-induced depolarization is larger in the smaller arteries might reflect the observation that inward rectifying K$^+$ channels are more abundant in smaller blood vessels (Nelson and Quayle, 1995).

In the presence of barium, the peak endothelium-dependent hyperpolarizations of the smooth muscle cells to prolonged acetylcholine exposures were not inhibited, and even increased in the small mesenteric arteries. The latter increase may be due to the enhanced driving force on intracellular K$^+$ ions after the barium-induced depolarization, or to the diminished total membrane conductance in the presence of barium, enlarging the impact of the hyperpolarizing mechanism on the cell membrane potential. Both these effects are expected to be larger with larger depolarization by barium and, therefore, in the smaller arteries. A similar increase in endothelium-dependent hyperpolarization has been observed in small mesenteric arteries of the rat after inhibition of the ATP-sensitive K^+ channels with glibenclamide (Vanheel and Van de Voorde, 1995). Similarly, in smooth muscle cells from guinea-pig coronary arteries, inhibition of the inward rectifier with 10^{-4} M barium increased the EDHF-induced hyperpolarization (Nishiyama *et al.*, 1998), while in cells of the intestinal submucosal and of mesenteric arterioles of the same species 5×10^{-4} M barium was used to depolarize the membrane potential away from the K^+ equilibrium potential in order to observe significant endothelium-dependent hyperpolarizations to acetylcholine (Hashitani and Suzuki, 1997; Yamamoto *et al.*, 1999).

An additional observation was that, both in main and small mesenteric arteries, the peak change in membrane potential caused by acetylcholine was reached after a longer delay during exposure to barium than under control conditions. The relevance of this finding was highlighted by the observation that changes in membrane potential induced by transient applications of acetylcholine were inhibited by barium. This may imply that the impact of the EDHF liberated by acetylcholine on the smooth muscle cells is altered by exposure to barium. However, both the decreased total conductance of the cell membrane and the enlarged driving force for K^+ efflux would tend to favor the opposite. Alternatively, these findings may suggest that barium somehow interferes with the liberation of EDHF by an action on the endothelial cells. A hampered liberation might indeed be manifested more in responses to transient than to more prolonged stimulation with acetylcholine. Since in endothelial cells the inward rectifier makes a substantial contribution to the resting membrane potential, the depolarization of these cells by barium (Daut *et al.*, 1994; Vaca *et al.*, 1996; Nilius *et al.*, 1997) could severely impair Ca^{2+} influx during stimulation by agonists. Moreover, barium directly inhibits the store operated channels of endothelial cells (Nilius, personal communication). Since increased Ca^{2+} levels are of primary importance for the release of EDHF (Chen and Suzuki, 1990), the impaired Ca^{2+} influx in the presence of barium would slow down EDHF release, as suggested by the present experiments.

The additional inhibition of the Na/K pump with ouabain (5×10^{-4} M) further depolarized the smooth muscle cells of the main and small mesenteric arteries, as expected from the loss of electrogenic pump activity. Since the K_d value of the ubiquitous low affinity α_1-isoform of the Na/K-ATPase in rat tissue is about 15×10^{-6} M (Noel and Godfraind, 1984), and 10^{-4} M of ouabain completely inhibits the dilatation of rat mesenteric arteries caused by readmission of K^+ (Adeagbo and Malik, 1990), it can be assumed that under the present conditions the pump is effectively inhibited by 5×10^{-4} M of the cardiotonic steroid. In the combined presence of barium and ouabain, the endothelium-dependent hyperpolarization induced by superfusion with acetylcholine was, although decreased, not abolished in the main mesenteric artery. In smaller arteries, additional exposure to ouabain did not affect the endothelium-dependent hyperpolarization. These observations suggest that in the main mesenteric artery and its second order branches neither the inward rectifier nor substantial Na/K pumping is involved in the response of the cell membrane of the smooth muscle to EDHF liberated by acetylcholine. Moreover, both transient and prolonged increases in extracellular K^+ concentration consistently depolarized the smooth muscle cells of main mesenteric and small mesenteric and gastric arteries. These experiments show that a putative increase in subendothelial K^+ concentration cannot cause hyperpolarization of these smooth muscle cells, excluding the possibility that K^+ represents EDHF in these preparations. In fact, an increase in interstitial K^+ activity could not be detected upon stimulation of the endothelial cells with a large concentration of acetylcholine, at least in superfused strips of the main mesenteric artery.

4. CONCLUSION

Combined application of barium and ouabain does not abolish endothelium-dependent hyperpolarization of the smooth muscle cells of the main and small mesenteric artery of the rat. In these arteries, as well as in small gastric arteries, increases in the extracellular concentration of K^+ depolarized the smooth muscle cells. These findings question the importance of the inward rectifier and Na/K pump in the phenomenon of endothelium-dependent hyperpolarization, at least in the studied arteries.

ACKNOWLEDGEMENTS

This work was supported by a grant from the National Fund for Scientific Research (FWO-Vlaanderen).

17 EDHF and potassium: blockade of chloride channels reveals relaxations of rat mesenteric artery to potassium

*Joanne M. Doughty, John P. Boyle
and Philip D. Langton*

K^+ has been proposed to be EDHF in small arteries. Acetylcholine-stimulated, EDHF-mediated dilatation/relaxation was compared with raised $[K^+]_o$ in rat mesenteric arteries. In pressurised arteries, acetylcholine (10^{-5} M) dilated all arteries. Raising $[K^+]_o$ from 5.88 to 10.58 mM only dilated a third of arteries tested. Ba^{2+} (3×10^{-5} M) did not affect dilatation to acetylcholine, but abolished those dilatations to raised $[K^+]_o$ in some but not all arteries tested. In arteries suspended for isometric recording of force, acetylcholine (10^{-6} M) relaxed endothelium intact arteries, but not arteries without endothelium. Raising $[K^+]_o$ from 5.9 to 10.9 mM failed to relax arteries in most cases. Under both isometric and pressurised conditions, relaxation and dilatation to raised $[K^+]_o$ was observed in the presence but not the absence of 5-nitro-2-(3-phenylpropylamino) benzoic acid (NPPB), in preparations previously shown to be refractory to raised $[K^+]_o$. The effect was reversible, concentration- and endothelium-dependent. Under both pressurised and isometric conditions, the relaxation to elevated $[K^+]_o$ in the presence of NPPB was completely reversed by Ba^{2+} (3×10^{-5} M). In presence of elevated $[K^+]_o$, NPPB and Ba^{2+}, acetycholine (10 µM) fully relaxed all arteries. Under isometric conditions, relaxations to elevated $[K^+]_o$ could be revealed by hyperosmotic (plus 60 mM sucrose) superfusion. This effect was endothelium-dependent and was reversed by Ba^{2+} (3×10^{-5} M).

These observations suggest that blockade of a volume-sensitive Cl conductance by NPPB or hyperosmotic superfusion can reveal a Ba^{2+}-sensitive dilatation or relaxation of rat mesenteric arteries to elevated $[K^+]_o$.

The nitric oxide synthase- and prostacyclin-independent relaxation that is accompanied by an endothelium-dependent hyperpolarization of the vascular smooth muscle currently defines the involvement of an endothelium-derived hyperpolarizing factor (EDHF) (Chen *et al.*, 1988; Taylor and Weston, 1988; Félétou and Vanhoutte, 1988; Corriu *et al.*, 1996; Ohlmann *et al.*, 1997; Zygmunt *et al.*, 1997). The identity of EDHF, and its mechanism of action remain elusive. EDHF may be potassium (Edwards *et al.*, 1998), and elevating extracellular potassium can mimic the effects of EDHF in rat hepatic and mesenteric arteries. In contrast, potassium does not mimic the effects of EDHF in porcine coronary and guinea-pig carotid arteries (Quignard *et al.*, 1999; Lacy *et al.*, 2000; Doughty *et al.*, 2000).

According to one model for EDHF, K^+ efflux from the endothelium through apamin- and charybdotoxin-sensitive channels is sufficient to raise K^+ in the myoendothelial space (Edwards *et al.*, 1998), leading to hyperpolarization and relaxation of the smooth muscle by stimulation of inward rectifier K^+ channels (Edwards *et al.*, 1988; Knot *et al.*, 1996; McCarron and Halpern, 1990) and/or the electrogenic Na^+/K^+-ATPase (Prior *et al.*, 1998).

An obvious test of this model is that raised extracellular potassium ($[K^+]_o$) should produce an endothelium-independent, relaxation with the characteristics of an EDHF-mediated relaxation. However, relaxations to raised $[K^+]_o$ are inconsistent and endothelium-dependent (Lacy *et al.*, 2000; Doughty *et al.*, 2000). The present study investigates the mechanism underlying the relaxation to raised $[K^+]_o$ in rat mesenteric arteries in order to explain the endothelium-dependence and inconsistent nature of the responses.

1. METHODS

200–300 g male Wistar rats were killed by stunning and cervical dislocation. Third order superior mesenteric arteries were dissected in physiological saline solution containing (mM): NaCl 119, KCl 4.7, NaHCO$_3$ 25, KH$_2$PO$_4$ 1.18, CaCl$_2$ 1.8, MgSO$_4$ 1.2, glucose 11, EDTA 0.027, N$^\omega$-nitro-L-arginine methyl ester (L-NAME) 0.1, indomethacin 0.0028. The pH was 7.4 when gassed with 95% O$_2$/5% CO$_2$.

1.1. Pressure myography

Leak-free segments of artery of at least 1 mm in length were mounted between two glass cannulae in an arteriograph (Living Systems Instrumentation, Burlington, VT, USA) at room temperature (18–21 °C) and pressurised to 80 mmHg, under conditions of no lumenal flow. The artery lumen was filled with the standard physiological saline solution (see above). Constant pressure was maintained via a pressure servo control system (PS200, Living Systems Instrumentation). Pressure transducers at both ends of the artery allowed continual monitoring of the intralumenal pressure. Arteries were viewed through a Nikon TMS inverted microscope and a measurement of the internal diameter was made from a video image using a video dimension analyser (V91, Living Systems Instrumentation). The arteriograph was continually superfused with the standard physiological saline solution (see above) at a rate of 25 ml/min. The superfusing physiological saline solution was warmed to 37 °C and no myogenic constriction of arteries was seen. Therefore, arteries were constricted with 3×10^{-7}–10^{-6} M phenylephrine applied to the superfusate. Pressure and diameter measurements were recorded to computer via a Digidata 1200B interface using Axoscope software version 7 (Axon Instruments, CA, USA). *Intraluminal Solutions*: During all experiments, the physiological saline solution contained 10^{-4} M L-NAME and 2.8×10^{-6} M indomethacin.

1.2. Wire myography

Segments of mesenteric artery were mounted in physiological saline solution in a Mulvany-Halpern wire myograph for the recording of isometric tension. The artery segments were sequentially stretched until the wall tension was equivalent to a transmural pressure of 100 mmHg (Mulvany and Halpern, 1977). The diameter was calculated and set to 90% of this value and the tissue allowed to equilibrate for 45 min. Arterial segments were first constricted with phenylephrine (10^{-8}–10^{-5} M) and subsequent contractions to phenylephrine were titrated to give 70% of maximal response.

Force is expressed as percentage of the contraction to phenylephrine (70% of maximal response).

1.3. Drugs

All drugs were made up as stock solutions in milli-Q water, unless otherwise stated, diluted in the experimental solution and applied in the superfusate. 5-nitro-2-(3-phenylpropylamino) benzoic acid (NPPB) was dissolved in dimethylsulphoxide (DMSO) such that the concentration of DMSO did not exceed 0.1% in the final solution. Indomethacin was dissolved in 2% Na_2CO_3 or ethanol. All drugs were supplied by Sigma (Poole, Dorset, UK).

1.4. Statistics

All data are expressed as mean values $\pm$ SEM for n experiments. Statistical significance was tested using a Student's t-test on paired data, unless stated otherwise. p less than .05 was regarded as significant.

2. RESULTS

2.1. Acetylcholine and potassium

Acetylcholine (10^{-5} M) dilated all pressurised arteries tested to their passive diameter (passive: $283 \pm 6.9\,\mu m$; level of tone: $170 \pm 8.2\,\mu m$; acetylcholine: $283 \pm 6.7\,\mu m$) ($n = 30$), whereas raising extracellular potassium ($[K^+]_o$) in the superfusing physiological saline solution from 5.88 mM physiological saline solution (normal) to 10.58 mM (high), by doubling the concentration of KCl in the standard physiological saline solution, fully dilated only nine out of thirty arteries to their passive diameter. In the remaining twenty-one arteries raising $[K^+]_o$ produced a weak dilatation ($n = 5$), or a, small constriction ($n = 16$) (Figure 17.1)

The ability of raised $[K^+]_o$ to produce dilatation in rat mesenteric arteries was not correlated with the artery diameter over the range tested (200–400 μm) (Figure 17.1). Arteries that did not dilate on raising the extracellular concentration of K^+ from 5.88 to 10.58 mM could not be dilated by further increases in $[K^+]_o$. Indeed, increases to 19.98 mM resulted in constriction ($n = 3$) (data not shown). Increasing $[K^+]_o$ in the lumen was not more effective at eliciting dilatation. If high $[K^+]_o$ in the superfusate failed to produce dilatation, then it also failed to produce dilatation when applied simultaneously in the lumen ($n = 3$).

2.2. Chloride channel blockade

In previous experiments, using pressurized arteries, constriction to Ba^{2+} (3×10^{-5} M) under control conditions was positively correlated with dilatation to raised extracellular potassium in those vessels (Doughty et al., 2000). The benzoate Cl channel blocker, 5-nitro-2-(3-phenylpropylamino) benzoic acid (NPPB) hyperpolarizes pressurized myogenic arteries (Nelson et al., 1997). Where elevating $[K^+]_o$ from 5.88 to 10.58 mM failed to dilate, application of a low concentration of NPPB (2×10^{-5} M)

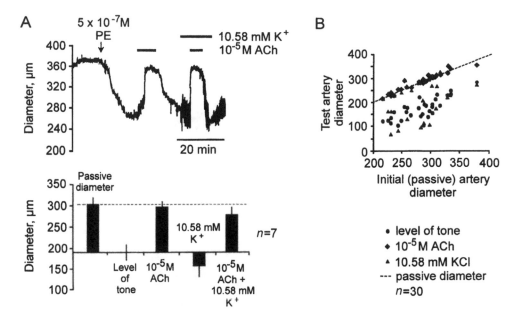

Figure 17.1 Dilatation to acetylcholine(ACh) and K^+ in rat mesenteric arteries. (A) Original recording in a pressurized artery that failed to dilate to on stepping from normal (5.88 mM) to high (10.58 mM) K^+. Acetylcholine (ACh; 10^{-5} M) dilated this blood vessel to close to its passive diameter both under control conditions (5.8 mM K^+) and in high K^+. Mean data ($\pm$SEM) are from seven similar experiments. The dashed line shows the passive diameter of the artery. (B) Scatter plot showing the relationship between the initial (passive) artery diameter (x-axis) and the level of tone of the arteries after constriction to phenylephrine (PE) (diamonds) and in the presence of 10^{-5} M acetylcholine (ACh; squares) and high $[K^+]$ (filled triangles). In all arteries tested ($n = 30$) acetylcholine dilated to the passive diameter, whereas high $[K^+]$ only dilated to the passive diameter in nine arteries. The failure of high $[K^+]$ to dilate was not related to the diameter of the artery.

produced partial reduction of tone. Subsequent elevation of $[K^+]_o$, from 5.88 to 10.58 mM, in the continued presence of NPPB, resulted in dilatation of all vessels tested. On washout of NPPB, raising $[K^+]_o$ did not result in dilatation ($n = 5$). The ability of NPPB to reveal dilatation to raised $[K^+]_o$ was abolished on removal of the endothelium ($n = 3$) (Figure 17.2).

In recordings of phenylephrine-induced contractions, less than one in twenty arteries with endothelium relaxed to raised $[K^+]_o$ in the absence of NPPB. In the presence of NPPB (10^{-5} M) raising $[K^+]_o$ fully relaxed all arteries tested ($n = 8$) (Figure 17.3). The relaxation to raised $[K^+]_o$ in the presence of NPPB was reversed by Ba^{2+} (3×10^{-5} M) (Figure 17.3). In the continued presence of raised $[K^+]_o$, NPPB and Ba^{2+}, subsequent addition of acetylcholine (10^{-5} M) resulted in full relaxation (Figure 17.3). The ability of NPPB to reveal relaxations to raised $[K^+]_o$ was lost after removal of the endothelium. Removal of the endothelium was achieved by abrasion using a hair and was confirmed by loss of the response to acetylcholine (data not shown).

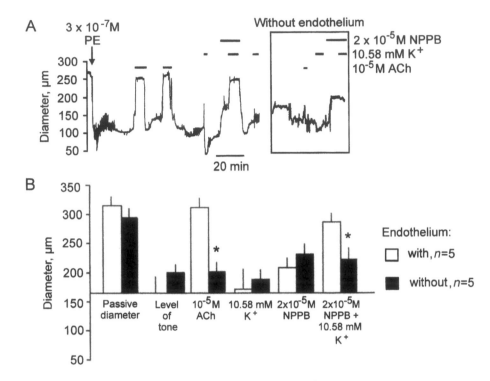

Figure 17.2 The effect of NPPB on dilatations to K^+ in pressurized arteries. (A) In arteries where stepping $[K^+]_o$ from 5.88 to 10.58 mM failed to produce dilatation, the response was induced in the presence of NPPB (2×10^{-5} M). The effect of NPPB on the ability of K^+ to dilate was fully reversible on washout. The gap in the data trace indicates a period of removal of the endothelium with an air bubble. In the absence of an endothelium, the effects of NPPB were abolished. (B) Mean data ($\pm$SEM, $n = 5$). The asterisks show statistical significance ($p < .05$; Student's t-test for unpaired observations). ACh = acetylcholine, 10^{-5} M; PE = phenylephrine, 3×10^{-7} M.

2.3. Concentration-dependence of NPPB-induced relaxations to raised $[K^+]_o$

Phenylephrine-induced (70% maximum) contractions from arteries with endothelium were used to determine the concentration-dependence of NPPB effects on: (1) control contractions; (2) control plus raised $[K^+]_o$; and (3) control plus raised $[K^+]_o$ plus Ba^{2+} (3×10^{-5} M).

NPPB relaxed phenylephrine-induced contractions ($IC_{50} = 7.2 \times 10^{-6}$ M, $n = 6$). In the presence of raised $[K^+]_o$ the NPPB concentration-effect curve was shifted leftward ($IC_{50} = 1.2 \times 10^{-6}$ M, $n = 10$). This leftward shift was inhibited in the presence of 3×10^{-5} M Ba^{2+} ($IC_{50} = 4.7^{-6}$ M, $n = 6$) (Figure 17.4).

2.4. Effect of anisosmotic solutions on responses to raised $[K^+]_o$

In recordings of isometric force, raised $[K^+]_o$ reduced phenylephrine-induced contractions only very rarely. Increasing the osmolarity of the superfusate by the addition

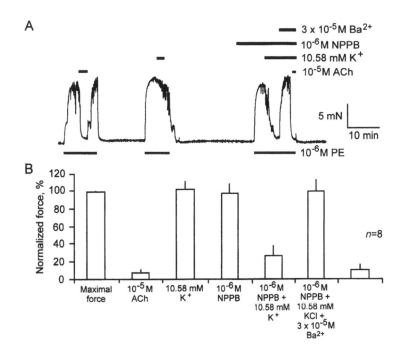

Figure 17.3 The effect of NPPB on dilatations to K^+ in arteries mounted for isometric measurement of force. (A) In arteries where stepping $[K^+]_o$ from 5.88 to 10.58 mM failed to produce relaxation, such response was induced in the presence of NPPB (10^{-6} M). This effect was reversed by Ba^{2+} (3×10^{-5} M). (B) Mean data ($\pm$SEM, $n = 8$). Acetylcholine (ACh; 10^{-5} M) was still able to relax fully in the presence of Ba^{2+}.

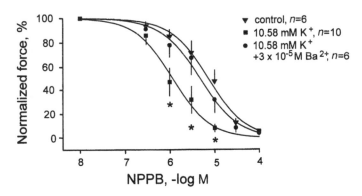

Figure 17.4 The concentration-effect curve for NPPB in arteries mounted for isometric measurement of force. NPPB relaxed isometric arteries with an IC_{50} of 7.2×10^{-6} M (triangles) ($\pm$SEM, $n = 6$). In the presence of 10.58 mM K^+ (squares), the concentration-effect curve for relaxation of arteries by NPPB was shifted to the left (IC_{50}: 1.1×10^{-6} M) ($\pm$SEM, $n = 10$). This leftward shift was inhibited in the presence of Ba^{2+} (3×10^{-5} M) (circles, IC_{50}: 4.69×10^{-6} M; $\pm$SEM, $n = 6$). Data shown as means $\pm$ SEM. The asterisks show significant difference from the control curve ($p < .05$; Student's t-test for unpaired observations).

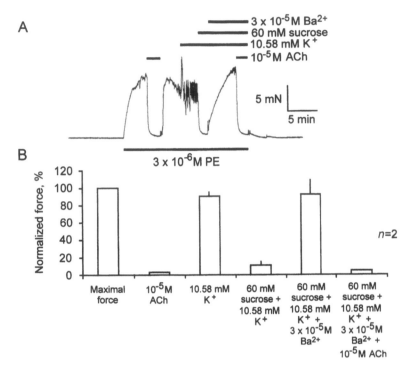

Figure 17.5 Hyperosmotic stress mimics the effects of NPPB to reveal relaxation of isometric arteries to K^+. (A) In arteries where stepping $[K^+]_o$ from 5.88 to 10.58 mM failed to produce relaxation, such response was induced in the presence of a hyperosmotic solution (60 mM sucrose added). This effect was reversed by Ba^{2+} $(3 \times 10^{-5} M)$. (B) Mean data ($\pm$SEM, $n = 2$). Acetylcholine (ACh; 10^{-5} M) was still able to relax fully in the presence of Ba^{2+}.

of 60 mM sucrose partially reduced control phenylephrine-induced contractions. In the presence of raised $[K^+]_o$, the addition of 60 mM sucrose resulted in full relaxation that could be reversed by Ba^{2+} $(3 \times 10^{-5} M)$ (Figure 17.5). In arteries without endothelium, the partial relaxation to sucrose but not the Ba^{2+}-sensitive relaxation to raised $[K^+]_o$ was observed (data not shown).

A small number of arteries exhibited relaxations to raised potassium under control conditions (Figure 17.6). Reduction of osmolarity by approximately 80 mosM (omission of 40 mM NaCl) prior to inducing the contraction to phenylephrine partially depressed the contraction but abolished the relaxation to raised $[K^+]_o$. Returning osmolarity to normal in the presence of raised $[K^+]_o$ resulted in relaxation.

3. DISCUSSION

3.1. Inwardly rectifying potassium channels – the endothelium

The investigation of the mechanism of relaxation to raised $[K^+]_o$ was impeded, initially, by the absence of a response to raised $[K^+]_o$, that was in stark contrast to the

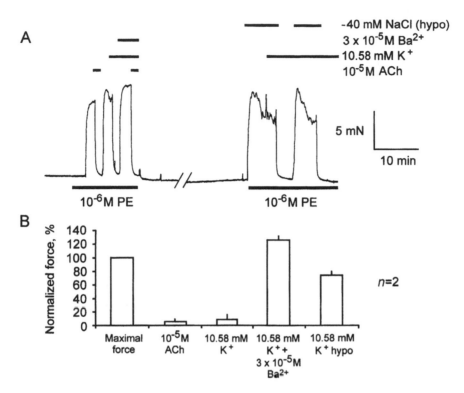

Figure 17.6 Hypoosmotic stress prevents relaxation of isometric arteries to K^+. (A) In arteries where stepping $[K^+]_o$ from 5.88 to 10.58 mM produced relaxation, that response was abolished in the presence of Ba^{2+} (3×10^{-5} M) or a hyposmotic solution (40 mMNaCl omitted). (B) Mean data ($\pm$SEM, $n = 2$).

robust relaxation to acetylcholine. In pressurized arteries, dilatations to raised $[K^+]_o$ could be blocked by low concentrations of Ba^{2+} alone, suggesting that hyperpolarization by members of the inward rectifier potassium channel family can be sufficient to account for K^+-induced dilatation (Nelson and Quayle, 1995). The Ba^{2+}-sensitivity was absent in arteries without endothelium, suggesting that the inward rectifier potassium channels are present on the endothelial cells and not the smooth muscle. A similar distribution of inward rectifier potassium channels may underlie the relaxation of mesenteric arteries in response to hypercapnia (Okazaki *et al.*, 1998). The variability of Ba^{2+}-sensitive dilatations to raised $[K^+]_o$ may reflect different densities of inward rectifier potassium channels throughout the mesenteric bed. In the coronary circulation, the density of inward rectifier potassium channels is inversely related to artery size. This is interpreted to reflect that mechanisms dependent upon the activation of inward rectifier potassium channels become increasingly important in smaller arteries (Quayle *et al.*, 1996; Quayle *et al.*, 1993). This interpretation would be consistent with the hypothesis that EDHF becomes progressively more important as arterial diameter decreases (Shimokawa *et al.*, 1996). However, the present data show no correlation between arterial diameter and the ability of K^+ to produce Ba^{2+}-sensitive dilatation.

3.2. Inwardly rectifying potassium channels – smooth muscle

Evidence for inward rectifier potassium channels in mesenteric artery myocytes is lacking, despite several attempts to demonstrate their presence (Nelson and Quayle, 1995). Messenger RNA encoding an inwardly rectifying K^+ channel family (K_{ir} 2.1) is present in rat mesenteric cells (Bradley *et al.*, 1999). However, no recordings of the native conductance in isolated mesenteric smooth muscle cells are available. Indeed, inward rectifier potassium channels have only been identified in one voltage-clamp study of intact mesenteric arterioles of the guinea-pig (Edwards and Hirst, 1988), and it is possible that the recorded currents were generated by the endothelium as well as the smooth muscle. Evidence for inward rectifier potassium channels is also limited in other arterial smooth muscle that respond to EDHF (Quignard *et al.*, 1999; Quayle *et al.*, 1997). A major source of Ba^{2+}-sensitive hyperpolarizing current/factor is the endothelium, and this is transmitted to smooth muscle by gap junctions (Doughty *et al.*, 2000). Increases in $[K^+]_o$ generated by K^+ flux through toxin-sensitive K^+ channels could play a supporting role in this mechanism, by causing endothelial hyperpolarization via activation of the inward rectifier and by actions on the smooth muscle Na^+/K^+-ATPase. Although, inward rectifier potassium channels have not been measured in mesenteric endothelial cells, evidence from endothelial cells obtained from other blood vessels shows that inward rectifier potassium channels are a major determinant of membrane potential (Voets *et al.*, 1996; Nilius *et al.*, 1997).

3.3. Membrane potential and inwardly rectifying potassium channel current

A possible explanation for the apparent absence of relaxation to raised $[K^+]_o$ or Ba^{2+}-sensitivity in some arteries might be found in a study on endothelial cells (Voets *et al.*, 1996), which demonstrated that the majority of cultured pulmonary endothelial cells were more depolarized than $-26\,mV$ and showed no effect of external Ba^{2+}, suggesting that inward rectifier potassium channels had little influence on membrane potential. Inward rectifier potassium channels pass more outward current in the voltage range just positive to E_K than at more depolarized potentials (Hille and Schwarz, 1978). Thus, it is possible that cells that are less than $30\,mV$ positive to E_K will pass more Ba^{2+}-sensitive outward current compared with those that are more than $30\,mV$ positive to E_K. The shift in the current–voltage relation of inward rectifier potassium channels current on raising $[K^+]_o$ will tend to hyperpolarize only those cells whose membrane potential was positive to the new, more depolarized, E_K but not so positive as to minimize inward rectifier potassium channels conductance. If the endothelial cells membrane potential is dominated by a chloride conductance, E_{Cl} is approximately $40\,mV$ positive to E_K in these experiments, there will be little or no outward current through inward rectifier potassium channels.

The failure of mesenteric arteries to constrict to Ba^{2+} or dilate to raised $[K^+]_o$ may be explained if endothelial cells in rat mesenteric arteries exhibit similar distributions of membrane potential. This hypothesis is supported by the data with the chloride channel blocker, NPPB. Arteries that failed to dilate to raised $[K^+]_o$ under control conditions, consistently dilated to it in the presence of a low concentration NPPB. This effect of NPPB was dependent on an intact endothelium and reversible on washout. NPPB can have non-specific effects in resistance arteries (Kato *et al.*, 1999), and may cause relaxation by blocking L-type calcium channels (Doughty *et al.*, 1998). However, at the concentration used, it is unlikely that the observed effects of NPPB are dependent on calcium channel blockade. As an alternative to NPPB block, the effect of anisomotic solutions was investigated. The endothelial chloride conductance is activated by hyposmotic stimuli (Voets *et al.*, 1996). In recordings of isometric force, superfusion by physiological saline solution made hyperosmotic by the addition of 60 mM sucrose had little effect on constrictions to phenylephrine but revealed relaxations to raised $[K^+]_o$ in arteries that had previously been refractory to the ion. This relaxation to raised potassium in the presence of hyperosmotic solutions was reversed by 10^{-5} M Ba^{2+} suggesting that relaxation depends upon the inward rectifier potassium channel. The small number of arteries that exhibited relaxations to raised potassium under control conditions allowed the effect of hyposomotic physiological saline solution to be tested. Under control conditions both acetylcholine and raised $[K^+]_o$ resulted in relaxation. Reduction of osmolarity (by approximately 80 mosM) partially depressed the constriction but abolished the relaxation to raised $[K^+]_o$. Subsequent restoration of normal osmolarity resulted in a prompt relaxation to the sustained raised $[K^+]_o$ that was reversed by a return to hyposmotic physiological saline solution. Together, these data suggest that Ba^{2+}-sensitive relaxations to raised $[K^+]_o$ depend upon the relative levels of volume- and NPPB-sensitive chloride and inwardly rectifying potassium currents.

3.4. Other models of EDHF

Even if K^+ is not EDHF, EDHF-mediated relaxation may be fundamentally dependent on hyperpolarization of the endothelium by toxin-sensitive K^+ conductances. Endothelial hyperpolarization may lead to hyperpolarization of smooth muscle if functional myoendothelial gap junctions coupling exists. Gap junction inhibitors are effective inhibitors of EDHF (Chaytor *et al.*, 1998; Dora *et al.*, 1999; Taylor *et al.*, 1998; Doughty *et al.*, 2000).

The possibility remains that a diffusable factor, independent of K^+ efflux from the endothelium, may contribute a component to endothelium-dependent hyperpolarization, but this would also need to be directly or indirectly toxin-sensitive. Compelling evidence that EDHF is likely to include a humoral factor that is not explained by K^+ comes from the experiments using sandwich (or donor) preparations (Chen *et al.*, 1991; Mombouli *et al.*, 1996). Possible candidates for this factor include epoxyeicosatrienoic acids, cannabinoids, such as anandamide, and residual NOS inhibitor-insensitive NO production (Vanhoutte, 1998).

4. CONCLUSIONS

Endothelium-dependent and Ba^{2+}-sensitive dilatations (and relaxations) to raised $[K^+]_o$ could be recorded from rat mesenteric artery only following reduction in chloride channel activity using NPPB or hyperosmotic physiological saline solution. The interpretation is that inwardly rectifying potassium channels are expressed on the endothelium and that the membrane potential of endothelium is critically important for responses to raised $[K^+]_o$ in this preparation.

ACKNOWLEDGEMENTS

The authors wish to thank Paul Kendrick for technical support. This work was supported by British Heart Foundation grant number PG/97182 (JMD and PDL) and Medical Research Council grant number G9609076 (JPB).

18 Cytochrome P450 2C – a source of EDHF and reactive oxygen species in the porcine coronary artery

B. Fisslthaler, D. Bredenkötter, Ralf P. Brandes,
U.R. Michaelis, Rudi Busse and Ingrid Fleming

In most arterial beds pulsatile stretch, shear stress and receptor-dependent agonists can induce endothelium-dependent relaxations, which are insensitive to the simultaneous inhibition of nitric oxide synthase and cyclooxygenase. This relaxation is attributed to the generation and release of an endothelium-derived hyperpolarizing factor (EDHF). Cytochrome P450 2C epoxygenases play a central role in EDHF-mediated responses in the porcine coronary artery. Specific inhibition of cytochrome P450 2C9 using sulfaphenazole or down-regulation of the cytochrome P450 2C protein with anti-sense oligonucleotides attenuates EDHF-mediated responses. However this approach also induces a significant leftward shift in the bradykinin-induced, NO-mediated, relaxation–response curve. A similar effect was observed in segments incubated with the oxygen radical scavenger Tiron or the antioxidant nordihydroguaretic acid. In microsomes purified from cells over-expressing cytochrome P450 2C9, a sulfaphenazole-sensitive production of reactive oxygen species could be demonstrated. This compound did not impair the activity of either the NADPH oxidase or xanthine oxidase. Enhancing cytochrome P450 2C levels in endothelial cells, either by over-expressing cytochrome P450 2C9 or by using β-naphthoflavone and nifedipine to induce cytochrome P450 expression, increased the generation of reactive oxygen species. These observations suggest that the expression of cytochrome P450 2C in coronary artery endothelial cells is not only essential for the production of EDHF, but also significantly contributes to the level of oxidative stress within the arterial wall.

Following inhibition of cycloxygenase and nitric oxide synthase, in human, porcine, canine and bovine coronary arteries, receptor-dependent agonists, such as bradykinin, induce almost complete relaxation. This residual relaxation is however sensitive to inhibitors of cytochrome P450 epoxygenases (Rosolowsky and Campbell, 1993; Hecker et al., 1994; Miura and Gutterman, 1998; Nishikawa et al., 1999), is preceded by a hyperpolarization of vascular smooth muscle cells, and can be attributed to endothelium-derived hyperpolarizing factor (EDHF). In coronary arteries, several regio-isomers of epoxyeicosatrienoic acid, which are products of cytochrome P450 epoxygenases, evoke both hyperpolarization and relaxation of vascular smooth muscle cells (Campbell et al., 1996). In the porcine coronary artery, the cytochrome P450 epoxygenase isoform which is crucial for the initiation of EDHF-mediated responses belongs to the 2C family and is homologous to cytochrome P450 2C8/9 (Fisslthaler et al., 1999).

NO and superoxide anions react rapidly *in vivo*, such that the bioavailability of NO and, as a consequence, NO-mediated relaxation is attenuated by an increase in the production of superoxide anions within the vascular wall (Rubanyi and Vanhoutte, 1986). Enzymes capable of generating reactive oxygen species within endothelial and smooth muscle cells include eNOS, cyclooxygenase, xanthine oxidase, NADPH oxidase and cytochrome P450 enzymes (Wolin, 2000). It is difficult to determine the enzymatic source of reactive oxygen species produced within the vasculature since the available inhibitors are relatively non-specific.

Superoxide anions and hydrogen peroxide are generated during the P450 reaction cycle when the electrons for the reduction of the central heme iron are transferred on the activated bound oxygen molecule. Since endothelial cells contain cytochrome P450 enzymes of the 2C and 2J families (Lin *et al.*, 1996; Fisslthaler *et al.*, 1999; Fisslthaler *et al.*, 2000; Node *et al.*, 1999), these enzymes may contribute to the generation of reactive oxygen species within the vascular wall.

1. METHODS

1.1. Cell culture

Human umbilical vein endothelial cells were isolated (Popp *et al.*, 1996). For transfection, cells were purchased from Cell Systems/Clonetics (Solingen). Confluent cells were incubated with nifedipine (10^{-7} M, 18 hours) or β-naphthoflavone (3×10^{-6} M, 48 hours). Subconfluent cultures (60–80% confluent) of endothelial cells were transfected with plasmids encoding cytochrome P450 2C9 using cationic liposomes (Superfect, Qiagen).

1.2. Detection of reactive oxygen species *in vitro*

The generation of oxygen-derived free radicals was analysed in microsomes prepared from insect cells over-expressing cytochrome P450 2C9 together with the P450 reductase and cytochrome b_5 (Natutec, Frankfurt, Germany), with purified xanthine oxidase (Sigma, Heidelberg, Germany) or in isolated human leukocytes, which contain NADPH oxidase. Reactive oxygen species in microsomal preparations were detected by the oxidation of 2′,7′-dichlorodihydrofluorescein (Oxyburst, Molecular Probes) to the fluorescent product 2′,7′-dichloroflurescein, whereas lucigenin-enhanced chemiluminescence was used to evaluate the generation of oxygen-derived free radicals by the NADPH oxidase and xanthine oxidase.

Free radical production in cultured endothelial cells loaded with 2′,7′-dichlorodihydrofluorescein diacetate was assessed as the intracellular conversion to the fluorescent product 2′,7′-dichlorofluorescein and visualized by *en face* confocal microscopy.

1.3. Organ chamber experiments

Epicardial arteries from freshly slaughtered pigs were used either directly after preparation, or following transfection with cytochrome P450 2C specific oligonucleotides. For transfection, thioate modified oligonucleotides (2.5 µg/ml, sequence of oligonucleotide, sense orientation: 5′CTCCCTCCTGGCCCACTCCTC3′) were incubated with $10\,\mu l$ superfect in minimal essential medium containing foetal calf serum (10%). The transfected blood vessels were perfused (5 ml/hr, 18 hours) with culture medium containing foetal calf serum (2%), streptomycin ($50\,\mu g/ml$), penicillin (50 u/ml) and polymyxin B ($1\,\mu g/ml$). Coronary artery rings were contracted with the thromboxane mimetic U46619 ($10^{-7}-10^{-6}$ M) to 80% of the maximal contraction and the relaxation in response to bradykinin was determined in the presence of diclofenac (10^{-5} M).

1.4. Statistical analysis

Data are expressed as means $\pm$ SEM. Statistical evaluation was performed using Student's t-test for unpaired data, one-way analysis of variance (ANOVA) followed by a Bonferroni t-test, or ANOVA for repeated measures where appropriate. Values of p less than .05 were considered to indicate statistically significant differences.

2. RESULTS

After treatment of porcine coronary artery rings with sulfaphenazole or transfection with anti-sense oligonucleotides directed against cytochrome P450 2C, the bradykinin-induced, NO-mediated relaxations were enhanced significantly (Table 18.1). A similar, although less pronounced leftward shift in the concentration–relaxation curve to bradykinin was observed in segments incubated with the O_2^- scavengers Tiron (10^{-5} M) and tempo (10^{-4} M) or the antioxidant nordihydroguaretic acid (3×10^{-5} M, Table 18.1).

Sulfaphenazole had no significant effect on the generation of oxygen-derived free radicals by a purified preparation of xanthine oxidase, or on the basal and phorbol 12-myristate, 13-acetate-induced activity of a leukocyte preparation containing NADPH oxidase. The generation of free radicals detected by the oxidation of

Table 18.1 Effects of down-regulation and inhibition of cytochrome P450 2C and of antioxidants on the bradykinin-induced, NO-mediated relaxation of rings of porcine coronary artery

Treatment	$R_{max}(\%)$	pEC_{50}	Treatment	$R_{max}(\%)$	pEC_{50}
Solvent	99.4 ± 3.0	8.22 ± 0.10	As CYP 2C	92.9 ± 2.7	$9.07 \pm 0.03^*$
Tiron	98.0 ± 0.7	$8.62 \pm 0.08^*$	Se CYP 2C	100 ± 4.0	8.26 ± 0.46
Tempo	99.5 ± 0.1	$8.40 \pm 0.07^*$	Solvent	95.2 ± 3.0	7.70 ± 0.06
NDGA	98.0 ± 1.3	$8.72 \pm 0.08^*$	Sulfaphenazole	100 ± 6.0	$8.52 \pm 0.03^*$

Notes
Endothelium-dependent, bradykinin-induced relaxations were determined in organ chambers using rings from porcine coronary arteries contracted with U46619 in the absence and presence of the antioxidants Tiron (10^{-5} M), tempo (10^{-4} M) and nordihydroguaretic acid (NDGA, 3×10^{-5} M), or the cytochrome P450 inhibitor sulfaphenazole (10^{-5} M). In some experiments, coronary arteries were transfected with either sense or antisense cytochrome P450 2C (CYP 2C) oligonucleotides over a period of 18 hours. R_{max} represents the maximal bradykinin-induced relaxation and pEC_{50} values were calculated by non-linear regression of the concentration–response curves. The data presented represent the means $\pm$ SEM from nine to twelve independent experiments. The asterisks indicate statistically significant ($p < .05$) differences with the respective control group.

Table 18.2 Effects of sulfaphenazole on the generation of reactive oxygen species by cytochrome P450 2C9, xanthine oxidase and leukocyte NADPH oxidase

	CYP 2C9 (% control signal)	Xanthine Oxidase (CPM)	NADPH-Oxidase ($CPM \times 10^3$)	
			Basal	PMA
Solvent	100	317 ± 24	10 ± 2	198 ± 33
Sulfaphenazole	$3 \pm 0.4^*$	311 ± 24	11 ± 1	196 ± 24

Notes
Radical generation by microsomes prepared from cells over-expressing cytochrome P450 2C9 (CYP 2C9) was determined using 2′,7′-dichloroflurescein fluorescence whereas lucigenin-enhanced chemiluminescence was used to evaluate the generation of oxygen-derived free radicals by a purified preparation of xanthine oxidase (1 mU/ml) and xanthine (10^{-4} M) as well as from a human leukocyte preparation containing NADPH oxidase. Experiments were performed in the absence (solvent) and presence of sulfaphenazole (10^{-5} M). Data presented are means $\pm$ SEM from four to six independent experiments. The asterisks indicate statistically significant ($p < .05$) differences with the respective control group.

2′,7′-dihydrochloroflurescein to 2′,7′-dichloroflurescein in microsomal preparations enriched in cytochrome P450 2C9 was nearly abolished by sulfaphenazole (10^{-5} M, Table 18.2), while the formation of oxygen-derived free radicals in microsomes prepared from cells over-expressing cytochrome P450 3A4 or 2C8 was not affected by the drug (data not shown).

The generation of reactive oxygen species by cytochrome P450 2C, was determined in cultured human endothelial cells, either under control conditions, or following the induction of cytochrome P450 enzymes by nifedipine (10^{-7} M, 18 hours) or β-naphthoflavone (3×10^{-6} M, 48 hours). In control cells, a low level of 2′,7′-dichloroflurescein fluorescence was detected, partially attributed to the auto-oxidation of the fluorescent dye. In nifedipine- and β-naphthoflavone-treated endothelial cells, in which there was a marked increase in the expression of cytochrome P450 2C, a significant increase in the 2′,7′-dichloroflurescein signal was recorded (Figure 18.1). The generation of reactive oxygen species, both under basal conditions and following pharmacological induction of cytochrome P450 2C, was abolished in the presence of the cytochrome P450 2C9 inhibitor sulfaphenazole (data not shown).

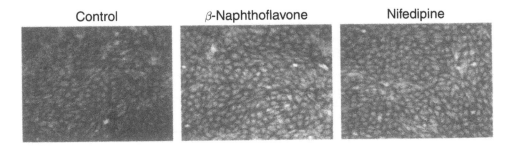

Figure 18.1 Induction of cytochrome P450 by nifedipine and β-naphthoflavone increases the generation of oxygen-derived free radicals in human endothelial cells. Endothelial cells were cultured in the presence and absence of nifedipine (10^{-7} M, 18 hours) or β-naphthoflavone (3×10^{-6} M, 48 hours) before incubation with 2′,7′-dichlorodihydrofluorescein diacetate (5×10^{-6} M, 1 hour). 2′,7′-Dichlorofluorescein fluorescence was monitored by confocal microscopy. Identical results were obtained using six separate cell batches. (*see Color Plate 7*)

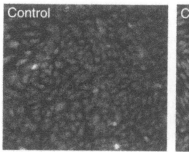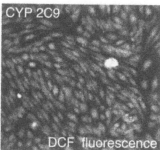

Figure 18.2 Over-expression of cytochrome P450 2C9 increases the generation of oxygen-derived free radicals in human endothelial cells. After transfection with pcDNA3.1 (control), or a cytochrome P450 2C9 expression plasmid, endothelial cells were maintained for an additional 24 hours prior to incubation with $2',7'$-dichlorodihydrofluorescein diacetate (5×10^{-6} M, 1 hour). $2',7'$-Dichlorofluorescein fluorescence was monitored by confocal microscopy. Identical results were obtained using five separate cell batches. (*see Color Plate 8*)

Cultured endothelial cells were transfected with plasmids encoding cytochrome P450 2C9. Western-blot analysis of the transfected cells showed that the cytochrome P450 2C9 protein levels reached a maximum at 24 hours after transfection (data not shown). Reactive oxygen species generation at this time point was significantly greater in the cytochrome P450 2C9 over-expressing cells than in cells transfected with an empty control vector (Figure 18.2). This increase in fluorescence was prevented in the presence of sulfaphenazole (data not shown).

3. DISCUSSION

The data summarized in this chapter highlight the fact that the cytochrome P450 2C expressed in endothelial cells of the porcine coronary artery not only is crucial for the generation of EDHF-mediated responses but also contributes significantly to the formation of reactive oxygen species within the vascular wall. One functional consequence of the down-regulation or inhibition of cytochrome P450 2C in porcine coronary arteries was a marked leftward shift in the concentration–relaxation curve to bradykinin, which under the experimental conditions employed is mediated exclusively by NO.

Homology among the different cytochrome P450 2C isoforms is high. However, sulfaphenazole selectively inhibits cytochrome P450 2C9 (Sai *et al.*, 2000). In the present study, sulfaphenazole inhibited the generation of reactive oxygen species by microsomes containing cytochrome P450 2C9 but was without effect on either the activity or generation of reactive oxygen species by the cytochrome P450 isoforms 2C8 and 3A4. The most frequently studied sources of reactive oxygen species in endothelial cells are the NADPH oxidase, xanthine oxidase, cycloxygenase and eNOS, especially in the absence of the cofactor tetrahydrobiopterin (Cosentino and Katusic, 1995). Diphenyleneiodonium has been used to characterise the enzymatic system(s) responsible for the generation of reactive oxygen species within the vasculature.

Diphenyleneiodonium is however, a non-selective inhibitor of flavin-dependent enzymes and completely inhibits the activity of all isoforms of P450 enzymes as well as that of eNOS (Xia *et al.*, 1998), xanthine oxidase (Sanders *et al.*, 1997) and NADPH oxidase (Cross and Jones, 1986). Thus, this compound does not permit the identification of the enzymatic source of oxygen-derived free radicals.

The contribution of cycloxygenase and eNOS to the formation of reactive oxygen species was excluded in the present study, since all experiments were performed in the presence of diclofenac and N^ωnitro-L-arginine. Moreover, the increase in the NO-mediated relaxation observed in the presence of sulfaphenazole rules eNOS out as a major source of oxygen-derived free radicals in the porcine coronary artery. In *in vitro* assays, neither NADPH oxidase, xanthine oxidase, cytochrome P450 2C8, nor 3A4 were sensitive to sulfaphenazole, leaving cytochrome P450 2C9 as the only possible candidate for the sulfaphenazole-sensitive synthesis of reactive oxygen species in endothelial cells.

Cytochrome P450 enzymes can generate superoxide anions in isolated rat hepatic microsomes (Bondy and Naderi, 1999; Puntarulo and Cederbaum, 1998). Cytochrome P450 enzymes are present both in endothelial (Lin *et al.*, 1996; Fisslthaler *et al.*, 1999; Node *et al.*, 1999) and in vascular smooth muscle cells (Gebremedhin *et al.*, 2000; Node *et al.*, 1999). Not only do cytochrome P450 epoxygenases generate vasoactive metabolites of arachidonic acid but the present study demonstrates these enzymes also can produce reactive oxygen species in amounts sufficient to compromise the bioavailability of NO. Indeed, the increased expression of cytochrome P450 2C in endothelial cells, following cytochrome P450 induction by nifedipine and β-naphthoflavone or transfection with plasmids encoding cytochrome P450 2C9, was associated with an increased intracellular generation of reactive oxygen species. However, the most convincing evidence suggesting that cytochrome P450 2C is a physiologically relevant source of superoxide anions and/or hydrogen peroxide in the coronary artery, is that treatment of endothelial cells of this artery with antisense oligonucleotides to attenuate the expression of cytochrome P450 2C protein enhanced NO-mediated relaxations. The activity of a related epoxygenase may therefore also underlie the arachidonic acid-consuming, cytochrome P450-dependent process previously reported to generate oxygen-derived free radicals in the rat heart (Fulton *et al.*, 1997).

4. CONCLUSION

Taken together, the results discussed in this chapter suggest that cytochrome P450 2C9, expressed in endothelial cells, not only is crucial for the generation of EDHF-mediated responses but is a potential major source of reactive oxygen species within the vascular wall.

ACKNOWLEDGEMENTS

The authors are indebted to Isabel Winter and Stergiani Hauk for expert technical assistance.

19 Cortisol increases EDHF-mediated relaxations in porcine coronary arteries and up-regulates the expression of cytochrome P450 2C9

J. Bauersachs, M. Christ, G. Ertl,
B. Fisslthaler, Rudi Busse and Ingrid Fleming

In addition to nitric oxide (NO) and prostacyclin, endothelium-dependent dilations in some vascular beds can be mediated by the endothelium-derived hyperpolarizing factor (EDHF). In the coronary circulation EDHF has been pharmacologically characterized as a cytochrome P450 (CYP)-derived metabolite of arachidonic acid. Moreover, an epoxygenase homologous to CYP 2C8/9 has been identified as an EDHF synthase. As the promotor region of CYP 2C8/9 contains consensus sequences for glucocorticoid response elements, the effect of cortisol on EDHF-mediated relaxations of isolated porcine coronary rings was determined, as well as on the expression of CYP 2C in endothelial cells. Cortisol treatment did not affect the endothelium-independent relaxation induced by sodium nitroprusside. NO-mediated relaxation induced by brady-kinin following constriction with KCl was slightly attenuated following exposure to cortisol. However, following incubation with cortisol, bradykinin-induced, NO syn-thase/cyclo-oxygenase-independent relaxations were enhanced. Acute incubation with cortisol did not alter vascular reactivity. In addition, in endothelial cells, the expression of CYP 2C9 was enhanced following incubation with cortisol. These results demonstrate the concomitant upregulation of EDHF-mediated relaxations and CYP 2C9 expression by long-term treatment with cortisol. These observations support the concept that an epoxygenase homologous to CYP 2C8/9 plays a crucial role in the generation of EDHF-mediated responses the in the coronary endothelium.

In addition to nitric oxide (NO) and prostacyclin, endothelial cells release an endothelium-derived hyperpolarizing factor (EDHF), which induces relaxation by hyperpolarizing vascular smooth muscle cells. In the coronary circulation EDHF has been pharmacologically characterized as a cytochrome P450 (CYP)-derived meta-bolite of arachidonic acid (Hecker *et al.*, 1994; Bauersachs *et al.*, 1994; Fulton *et al.*, 1995; Campbell *et al.*, 1996; Popp *et al.*, 1996; Popp *et al.*, 1998), and an epoxygenase homologous to CYP 2C8/9 has been identified as an EDHF synthase by experiments using anti-sense-oligonucleotides (Fisslthaler *et al.*, 1999). CYP 2C8 and 9 are highly homologous, and the promotor region of both enzymes contains consensus sequences for glucocorticoid response elements (Ged and Beaune, 1991; Morais *et al.*, 1993). Therefore, in the present study, the effect of cortisol on the expression of CYP 2C in endothelial cells and on EDHF-mediated relaxation of isolated rings of the porcine coronary artery was investigated.

1. METHODS

1.1. Organ culture and vascular reactivity studies

Porcine coronary arteries (obtained from the local slaughterhouse) were cleaned of connective tissue and cut into segments (3–4 mm in length). Segments were cultured in Medium 199 (cc pro, Neustadt, Germany) containing polymyxin B. Rings were incubated with cortisol (10^{-7} M) or vehicle for 24 h. Thereafter, rings were mounted in an organ bath (Föhr Medical Instruments, Seeheim, Germany) for isometric force measurement as described (Bauersachs *et al.*, 1997). Rings were equilibrated for 30 min under a resting tension of 3 g in oxygenated (95% O_2, 5% CO_2) Krebs–Henseleit solution (pH 7.4, 37 °C) of the following composition: NaCl 118 mmol/l, KCl 4.7 mmol/l, $MgSO_4$ 1.2 mmol/l, $CaCl_2$ 1.6 mmol/l, K_2HPO_4 1.2 mmol/l, $NaHCO_3$ 25 mmol/l, glucose 12 mmol/l, and the cycloxygenase inhibitor diclofenac (10^{-6} M). Rings were repeatedly contracted by KCl (100 mM) until reproducible responses were obtained. Thereafter, the rings were preconstricted with the thromboxane mimetic U46619 ($10^{-8} - 10^{-7}$ M) to about 70% of the maximal constriction and the relaxation to cumulative doses of bradykinin ($10^{-10} - 10^{-6}$ M) and to sodium nitroprusside ($10^{-9} - 10^{-6}$ M) was assessed with or without prior inhibition of NO synthase using N^{ω}-nitro-L-arginine (L-NA, 3×10^{-4} M, 30 min). For the determination of short-term effects, cortisol was applied to the organ chamber for 30 min.

1.2. Expression studies

Porcine epicardial artery segments (40 mm long) were excised, side branches were sealed with surgical clips, and the segment was cannulated at both ends and placed into vessel chambers (Fisslthaler *et al.*, 2000). After equilibration, coronary arteries were perfused with MEM containing cortisol (10^{-7} M, 18–24 h). Endothelial cells or total RNA was isolated through intraluminal incubation with either dispase (2.4 U/ml) or guanidine isothiocyanate. Random hexanucleotide primers were used for reverse transcription (RT) of equal amounts of RNA as described (Fisslthaler *et al.*, 2000). The oligonucleotides used for polymerase chain reaction (PCR) were derived from a porcine CYP 2C34 sequence (genebank accession no.: U35843), upstream primer: AGA-CAACGAGCACCACTCTG, downstream primer: CTTGGGGATGAGGTAGTTT which exhibited a high homology to the human 2C8 sequence (genebank accession no.: Y00498). CYP 2B2 upstream primer: TGGTGGAGGARCTGCGGAATCC, downstream primer: TGCCTTCGCCAAGACAAAYGCG (genebank accession no.: M34452); CYP 2J2 upstream primer: CCCTCAYTTCAAGATCAACA, downstream primer: GCAGATGAGGTTTTCTTCAT (genebank accession no.: U37143) and elongation factor (EF) upstream primer: GACATCACCAAGGGTGTGCAG, downstream primer: GCGGTCAGCACACTGGCATA.

PCR products were separated on an agarose gel and visualized by staining with ethidiumbromide. For the verification of the DNA fragment the PCR-products were transferred to nylon membranes and hybridized with ^{32}P-labelled DNA fragments derived from a plasmid containing the coding sequence of CYP 2C8, CYP 2B or CYP 2J2. Phenol-soluble protein or microsomal fractions (100,000 g pellets) prepared from isolated porcine coronary endothelial cells were subjected to SDS-PAGE (8%) and Western blotting using two different CYP 2C11 polyclonal antibodies (kindly provided by Dr E. Morgan, Atlanta, or purchased from Daiichi Pure Chemicals).

1.3. Materials

All biochemicals were obtained in the highest purity available from Sigma (Deisenhofen, Germany).

1.4. Statistics

Relaxations are given as percentage of the response to U46619. All data in the figures and in the text are expressed as mean ± SEM of n experiments with segments from different arteries. Statistical analysis was performed by one-way analysis of variance (ANOVA) followed by a Bonferroni t-test or by the two-tailed Student's t-test for unpaired data, where appropriate. Differences were considered to be statistically significant when p was less than .05.

2. RESULTS

2.1. Vasodilator responses

In coronary rings constricted with U46619, sodium nitroprusside elicited a concentration-dependent relaxation which was not affected by cortisol treatment (24 h) (Figure 19.1).

During contractions to U46619, bradykinin induced relaxations, which were slightly enhanced in rings exposed to cortisol for 24 h (Figure 19.2). Bradykinin-induced relaxations in the presence of L-NA were markedly enhanced following exposure to cortisol (Figure 19.2). In contrast, during contractions with KCl (30 mM) the bradykinin-induced relaxation was slightly diminished by 24 h incubation with cortisol (Figure 19.2).

Short-term exposure to cortisol (10^{-7} M, 30 min) did not affect relaxations elicited by sodium nitroprusside or bradykinin (Figure 19.3).

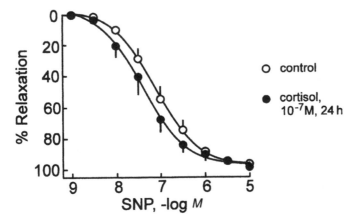

Figure 19.1 Sodium nitroprusside (SNP)-induced relaxations of porcine coronary arteries constricted with the thromboxane mimetic U46619. The rings were incubated for 24 h either with cortisol (10^{-7} M, ●), or with control medium (○). The results are expressed as the mean ± SEM from eight to ten separate experiments.

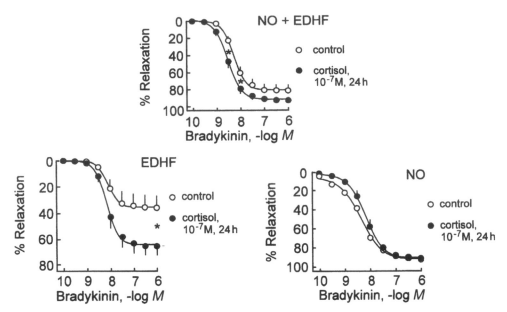

Figure 19.2 Bradykinin-induced relaxations of porcine coronary arteries during contractions to U46619 in control solution (A, NO- plus EDHF-mediated relaxation), in the presence of N^G-nitro-L-arginine (B, EDHF-mediated relaxation) and during constriction with KCl (C, NO-mediated relaxation). The rings were incubated for 24 h either with cortisol (10^{-7} M, ●), or with control medium (○). The results are expressed as the mean ± SEM from eight to ten separate experiments. The asterisk indicates statistically significant differences with control ($p < .05$).

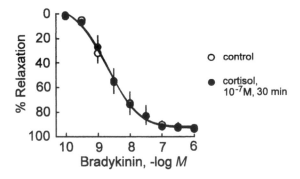

Figure 19.3 Bradykinin-induced, EDHF-mediated relaxation of porcine coronary arteries constricted with the thromboxane mimetic U46619 in the presence of N^G-nitro-L-arginine (3×10^{-4}, 30 min). The rings were either incubated for 30 min with cortisol (10^{-7} M, ●), or with vehicle (○). The results are expressed as the mean ± SEM from six to eight separate experiments.

2.2. Expression of cytochrome P450

Porcine coronary arteries were incubated with cortisol (10^{-7} M) for 18–24 h. Cortisol significantly enhanced the expression of CYP 2C RNA and CYP 2C9 protein (Figure 19.4).

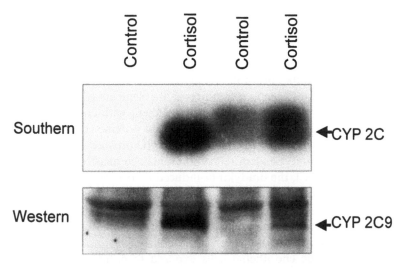

Figure 19.4 Expression of CYP 2C in native porcine coronary artery segments incubated for 18 h either with cortisol (10^{-7} M), or with control medium.

3. DISCUSSION

In response to agonists as well as physical stimuli, endothelial cells from different species and vascular beds release an L-NA/diclofenac insensitive factor which hyperpolarizes and relaxes vascular smooth muscle cells by activating Ca^{2+}-dependent K^+ channels (Nagao and Vanhoutte, 1992; Hecker *et al.*, 1994; Fulton *et al.*, 1994; Zygmunt and Högestätt, 1996). However, there is considerable controversy about the identity of EDHF, and the mechanisms which are involved in the transmission of endothelium-dependent hyperpolarization (for review see Mombouli and Vanhoutte (1997)). The term EDHF comprises more than one factor, since the hyperpolarizing factor released from the guinea pig carotid, and rat mesenteric and hepatic arteries exhibits pharmacological characteristics very different from those of the EDHF in the coronary system (Zygmunt *et al.*, 1996; Corriu *et al.*, 1996; Fukao *et al.*, 1997).

Pharmacological characterization of the EDHF derived from agonist-stimulated porcine coronary endothelium suggests that this factor may be a cytochrome P450-dependent metabolite of arachidonic acid such as an epoxyeicosatrienoic acid (Rubanyi and Vanhoutte, 1987; Rosolowsky and Campbell, 1993; Bauersachs *et al.*, 1994; Fulton *et al.*, 1995; Campbell *et al.*, 1996; Popp *et al.*, 1996, 1998). However, most of the pharmacological cytochrome P450 inhibitors available exert nonselective effects on K_{Ca}^+ channel activity and endothelial Ca^{2+} signaling (Alvarez *et al.*, 1992; Graier *et al.*, 1995). Therefore alternative approaches for the selective inhibition of cytochrome P450 oxygenases have been chosen. Using transfection with antisense oligonucleotides against the coding region of CYP 2C8/9, EDHF-mediated relaxation and hyperpolarization could be markedly attenuated in porcine coronary arteries and in resistance arteries from hamster gracilis muscle, suggesting that this enzyme may be an EDHF synthase (Fisslthaler *et al.*, 1999; Bolz *et al.*, 2000). RT-PCR was used to screen native

porcine coronary artery endothelial cells and cultured human coronary artery endothelial cells. Of the CYP epoxygenases investigated isozymes homologous to 2C8/9
and 2J2 were expressed in both human and porcine coronary artery endothelial cells
(Fisslthaler *et al.*, 2000). Only the globally expressed CYP 2C family fitted the
criteria of an EDHF synthase, since its expression was consistently enhanced by
β-naphthoflavone in all of the endothelial cell types studied (Fisslthaler *et al.*, 1999;
Fisslthaler *et al.*, 2000). As the promotor regions of CYP 2C8 and CYP 2C9
contain consensus sequences for glucocorticoid response elements (Ged and Beaune,
1991; Morais *et al.*, 1993), the effect of long-term treatment with cortisol was determined on the generation of EDHF-mediated responses in porcine coronary arteries.

Long-term incubation with cortisol enhanced NO/prostacyclin-independent
relaxation, while endothelium-independent relaxation remained unaffected. In contrast,
following constriction with KCl, the bradykinin-induced relaxation which is mediated
exclusively by NO was slightly attenuated by cortisol treatment. This effect may be a
consequence of a reduced expression of the endothelial NO synthase, as also observed
in rats with glucocorticoid-induced hypertension after being given dexamethasone for
seven days (Wallerath *et al.*, 1999). However, endothelial NO synthase activity was
not affected in porcine aortic endothelial cells exposed to either cortisol or dexamethasone, which is in contrast to above mentioned findings (Radomski, 1990; Christ
et al., 1999). Furthermore, the bioavailability of NO may be reduced through
enhanced production of reactive oxygen species as has been observed following
up-regulation of CYP 2C8/9 in endothelial cells by β-naphthophlavone or nifedipine
(Fisslthaler *et al.*, chapter 18, this volume).

During contraction to U46619 in the presence of diclofenac, the bradykinin-induced
relaxation is mediated by both NO and EDHF, it is however almost impossible to
quantify the percentage contribution of each autacoid. Since the pure NO-mediated
response was attenuated by cortisol, the slight enhancement of the combined NO/
EDHF-mediated relaxation following exposure to cortisol suggests that the relative
contribution of EDHF to this response in porcine coronary arteries is more important
than that of NO.

The present results indicate that there is a selective up-regulation of EDHF-mediated responses following prolonged treatment with cortisol. Moreover, cortisol
enhanced the expression of CYP 2C mRNA and protein in endothelial cells, an effect
similar to that of nifedipine, which induced a parallel increase in the expression of
cytochrome P450 2C and EDHF-mediated responses (Fisslthaler *et al.*, 2000).
In contrast, the *acute* addition of cortisol to arterial rings in the organ chamber
was without effect on EDHF-mediated relaxation. Steroids possess both genomic
and non-genomic cardiovascular actions (Christ and Wehling, 1998). However,
the lack of acute effects of cortisol on vascular reactivity implies that the increase in
CYP 2C expression is mediated by genomic actions via the glucocorticoid response
elements in the promotor regions of CYP 2C (Ged and Beaune, 1991; Morais *et al.*,
1993).

4. CONCLUSION

The present findings demonstrate the concomitant upregulation of EDHF-mediated
relaxation and CYP 2C8/9 expression by prolonged treatment with cortisol. These

observations support the concept that an epoxygenase homologous to CYP 2C8/9 plays a crucial role in the generation of EDHF-mediated responses in the coronary endothelium.

ACKNOWLEDGEMENTS

The authors wish to thank Claudia Liebetrau for expert technical assistance.

20 An arachidonic acid metabolite(s) produced by the endothelial cytochrome P450 isoform, CYP3A4, relaxes the lingual artery of the monkey via K$^+$ channel opening

K. Ayajiki, H. Fujioka, N. Toda, S. Okada,
Y. Minamiyama, S. Imaoka, Y. Funae
and T. Okamura

In strips of lingual arteries of the monkey, acetylcholine produced endothelium-dependent relaxations which were not or only slightly attenuated by indomethacin, and significantly attenuated by N^G-nitro-L-arginine (L-NA). The response to acetylcholine resistant to L-NA and indomethacin was abolished in the strips exposed to high K$^+$. Glibenclamide, iberiotoxin or apamin alone did not affect the relaxation, but charybdotoxin partially inhibited it, while the remaining relaxation was abolished by additional treatment with apamin. The acetylcholine-induced relaxation resistant to L-NA and indomethacin was inhibited by non-selective cytochrome P450 monoxygenase (CYP) inhibitors (metyrapone, proadifen and 17-octadecynoic acid) and selective CYP3A inhibitors (ketoconazole and progesterone). Selective inhibitors of other CYP isoforms (debrisoquine, lauric acid and sulfaphenazole) did not reduce the response to acetylcholine. Filtrate of the reaction mixture containing human liver microsomes rich in CYPs, arachidonic acid and NADPH incubated at 37 °C relaxed arteries without endothelium, used as bioassay tissues. The relaxation was abolished by high K$^+$, and was suppressed by the combined treatment with charybdotoxin plus apamin, but not with iberiotoxin. Further, the relaxations were markedly inhibited by incubation with ketoconazole, progesterone or anti-CYP3A4 antibody. The presence of CYP3A4 was detected immunohistochemically in the endothelium of the monkey lingual artery. In conclusion, the endothelium-dependent relaxation of the monkey lingual artery is mediated mainly by NO and by a charybdotoxin plus apamin-sensitive calcium-dependent K$^+$ channel opening substance(s) that may be a CYP3A4-derived metabolite(s) of arachidonic acid.

Endogenous relaxing substances derived from the endothelium include endothelium-derived hyperpolarizing factor (EDHF), vasodilator prostanoids (Vanhoutte and Mombouli, 1996) and nitric oxide (NO) (Moncada *et al.*, 1991). EDHF is defined as a substance(s) from the endothelium that hyperpolarizes cell membrane and induces relaxation of smooth muscle. The K$^+$ channel subtypes involved in the EDHF-mediated responses are different depending on the blood vessel, the species and the EDRF-releasing agonist used, suggesting that EDHF is not a single molecule but includes various substances responsible for different modes of action. Although in some blood vessels, NO reportedly acts as a hyperpolarizing factor (Cohen *et al.*,

1997), a considerable amount of data suggests that EDHF is a substance(s) other than NO and prostanoids. Metabolites of arachidonic acid derived from cytochrome P450 monoxygenase (CYP) could be EDHF (Campbell *et al.*, 1996; Fisslthaler *et al.*, 1999). However, EDHF(s) is not an epoxyeicosatrienoic acid (Chataigeau *et al.*, 1998; Eckman *et al.*, 1998). Although K^+ (Edwards *et al.*, 1998) and endogenous cannabinoids may contribute to EDHF-mediated responses, this hypothesis is not generally accepted (Hecker, 2000; Mombouli and Vanhoutte, 1997). Therefore, the identity of EDHF appears to differ among vascular beds and animal species.

Since little information is available about EDHF in primate arteries, various isolated arteries of the monkey were screened and the lingual arteries were found to respond to acetylcholine with endothelium-dependent relaxations mediated in part by a substance other than NO and prostanoids. The present study therefore aimed to determine the mechanisms of action of acetylcholine, with reference to K^+ channels, to analyze the nature of substance(s) liberated from the endothelium using inhibitors of CYP isoforms and to elucidate whether or not human liver microsomes rich in CYPs can synthesize a vasodilator substance(s) that is responsible for K^+ channel opening.

1. MECHANICAL RESPONSES

1.1. Acetylcholine-induced relaxation sensitive to indomethacin or L-NA

Japanese monkeys were killed by exanguination from the common carotid arteries under deep anesthesia. The tongue was removed rapidly. The deep lingual artery was isolated and cut into helical strips, taking special care to preserve the endothelium. The strips were suspended vertically between hooks in a muscle chamber containing a modified Ringer–Locke solution, maintained at $37 \pm 0.3\,^\circ$C and aerated with a mixture of 95% O_2 and 5% CO_2. Isometric contractions and relaxations were displayed on an ink-writing oscillograph. The integrity of endothelial function was determined by a relaxant response to 10^{-7} M of Ca^{2+} ionophore A23187.

In strips contracted with prostaglandin $F_{2\alpha}$ ($10^{-7}-10^{-6}$ M), the addition of acetylcholine ($10^{-8}-10^{-5}$ M) induced a concentration-related relaxation. Mechanical removal of the endothelium abolished the response but did not inhibit the relaxation caused by sodium nitroprusside (Ayajiki *et al.*, 1999). Treatment with indomethacin (10^{-6} M) did not, or only slightly reduced the acetylcholine-induced relaxation. In strips treated with indomethacin, acetylcholine-induced relaxations were attenuated by treatment with L-NA (10^{-5} M), and L-arginine (10^{-3} M) reversed the inhibition. Two-(4-carboxyphenyl)-4,4,5,5-tetramethylimidazole-1-oxyl 3-oxide, sodium salt (carboxy PTIO, 3×10^{-4} M), a NO-scavenger (Akaike *et al.*, 1993), failed to inhibit further the response to acetylcholine in strips treated with 10^{-4} M L-NA- and 10^{-6} M indomethacin (Ayajiki *et al.*, 1999). These findings indicate that the monkey lingual arteries respond to acetylcholine with concentration-dependent relaxations only when the endothelium is intact. The response caused by acetylcholine was mediated minimally by prostacyclin and moderately by NO. However, large magnitude of the acetylcholine-induced relaxation was observed under combined treatment with indomethacin and L-NA, indicating that it is due to the release of endothelium-derived hyperpolarizing factor (EDHF).

1.2. Acetylcholine-induced relaxation resistant to L-NA and indomethacin

In the L-NA- and indomethacin-treated strips, acetylcholine-induced relaxations were abolished by exposure to high K^+ solutions (2×10^{-2} M in final), but were not affected by treatment with glibenclamide (10^{-6} M), an ATP-sensitive K^+ channel inhibitor. Treatment with iberiotoxin (10^{-7} M) or apamin (10^{-6} M) alone failed to inhibit the response, which was attenuated significantly by charybdotoxin (3×10^{-8} M). The charybdotoxin-resistant relaxation was abolished by additional treatment with apamin (10^{-6} M). Sodium nitroprusside-induced relaxations and the basal tone were not affected by the K^+ channel inhibitors used (Ayajiki *et al.*, 1999). These findings suggest that the relaxation caused by acetylcholine is due to activation of calcium-dependent K^+ channels with small or intermediate conductance, but not with large conductance. A similar profile has also been reported for the acetylcholine-induced relaxations of rabbit coronary arteries (Dong *et al.*, 1997), and rat hepatic arteries (Zygmunt *et al.*, 1997).

In addition, metyrapone (10^{-3} M) and proadifen (10^{-5} M) (Ayajiki *et al.*, 1999), and 17-octadecynoic acid (3×10^{-6} M) (Figure 20.1), non-specific inhibitors of cytochrome P450, almost abolished the relaxation induced by acetylcholine. Neither lauric acid (10^{-6} and 10^{-5} M), an inhibitor of CYP4A1 (Lawson *et al.*, 1991), nor debrisoquine (10^{-6} and 10^{-5} M), an inhibitor of CYP2D6 (Marre *et al.*, 1992), affected the response to acetylcholine (Ayajiki *et al.*, 1999). Sulfaphenazole, an inhibitor of CYP2C (Fisslthaler *et al.*, 1999), did not affect the response either (Figure 20.1). Treatment with ketoconazole (10^{-5} M) (Ayajiki *et al.*, 1999) and progesterone (10^{-5} M), selective inhibitors of CYP3A family (Maurice *et al.*, 1992; Jang *et al.*, 1996; Waxman *et al.*, 1991), significantly impaired the actions of acetylcholine (Figure 20.1). The concentrations of these CYP3A inhibitors are reportedly ineffective on calcium-dependent K^+ channel function (Ishii *et al.*, 1997). Sodium nitroprusside-induced

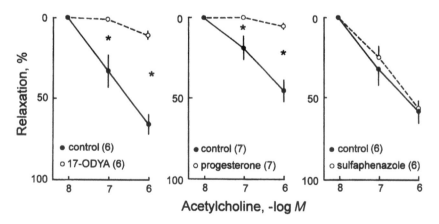

Figure 20.1 Modifications by 17-octadecynoic acid (17-ODYA, 3×10^{-6} M), progesterone (10^{-5} M) and sulfaphenazole (10^{-5} M) of relaxations induced by acetylcholine in monkey lingual arteries with intact endothelium (E+) in the presence of indomethacin (10^{-6} M) and N^G-nitro-L-arginine (10^{-4} M). Numbers in parenthesis indicate the number of strips from individual monkeys. Data shown as means ± SEM. The asterisks indicate statistisically significant differences from control (Student's *t*-test for unpaired obsevations; $p < .05$).

relaxations and the basal tone were not affected by the cytochrome P450 inhibitors used. These findings indicate that, as far as monkey lingual arteries are concerned, CYP3A is responsible for the production of the endothelium-derived vasodilator substance which opens K^+ channels. Metabolites of arachidonic acid produced by cytochrome P450 may be candidates for EDHF, since relaxations caused by brady-kinin of swine coronary arteries treated with L-NA are inhibited by apamin and proadifen, and an epoxide, an arachidonate metabolite produced by cytochrome P450, is involved in the response (Hecker *et al.*, 1994). CYP2C may be an EDHF-synthase in swine coronary artery (Fisslthaler *et al.*, 1999). However, this is not the case for the monkey lingual artery, since the CYP2C inhibitor, sulfaphenazole, did not affect the acetylcholine-induced relaxation resistant to inhibitors of NO synthase and cyclooxygenase. Therefore, CYP isozymes responsible for EDHF production may differ among species.

1.3. Anandamide and K^+

Anandamide (10^{-6} M), in a concentration sufficient to produce relaxation in rat isolated mesenteric arteries (White and Hiley, 1997; Plane *et al.*, 1997), did not change arterial tone, and relaxations induced at a ten times higher concentration were clearly slower than those caused by an equipotent concentration (10^{-8} M) of acetylcholine. Therefore, this substance does not seem to be involved in the endothelium-dependent, L-NA-resistant relaxation in monkey lingual arteries (Ayajiki *et al.*, 1999).

In the rat hepatic artery, EDHF may be K^+ released from endothelial cells through charybdotoxin- and apamin-sensitive K^+ channels, whereby the increase in myoendo-thelial K^+ concentration hyperpolarizes and relaxes adjacent smooth muscle cells by activating Ba^{2+}-sensitive K^+ channels and Na^+/K^+-ATPase (Edwards *et al.*, 1998). However, this is not the case for the monkey lingual artery because the addition of 5×10^{-3} M K^+ contracted the artery without endothelium treated with L-NA and indomethacin. The same concentration of K^+ induces relaxations in cerebral arteries (Toda, 1974).

2. BIOASSAY OF PRODUCTS OF CYTOCHROME P450

A cytochrome P450-rich microsome fraction from the human liver was prepared (Imaoka *et al.*, 1990). Briefly, 0.25 ml of reaction mixture containing human liver microsomes (200 µg protein), 8×10^{-4} M reduced form of nicotinamide-adenine di-nucleotide phosphate (NADPH) and 10^{-5} M arachidonic acid in 5×10^{-2} M sodium phosphate buffer (pH 7.5) was incubated at 37 °C for 30 min. After incubation with or without ketoconazole (10^{-5} M), progesterone (10^{-5} M), or anti-CYP3A4 antibody (1:1, 15 µl), the reaction mixture was filtered with microcon 30 (Amicon, Inc., Beverly, MA, USA), and 50 µl of the filtrate was used for bioassay. The anti-CYP3A4 antibody at the concentration used inhibits testosterone hydroxylation by CYP3A4 more than 80%. The filtrate was applied directly to the bathing media (10 ml) and the mechanical response was obtained in lingual arterial strips without endothelium treated with indomethacin (10^{-6} M) and L-NA (10^{-4} M) and contracted with prostaglandin $F_{2\alpha}$ (10^{-7}–10^{-6} M). The filtered reaction mixture, when applied to the L-NA- and in-domethacin-treated lingual arterial strips without endothelium, used as a bioassay tissue, elicited relaxation whereas acetylcholine did not change arterial tone. Removal of NADPH or the enzyme preparation from the mixture abolished the ability of the filtrate to relax the bioassay tissue. The relaxations were abolished in the strips exposed to high K^+ solution. Combined treatment of the assay tissue with charybdotoxin (3×10^{-8} M) plus apamin (10^{-6} M) suppressed the relaxation, while treatment with iberiotoxin (10^{-7} M) did not influence the response (Ayajiki et al., 1999). The relaxations induced by the reaction mixture were almost abolished by incubation with ketoconazole (10^{-5} M; final concentration in the organ bath, 5×10^{-8} M) (Figure 20.2), or progesterone (10^{-5} M), ($18.2 \pm 2.8\%$ relaxation without treatment versus $1.9 \pm 1.3\%$ relaxation under treatment with 10^{-5} M progesterone, $n = 6$, $p < .05$, unpaired t-test). These findings indicate that the relaxation could be induced by CYP3A products responsible for calcium-dependent K^+ channel opening, and that the same occurs during acetylcholine-induced relaxation in the arteries with endothelium. This hypothesis is supported by the finding that incubation with specific antibodies raised against purified human liver CYP3A4 (Imaoka et al., 1996) inhibits the relaxations induced by the filtered media.

Epoxyeicosatrienoic acids, CYP products, may be EDHFs in bovine coronary arteries stimulated by methacholine (Campbell et al., 1996), and 11,12-epoxyeicosatrienoic acid in swine coronary arteries (Fisslthaler et al., 1999). Responses to the epoxides were not tested in the present study. However, 11,12-epoxyeicosatrienoic

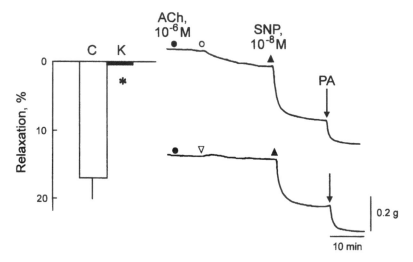

Figure 20.2 Summary data (left panel, $n = 6$) and original recording (right) of the responses to products of cytochrome P450 of monkey lingual arteries without endothelium in the presence of indomethacin (10^{-6} M) and N^G-nitro-L-arginine (10^{-4} M) as affected by treatment of the reaction mixture with ketoconazole (K, 10^{-5} M). Left panel: The ordinate denotes relaxations relative to those induced by papaverine (PA, 10^{-4} M). 'C' denotes the response to the reaction mixture with full components (liver microsomes as enzyme preparation, arachidonic acid and NADPH). Right panel: ACh ●, acetylcholine (10^{-6} M); ○, products of cytochrome P450; ▽, products of cytochrome P450 incubated with ketoconazole (10^{-5} M); SNP ▲, sodium nitroprusside (10^{-8} M). Data shown as means $\pm$ SEM. The asterisks indicate statistisically significant differences from control (Student's t-test for unpaired obsevations; $p < .05$).

acid-induced relaxation is inhibited by iberiotoxin in the guinea-pig coronary artery (Eckman *et al.*, 1998). Since the relaxation induced by products of cytochrome P450 in the monkey lingual artery is not sensitive to iberiotoxin, it is unlikely that 11,12-epoxyeicosatrienoic acid is EDHF in monkey arteries.

3. HISTOCHEMICAL STUDY

Using an immunohistochemical technique (Minamiyama *et al.*, 1999), the presence of CYP3A4 was examined in monkey lingual arteries. A CYP3A4-specific antibody, but not the preimmune serum, gave positive stainings of the endothelial cells together with smooth muscle cells of the artery.

4. CONCLUSION

An endothelium-derived vasodilator substance(s) other than NO and prostanoids appears to be a CYP3A4-product(s) other than 11,12-epoxyeicosatrienoic acid. This

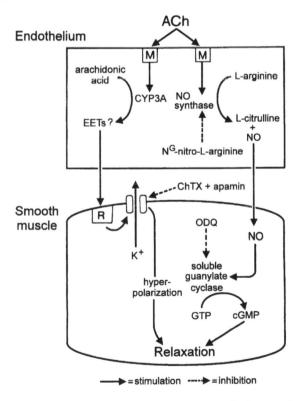

Figure 20.3 Schematic representation of the mechanisms underlying the relaxation induced by acetylcholine in monkey lingual arteries with intact endothelium. ACh, acetylcholine; M, muscarinic receptor; EETs, epoxyeicosatrienoic acids; NO, nitric oxide; CYP3A, cytochrome P450 3A subtype; ChTX, charybdotoxin; R, postulated receptor of CYP3A product(s) from arachidonic acid; ODQ, 1H[1,2,4]oxadiazolo[4,3-a]quinoxalin-1one; cGMP, cyclic GMP, cyclic GMP.

metabolite(s) of arachidonic acid opens the charybdotoxin- and apamin-sensitive calcium-dependent K^+ channels with small or intermediate conductance on the smooth muscle, resulting in relaxation. Monkey lingual arteries are expected to relax in response to acetylcholine mainly by the release of NO and the CYP3A4-derived arachidonic acid metabolite(s) from the endothelium (Figure 20.3).

21 EDHF-mediated responses induced by bradykinin in the porcine coronary artery

T. Chataigneau, Ingrid Fleming and Rudi Busse

Hyperpolarization and relaxation mediated by endothelium-derived hyperpolarizing factor (EDHF) in the porcine coronary artery involve a cytochrome P450-epoxygenase-derived metabolite. To further characterize the cellular mechanisms underlying EDHF-mediated hyperpolarization and relaxation of the porcine coronary artery, the effects of inhibitors of cytochrome P450-epoxygenase enzymes, potassium channels and gap junctional communication were compared. Sulfaphenazole, a selective cytochrome P450 2C9 inhibitor, attenuated EDHF-mediated hyperpolarizations and relaxations. In the presence of Δ^9-tetrahydrocannabinol, previously reported to inhibit EDHF production, both EDHF-mediated responses were also blocked to the same extent. The combination of barium plus ouabain had no effect on EDHF-mediated hyperpolarization, but the combination of charybdotoxin plus apamin abolished both the EDHF-mediated hyperpolarization and relaxation. Iberiotoxin, an inhibitor of large conductance Ca^{2+}-dependent K^+ channels, and 18α-glycyrrhetinic acid, a gap junction uncoupling agent, failed to significantly affect EDHF-mediated responses in bicarbonate-buffered physiological salt solution, but inhibited those recorded in bicarbonate-free solution. These results confirm the crucial role of products of cytochrome P450-epoxygenase in EDHF-mediated responses in the porcine coronary artery. They also indicate that the Na^+/K^+ ATPase, inwardly rectifying potassium channels and gap junctional communication play little or no role in mediating these responses. Moreover, EDHF-mediated hyperpolarization can be rendered sensitive to iberiotoxin and 18α-glycyrrhetinic acid by the removal of extracellular bicarbonate.

The production of vasoactive substances such as nitric oxide (NO; Furchgott and Zawadzki, 1980; Palmer *et al.*, 1987), prostacyclin (Moncada and Vane, 1979) and endothelium-derived hyperpolarizing factor (EDHF; Chen *et al.*, 1988; Félétou and Vanhoutte, 1988; Huang *et al.*, 1988; Taylor and Weston, 1988) by endothelial cells contributes to the local regulation of vascular tone. EDHF-mediated hyperpolarizations and relaxations of the porcine coronary artery depend on the generation of a cytochrome P450-epoxygenase-derived product, most probably an epoxyeicosatrienoic acid (EET) (Popp *et al.*, 1996; Fisslthaler *et al.*, 1999, 2000). Although experiments using superfusion bioassay models demonstrate that the cytochrome P450-epoxygenase-derived EDHF can exist as a distinct and transferable factor (Popp *et al.*, 1996; Gebremedhin *et al.*, 1998), the intercellular transfer of EDHF or the vascular effects of EDHF may require functional gap junctional communication. Gap junction uncoupling agents inhibit EDHF-mediated hyperpolarization and relaxation in several vascular beds (Chaytor *et al.*, 1998; Taylor *et al.*, 1998; Dora *et al.*, 1999; Edwards *et al.*, 1999a; Fukuta *et al.*, 1999), suggesting that an active intercellular communication is a prerequisite for at least some EDHF-mediated responses. Therefore, the effects of a gap junction inhibitor, 18α-glycyrrhetinic acid, were investigated on the bradykinin-induced hyperpolarization and relaxation of the porcine coronary arteries. The effects of potassium channel blockers as well as those of Δ^9-tetrahydrocannabinol, a cannabinoid CB_1 receptor agonist, were investigated also.

1. MATERIALS AND METHODS

1.1. Preparations

Porcine hearts were obtained from a local slaughterhouse and placed into ice-cold HEPES-Tyrode of the following composition (in mM): NaCl 137, KCl 2.7, $CaCl_2$ 1.8, $MgCl_2$ 0.5, NaH_2PO_4 0.36, HEPES 10, glucose 5 (pH 7.4, 4 °C) during the transport to the laboratory. Thereafter, the coronary epicardial arteries (about 50 mm length, about 2.5 mm mean external diameter) were excised, cleaned of adherent fat and connective tissues, and stored at 4 °C until use.

1.2. Intracellular microelectrodes

Segments of porcine coronary arteries were slit open longitudinally, pinned to the sylgard base of a heated organ chamber with the intimal side upward, then superfused (5 ml/min) with HEPES-Tyrode solution.

The membrane potential of smooth muscle cells was recorded with glass capillary microelectrodes (tip resistance of 80–120 MΩ) filled with KCl (3 M) and connected to the headstage of a high impedance amplifier (intra 767, WPI). The reference electrode (Dri-Ref reference electrodes, WPI), also filled with KCl, but exhibiting low electrolyte leakage and immersed into the bathing solution, was directly connected to the amplifier. The signal was continuously monitored on an oscilloscope and simultaneously recorded on paper. Impalement of smooth muscle cells was performed from the intimal side. Successful impalements were indicated by a sudden negative drop in potential from the baseline (zero potential reference) followed by a stable negative potential for at least 2 min. Bradykinin and cromakalim were applied as bolus injections into the organ chamber to obtain the required concentration.

In some experiments, segments were superfused with a modified Tyrode's solution of the following composition (in mM): NaCl 132, KCl 4, $CaCl_2$ 1.6, $MgCl_2$ 1.2, NaH_2PO_4 0.36, $NaHCO_3$ 23.8, Ca^{2+}-EDTA 0.05, glucose 10 (aerated with a gas mixture of 75% N_2/20% O_2/5% CO_2, PO_2 140 mmHg, PCO_2 38–40 mmHg, pH 7.4).

All experiments were performed in the presence of N^ω-nitro-L-arginine (3×10^{-4} M), diclofenac (10^{-5} M) and U46619 (10^{-6} M). The preparations were superfused for at least 45 min prior to measuring membrane potential.

1.3. Vascular reactivity

Rings were suspended in organ chambers for the measurement of isometric force. Experiments were performed in Krebs–Henseleit solution of the following composition (in mM): NaCl 119, KCl 4.7, $CaCl_2$ 1.6, $MgSO_4$ 1.2, KH_2PO_4 1.2, $NaHCO_3$ 25, Ca^{2+}-EDTA 0.026, glucose 12 (gassed with 95% O_2/5% CO_2, pH 7.4). The passive tension was adjusted to 5 g. Thereafter, the rings were repeatedly exposed to a high KCl (80 mM) Krebs–Henseleit solution until stable contractions were obtained. After washing, the rings were contracted using U46619 (10^{-7}–10^{-6} M) to approximately 80% of the maximal response to KCl and concentration–response curves were obtained in response to cumulative concentrations of bradykinin (10^{-10}–3×10^{-6} M).

All experiments were performed in the presence of N^{ω}-nitro-L-arginine (3×10^{-4} M) and diclofenac (10^{-5} M).

1.4. Drugs

N^{ω}-nitro-L-arginine, diclofenac; sulfaphenazole, Δ^9-tetrahydrocannabinol; 18α-glycyr-rhetinic acid; ouabain and apamin were purchased from Sigma-Aldrich (Steinheim, Germany). Bradykinin, charybdotoxin, and iberiotoxin were provided by Bachem Biochemica GmbH (Heidelberg, Germany). N-2-hydroxyethylpiperazine-N'-2-ethanesulphonic acid (HEPES) was from SERVA (Heidelberg, Germany). U46619 (9,11-dideoxy-11α,9α-epoxymethano-prostaglandin $F_{2\alpha}$) was obtained from Upjohn (Ann Arbor, MI, USA). Barium (Ba^{2+}) was from Merck (Darmstadt, Germany). Cromakalim was a generous gift from Aventis (Frankfurt am Main, Germany).

1.5. Statistical analysis

Data are shown as means $\pm$ SEM; n indicates the number of vascular segments (animals) examined. Statistical analysis was performed using Student's t-test for paired or unpaired observations. Differences were considered to be statistically significant when p was less than .05.

2. RESULTS

2.1. P450 inhibitor and cannabinoid CB$_1$ receptor agonist

In isolated segments of porcine coronary arteries, bradykinin (10^{-6} M) induced an endothelium-dependent hyperpolarization which was inhibited significantly by the selective cytochrome P450 2C9 inhibitor sulfaphenazole (10^{-5} M; -16.5 ± 2.9 mV in control versus -6.9 ± 2.3 mV in the presence of sulfaphenazole, $n = 7$–11). In isolated rings, bradykinin (10^{-9}–3×10^{-6} M) elicited concentration-dependent relaxations which were attenuated significantly in the presence of sulfaphenazole (10^{-5} M; maximal relaxation, R_{max}: $75 \pm 6\%$ in control versus $30 \pm 6\%$ in sulfaphenazole-treated rings, $n = 6$).

Δ^9-tetrahydrocannabinol (3×10^{-5} M), a cannabinoid CB$_1$ receptor agonist, significantly inhibited the bradykinin-induced hyperpolarization and almost abolished the bradykinin-induced relaxation (Figure 21.1).

2.2. Potassium channel blockers and Na$^+$/K$^+$ ATPase-inhibitor

Exposure to Ba^{2+} (3×10^{-5} M) and ouabain (10^{-6} M), to inhibit inwardly rectifying K^+ channels and Na$^+$/K$^+$ ATPase, respectively, induced a significant depolarization of the smooth muscle cells (resting membrane potential: -47.2 ± 2.4 mV and -34.5 ± 1.3 mV, in the absence and presence of the inhibitors, respectively, $n = 4$–6). Ba^{2+} and ouabain did not affect significantly the bradykinin-induced, EDHF-mediated

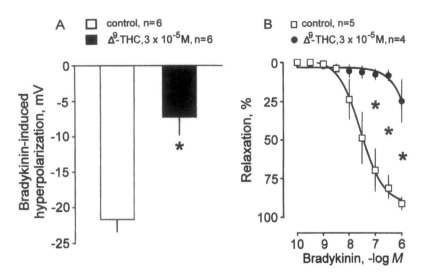

Figure 21.1 Effects of the CB_1 receptor agonist Δ^9-tetrahydrocannabinol (Δ^9-THC, 3×10^{-5} M) on bradykinin (BK)-induced hyperpolarization (A, bargraph, 10^{-6} M BK, HEPES-Tyrode) and relaxation (B, concentration–relaxation curves, Krebs–Henseleit), in the presence of N^ω-nitro-L-arginine (3×10^{-4} M), diclofenac (10^{-5} M) and U46619 (10^{-7}–10^{-6} M). Data are shown as means ± SEM. The asterisks indicate stastically significant ($p < .05$) differences from control.

hyperpolarization of the porcine coronary artery (Figure 21.2). The bradykinin-induced, EDHF-mediated hyperpolarization was nearly abolished in the combined presence of charybdotoxin (10^{-7} M) plus apamin (10^{-7} M; -21.5 ± 1.7 mV in control versus -3.5 ± 1.3 mV in the presence of the two toxins, $n = 5$). The combination of charybdotoxin plus apamin abolished the bradykinin-induced, EDHF-mediated relaxation (R_{max}: $63 \pm 7\%$ in control versus $2 \pm 1\%$ in the presence of charybdotoxin and apamin, $n = 7$).

The effect of iberiotoxin, an inhibitor of large conductance calcium-dependent potassium channels (BK_{Ca}) on the bradykinin-induced, EDHF-mediated hyperpolarization was investigated in two different physiological salt solutions (Figure 21.3). When the vascular segments were superfused with HEPES-Tyrode, iberiotoxin (10^{-8} or 10^{-7} M for at least 60 min) did not significantly modify the resting smooth muscle membrane potential. Under these experimental conditions, the bradykinin (10^{-6} M)-induced hyperpolarization was not altered significantly by 10^{-8} M iberiotoxin (-18.7 ± 2.8 mV in control versus -19.3 ± 5.7 mV in iberiotoxin-treated segments, $n = 3$) but was abolished by 10^{-7} M of the toxin (-21.8 ± 2.1 mV in control versus -0.4 ± 3.0 mV iberiotoxin-treated segments, $n = 5$). In contrast, in modified Tyrode's solution, iberiotoxin (10^{-7} M) slightly depolarized the smooth muscle cells (resting membrane potential: -46.8 ± 4.3 mV and -38.0 ± 2.4 mV, in the absence and presence of iberiotoxin, respectively, $n = 5$), and slightly but not significantly reduced the bradykinin-induced hyperpolarization (-23.4 ± 3.1 mV and -12.8 ± 3.7 mV, in the absence and presence of iberiotoxin, respectively, $n = 5$).

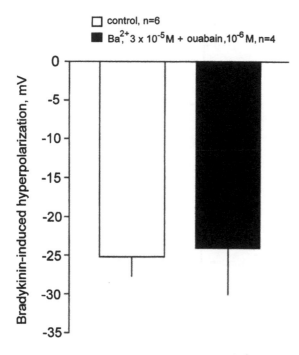

Figure 21.2 Effect of the combination of Ba^{2+} (3×10^{-5} M) and ouabain (10^{-6} M) on the bradykinin (BK, 10^{-6} M)-induced hyperpolarization (bargraph, HEPES-Tyrode) in porcine coronary arteries, in the presence of N^{ω}-nitro-L-arginine (3×10^{-4} M), diclofenac (10^{-5} M) and U46619 (10^{-6} M). Data are shown as means $\pm$ SEM. The combination of Ba^{2+} plus ouabain had no statistically significant effect.

2.3. Gap junction inhibitor

18α-glycyrrhetinic acid (10^{-4} M) significantly inhibited the bradykinin-induced hyperpolarization recorded in HEPES-Tyrode (Figure 21.4) without altering that induced by cromakalim (-26.5 ± 4.3 mV and -27.8 ± 3.6 mV, in the absence and presence of 18α-glycyrrhetinic, respectively, $n = 4$). However, in Krebs–Henseleit solution, the bradykinin-induced hyperpolarization was not modified by 18α-glycyr-rhetinic acid (Figure 21.4). The EDHF-mediated relaxation to bradykinin was not affected significantly by 18α-glycyrrhetinic acid (R_{max}: $88 \pm 2\%$ and $84 \pm 4\%$ and pD_2: 7.93 ± 0.08 and 7.42 ± 0.19, in the absence and presence of 18α-glycyrrhetinic, respectively, $n = 5$).

3. DISCUSSION

The results of the present study further highlight the role of products of cytochrome P450 in EDHF-mediated responses. They imply that inwardly rectifying potassium channels and Na^+/K^+ ATPase do not mediate the bradykinin-induced hyperpolarization of the porcine coronary artery. Furthermore, functional gap junctional communications do not seem to be a prerequisite for EDHF-mediated relaxation in this artery.

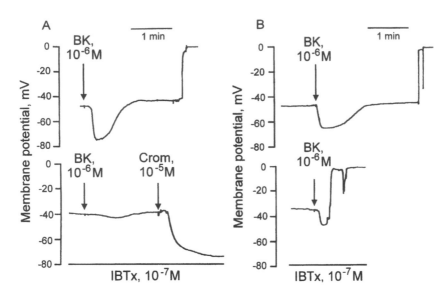

Figure 21.3 Original recordings illustrating the effect of iberiotoxin (IBTx, 10^{-7} M), blocker of the large conductance calcium-activated potassium channel, on bradykinin (BK, 10^{-6} M)-induced hyperpolarization of the porcine coronary artery in HEPES-Tyrode (A) and modified Tyrode (B), in the presence of N^ω-nitro-L-arginine (3×10^{-4} M), diclofenac (10^{-5} M) and U46619 (10^{-6} M). The control recordings are shown in the upper panels and the tracings recorded in the presence of iberiotoxin are shown in the lower panels. EDHF-mediated hyperpolarization was abolished by 10^{-7} M iberiotoxin in HEPES-Tyrode whereas cromakalim (Crom, 10^{-5} M) was still able to induce a complete hyperpolarization. In contrast, iberiotoxin did not significantly alter the EDHF-mediated hyperpolarization recorded in modified Tyrode, a bicarbonate-buffered physiological salt solution.

In accordance with the previous conclusion that an epoxygenase of the cytochrome P450 2C family fulfills certain characteristics of an EDHF synthase, sulfaphenazole, a selective CYP 2C9 inhibitor, attenuated bradykinin-induced, EDHF-mediated hyperpolarizations and relaxations (Popp *et al.*, 1996; Fisslthaler *et al.*, 1999, 2000). These results further highlight the central role of a cytochrome P450-epoxygenase-derived metabolite in the generation of EDHF-mediated responses in the porcine coronary artery. EDHF-mediated hyperpolarization and relaxation were also inhibited by the cannabinoid receptor agonist, Δ^9-tetrahydrocannabinol, an effect which is best explained by an inhibition of the production and/or the action of EDHF and may be related to a modulation of phospholipase A_2 activity (Evans *et al.*, 1987), a process which may deplete cytochrome P450-epoxygenase of substrate.

Given that a cytochrome P450 enzyme appears to play a central role in the generation of EDHF-mediated responses, products of cytochrome P450, such as 5,6-, 8,9- or 11,12-EET may act directly as an EDHF. Indeed, the exogenous application of EETs to isolated arteries elicits both hyperpolarization and relaxation of vascular smooth muscle and thus vasodilatation (Campbell *et al.*, 1996; Oltman *et al.*, 1998); these responses were inhibited by iberiotoxin. While EDHF-like, iberiotoxin-sensitive responses have been described (Nishikawa *et al.*, 1999; Huang *et al.*, 2000), in almost

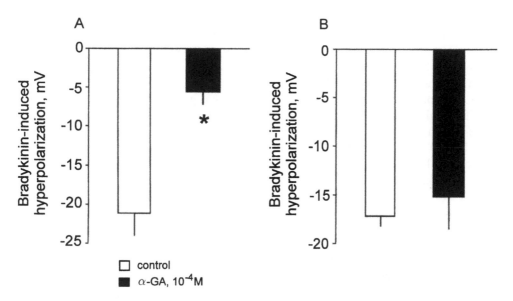

Figure 21.4 Effects of the gap junction inhibitor 18α-glycyrrhetinic acid (α-GA, 10^{-4} M) on bradykinin (BK, 10^{-6} M)-induced hyperpolarization in HEPES-Tyrode (A) and Krebs–Henseleit (B), in the presence of N^{ω}-nitro-L-arginine (3×10^{-4} M), diclofenac (10^{-5} M) and U46619 (10^{-6} M). Data are shown as means ± SEM ($n = 6$–9). The asterisks indicate stastically significant ($p < .05$) differences from control.

all vascular preparations studied to date, EDHF-mediated responses are abolished by the combination of charybdotoxin plus apamin and are unaffected by BK_{Ca} inhibitors such as iberiotoxin. Exactly how the combination of charybdotoxin plus apamin inhibits EDHF-induced hyperpolarizations and relaxations is unclear. However, charybdotoxin and apamin likely act on endothelial cells (Edwards *et al.*, 1998, 2000; Doughty *et al.*, 1999; Ohashi *et al.*, 1999; Quignard *et al.*, 2000) which implies that hyperpolarization of the endothelial cells, supposedly due to the activation of intermediate- and small-conductance calcium-activated potassium channels (IK_{Ca} and SK_{Ca}, respectively), is a prerequisite for that of the vascular smooth muscle cells (Edwards *et al.*, 1999b; Andersson *et al.*, 2000). In the present study, iberiotoxin inhibited the EDHF-mediated hyperpolarization of coronary artery smooth muscle cells, but only when tissues were maintained in a bicarbonate-free buffer. No significant inhibition of hyperpolarization was recorded in bicarbonate-buffered physiological salt solution. These observations imply that the activation of BK_{Ca} is not an essential component of the EDHF-induced hyperpolarization of the porcine coronary artery, but that these channels can be activated and can contribute to EDHF-mediated hyperpolarization, under certain conditions.

In response to agonists, K^+ ions may leave the endothelial cells through K_{Ca} channels and accumulate in the myoendothelial space in a concentration sufficient to activate inwardly rectifying potassium channels and Na^+/K^+ ATPase in smooth muscle cells. K^+ may represent EDHF in rat hepatic and mesenteric arteries (Edwards *et al.*, 1998, 1999b). However, the EDHF generated in the porcine coronary artery is different in that the EDHF-mediated hyperpolarization in this artery is insensitive to the combination of Ba^{2+} plus ouabain. These findings confirm that the activation of inwardly rectifying potassium channels and/or the Na^+/K^+ ATPase are not an integral component of EDHF-mediated hyperpolarization of vascular smooth muscle in this artery (Quignard *et al.*, 1999; Edwards *et al.*, 2000).

Functional gap junctional communication between endothelial and smooth muscle cells may be essential for EDHF-mediated responses (Chaytor *et al.*, 1998; Dora *et al.*, 1999). This proposal is based on the observation that gap junction uncoupling agents inhibit the nitric oxide and prostaglandin-independent relaxation in several arteries. In the present study, the gap junction uncoupler 18α-glycyrrhetinic acid, almost abolished EDHF-mediated hyperpolarization in the absence of bicarbonate. Under more physiological conditions, in the presence of the latter, 18α-glycyrrhetinic acid did not affect bradykinin-induced, EDHF-mediated hyperpolarizations and relaxations of the porcine coronary artery, suggesting that myoendothelial and/or homocellular gap junctional communication does not play a major role in EDHF-mediated responses in this blood vessel. These results contrast with the fact that 18α-glycyrrhetinic acid inhibits EDHF-mediated relaxations of the iliac artery and jugular vein of the rabbit (Taylor *et al.*, 1998; Griffith and Taylor, 1999) and the EDHF-mediated dilatation of the rat mesenteric artery (Doughty *et al.*, 2000). However, all of EDHF-mediated responses recorded in the arteries listed above are insensitive to inhibitors of cytochrome P450, and thus the EDHF in these arteries markedly differs from cytochrome P450-derived EDHF.

4. CONCLUSION

Taken together, the present results confirm that, in the porcine coronary artery, bradykinin-induced, EDHF-mediated hyperpolarizations and relaxations are dependent on the activity of cytochrome P450. No evidence was obtained to suggest that either inwardly rectifying potassium channels, Na^+/K^+ ATPase or active homo-/hetero-cellular gap junctional communication modulate EDHF-mediated responses in this artery.

A novel aspect of the present study is the differential sensitivity of EDHF-mediated responses to pharmacological inhibitors in the presence and absence of bicarbonate. The critical cellular mechanism which renders EDHF-mediated hyperpolarization sensitive to 18α-glycyrrhetinic acid and iberiotoxin in the absence of bicarbonate is unknown. Factors that may be activated differentially under the two conditions include differences in intracellular pH, the activity of chloride channels or the existence of as yet unidentified K^+ channels.

22 Epoxyeicosatrienoic acid release mediates nitric oxide-independent dilatation of rat mesenteric vessels

*Ayotunde S.O. Adeagbo, Adebayo O. Oyekan,
Irving G. Joshua, K. Cameron Falkner,
Russell A. Prough and William M. Pierce Jr.*

The vasodilatation of the isolated, perfused mesenteric bed of the rat to acetylcholine is mostly independent of nitric oxide and prostanoids. This nitric oxide-/prostanoid-independent vasodilatation is blocked by inhibitors of Ca^{2+}-activated potassium channels and thus presumably is mediated by endothelium-derived hyperpolarizing factor (EDHF). The hypothesis was tested that epoxyeicosatrienoic acid (EET), is the EDHF responsible. Vascular responses to acetylcholine were studied in isolated mesenteric beds perfused with physiological salt solutions containing N^ω-nitro-L-arginine methyl ester and indomethacin to block the synthesis of nitric oxide and prostanoids, respectively. The following were determined: (a) NADPH-dependent metabolism of radio-labeled arachidonic acid in homogenates of, and microsomes from, mesenteric blood vessels by a reverse-phase high performance liquid chromatography (HPLC); (b) EET release from the mesenteric vascular bed by an HPLC-coupled, electrospray ionization tandem mass spectrometry (HPLC-MS-MS). Acetylcholine elicited dilatation of the mesenteric vascular bed accompanied by release of ^{14}[C]-arachidonic acid (after labeling) during constrictions caused by an α_1-adrenoceptor agonist. Both effects of acetylcholine were blocked by compounds $AACOCF_3$ and U73122, inhibitors of phospholipase A_2 and C, respectively. Vascular homogenates, or microsomes converted ^{14}[C]-arachidonic acid to EETs (determined by HPLC profiles) in the presence of NADPH and molecular oxygen. Infusion of acetylcholine, but not pinacidil or sodium nitroprusside, to constricted blood vessels released a substance identified positively by HPLC-MS-MS as an EET. Authentic 5,6-EET elicited vasodilatation, which like that to acetylcholine, was attenuated by tetrabutylammonium, apamin plus charybdotoxin, or by 80 mM K^+. These data strongly suggest that an EET is the mediator of the nitric oxide-/prostanoid-independent dilatation in response to acetylcholine, and thus that an EET probably is EDHF in the rat mesenteric vascular bed.

Endothelium-dependent dilatation of the isolated, perfused rat mesenteric bed in response to acetylcholine (Adeagbo and Triggle, 1993), or of the perfused rat heart (Fulton *et al.*, 1995) and the porcine coronary artery to bradykinin (Cowan and Cohen, 1991), is mostly independent of the release of nitric oxide or the synthesis of prostanoids. The nitric oxide-/prostanoid-independent vasodilatation is blunted by tetrabutyammonium (a non-selective K^+ channel blocker) and a combination of apamin plus charybdotoxin (small- and large/intermediate-conductance K^+ channel blockers, respectively). Thus, the endothelium of these vascular beds release a factor(s), termed endothelium-derived hyperpolarizing factor (EDHF), which is distinct from nitric oxide and prostanoids and which hyperpolarizes the arterial smooth muscle cells through an increase in potassium conductance (Doughty, *et al.*, 1999; Félétou and Vanhoutte, 1999).

There is no agreement on the chemical identity of EDHF. In bovine and porcine coronary arteries EDHF may be a cytochrome P450 metabolite such as an epoxy-eicosatrienoic acid (EET) (Hecker *et al.*, 1994; Popp *et al.*, 1996; Li and Campbell, 1997; Fisslthaler *et al.*, 1999). Evidence in support of this include: (a) cytochrome P450 enzymes are abundant in the endothelium (Abraham *et al.*, 1985; McGiff *et al.*, 1996) and mediate the formation of an EET(s) (Harder *et al.*, 1995); (b) EETs relax contracted coronary or cerebral arteries with endothelium, but are ineffective in blood vessels bathed with excess K^+ (Campbell *et al.*, 1996; Gebremedhin *et al.*, 1992); and (c) EETs can open large-conductance calcium-activated K^+ (BK_{Ca}) channels and hyperpolarize smooth muscle cells in the cell-attached patch-clamp configuration (Li and Campbell, 1997; Campbell *et al.*, 1996; Gebremedhin *et al.*, 1992). This supportive evidence is challenged by the observation that EETs do not relax some blood vessels (Zygmunt *et al.*, 1996) and that EET and EDHF-mediated responses are blocked by different potassium channel blockers (Fukao *et al.*, 1997). The situation is further compounded by the fact that some cytochrome P450 blockers do not inhibit EDHF-mediated responses (Zygmunt *et al.*, 1996; Fukao *et al.*, 1997; Corriu *et al.*, 1996; Ohlmann *et al.*, 1997). In addition, cytochrome P450 inhibitors that block EDHF responses such as proadifen (SKF 525A), 7-ethoxyresorufin, clotrimazole, ketoconazole and miconazole exhibit a wide array of non-selective actions (Quilley *et al.*, 1997). For example, SKF 525A acts at muscarinic receptors (Choo *et al.*, 1986); 7-ethoxyresorufin inhibits nitric oxide synthase (Bennett *et al.*, 1992) while the imidazole compounds inhibit responses to K^+ channel openers (Zygmunt *et al.*, 1996; Fukao *et al.*, 1997; Graier *et al.*, 1996; Edwards *et al.*, 1996; Vanheel and Van de Voorde, 1997), nitric oxide synthase (Dudek *et al.*, 1995), and intracellular Ca^{2+}/calmodulin (Wolff *et al.*, 1993). Furthermore, EDHF-mediated responses are observed in blood vessels such as aorta and carotid arteries of the rabbit that do not produce metabolites of arachidonic acid by the cytochrome P450 pathway (Pfister *et al.*, 1991), suggesting that other factors must mediate the endothelium-dependent hyperpolarization and relaxation.

An alternative view, based on studies in rat hepatic and mesenteric arteries, is that EDHF may be K^+ ions released as a consequence of the opening of endothelial cell K^+ channels and the subsequent hyperpolarization (Edwards *et al.*, 1998). However, increases in extracellular K^+ do not hyperpolarize porcine coronary arterial smooth muscle cells (Quignard *et al.*, 1999). Second, in small mesenteric arteries of the rat K^+ ions do not mimic EDHF released by acetylcholine (Lacy *et al.*, 2000). These studies support the concept of multiple EDHFs and the notion that the chemical nature of EDHF varies with the vascular bed.

Observations with inhibitors of cytochrome P450 on EDHF mediated responses in the rat mesenteric artery yield controversial results. Thus, inhibitors can block the relaxations (Hecher *et al.*, 1994; Adeagbo, 1997) and hyperpolarizations (Chen and Cheng, 1996) elicited by acetylcholine, and the induction of cytochrome P450 enhances these effects (Chen and Cheng, 1996). In other studies, P450 inhibitors do not alter acetylcholine-induced relaxations or hyperpolarization (Vanheel and Van de Voorde, 1997). None of these studies performed biochemical investigations of the metabolism of arachidonic acid.

The present study was designed to test the hypothesis that EDHF is a cytochrome P450 metabolite of arachidonic acid in the mesenteric vascular bed. It demonstrates that acetylcholine can liberate arachidonic acid from radio-labeled vascular stores and can release, upon infusion into mesenteric vascular beds, a substance identified positively by mass spectrometry as an EET. The study also demonstrates that homogenates of, or microsomes obtained from, mesenteric blood vessels convert ^{14}[C]-arachidonic acid to products with HPLC profiles of EET.

1. METHODS

1.1. Isolation and perfusion of mesenteric vascular beds

Mesenteric vascular beds of rats were excised under pentobarbitone (60 mg/kg, intra-peritoneally) anesthesia and perfused (5 ml/min; Masterflex peristaltic pump) *in vitro* with physiological salt solution at 37 °C. The perfusing solution had the following composition (in mM): NaCl 118, KCl 4.7, $CaCl_2$ 2.5, KH_2PO_4 1.2, $MgSO_4$ 1.2, $NaHCO_3$ 12.5 and glucose, 11.1. Depolarizing (80 mM K^+) solution was made by substituting an equimolar amount of K^+ for Na^+. The pH of all solutions after bubbling with 95% O_2, 5% CO_2 gas mixture was 7.4. Vascular beds were routinely perfused with salt solution containing N^ω-nitro-L-arginine methyl ester (L-NAME, 1×10^{-4} M) plus indomethacin (5×10^{-6} M) to block the synthesis of nitric oxide and prostanoids, respectively. Perfusion pressures were recorded with Statham pressure transducers coupled to a Grass polygraph (model 7H). In order to demonstrate dilatation to agonists, vascular tone was augmented by the infusion of an α_1-adrenoceptor agonist, cirazoline (0.2–0.5×10^{-7} M). Acetylcholine or 5,6-EET was injected into the perfusate in bolus doses in the absence, or during infusion of tetrabutylammonium (1×10^{-3} M), or apamin (0.5×10^{-6} M) plus charybdotoxin (1×10^{-7} M).

1.2. Release of putative precursor

Endogenous labeling of the phospholipid pool was achieved by perfusion for 25 min with a re-circulating physiological salt solution that contained 1% bovine serum albumin and a mixture of ^{14}[C]- (0.7 µCi/ml) and cold-arachidonic acid (1 µg/ml). Unincorporated arachidonic acid was washed off for 10 min, following which cira-zoline (5×10^{-6} M) was added to the perfusion medium to generate vascular tone. Perfusate samples were collected every 4 min prior to (BASAL), and following bolus applications of acetylcholine (1×10^{-5} M), histamine, or pinacidil (1×10^{-4} M) in the absence, and in the presence of compounds $AACOCF_3$ (3×10^{-6} M, a phospholipase A_2 inhibitor), U73122 (3×10^{-6} M, a phospholipase C inhibitor), or U73343 (3×10^{-6} M, negative control). Samples were counted for radioactivity (^{14}[C] counts) with a β-scintillation Beckman radioactivity counter (model LS 1801). Release of radioactivity and vasodilatation by each of the dilator agents were calculated as a % of basal counts and as a % of cirazoline-induced tone, respectively.

1.3. Measurement of epoxides

Mesenteric vascular beds were set up, perfused with physiological salt solution and allowed to equilibrate for 45 min following which, a 20 min perfusate sample (100 ml total volume) was collected. Cirazoline (1×10^{-6} M) was then added to the perfusate to constrict the vessels and upon attaining a stable tone, another 20 min perfusate sample was collected. Thereafter, acetylcholine (1×10^{-5} M) was infused together with cirazoline and a third perfusate sample was collected during the dilatation response to acetylcholine. A parallel series of experiments was performed on blood vessels denuded of endothelium by infusion of aerated distilled water for 10 min. Samples were collected as described above, except that additional perfusate samples were obtained during the infusion of the endothelium-independent vasodilators sodium nitroprusside (1×10^{-5} M), or pinacidil (1×10^{-5} M).

Deuterium-labeled ($\pm$) 11,12-EET-d_8 (10 ng/ml) was added to all perfusate samples to serve as an internal standard for epoxide detection and as a reflector for the recovery of the eicosanoid through the concentration process. Each sample was passed through a C-18 resin column to adsorb any constituent EETs, then, rinsed with 4 ml 90% methanol in water. The eluates were collected and concentrated by evaporating the methanol under a slow stream of N_2 gas. The concentrated samples were applied to the mass spectrometer for mass to charge analysis.

1.4. Vessel homogenates and microsomes

Mesenteric vessels were minced with a sharp pair of scissors in a beaker containing 20 ml 0.1 M phosphate plus 0.15% KCl buffer (homogenization buffer, pH 7.4). The buffer contained phenylmethylsulfonyl fluoride and a cocktail of six other protease inhibitors with broad specificity for the inhibition of aspartic, cysteine, and serine proteases as well as aminopeptidases. The homogenate was either used to study ^{14}[C]-arachidonic acid metabolism (preliminary HPLC studies), or processed for preparation of microsomal pellets. To prepare mesenteric vessel microsomes, the homogenates were centrifuged for 15 min at 20,000 g; the supernatant layer was retained while the tissue debris (bottom) and floating fat (top) layers were discarded. The supernatant was centrifuged further for one hour at 100,000 g. The cytosolic (top) layer was discarded while the microsomal pellets (bottom portion) was reconstituted in 0.5 ml homogenization buffer containing 15% glycerol (to preserve their functional integrity). This was eventually dispersed evenly with a glass pestle and aliquoted into three or four batches for the desired experiments, or stored at $-80\,^{\circ}$C. The total protein content of the homogenates, or the microsomal fractions was estimated (Lowry *et al.*, 1951).

The vessel homogenates and the microsomes were used to study the conversion of ^{14}[C]-arachidonic acid to EETs. Three reaction tubes, each containing KHPO$_4$ buffer (0.01 mM, pH 7.4), were set up as follows: (a) 1 mg homogenate/microsomal protein plus 0.5 μCi ^{14}[C]-arachidonic acid plus 0 mM reduced nicotinamide adenine dinucleotide phosphate (NADPH, negative control); (b) 1 mg homogenate/microsomal protein plus 0.5 μCi ^{14}[C]-arachidonic acid plus 1 mM NADPH; and (c) 1 mg homogenate/microsomal protein plus 0.5 μCi ^{14}[C]-arachidonic acid plus 1 mM NADPH plus 5 μM clotrimazole. Indomethacin (1×10^{-5} M) was added to each of the tubes. The tubes were incubated in a shaking water bath (200 rpm) at 37 °C under a stream of 95% O_2–5% CO_2 gas mixture to provide adequate oxygenation. At the end of 30 min incubation, the reactions were terminated by acidification with 0.1 M formic acid (pH 3.5). Thereafter, arachidonic acid metabolites were extracted with two volumes of ethyl acetate and the organic phase evaporated to dryness with N_2 gas. The extract was reconstituted with ethanol followed by product separation by reverse phase

HPLC using a linear gradient of 1.25%/min from acetonitrile:water:acetic acid (50:50:0.1, v/v) to acetonitrile:acetic acid (100:0.1, v/v) solvent phase over a 25 min period at a flow rate of 1.0 ml/min. The elution profile of the radioactive metabolites of arachidonic acid was detected and counted using an on-line radioactive detector (Radiomatic Instruments & Chem. Co., Meriden, CT, USA). The identity of each metabolite was confirmed by its co-migration with authentic standards.

1.5. Drugs

Acetylcholine hydrobromide, arachidonic acid, clotrimazole, histamine dihydro-chloride, NADPH, N^{ω}-nitro-L-arginine methyl ester, indomethacin, and tetrabutyl-ammonium bromide were purchased from Sigma Chem. Co. (St. Louis, MO, USA). Cirazoline hydrochloride, pinacidil, U-73122 and U-73343 were purchased from Research Biochem. (Natick, MA, USA) while AACOCF$_3$, 5,6-EET and ($\pm$) 11,12-EET-d$_8$ were purchased from Biomol Res. Labs., Plymouth Meeting, PA, USA. The Protease Inhibitor Cocktail Set III and phenylmethylsulfonyl fluoride were purchased from Calbiochem-Novabiochem Corp. (La Jolla, CA, USA).

1.6. Data analysis

Changes in perfusion pressure were expressed as a percentage of the arterial perfusion pressure before the administration of a vasodilator agent. Values are expressed as mean $\pm$ SEM, and differences between the mean values were compared using either Student's *t*-test for paired observations, or ANOVA (multiple comparisons). The difference between means was considered significant when p was less than .05.

2. RESULTS

2.1. Vasodilatation to acetylcholine and 5,6-EET

The basal perfusion pressure of mesenteric vascular beds perfused with normal phy-siological salt solution was 22.6 ± 0.3 mmHg ($n = 58$). The continuous infusion of cirazoline (5×10^{-7} M) produced increases in perfusion pressure to a sustained level of 108.0 ± 5.1 mmHg. Bolus applications of acetylcholine (1×10^{-10}–1×10^{-5} mole), 5,6-EET (1×10^{-4} and 3×10^{-4} mole), histamine (1×10^{-5}–1×10^{-3} mole) or pinacidil (1×10^{-4} mole) initiated dose-dependent decreases in perfusion pressure. Tetrabutylammonium (TBA, 1×10^{-3} M) abolished the responses to 5,6-EET and markedly reduced that to acetylcholine (Figure 22.1). In vascular beds perfused with 80 mM K$^+$ physiological salt solution, the acetylcholine-evoked vasodilator responses were nearly abolished. Similarly, decreases in perfusion pressure in response to 1×10^{-4} and 3×10^{-4} mole 5,6-EET were abolished during perfusion with 80 mM K$^+$ depolarizing salt solution. The responses to acetylcholine were abolished by the combination of apamin (0.5×10^{-6} M) plus charybdotoxin (1×10^{-7} M) (Figure 22.2). These combination of antagonists nearly abolished dilator responses elicited by either 3×10^{-4} mole 5,6-EET, or by 1×10^{-4} mole histamine, but failed to sig-nificantly alter the vasodilatation elicited by 1×10^{-6} mole sodium nitroprusside (Figure 22.2).

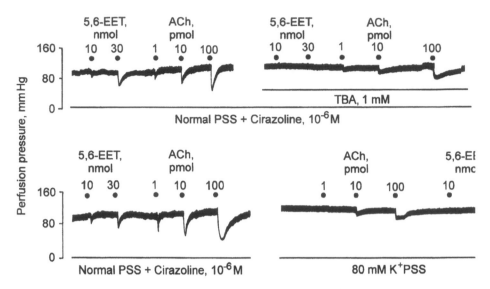

Figure 22.1 Original recording of the effects of tetrabutylammonium (TBA, 1×10^{-3} M) and 80 mM K^+ depolarizing salt solution on vasodilatation elicited by 5,6-EET and acetylcholine. Tetrabutylammonium was tested on vascular beds constricted with cirazoline (0.3–1×10^{-6} M).

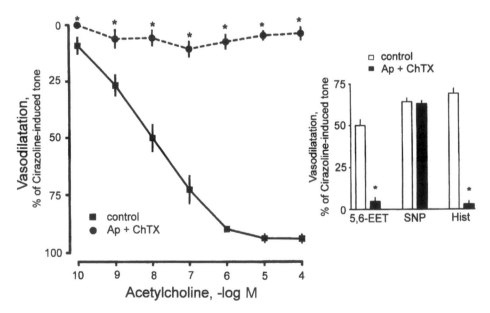

Figure 22.2 Dose–responses to acetylcholine and their attenuation by apamin (AP, 0.5×10^{-6} M) plus charybdotoxin (ChTx, 1×10^{-7} M). The bar graph (insert) indicate vasodilator responses to 5,6-EET (3×10^{-4} mole), sodium nitroprusside (SNP, 1×10^{-6} mole) and histamine (HIST, 1×10^{-4} mole) before (hatched bars) and during infusion (solid bars) of 0.5×10^{-6} M apamin plus 1×10^{-7} M charybdotoxin (AP + ChTx). Each point on the graph represents the mean ± SEM. ($n = 8$); each bar column represents the mean ± SEM ($n = 5$). The asterisks (*) denote statistically significant differences ($p < .05$).

2.2. Release of ^{14}[C]-arachidonic acid

Acetylcholine (1×10^{-5} mole), histamine (1×10^{-4} mole), or pinacidil (1×10^{-4} mole) elicited dilatation of about similar magnitudes. The dilatations to acetylcholine and histamine, but not pinacidil, were accompanied by the release of ^{14}[C]-arachidonic acid. Both the vasodilator and the ^{14}[C]-arachidonic acid releasing effects of acetylcholine

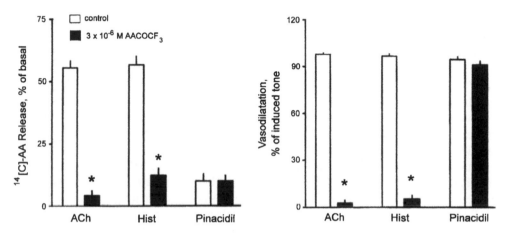

Figure 22.3 Effect of AACOCF$_3$, a phospholipase A$_2$ blocker, on the release of ^{14}[C]-(AA) from radiolabeled phospholipid pool (left), and on vasodilatation (right) elicited by acetylcholine (ACH), histamine (HIST) or pinacidil. The open (□) and solid (■) bars represent the responses in the absence, and during infusion of 3×10^{-6} M AACOCF$_3$, respectively. Each bar column represents the mean ± SEM of six experiments. The asterisks (*) denote statistically significant differences ($p < .05$).

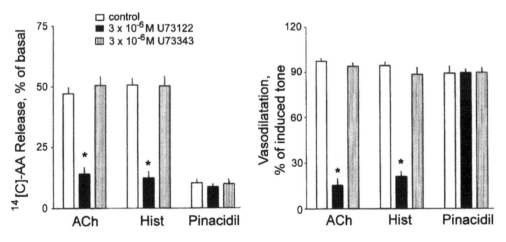

Figure 22.4 Effect of U73122, a phospholipase C blocker, and its negative control compound U73343, on the release of ^{14}[C]-(AA) from radiolabeled phospholipid pool (left), and on vasodilatation (right) elicited by acetylcholine (ACH), histamine (HIST) or pinacidil. The open (□), solid (■) and hatched bars represent the responses in the absence, and during infusion 3×10^{-6} M of U73122 and U73343, respectively. Each bar column represents the mean ± SEM of six experiments. The asterisks (*) denote statistically significant differences ($p < .05$).

and histamine were blocked by compounds AACOCF$_3$ (Figure 22.3) and U73122 (Figure 22.4), inhibitors of phospholipase A$_2$ and C, respectively. Compound U73343, the negative control for U73122, had no effects on vasodilatation and ^{14}[C]-arachidonic acid release (see Figure 22.4).

2.3. Epoxide formation and release

Vascular homogenates or microsomes metabolized ^{14}[C]-arachidonic acid to products with a retention times (R_Ts) of 8–9 min and 12–14 min on the reverse phase HPLC chromatogram (Figure 22.5A). These R_Ts correspond to those of authentic 20-hydroxyeicosa-tetraenoic acid (20-HETE) and EETs, respectively. The metabolism of ^{14}[C]-arachidonic acid to such products occurred in the presence of NADPH and was blocked by incubating the homogenates or microsomes with 5×10^{-6} M clotrimazole (Figure 22.5B). In homogenates or microsomes incubated with ^{14}[C]-arachidonic acid in the absence of NADPH, the peak of the products with R_T of 12–14 min was absent.

An electrospray ionization tandem mass spectrometry (MS-MS) was used to detect endogenous epoxide(s) released into mesenteric bed perfusate samples to which a deuterium-labeled ($\pm$) 11,12-EET-d$_8$ (10 ng/ml) was added as an internal standard. The EET-d$_8$ was fragmented with argon and its molecular mass and those of its various products were determined. Based on the molecular mass patterns of the internal standard, the data indicate that acetylcholine infusion released an EET from the

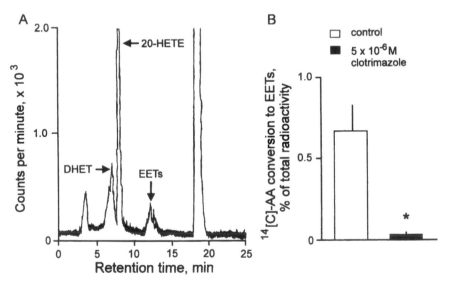

Figure 22.5 (A) A representative reverse-phase HPLC chromatogram indicating the products formed from NADPH-dependent microsomal metabolism of ^{14}[C]-(AA). Identified metabolite peaks are: dihydroxyeicosatrienoic acid (DHET), epoxyeicosatrienoic acids (EETs), and 20-hydroxyeicosatetraenoic acid (20-HETE). (B) NADPH-dependent metabolism of ^{14}[C]-(AA) in control microsomes of rat mesenteric blood vessels ($\square$) and microsomes treated with clotrimazole (5×10^{-6} M; $\blacksquare$). Each bar column represents the mean $\pm$ SEM ($n = 7$); the asterisk (*) denotes statistically significant difference ($p < .05$).

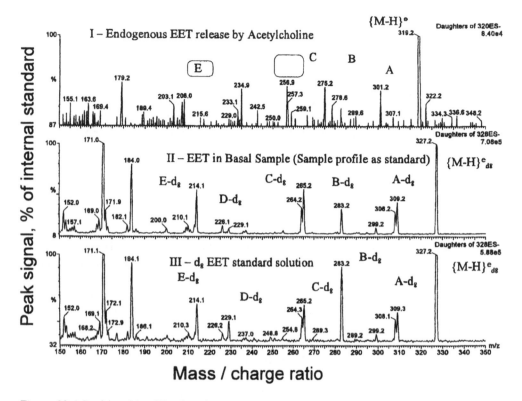

Figure 22.6 Positive identification by mass spectrometry of EET released by infusion of acetylcholine (1 nmol) into a perfused rat mesenteric arterial bed. Note the molecular mass 319.2 (endogenous) versus 327.2 of the internal standard {(±) 11,12-EET-d_8}. The difference of 8 equals the molecular mass of deuterium.

endothelium into the mesenteric vascular perfusates. The molecular mass of the substance found in basal unstimulated samples was 327.2, which correlated to the mass of the internal standard. However, the mass of the substance released by acetylcholine into the perfusate was 319.2 (Figure 22.6). The difference of eight from the molecular mass of the internal standard is the mass of deuterium. Conversely, only the internal standard (molecular mass of 327.2) was detectable in perfusate samples collected during the infusion of pinacidil or sodium nitroprusside to constricted blood vessels.

3. DISCUSSION

The rat mesenteric vascular bed undoubtedly releases a non-nitric oxide, non-prostanoid endothelial factor that hyperpolarizes the vascular smooth muscle cells to bring about their relaxation. In mesenteric arteries, or the mesenteric vascular bed of the rat, there are three distinct candidates as EDHF: (a) a labile metabolite (Chen and Cheng, 1996; Adeagbo, 1997); (b) an endogenous cannabinoid, arachidonoyl-ethanolamide (anandamide) (Randall *et al.*, 1996), and (c) potassium ions effluxed from endothelial cells (Edwards *et al.*, 1998). The present study presents evidence that a product, namely an EET(s), is probably the EDHF secreted by the endothelium of the perfused mesenteric arterial bed of the rat.

In order for EET(s) to be an EDHF, it must fulfil some criteria. First, the authentic EET must mimic nitric oxide-/prostanoid-independent relaxations both in terms of sensitivities to K^+ channel blockers and to excess potassium. The present data show that acetylcholine, or 5,6-EET elicited dilatation of perfused rat mesenteric arterial bed. The dilator effects of both compounds were blocked by tetrabutylammonium (a non-selective K^+ channel antagonist), and by a combination of apamin plus charybdotoxin (a small- and intermediate/large-conductance K_{Ca} channel blocker, respectively). Dilator responses to either acetylcholine or 5,6-EET were also attenuated in vascular beds perfused with 80 mM K^+ depolarizing salt solution. These results suggest that acetylcholine and 5,6-EET dilate the perfused rat mesenteric arterial bed by promoting the movement of potassium through K_{Ca} channels. Second, there must be a system for the formation of the putative factor within the vascular bed in question. This must include the presence of a precursor and a demonstrable capacity of the vascular bed to convert the precursor to the putative EDHF (EETs). The endogenous lipid pool of the rat mesenteric arterial bed was labeled with [14][C]-arachidonic acid and the endothelium-dependent vasodilatation in response to acetylcholine and histamine, but not endothelium-independent responses to pinacidil, were accompanied by the release of radio-labeled arachidonic acid into the perfusate. In mesenteric arteries without endothelium, acetylcholine did not dilatate and also failed to increase [14][C] release above basal levels. The latter observation, taken together with the lack of [14][C] release by pinaciil, indicate that [14][C] was mostly incorporated into the membrane lipids of the endothelial cells and was releasable by activators of these cells. Phospholipases liberate arachidonic acid from membrane-bound phospholipids in vascular tissues and other cell types (Capdevila *et al.*, 1992). Thus, the effects of inhibition of phospholipases A_2 and C with AACOCF$_3$ and U73122, respectively, were examined on acetylcholine-induced relaxations and the release of radioactivity. The dilatation to acetylcholine and the associated [14][C]-arachidonic acid release were blocked by AACOCF$_3$ or U73122. However, the negative control for U73122, compound U73343, did not alter those responses. These results suggest that the release of [14][C]-arachidonic acid that accompanies acetylcholine or histamine relaxations involved both phospholipase A_2 and phospholipase C pathways.

Furthermore, the present study demonstrates that rat mesenteric arteries can convert radio-labeled precursor ([14][C]-arachidonic acid) to EETs in an NADPH-dependent manner. Arterial homogenates or microsomes metabolize [14][C]-arachidonic acid to products with a retention time similar to that of authentic EETs. Additional evidence that the EDHF secreted by the endothelium of the rat mesenteric vascular bed is a cytochrome P450 product is provided by the fact that clotrimazole, an inhibitor of epoxygenases, blocks the conversion of [14][C]-arachidonic acid to EETs.

Third, release of EETs must accompany the relaxation elicited by an endothelium-dependent vasodilator such as acetylcholine. Infusion of acetylcholine to constricted vascular beds resulted in vasodilatation. Using mass spectrometry, a substance was detected with the molecular mass of an EET in perfusates of vascular beds collected during such acetylcholine-induced dilatation. Only the internal standard, ($\pm$) 11,12-EET-d$_8$ was detectable in the absence of acetylcholine. In addition, no EETs were detectable in perfusate samples collected during vasodilatation with endothelium-independent agonists such as pinacidil and sodium nitroprusside. Taken together, these results indicate that the mesenteric endothelium is the source of EETs that is released into the perfusate by acetylcholine.

Based on the capacity to form cytochrome P450 products from arachidonic acid mammalian blood vessels have been classified into three types (Campbell and Harder, 1999). The first group, which comprises coronary, renal and cerebral arteries, convert arachidonic acid to products with EDHF properties. The products were identified by HPLC and mass spectrometry (Campbell *et al.*, 1996) and by bioassay (Gebremedhin *et al.*, 1998) as EETs. The rabbit aorta and carotid artery are in the second category. These blood vessels do not possess a cytochrome P450 pathway for the metabolism of arachidonic acid and EDHF in these vessels may well be another, unidentified substance. The third category of blood vessels comprises of rat mesenteric artery, hepatic arteries, portal vein, and guinea-pig carotid artery. In these blood vessels, the involvement of metabolites of arachidonic acid have not been determined biochemically. The present study documents unequivocally that rat mesenteric arteries can form EET(s) from arachidonic acid and that clotrimazole, an epoxygenase blocker, inhibits EET formation. The vascular bed also released an EET when challenged with the endothelium-dependent dilator agonist acetylcholine.

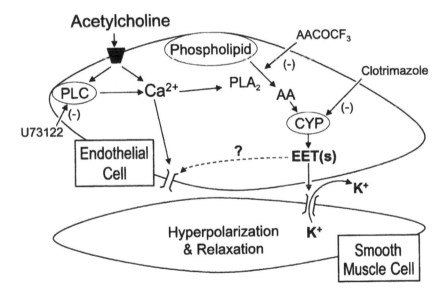

Figure 22.7 A schematic cascade of events that result in the synthesis of putative EDHF and its vascular action in the mesenteric arterial bed of the rat. Acetylcholine, or histamine, activates endothelial cell receptors leading to phospholipase C-mediated (can be blocked by U73122) increases in intracellular Ca^{2+} concentrations. Ca^{2+} activates cytosolic phospholipase A_2 (can be blocked by $AACOCF_3$) leading to cleavage of arachidonic acid from phospholipid membranes. Arachidonic acid is metabolized by cytochrome P450 epoxygenases in the endothelium to epoxyeicosatrienoic acids (can be blocked by clotrimazole). Epoxyeicosatrienoic acids (EETs) diffuse to underlying smooth muscle cells to activate K_{Ca} channels leading to smooth muscle cell hyperpolarization and relaxation. EETs might cause hyperpolarization of the endothelial cells through the activation of K^+ channels located on those cells.

The findings of the present study are consistent with the postulate that EDHF is a diffusible factor (Popp *et al.*, 1996; Gebremedhin *et al.*, 1998). The cascade of events that result in endothelium-dependent hyperpolarizations of rat mesenteric smooth muscle cells can be summarized in Figure 22.7: (a) endothelial cell receptor activation by acetylcholine or histamine leads to phospholipase C-mediated increases in intracellular $[Ca^{2+}]$; (b) Ca^{2+} activates cytosolic phospholipase A_2 leading to cleavage of arachidonic acid from phospholipid membranes; (c) arachidonic acid is metabolized by cytochrome P450 epoxygenases in the endothelium to EET(s); and (d) EET(s) diffuse to underlying smooth muscle cells to activate K_{Ca} channels leading to smooth muscle cell hyperpolarization and relaxation. However, the possibility cannot be ignored that EETs might cause endothelial cell hyperpolarization through the activation of K^+ channels located on those cells (Edwards *et al.*, 1998). The use in the present study of apamin plus charybdotoxin did not reveal the probable location (endothelium and/or smooth muscle) of the K^+ channels activated by EETs. Apamin is a selective blocker of the small conductance K_{Ca}, but charybdotoxin is non-specific, as it blocks large/intermediate K_{Ca} as well as some voltage-dependent potassium channels (Félétou and Vanhoutte, 1999). EETs produced by endothelial cells could possibly augment the intracellular calcium concentration and thus foster a positive feedback for vascular relaxation through the release of EDHF and nitric oxide (Graier *et al.*, 1995).

4. CONCLUSION

The present study, though limited in terms of the mechanism(s) by which EETs elicit relaxation of vascular smooth muscle, is strong in establishing that mesenteric blood vessels of the rat have the capacity to produce EETs through the cytochrome P450 epoxygenases, and can release the metabolite in response to endothelium-dependent vasodilators such as acetylcholine.

ACKNOWLEDGEMENTS

This research was made possible through a grant of the Jewish Hospital Foundation, Louisville, KY and the American Heart Association, Ohio Valley Affiliate to ASOA, and NIH grants NHL59884, HL03674 and the Established Investigator Award of the AHA to AOO. We are grateful to Mr. Ned Smith for his skillful assistance with the mass spectrometric (MS-MS) analysis of the mesenteric perfusate samples.

23 Epoxyeicosatrienoic acid and endothelium-dependent hyperpolarization in porcine coronary arteries

A.H. Weston, G. Edwards, C. Thollon,
M.J. Gardener, J.-P. Vilaine,
Paul M. Vanhoutte and Michel Félétou

11,12-epoxyeicosatrienoic acid was proposed to be the hyperpolarizing factor in porcine coronary arteries (Fisslthaler *et al.*, 1999). To test this hypothesis, the pharmacology of the hyperpolarizing effects of 11,12-epoxyeicosatrienoic acid and the endothelium-derived hyperpolarizing factor (elicited with substance P) in the porcine coronary artery were compared using sharp micro-electrode techniques. The hyperpolarizations of smooth muscle induced either by substance P or by 11,12-epoxyeicosatrienoic acid in intact porcine coronary arteries were abolished by charybdotoxin plus apamin but only moderately inhibited by iberiotoxin plus apamin. However, in coronary arteries without endothelium the hyperpolarization induced by 11,12-epoxyeicosatrienoic acid was abolished by iberiotoxin alone. In intact arteries, 11,12-epoxyeicosatrienoic acid induced an iberiotoxin-insensitive hyperpolarization of the endothelial cells. These results collectively suggest that 11,12-epoxyeicosatrienoic acid is not an endothelium-derived hyperpolarizing factor in the porcine coronary artery. Instead it seems that this eicosanoid has two basic effects. One of these is to hyperpolarize coronary artery smooth muscle directly via the opening of an iberiotoxin-sensitive potassium channel (presumably BK_{Ca}) in these cells. The other is hyperpolarization of the endothelium, an action involving the opening of both apamin- and charybdotoxin- (but not iberiotoxin-) sensitive potassium channels (presumably SK_{Ca} and IK_{Ca}, respectively).

In bovine and porcine coronary arteries, endothelium-derived hyperpolarizing factor (EDHF) could be a cytochrome P450 metabolite, such as an epoxyeicosatrienoic acid (EET) (Rubanyi and Vanhoutte 1987; Komori and Vanhoutte 1990; Hecker *et al.*, 1994; Popp *et al.*, 1996; Li and Campbell, 1997; Fisslthaler *et al.*, 1999). Indeed, EETs are produced from coronary artery endothelial cells (Rosolowsky *et al.*, 1990; Campbell *et al.*, 1996; Rosolowsky and Campbell, 1996) and can hyperpolarize vascular smooth muscle (Campbell *et al.*, 1996; Eckman *et al.*, 1998, Fisslthaler *et al.*, 1999). Inhibitors of the cytochrome P450 monoxygenase and antisense oligonucleotides suppress EDHF-mediated responses in coronary arteries from various species (Rosolowski and Campbell, 1993; Bauersachs *et al.*, 1994; Hecker *et al.*, 1994; Fulton *et al.*, 1995; Graier *et al.*, 1996; Miura and Gutterman, 1998; Fisslthaler *et al.*, 1999; Bolz *et al.*, 2000). In those blood vessels, EETs increase the activity of calcium-activated potassium channels sensitive to tetraethylammonium, charybdo-toxin or iberiotoxin (Gebremedhin et al., 1992; Hu and Kim, 1993; Campbell et al., 1996; Li et al., 1997; Eckman et al., 1998; Gebremedhin et al., 1998; Hayabushi et al., 1998). However, from these inhibitors only iberiotoxin is selective for the large-conductance calcium-sensitive K^+ channel (BK_{Ca}: Kuriyama et al., 1995; Kaczorowski et al., 1996) indicating that the potassium conductance opened by EETs in coronary artery smooth muscle cells is still uncertain. In contrast, iberiotoxin has little, if any, effect on EDHF-mediated responses in various blood vessels (Zygmunt and Högestätt, 1996; Corriu et al., 1996; Chataigneau et al., 1998; Eckman et al., 1998; Quignard et al., 1999).

The aim of the present study was to characterize in the isolated porcine coronary artery the electrophysiological aspects of the response to EDHF and to compare it to those of 11,12-EET.

1. METHODS

Porcine left descending coronary arteries were obtained either from the local slaughterhouse and transported to the laboratory in ice-cold Krebs solution or from Large-White pigs (male or female, 25 kg) anaesthetized with a mixture of tiletamine plus zolazepam, (intramuscularly, each 20 mg/kg). The isolated coronary arteries were pinned to the Sylgard base of a heated organ chamber and superfused (10 ml/min), at 37 °C, with Krebs solution containing N^{ω}-L-nitro-arginine (3×10^{-4} M) and indomethacin (10^{-5} M). Smooth muscle cells were impaled from the adventitial side and endothelial cells from the intimal side, using microelectrodes filled with 3 M KCl (resistance 40–80 MΩ). In some experiments the endothelial layer was removed by gentle rubbing, and the lack of endothelium in each blood vessel segment was confirmed by the absence of a response to substance P.

Drugs were added as bolus injections directly into the organ chambers in quantities calculated to give (transiently) the final concentrations indicated. The K^+-channel inhibitors were added to the reservoir of Krebs superfusing the bath. In some experiments the coronary arterial segments were superfused continuously with bradykinin so that responses were observed under equilibrium conditions.

1.1. Drugs and solutions

Krebs solution comprised (mM): Na^+ 143, K^+ 4.6, Ca^{2+} 2.5, Mg^{2+} 1.2, Cl^- 126.4, $H_2PO_4^-$ 1.2, SO_4^{2-} 1.2, HCO_3^- 25, glucose 11.1 and was bubbled with 95% O_2 and 5% CO_2.

The following substances were used: bradykinin, N^{ω}-L-nitro-arginine, NS1619 (1,3-dihydro-1-(2-hydroxy-5-(trifluoromethyl)phenyl)-5-(trifluoromethyl)-2H-benzimidazol-2-one) and substance P (RBI/Sigma, Poole, UK), apamin, synthetic charybdotoxin and iberiotoxin (Latoxan, Valence, France), (±) 11,12-epoxyeicosa-5Z,8Z14Z-trienoic acid (11,12-EET, Affinity Research Products Ltd, Golden, CO, USA), indomethacin, levcromakalim (SmithKline Beecham, Harlow, UK). 11,12-EET was dissolved in ethanol. The bolus injection of this vehicle (10 μl of ethanol) produced a small but significant hyperpolarization (-3 to -5 mV) of both smooth muscle and endothelial cells.

1.2. Statistics

Student's *t*-test (paired or unpaired as appropriate) was used to assess the probability that differences between mean values had arisen by chance. Differences were considered to be statistically significant when *p* was less than .05.

2. RESULTS

2.1. Membrane potential of smooth muscle cells

2.1.1. Continuous superfusion

Under control conditions and in the presence of the endothelium, the membrane potential of porcine coronary artery smooth muscle cells was -58.4 ± 1.8 mV ($n = 11$). The addition of N^{ω}-L-nitro-arginine (L-NA, 3×10^{-5} M) plus indomethacin (10^{-4} M) provoked a significant depolarization (membrane potential: -51.0 ± 1.1 mV, $n = 11$). Under these conditions, bradykinin (3×10^{-8} M) produced an endothelium-dependent hyperpolarization of -19.9 ± 1.0 mV ($n = 11$). In the presence of L-NA and

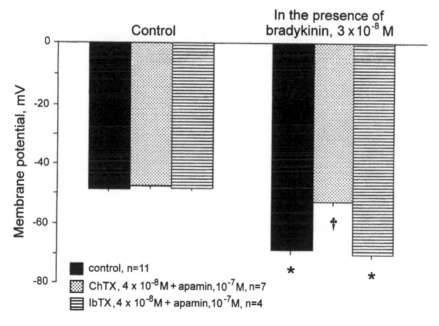

Figure 23.1 Membrane potential of smooth muscle cells from isolated porcine coronary artery with endothelium in the presence of a continuous superfusion of Krebs solution containing L-nitro-arginine (3×10^{-6} M) and indomethacin (10^{-5} M). Effects of the combination of two inhibitors of calcium-activated potassium channels charybdotoxin (ChTX, 4×10^{-8} M) plus apamin (10^{-7} M) and iberiotoxin (IbTX, 4×10^{-8} M) plus apamin on bradykinin- (3×10^{-8} M) induced endothelium-dependent hyperpolarization. Data are shown as means $\pm$ SEM. The asterisks indicate a statistically significant difference induced by the addition of bradykinin. The dagger indicates a statistically significant difference induced by the combination of charybdotoxin plus apamin.

indomethacin, the addition of charybdotoxin (8×10^{-8} M, $n = 3$), apamin (10^{-7} M, $n = 3$), the combination of charybdotoxin (4×10^{-8} M) plus apamin (10^{-7} M, $n = 7$) or the combination of iberiotoxin (4×10^{-8} M) plus apamin (10^{-7} M, $n = 4$) did not significantly affect the resting membrane potential. Bradykinin-induced hyperpolarization was abolished by the combination of charybdotoxin plus apamin but was not significantly influenced by the toxins individually or by the combination of iberiotoxin and apamin (Figure 23.1).

2.1.2. Bolus injections

2.1.2.1. With endothelium

In the presence of L-NA (3×10^{-4} M) and indomethacin (10^{-5} M), the resting membrane potential of the porcine coronary artery smooth muscle was 51.6 ± 0.2 mV, ($n = 15$). Substance P (10^{-7} nM) hyperpolarized the smooth muscle cells of intact arteries by 28.4 ± 0.8 mV ($n = 8$). Iberiotoxin (10^{-7} M) did not affect the responses to substance P. In contrast the hyperpolarization to NS1619 (3.3×10^{-5} M) was abolished by iberiotoxin (data not shown). Charybdotoxin (10^{-7} M) alone or the combination of iberiotoxin plus apamin (10^{-7} M) produced a small but statistically significant inhibition of the hyperpolarization produced by substance P. The combination of charybdotoxin plus apamin virtually abolished the hyperpolarization to substance P (Figure 23.2). The hyperpolarization produced by cromakalim (10^{-5} M) was unaffected by these toxins, alone or in combination.

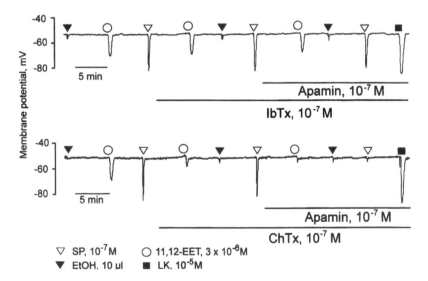

Figure 23.2 Membrane potential of smooth muscle cells from an isolated porcine coronary artery with endothelium in the presence of L-nitro-arginine (3×10^{-4} M) plus indomethacin (10^{-5} M) Original traces showing the inhibitory effects of inhibitors of calcium-activated potassium channels charybdotoxin (ChTX, 10^{-7} M), apamin (10^{-7} M) and iberiotoxin (IbTX, 10^{-7} M) on the responses to bolus infusion of substance P (SP, 10^{-7} M), ethanol (EtOH, solvent of 11,12-EET, 10 µl), 11,12-EET (3×10^{-6} M) and levcromakalim (LK, a selective opener of K-ATP channels, 10^{-5} M).

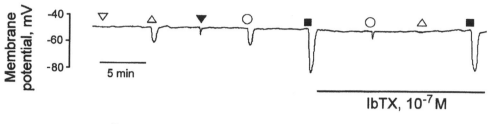

Figure 23.3 Membrane potential of a smooth muscle cell from isolated porcine coronary artery without endothelium in the presence of L-nitro-arginine (3×10^{-4} M) plus indomethacin (10^{-5} M). Original trace showing the inhibitory effects of the inhibitor of large conductance calcium-activated potassium channel iberiotoxin (IbTX, 10^{-7} M) on the bolus infusion of substance P (SP, 10^{-7} M), NS1619 (a selective activator of BK_{Ca}, 3.3×10^{-5} M), ethanol (EtOH, solvent of 11,12-EET, 10 μl), 11,12-EET (3×10^{-6} M) and levcromakalim (LK, a selective opener of K-ATP channels, 10^{-5} M).

11,12-EET (3×10^{-6} M) hyperpolarized the smooth muscle cells by 18.6 ± 0.8 mV ($n = 8$). Iberiotoxin induced a small but significant inhibition of the hyperpolarization produced by 11,12-EET, that was not modified by the addition of apamin. In contrast, charybdotoxin induced a significantly larger inhibition of the hyperpolarization, with abolition of the residual hyperpolarization by apamin (Figure 23.2).

2.1.2.2. *Without endothelium*

In blood vessels without endothelium, the smooth muscle cells were slightly but significantly depolarized when compared to controls (-50.0 ± 0.3 mV, $n = 5$). In the absence of the endothelium, substance P did not produce any significant changes in membrane potential while 11,12-EET hyperpolarized the smooth muscle by 12.6 ± 0.3 mV ($n = 4$), a value that was significantly less than in the presence of the endothelium. The hyperpolarizations to both 11,12-EET and NS1619 were abolished by iberiotoxin. In contrast the hyperpolarization produced by cromakalim was unaffected by the toxin (Figure 23.3).

2.2. Membrane potential of endothelial cells

In intact porcine coronary artery, the resting membrane potential of endothelial cells was -47.9 ± 0.3 mV ($n = 8$). Both substance P and 11,12-EET hyperpolarized the endothelial cells. For both substances, the amplitude of the endothelial hyperpolarization was significantly larger than that observed in smooth muscle cells. Iberiotoxin did not influence the hyperpolarizations produced by either substance P or 11,12-EET. In contrast, charybdotoxin produced a significant and partial inhibition of the hyperpolarization induced by both mediators. The charybdotoxin-sensitive

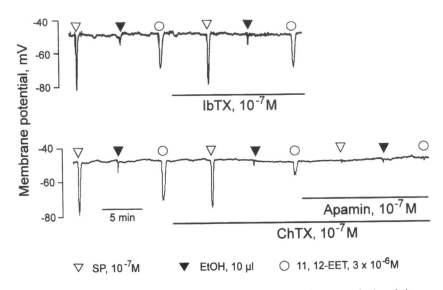

Figure 23.4 Membrane potential of endothelial cells from an isolated intact porcine coronary artery in the presence of L-nitro-arginine (3×10^{-4} M) and indomethacin (10^{-5} M). Original traces showing the inhibitory effects of inhibitors of calcium-activated potassium channels charybdotoxin (ChTX, 10^{-7} M), apamin (10^{-7} M) and iberiotoxin (IbTX, 10^{-7} M) on the bolus infusion of substance P (SP, 10^{-7} M), ethanol (EtOH, solvent of 11,12-EET, $10\,\mu$l) and 11,12-EET (3×10^{-6} M).

component was significantly larger for the hyperpolarization produced by 11,12-EET than the one produced by substance P. The addition of apamin abolished the remaining hyperpolarizations in both cases (Figure 23.4).

3. DISCUSSION

Substance P and bradykinin produced endothelium-dependent smooth muscle hyperpolarizations which showed the axiomatic features of 'EDHF' (Mombouli and Vanhoutte, 1997; Edwards and Weston, 1998; Félétou and Vanhoutte, 1999). Substance P- and bradykinin-induced increases in membrane potential were observed in the presence of inhibitors of both cycloxygenase and nitric oxide synthase. They were not inhibited by the combination of the two toxins iberiotoxin and apamin but was abolished by the combination of charybdotoxin plus apamin. In vascular preparations, iberiotoxin selectively inhibits smooth muscle BK_{Ca} channels but does not inhibit endothelial cell IK_{Ca} channels, whereas charybdotoxin inhibits both channel types (Edwards *et al.*, 1999b; Kaczorowski and Garcia, 1999). These results confirm that IK_{Ca} and SK_{Ca} are involved in the EDHF responses but not BK_{Ca} (Garland and Plane 1996; Zygmunt and Hoggestatt, 1996; Corriu *et al.*, 1996; Chen and Cheung, 1997; Hashitani and Suzuki, 1997; Petersson *et al.*, 1997; Zygmunt *et al.*, 1998; Edwards *et al.*, 1998, 1999; Chataigneau *et al.*, 1998; Yamanaka *et al.*, 1998; Quignard *et al.*, 1999). The vascular K$^+$ channels inhibited by the combination of charybdotoxin

(IK$_{CA}$) plus apamin (SK$_{CA}$) are most likely situated on the endothelial cells. Indeed, calcium-activated potassium channels are expressed in endothelial cells (Marchenko and Sage, 1996). In the rat hepatic artery, the rabbit aortic valve and the porcine coronary artery (present study) the combination of charybdotoxin plus apamin inhibits endothelial cell hyperpolarization (Edwards *et al.*, 1998; Ohashi *et al.*, 1999). Furthermore, in rat mesenteric artery, charybdotoxin and apamin block EDHF responses if selecively applied to the endothelium (Doughty *et al.*, 1999). Finally, a conductance specifically sensitive to the combination of charybdotoxin plus apamin, and which was distinct from BK$_{Ca}$, could not be detected in isolated smooth muscle cells from the rat hepatic and the guinea-pig carotid artery (Zygmunt *et al.*, 1997; Quignard *et al.*, 2000). Thus, the results of the present study indicate that the opening of these endothelial potassium channels is also a critical step in the endothelium-dependent hyperpolarizations.

In the porcine coronary artery with endothelium, 11,12-EET produced an hyperpolarization of the smooth muscle that was abolished by the combination of apamin plus charybdotoxin but barely affected by that of iberiotoxin plus apamin, in this respect mimicking the EDHF-mediated response. In preparations without endothelium, 11,12-EET also hyperpolarized the smooth muscle although the magnitude of the response was smaller than in intact blood vessels. However, this effect was essentially abolished by iberiotoxin at a concentration that also abolished hyperpolarizations to the BK$_{Ca}$ opener, NS1619 indicating that 11,12-EET opened BK$_{Ca}$ channels on the myocytes. In studies using isolated coronary arterial smooth muscle cells, the potassium channel opened by exogenous EETs, including 11,12-EET, has a large unitary conductance. Since it is inhibited by iberiotoxin (Gebremedhin *et al.*, 1992, 1998; Li and Campbell, 1997; Hayabuchi *et al.*, 1998), it is likely to be BK$_{Ca}$ (Kaczorowski *et al.*, 1996) and this conclusion is consistent with the results of the present study. However, since the EDHF response is inhibited by the combination of apamin plus charybdotoxin and not by apamin plus iberiotoxin it seems unlikely that an 11,12-EET *per se* can account for the effects usually attributed to EDHF.

The 11,12-EET-induced hyperpolarization of either smooth muscle or endothelial cells of intact vessels was more sensitive to charybdotoxin alone than was the effect of substance P. EETs are believed to stimulate endothelial cell calcium influx via calcium release-activated channels (CRAC) (Hoebel *et al.*, 1997; Mombouli *et al.*, 1999). Speculatively, the primary effect of 11,12-EET may thus be to stimulate calcium influx via endothelial CRAC at a site closely associated with IK$_{Ca.}$. In the absence of the endothelial cell layer, the effect of 11,12-EET may result from the stimulation of calcium influx via smooth muscle CRAC channels which results in the opening of BK$_{Ca}$ channels and a smaller hyperpolarization.

In conclusion, the present study confirms that during EDHF-mediated responses, hyperpolarizations of vascular smooth muscle cell are initiated by the hyperpolarization of endothelial cells. It demonstrates that although 11,12-EET could be an essential component of the endothelial signal transduction in EDHF-mediated responses, the cytochrome P450 metabolite *per se* is not a diffusible hyperpolarizing factor released by endothelial cells.

24 Lipoxygenase-derived metabolites of arachidonic acid are not involved in the endothelium-dependent hyperpolarization to acetylcholine in the carotid artery of the guinea-pig

J.F. Quignard, T. Chataigneau, Catherine Corriu, Michel Félétou and Paul M. Vanhoutte

The present study was designed to determine whether or not lipoxygenase-dependent metabolites of arachidonic acid are involved in the endothelium-dependent hyperpolarization of the carotid artery of the guinea-pig. The specific 12-lipoxygenase inhibitor cinnamyl-3,4 dihydroxy-α-cyanocinnamate (CDC), the non-specific inhibitor of lipoxygenase, cycloxygenase and cytochrome P450 eicosatetraynoic acid (ETYA), and the inhibitors of phospholipase A2 AACOCF3 and quinacrine did not significantly affect the membrane potential of the vascular smooth muscle cells while the 5-lipoxygenase inhibitor AA861 produced a significant hyperpolarization. Acetylcholine-induced hyperpolarizations were not significantly affected by AACOCF3, ETYA and quinacrine. In contrast, CDC at 10^{-5} M (but not at 10^{-6} M) and AA861 (10^{-6} and 10^{-5} M) produced a partial but significant inhibition of the hyperpolarization. ($\pm$)12-Hydroxy-eicosatetraenoic acid (12-HETE, 10^{-6} M) and 12(S)-hydroperoxy-eicosatetraenoic acid (12(S)-HpETE, 3×10^{-6} M) did not induce significant changes in membrane potential. In isolated vascular smooth muscle cells, CDC inhibited voltage-gated potassium currents sensitive to 4-aminopyridine and increased calcium-activated potassium currents sensitive to charybdotoxin while AA861 inhibited both potassium currents. These results suggest that lipoxygenase-dependent metabolites of arachidonic acid are unlikely to be involved in the acetylcholine-induced endothelium-dependent hyperpolarization of the carotid artery of the guinea-pig.

Arachidonic acid metabolites may play a role in the endothelium-dependent hyperpolarizations (EDHF) that are resistant to inhibitors of cycloxygenase and nitric oxide synthase (Rubanyi and Vanhoutte, 1985; Campbell *et al.*, 1996; Popp *et al.*, 1996; Pfister *et al.*, 1998; Weintraub *et al.*, 1998; Fisslthaler *et al.*, 1999). In vascular tissue, arachidonic acid is released from the membrane lipids and can be metabolised not only by cyclooxygenase, but also by various other enzymes including cytochrome P450 monoxygenases and lipoxygenases (Greenwald *et al.*, 1979; Seed and Bass, 1999). In bovine, porcine and canine coronary arteries, epoxyeicosatrienoic acids, metabolites of the cytochrome P450 monoxygenase, may be implicated in endothelium-dependent hyperpolarizations (Campbell *et al.*, 1996; Popp *et al.*, 1996; Fisslthaler *et al.*, 1999). In addition, endothelium-derived eicosanoids (12 and 15 HpETE or HETE) produced by the lipoxygenase pathways relax various isolated arteries such as the rabbit aorta (Pfister *et al.*, 1998, 1999; Rosolowsky *et al.*, 1990) and activate potassium channels (Piomelli *et al.*, 1987; Buttner *et al.*, 1989). In the guinea-pig carotid artery, the involvement of a cytochrome P450 monoxygenase metabolite has been ruled out (Corriu *et al.*, 1996; Chataigneau *et al.*, 1998) but the role of lipoxygenase metabolites is unknown. Therefore, the present experiments were designed to assess the possible involvement of lipoxygenase in the genesis of endothelium-dependent hyperpolarization.

1. MATERIALS AND METHODS

1.1. Microelectrode studies

The internal carotid artery of the guinea-pig was dissected and cleaned of adherent connective tissues, pinned to the bottom of an organ chamber and superfused with a thermostated modified Krebs–Ringer bicarbonate solution of the following composition (in mM): NaCl 118.3, KCl 4.7, $CaCl_2$ 2.5, $MgSO_4$ 1.2, KH_2PO_4 1.2, $NaHCO_3$ 25, glucose 11.1 and EDTA 0.026 (buffered with 95% O_2/5% CO_2, pH 7.4). Transmembrane potential was recorded by using glass capillary microelectrodes (tip resistance of 30–90 MΩ) filled with KCl (3 M) and connected to the headstage of a recording amplifier (intra 767, WPI). Impalements of the smooth muscle cells were performed from the adventitial side. Successful impalements were signalled by a sudden negative drop in potential from the baseline (zero potential reference) followed by a stable negative potential for at least 3 min. All the experiments were performed in the presence of N^ω-nitro-L-arginine (10^{-4} M) and indomethacin (5×10^{-6} M) to inhibit nitric oxide synthase and cyclooxygenase, respectively (Corriu *et al.*, 1996).

1.2. Patch-clamp studies

Male Hartley guinea-pigs (250–300 g) were anaesthetised by intraperitoneal administration of pentobarbitone (200 mg/kg). The media of guinea-pig carotid arteries was dissected from cleaned arteries. The smooth muscle cells were enzymatically dissociated (see Quignard *et al.*, 1999). Whole-cell potassium currents were recorded at room temperature using the patch-clamp technique. The cells were superfused with a solution containing (in mM): NaCl 125, KCl 5, $CaCl_2$ 2, $MgCl_2$ 1.2, HEPES 10 and glucose 11 (pH 7.4 with NaOH). The intracellular solution had the following composition (in mM): KCl 130, $MgCl_2$ 2, ATP 3, GTP 0.5, HEPES 25, EGTA 1, $CaCl_2$ 0.5 mM and Glucose 11 (pH 7.2 with NaOH). Data were recorded with pClamp6 software (Axon Instruments, USA) through a RK-400 amplifier (Biologic, France).

1.3. Drugs

The following drugs were used: acetylcholine, indomethacin, N^ω-nitro-L-arginine, quinacrine (Sigma, La Verpillère, France); charybdotoxin (Latoxan, Rosans, France); cinnamyl-3,4 dihydroxy-α-cyanocinnamate (CDC), 2,3,5-Trimethyl-6-(12-hydroxy-5,10-dodecadiynyl)-1,4-benzoquinone (AA846), Arachidonyl trifluoromethyl ketone (AACOCF3) (Tebu, Paris, France); eicosatetraynoic acid (EYTA), (±)12-hydroxy-eicosatetraenoic acid (12-HETE) and 12(S)-hydroperoxy-eicosatetraenoic acid (12(S)-HpETE) (cayman chemical).

Indomethacin was dissolved in deionized water with an equimolar concentration of Na_2CO_3. CDC, AA861, 12(S)-HpETE, and 12-HETE were dissolved in a stock solution of ethanol. The other drugs were dissolved in water.

1.4. Statistics

Data are shown as mean $\pm$ SEM; n indicates the number of cells. Statistical analysis was performed using Student's t-test for paired or unpaired observations. Differences were considered to be statistically significant when p was less than .05.

2. RESULTS

2.1. Intracellular microelectrode studies

In a first set of experiment, the mean resting membrane potential of the smooth muscle cells of the guinea-pig isolated carotid artery averaged -57.6 ± 1.6 mV ($n = 35$) and acetylcholine (10^{-6} M) induced an endothelium-dependent hyperpolarization of -15.1 ± 1.1 mV ($n = 35$). In the presence of quinacrine (10^{-5} M) and ETYA (5×10^{-5} M), the resting membrane potential and the hyperpolarizations induced by acetylcholine were not significantly affected (Figure 24.1).

In a second set of experiments, the mean resting membrane potential was -52.0 ± 0.9 mV ($n = 74$). Acetylcholine (10^{-6} M) induced an endothelium-dependent

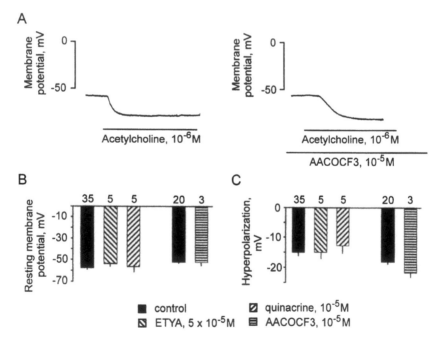

Figure 24.1 Inhibitors of phospholipase A2 and lipoxygenase and hyperpolarization induced by acetylcholine (10^{-6} M) in the isolated carotid artery of guinea-pig. (A) Recording of acetylcholine-induced hyperpolarization in absence (left) and presence (right) of AACOCF3 (10^{-5} M). (B) Effects of ETYA (5×10^{-5} M), quinacrine (10^{-5} M) and AACOCF3 (10^{-5} M) on the resting membrane potential. (C) Effects of ETYA (5×10^{-5} M), quinacrine (10^{-5} M) and AACOCF3 (10^{-5} M) on the amplitude of the acetylcholine-induced hyperpolarization. (B and C) Data are shown as means $\pm$ SEM. The numbers indicate the number of cells studied.

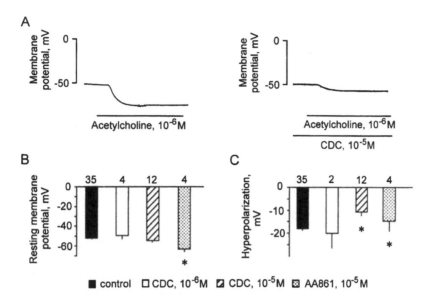

Figure 24.2 Inhibitors of lipoxygenase and hyperpolarization induced by acetylcholine (10^{-6} M) in the isolated carotid artery of guinea-pig. (A) Recording of acetylcholine-induced hyperpolarization in absence (left) and presence (right) of CDC (10^{-5} M). (B) Effects of CDC (10^{-6} M and 10^{-5} M) and AA861 (10^{-5} M) on the resting membrane potential. (C) Effects of CDC (10^{-6} M and 10^{-5} M) and AA861 (10^{-5} M) on the amplitude of the acetylcholine-induced hyperpolarization. (B and C) Data are shown as means ± SEM. The numbers indicate the number of cells studied.

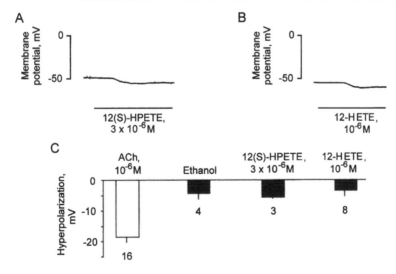

Figure 24.3 Effects of the lipoxygenase metabolites 12(S)-HpETE (3×10^{-6} M) and 12-HETE (10^{-6} M) on the membrane potential of vascular smooth muscle cells in the isolated carotid artery of the guinea-pig. (A and B) Recording of the membrane potential after bolus application of 12(S)-HpETE (3×10^{-6} M) and 12-HETE (10^{-6} M), respectively. (C) Summary bar-graph. Data are shown as means ± SEM. The numbers indicate the number of cells studied.

hyperpolarization (-18.2 ± 0.6 mV, $n = 55$). In the presence of AACOCF3 (10^{-5} M), the resting membrane potential and the acetylcholine-induced hyperpolarization were not significantly affected (Figure 24.1). CDC (10^{-6} and 10^{-5} M) did not alter the membrane potential, but at the highest concentration tested induced a significant inhibition of the acetylcholine-induced hyperpolarization (Figure 24.2). AA861 (10^{-6} and 10^{-5} M) hyperpolarized the smooth muscle cells. This effect was associated with a partial inhibition of the hyperpolarization induced by acetylcholine (Figure 24.2).

Bolus injection of 12(S)-HpETE (3×10^{-6} M, $n = 3$) and 12-HETE (10^{-6} M, $n = 8$) produced minor changes in membrane potential that were similar to those with solvent (5% v/v alcohol, $n = 4$) and significantly smaller than those produced by acetylcholine (Figure 24.3).

2.2. Patch-clamp studies

Freshly dissociated vascular smooth muscle cells from the guinea-pig carotid artery expressed voltage-gated and calcium-activated potassium channels (Quignard *et al.*, 2000). With a holding potential of -100 mV, both currents could be recorded. With a holding potential of 0 mV, only calcium-activated potassium current were recorded.

With a holding potential of -100 mV, in the presence of 10 mM of EGTA to chelate intracellular calcium, CDC (from 10^{-7} to 2×10^{-5} M) produced a concentration-dependent inhibition of the 4-aminopyridine-sensitive, voltage-dependent potassium current (Figure 24.4). With a holding potential of 0 mV, and with a high concentration of free intracellular calcium, CDC (from 10^{-7} to 2×10^{-5} M) induced an increase in the charybdotoxin-sensitive outward current ($+180 \pm 30\%$, $n = 4$ at $+60$ mV for the concentration of 2×10^{-5} M, Figure 24.4). In both conditions (holding potentials of -100 mV and 0 mV), the effects of CDC were also rapidly and completely reversible. AA861 (2×10^{-5} M) abolished the total outward potassium current recorded in response to a voltage step to $+40$ mV from a holding potential of -100 mV (Figure 24.5). This inhibition was reversible. In contrast, AACOCF3 (10^{-5} M) had no effect on the various potassium currents studied (Figure 24.5).

3. DISCUSSION

The present study suggests that, in the isolated carotid artery of the guinea-pig, the involvement of arachidonic acid and lipoxygenase metabolites in the endothelium-dependent hyperpolarization is unlikely.

Arachidonic acid is an intracellular second messenger that is released from the lipids of the plasma membrane, mainly by phospholipase A_2, and then metabolized into bioactive substances by several enzymes including lipoxygenases (Greenwald *et al.*, 1979). The acetylcholine-induced hyperpolarization was not affected by quinacrine and ETYA, two non-specific inhibitors of phospholipase A_2 (Chi *et al.*, 1982) as well as by AACOCF3, one of the most specific inhibitor of this enzyme (Ackerman *et al.*, 1995). These results indicate that in the guinea-pig carotid artery, the mobilization of arachidonic acid is not involved in EDHF-mediated responses confirming previous observations in this and other vascular tissues (Corriu *et al.*, 1996; Yamanaka *et al.*, 1998; Drummond *et al.*, 2000).

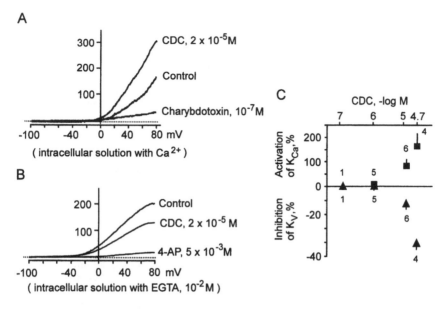

Figure 24.4 CDC and potassium channels in vascular smooth muscle cells of the guinea-pig carotid artery. (A) CDC (2×10^{-5} M) and calcium-activated potassium current elicited by a ramp depolarization (holding potential -100 mV, high intracellular free calcium). Note that this current was inhibited by charybdotoxin (10^{-7} M), voltage-gated potassium channels were inhibited by a holding potential of 0 mV prior to the ramp. (B) CDC (2×10^{-5} M) inhibited voltage gated potassium current elicited by a ramp depolarization (holding potential -100 mV, very low intracellular free calcium). The current was inhibited by 4-aminopyridine (4-AP, 5×10^{-3} M). (C) Concentration-dependent activation of the calcium-activated potassium current (K_{ca}) and concentration-dependent inhibition of the voltage-gated potassium (K_v) by CDC top and bottom panel, respectively). Data are shown as means $\pm$ SEM. The numbers indicate the number of cells studied.

Quinacrine, and ETYA compounds that are also non-specific inhibitors of lip-oxygenases (ETYA: Kd for 5-, 12- and 15-lipoxygenases: 10^{-5}, 3×10^{-7}, 2×10^{-7} M, respectively; Salari *et al.*, 1984) did not influence endothelium-dependent hyper-polarization. In contrast, both CDC, a poorly selective 12-lipoxygenase inhibitor (Kd: 2×10^{-6}, 6×10^{-8}, 3×10^{-6} M for 5-, 12- and 15-lipoxygenase, respectively; Cho *et al.*, 1991, and AA861, an inhibitor of 5-lipoxygenase (Kd for 5-, and 12-lipoxygenase: 10^{-7}, $>10^{-5}$ M, Ashida *et al.*, 1983), produced a partial but significant inhibition of the hyperpolarization evoked by acetylcholine. These results are in agreement with pre-vious studies showing an inhibitory effect of AA861 on acetylcholine-mediated relaxations in various vascular beds (Matsumoto *et al.*, 1992; Satake *et al.*, 1997; Obi *et al.*, 1991; Kanamaru *et al.*, 1987, 1989). However, the inhibitory effect of AA861 could be due a lack of specificity. Indeed, this compound *per se* produced a hyperpo-larization of the smooth muscle cells. This may explain the decrease in the amplitude of the acetylcholine-induced hyperpolarization, as the amplitude of the latter is negat-ively correlated with the absolute value of the resting membrane potential (Chataigneau *et al.*, 1998). Furthermore, the analysis of the potassium currents in the smooth muscle

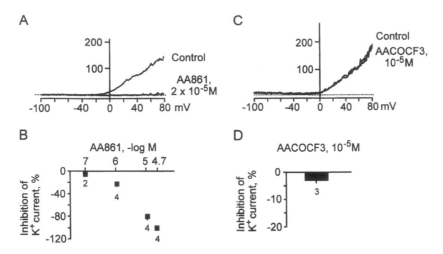

Figure 24.5 Potassium channels, AA861 and AACOCF3 in vascular smooth muscle cells of the guinea-pig carotid artery. (A) AA861 (2×10^{-5} M) inhibited potassium current elicited by a ramp depolarization (holding potential -100 mV, high intracellular free calcium). This current was inhibited by the combination of charybdotoxin (10^{-7} M) plus 4-AP (5×10^{-3} M) (data not shown). (B) Concentration-dependent inhibition of the potassium current by AA861. (C) AACOCF$_3$ (10^{-5} M) and potassium current elicited by a ramp depolarization (holding potential -100 mV, high intracellular free calcium). (D) Summary bar-graph of the effects of AACOCF$_3$. Data are shown as means $\pm$ SEM. The numbers indicate the number of cells studied.

cells of the guinea-pig carotid artery revealed non-specific effects of both CDC and AA861. Vascular smooth muscle cells of the guinea-pig carotid artery express different type of potassium channels (e.g., calcium-activated potassium channels sensitive to apamin and iberitoxin (K_{Ca}) and voltage gated potassium channels sensitive to 4-aminopyridine (K_V) (Quignard *et al.*, 2000)). CDC produced a concentration-dependent partial inhibition of the current but also increased the K_{Ca} current. The concentrations necessary to induce alterations of the potassium currents were in the same order of magnitude than those required to inhibit acetylcholine-induced hyperpolarization. Furthermore, the other inhibitor of lipoxygenase that significantly reduced endothelium-dependent hyperpolarization, AA861 also inhibited the two types of potassium currents studied (K_{Ca} and K_V). The non-specific effects of these drugs and especially interactions with ion channels have been described frequently. For example, nordihydroguaiaretic acid activates K_{Ca} current and inhibits K_V current and voltage-gated calcium channel, these effects being unrelated to the inhibition of lipoxygenase (Yamamura, 1999; Hatton and Peers, 1997). Interestingly, in the present study, the specific inhibitor of phospholipase A2 AACOCF3 did not affect the various potassium channels studied and did not influence either the resting membrane potential of smooth muscle cells or the acetylcholine-induced hyperpolarization.

Altogether these results cast some doubt on the participation of a lipoxygenase metabolite of arachidonic acid in the EDHF-mediated responses in the guinea-pig carotid artery. This hypothesis was definitively ruled out by the observation that 12(S)-HpETE, a product of lipoxygenase that can activate potassium channels

(Buttner *et al.*, 1989; Belardetti *et al.*, 1989), and its metabolite 12-HETE did not significantly affect the membrane potential of the smooth muscle cells of the guinea-pig carotid artery while, under the same experimental conditions, acetylcholine produced endothelium-dependent hyperpolarizations. The results of the present study are in agreement with earlier studies showing that 12-HETE did not relax isolated blood vessels (Masferrer and Mullane, 1988; Forstermann and Neufang, 1984).

25 Cytochrome P450 isoforms in the brain encode cell specific hyperpolarizing factors with a common mechanism of action

David R. Harder, Cindy C. Zhang,
Mohammad R. Taheri, Jayashree Narayanan,
Richard J. Roman, Chad E. Voskuil,
William B. Campbell and Meetha Medhora

Evidence has accumulated for the extra hepatic role of cytochrome P450 metabolites of arachidonic acid especially in the vasculature. Arachidonic acid is metabolized to hydroxyeicosatetraenoic acids (HETEs) and epoxyeicosatrienoic acids (EETs) by a family of cytochrome P450 isozymes. The distribution and expression of these isozymes is cell specific. These metabolites are emerging as important cellular second messengers and carry out numerous functions. HETEs play a role in the autoregulation of blood flow, and are involved in the regulation of membrane ion channels. EETs are emerging to be an important hyperpolarizing factor predominantly in the microvasculature. This chapter summarizes the current knowledge concerning the role of EETs in the cerebral circulation with respect to functional hyperemia.

Metabolites of arachidonic acid (AA) formed by extra hepatic cytochrome P450 can be released from both endothelial and parenchymal cells and help to regulate regional blood flow. Both hydroxyeicosatetraenoic acids (HETEs) and epoxyeicosatrienoic acids (EETs) not only function as signal transduction molecules regulating the excitability of vascular smooth muscle (Ellis *et al.*, 1990; Gebremedhin *et al.*, 1992; Komori *et al.*, 1993) but its mitogenic activity as well (Burns *et al.*, 1995, Chen *et al.*, 1998; Munzenmaier and Harder, 2000). These actions of HETEs and EETs are mediated by phosphorylation and regulation of membrane ion channel proteins, and by the induction of intracellular second messengers (Shivachar *et al.*, 1995; Lange *et al.*, 1997; Node *et al.*, 1999).

1. CELL SPECIFIC CYTOCHROME P450 ISOFORMS

In the brain, astrocytes express P450 genes coding for epoxygenase enzymes catalyzing the formation of EETs from arachidonic acid. Epoxygenases are also expressed in the endothelium through different cell-specific genetic isoforms. The principal metabolites in this regard appear to be 11,12- and 14,15-EETs. In the rat, parietal cortical astrocytes contain P450 2C11, whereas the endothelium generates these same metabolites through a different P450 gene, which has not yet been fully characterized in cerebral arteries (Campbell *et al.*, 1996; Quilley *et al.*, 1997; Mombouli *et al.*, 1997;

Gebremedhin *et al.*, 1998a; Fisslthaler *et al.*, 1999). There are over 232 cytochrome P450 genes in mammalian cells many of which make the same or similar metabolites. One of the actions of epoxygenated metabolites of arachidonic acid is to reduce arterial tone by hyperpolarizing and inhibiting the activation of vascular smooth muscle.

The multiplicity of genes (either splice variants of a given "family" or different genes encoding for similar enzymes) allows for an extreme diversity in function in a cell specific manner. This multiplicity of isoforms is much more diverse than for nitric oxide synthase or cycloxygenase isoforms in that there are only a few members in these cases as compared to the P450s. The large diversity of P450s allows controlled induction of specific isoforms resulting in a wide range of finely tuned vascular effects.

The expression of selective NOS isoforms is difficult to achieve experimentally, and may not be possible under certain physiological conditions. Conversely, the induction of P450 is cell and condition specific (Fisslthaler *et al.*, 1999). Examples of this include induction of omega-hydroxylase of the P450 4A family in vascular smooth muscle while leaving EETs production via a P450 2C in endothelium alone (Shatara *et al.*, 2000). Cytokines will increase in all cell types, and the induction of inducible nitric oxide synthase can be catastrophic in that induction is difficult to control from cell to cell. In the rat, astrocytes produce EETs via induction of 2C11. However EETs can be produced via a purinergic receptor mediated stimulation of endothelial cells (Campbell *et al.*, 1996). The EETs produced by astrocytes and endothelium are similar in their mode of action, yet induction is differentially regulated, as may be the physiological mode of action. Astrocytes produce at least two of the EET regioisoforms, however, the predominant one appears to be 14,15-EET, which not only increases microvascular blood flow but is mitogenic as well (Burns *et al.*, 1995). Preliminary data suggests that the predominant EET released from rat cerebral microvascular endothelial cells are 14,15-EET and 5,6-EET which have been shown to dilate cerebral arterioles, but the role of these on mitogenic activity has to be determined (Figure 25.1).

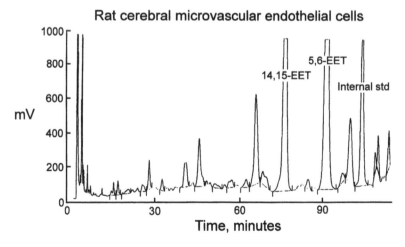

Figure 25.1 Reverse phase high performance liquid chromatographic separation of arachidonic acid metabolites in endothelial cells by fluorescent assay. Acidified ethyl acetate extracts of endothelial cells were derivatized with the fluorescent probe (2-(2,3-naphthalamino) ethyltrifluoromethanesulfonate), purified by C18 Sep-Pak chromatography and analyzed by high performance liquid chromatography (Maier *et al.*, 2000). EET = epoxyeicosatrienoic acid; std = standard.

2. PREPONDERENCE OF EETs IN THE MICROCIRCULATION

The enzymes producing EETs are expressed in the microvasculature. While this is commonly stated the data in support of it is somewhat indirect. Cytochrome P450 activity is expressed in the microcirculation of kidney, brain, heart, gut and skeletal muscle (Harder *et al.*, 2000). NOS activity is found in large and intermediate size vessels of most vascular beds, however, it is often difficult to find P450 activity in these same blood vessels. While it is not easy to measure NOS activity in the microcirculation via conventional arginine-citrulline assay systems, it may be more a problem of obtaining sufficient tissue rather than a lack of activity. However one can say with relative certainty, that P450 activity is a major factor in the regulation of the microcirculation (Harder *et al.*, 1995).

One of the major targets for the action of epoxygenated products of AA metabolized by P450 enzymes is the Ca^{2+} activated K channel K_{Ca} (Harder *et al.*, 1994). While exhaustive study excluding other K channel types has been published, the major K channel that is gated or exhibits an increase in outward current in vascular smooth muscle is the K_{Ca} (Nelson and Quayle, 1995). Increasing K_{Ca} activity hyperpolarizes, while inhibition of K_{Ca} depolarizes arterial muscle. It is a biological fact that a final common denominator of HETEs and EETs is their action on K_{Ca} (Gebremedhin *et al.*, 1992; Harder, 1994; Campbell *et al.*, 1996; Gebremedhin *et al.*, 1998a,b). In cerebral arteriolar smooth muscle, the omega-hydroxylase product of arachidonic acid – 20HETE inhibits K_{Ca} (Harder *et al.*, 1994). 20HETE helps to maintain autoregulation of cerebral blood flow in response to increasing arterial pressure (Gebremedhin *et al.*, 2000; Harder *et al.*, 2000). Maintenance of vessel caliber in the face of increasing arterial pressure requires either that intracellular Ca^{2+} rises or that sensitivity to Ca^{2+} increases. To keep the plasma membrane of arteriolar smooth muscle from hyperpolarizing and the vessel from dilating, K_{Ca} must be inhibited – an action which occurs via phosphorylation of K_{Ca} through a protein kinase C-dependent mechanism requiring the production of 20-HETE, and an increase in intracellular Ca^{2+} level (Gebremedhin *et al.*, 1998b).

3. MECHANISM UNDERLYING FUNCTIONAL HYPEREMIA IN THE BRAIN

One of the major P450 genes expressed in cortical astrocytes is 2C11. The EETs produced by rat cortical astrocytes are 14,15-EET and 11,12-EET, which are released from astrocytes by the excitatory neurotransmitter glutamate (Amruthesh *et al.*, 1992, 1993; Alkayed *et al.*, 1996). The production and release of EETs from astrocytes is blocked by both pharmacological inhibition of P450 epoxygenase activity and by antisense oligonucleotides against 2C11 (Harder *et al.*, 1998a). Using a fluorescent assay for EETs, the production of EETs can be demonstrated in primary cultures of astrocytes (Figure 25.2). EETs have also been detected in the cerebral spinal fluid (data not shown). Preliminary data suggest that EETs can be stored in astrocytes and released upon neural stimulation. Uniformly radio-labeled EETs were infused into the brains of anesthetized rats for 3 hours. These EETs were then localized in sections of the rat brain by means of a double-labeling technique with combination of immunohistochemistry to glial fibrillary acidic protein, a marker for astrocytes, and autoradiography.

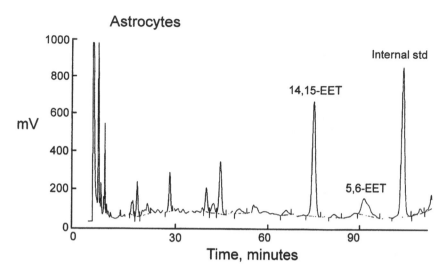

Figure 25.2 Reverse phase high performance liquid chromatographic separation of metabolites of arachidonic acid in primary cultures of astrocytes by fluorescent assay. EET = epoxyeicosatrienoic acid; std = standard.

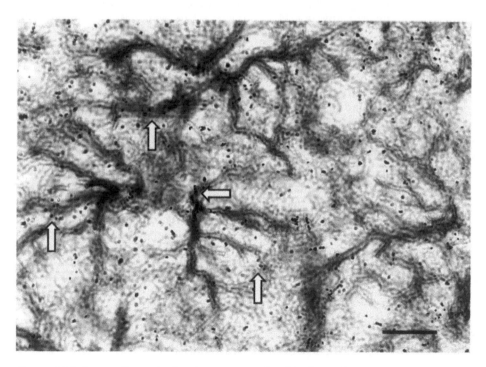

Figure 25.3 Autoradiograph showing an example of brain section that was infused with radiolabeled EET and immunohistochemically stained with glial fibrillary acidic protein (GFAP). Note the colocalization of radiolabeled EETs with GFAP-immunoreactive profiles (arrows). Scale bar, 30 µm. (*see Color Plate 9*)

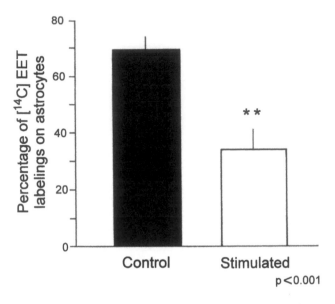

Figure 25.4 Quantitative analysis of the location of radiolabeled EETs in brain sections of control and barrel cortex-stimulated rats. About 70% of radiolabeled EETs were located in astrocytes in the control animals. There was decreased EET labelings on the astrocytes after intense whisker stimulation. Data shown as means $\pm$ SEM ($n = 14$). The double asterisk indicates a statistically significant ($p < .001$) difference.

This demonstrated localization of radiolabeled EETs in the astrocytes (Figure 25.3). Following intense neural stimulation of the whisker barrel cortex a decreased radioactive signal was found in the astrocytes (Figure 25.4). These data do, albeit preliminary, add further support to the hypothesis that EETs released from astrocytes in response to neural activity are responsible for the functional hyperemia observed in separate functional studies (Alkayed *et al.*, 1997).

The role of functional hyperemia in the brain is to provide sufficient nutrients to metabolically active neurons and thus support prolonged activity (Harder *et al.*, 2000). Previous hypotheses suggest that neurons release vasodilators (Garthwaite *et al.*, 1988). These hypotheses have been challenged, however, due to several factors including the distance from neurons to the cerebral microcirculation (Harder *et al.*, 1998b). A role for astrocytes and astrocytic derived hyperpolarizing factor is firmly supported by the available data (Amruthesh *et al.*, 1992, 1993; Alkayed *et al.*, 1996, 1997; Harder *et al.*, 1997, 1998a,b).

4. HYPERPOLARIZING FACTORS BLOCK AUTOREGULATORY MECHANISMS

In the brain, second to second autoregulation of blood flow is a fundamental property of the blood vessel wall. In cerebral arterial smooth muscle P450 mRNAs of the 4A family encode for omega-hydroxylases, which catalyze arachidonic acid into

20-HETE (Okamoto *et al.*, 2000). 20-HETE is an intracellular second messenger that regulates ion channel activity, phosphorylating the α-subunits of K_{Ca} and L-type Ca^{2+} channels to potently activate vascular smooth muscle (Lange *et al.*, 1997; Gebremedhin *et al.*, 1998b). The substrates and cofactors required to form 20-HETE are controlled by membrane phospholipases in the cell. These phospholipases are activated by an elevation of transmural pressure. Inhibition of K_{Ca} blocks all membrane hyperpolarization as intracellular Ca^{2+} increases, thereby, maintaining high levels of myogenic tone. Thus arterial caliber becomes smaller as arterial pressure increases. EETs released from astrocytes in response to excitatory transmitters during neuronal activity increase K_{Ca} activity, reversing autoregulatory behavior and hyperpolarizing arterial muscle. As a consequence, the arterial caliber increases, which redistribute blood, flow to metabolically active neurons, resulting in functional hyperemia (Harder *et al.*, 1998a, 2000). EETs and NO are also released from the endothelium, to add to this increase in cerebral blood flow. At this point it is not known if the purpose of endothelial hyperpolarizing influences are the same as those coming from astrocytes. However, the hyperpolarizing influences derived from astrocytes are also mitogenic in nature, and may, therefore, regulate capillary density. Thus, the chronic release of astrocytic EETs due to long term activation of specific nerves may enhance functional hyperemia by increasing capillary density (Munzenmaier and Harder, 2000). At this point we can only speculate that astrocytic mediated EET release enhances functional hyperemia, upon neural activation. This may function in task performance ability and perhaps learning capacity.

Currently, there is no indication that astrocytic and endothelial hyperpolarizing mechanisms are linked except to inhibit myogenic activity in cerebral arterioles, allowing blood flow to increase. It is clear, however, that the two mechanisms can occur independently and may be mediated by different P450 isoforms in the different cell types.

ACKNOWLEDGMENTS

This work was supported in part by NIH grant RO1 NS32321 and PO1 HL59996, and VA Merit Grant 3440. The authors also thank Rachel B. Kraemer for technical support.

26 Expression of recombinant cytochrome P450 epoxygenase in rat brain

Meetha Medhora, Hirotsugu Okamoto, Jayashree Narayanan, Chenyang Zhang, Xinnan Niu, Mohammad R. Taheri, Rachel Kraemer, Jorge Capdevila and David R. Harder

Epoxyeicosatrienoic acids (EETs) carry out a number of functions in brain tissue, some of which include vasodilatation of cerebral vessels and endothelial tube formation. The excitatory neurotransmitter glutamate, releases EETs from cultured astrocytes. Inhibition of EET synthesis in the whisker barrel cortex of the rat partially blocks functional hyperemia. To better understand these functions of EETs an attempt to overexpress cytochrome P450-epoxygenases in rat brain was made. This approach has been challenging because P450 enzymes need specific cofactors. Also gene delivery into brain *in vivo* is difficult due to the high cell density in the parenchyma. Recombinant genes have been successfully expressed in rat brain by infusion of adenoviral vectors into the lateral ventricle. When introduced in this way, viral coded genes showed abundant expression in the ependymal cells. In this study expression in the choroid plexus was also observed. The next step was to introduce a bacterial cytochrome P450 epoxygenase, BM-3 F87V, into cultured rat astrocytes. The recombinant BM-3 F87V cloned in an adenovirus genome, synthesized 14S, 15R-EET and its corresponding dihydroxyeicosatrienoic acids (DiHETEs) after infection into cultured astrocytes. The bacterial gene also increased growth of the astrocytes after stimulation with serum, as measured by radioactive thymidine incorporation assays. Expression of Ad5/BM-3 F87V in brain tissue was monitored by infusion of the virus into the rat brain ventricle followed by the substrate, ^{14}C-arachidonic acid, after 24 hours. Cellular lipids were extracted and resolved by reverse phase high performance liquid chromatography (rpHPLC). The results showed conversion of the arachidonic acid into 14,15-EET demonstrating potential for use of recombinant P450 enzymes for research as well as gene therapy in the brain.

The cytochrome P450 gene family consists of over 232 members (Harder *et al.*, 1994). The enzymes are often pleiotropic and redundant. For example multiple genes from the families A, B, C, D, E and J (Kempermann *et al.*, 1994; Montoliu *et al.*, 1995; Komori *et al.*, 1993; Medhora and Harder, 1998) that are present in the brain can epoxygenate the lipid arachidonic acid to produce epoxyeicosatrienoic acids (EETs). The functions of EETs have been deciphered using pharmacological inhibitors that can bind to members of other P450 families, complicating inferences. It has become evident that molecular tools are necessary to dissect the specificities of this system. However, classical loss of function approaches have fundamental limitations due the redundancy of the genes. In spite of this, antisense studies (Harder *et al.*, 1998;

Fisslthaler *et al.*, 1999) and gene knock outs have already yielded significant information. Overexpression of specific gene products is another tool that is available (Chen *et al.*, 1999; Fisslthaler *et al.*, 1999; Zeldin *et al.*, 1995; Waxman, 1984; Kronbach *et al.*, 1989). This study attempts to investigate epoxygenase function *in vivo*.

The EETs have numerous functions, particularly in the brain. There are four commonly described regioisomers, 5,6-, 8,9-, 11,12- and 14,15-EETs that have been tested for vasoreactivity (Gebremedhin *et al.*, 1992; Ellis *et al.*, 1990; Komori, 1993; Medhora and Harder, 1998). In addition, metabolites of EETs by the action of cyclooxygenase and hydrolase enzymes also show activity (Amruthesh *et al.*, 1993; Leffler *et al.*, 1997). The EETs were released from cultured astrocytes by the neurotransmitter glutamate (Alkayed *et al.*, 1997). Interest in these compounds has increased after their protective role in inflammation was observed (Node *et al.*, 1999) and by identification of EETs as the endothelium-derived hyperpolarizing factor (EDHF) in the coronary vasculature (Campbell *et al.*, 1996; Fisslthaler *et al.*, 1999; Quilley *et al.*, 1997; Mombouli *et al.*, 1997). Evidences for EETs in cerebral angiogenesis (Munzenmaier and Harder, 2000), growth (Chen *et al.*, 1998; Burns *et al.*, 1995) and intracellular signaling (Shivachar *et al.*, 1995; Node *et al.*, 1999), have further prompted use of the epoxygenases as candidates for gene transfer into the brain during stroke and other pathological states. Working towards this goal the mammalian gene 2C11 found in astrocytes, was cloned into an adenoviral vector (Medhora and Harder, 1998). In this study a bacterial epoxygense, BM-3 F87V (Graham-Lorence *et al.*, 1997) was used to test EET formation by gene transfer into the brain.

The bacterial gene derived from *Bacillus megaterium* has been engineered and specifically yields high levels of regio- and stereoselective 14S,15R-EET (Graham-Lorence *et al.*, 1997) The enzyme also contains a fused P450 reductase, necessary for EET formation. The presence of P450 reductase in various cell types of the brain is not well defined, making the bacterial enzyme attractive for transfer into brain cells that may have low levels of reductase. Adenovirus carrying the gene would facilitate rapid and relatively easy transfer of DNA to many types of cells in the brain (Ooboshi *et al.*, 1995; Muhonen *et al.*, 1997; Heistad and Faraci, 1996; Medhora and Harder, 1998). First, BM-3 F87V was tested for production of EETs and growth of astrocytes in cultured cells. The recombinant adenovirus was then injected into the lateral ventricle to monitor its ability to produce EET in the brain.

1. METHODS

1.1. Cell culture

Astrocytes were cultured from the hippocampi of 2–3-day-old Sprague-Dawley rat brains (Alkayed *et al.*, 1996). Briefly, the hippocampi were carefully dissected and cut into small pieces. The tissue was digested in serum free Dulbecco's modified Eagle's medium (DMEM) with 20 U/ml papain at 37 °C for 40 minutes with gentle agitation and washed three times in growth media consisting of DMEM supplemented with 10% heat inactivated fetal bovine serum (FBS) and antibiotics (1%). Tissue pieces were broken up by triturating with a narrow bore pipette and the cells were seeded at a density of 2×10^5/sq.cm (~ 2 hippocampi/T-75 flask) in the wash medium. The flasks were incubated in a tissue culture incubator at 37 °C under 5% CO_2 with 95% air. The medium was changed after two days and the cells were then fed twice a week. They were split for viral infection after they were 90% confluent.

1.2. Viral infection

The astrocyte cultures were passaged onto 100 mm tissue culture dishes until they were 80% confluent to obtain a homogenous cell population free of microglia. These cells were infected with Ad5/β-galactosidase or Ad5/BM-3 F87V by replacing the media with 4 ml of DMEM containing 2% FBS and required number of virus for each 100 mm dish (Medhora and Harder, 1998). The virus was diluted to the specific multiplicity of infection (MOI, which was usually 50, i.e., 50 plaque forming units (pfu) for every astrocyte in the dish) mentioned in each experiment. The mixture was rocked gently in a tissue culture incubator for 50 minutes. The media was removed and the virus neutralized with concentrated bleach. The cells were fed with growth media for 24 hours. To induce quiescence the media was replaced with DMEM supplemented with 0.1% bovine serum albumin (BSA, fatty acid and endotoxin free purchased from Sigma Chemicals, St. Louis, MO, USA) and antibiotics.

1.3. Western analysis

Astrocytes were infected with Ad5/BM-3 F87V (for amplification protocols see Foschi *et al.* (1997)) at increasing MOIs from 0, 6.25, 12.5, 25, 50 and 100. The cells were washed three times with phosphate buffered saline (PBS from Sigma) and scraped for preparation of microsomes by differential centrifugation (Alkayed *et al.*, 1996). Each 100 mm dish was homogenized in 300 µl sucrose buffer, which was used for electrophoresis on a 7.5% polyacrylamide gel (Alkayed *et al.*, 1996). The gel was transferred to nitrocellulose, developed with BM-3 specific polyclonal antibody and the bands detected by chemiluminescence. The experiments were repeated with astrocytes infected with Ad5/β-gal (prepared as described by Foschi *et al.* (1997)). No 130 kD BM-3 protein was seen in these blots (result not shown).

1.4. Lipid extraction from cultured astrocytes

Astrocytes were purified, seeded on 100 mm dishes and infected with a control recombinant adenovirus or Ad5/BM-3 F87V at a MOI of 50 as described above. The cells were made quiescent for 24 hours and then ^{14}C-arachidonic acid was added to the media (0.5 µCi/100 mm dish of specific activity of 57 mCi/mmol in the presence of cold arachidonic acid, which was added to give a final concentration of 25–30 µM arachidonic acid). The dishes were incubated at 37 °C for 30 minutes. The media was then removed and acidified with 1 M formic acid (80 µl/ml) to reach a pH below 4.0 (Alkayed *et al.*, 1996). It was extracted twice with equal volumes of ethyl acetate, back-extracted once with 1 ml of water and dried under pure nitrogen. The lipid residue was resuspended in a small volume of ethanol and counted. Equal counts from control virus and Ad5/BM-3 F87V media were resolved separately on a 2.1×25 cm C18 reverse phase high performance liquid chromatography (rpHPLC) column (Supelco LC-18) with a linear solvent gradient ranging from 30 volume acetonitrile/70 volume water/0.1 volume acetic acid to 100 volume acetonitrile/0.1 volume acetic acid, over 50 minutes at a flow rate of 0.5 ml/minute. The radioactive products were detected by an on-line radioactive flow detector.

1.5. Thymidine incorporation in astrocytes

Primary cultures of astrocytes were transferred into twenty-four well tissue culture clusters at a density of 50,000 cells/well. After 24 hours the wells were infected with control virus (Ad5/β-galactosidase) or Ad5/BM-3 F87V at a MOI of 50 and allowed to recover in growth medium (DMEM + 10% FBS + antibiotics). The media was removed after 24 hours, the cells were washed with PBS and placed in serum free media containing 0.1% fat-free BSA for 24 hours. They were treated with the same media containing 0.1% BSA (four wells for each virus) or stimulated with media containing 20% FBS (four wells/virus). After 18 hours ^{3}H-thymidine (2 µCi/well) was added and allowed to incorporate for 3 hours. The wells were washed three times with PBS and treated with ice-cold 15% trichloroacetic acid for 30 minutes at 0 °C to precipitate the macromolecules. The trichloroacetic acid was removed and the cells washed twice with distilled water and dried in a hood. Precipitates were solubilized with 0.5 ml/well of 1 N NaOH for 20 minutes at 37 °C. The NaOH was neutralized with an equal volume of HCl (1 M) and the contents quantitatively removed to scintillation tubes. Scintillation fluid (2.5 ml/ml solution of Ecoscint from National Diagnostics, Atlanta, GA, USA) was added to the samples which were counted for 5 minutes each. Results were pooled from three independent experiments. The means and standard errors were computed using Sigmastat 2.0 software and analyzed statistically in a *t*-test. There was a significant difference ($p < .05$) between serum stimulation of control virus infected astrocytes versus astrocytes infected with Ad5/BM-3 F87V.

1.6. Infusion of virus into rat brain

Rats (8–10-week-old Sprague-Dawley, 250 gm) were anesthetized with 0.5 ml nembutal (40 mg/kg IP) until all tail and feet pain reflexes were abolished. The animals were fitted in a stereotaxic apparatus on a heating pad. Temperature was monitored with a rectal thermometer. The head was shaved and a midline incision was made between the ears to expose the skull. A small hole was drilled above the co-ordinates 1.2 mm lateral and 0.7 mm posterior to Bregma. A 30 gauge needle was inserted at the same co-ordinates to a depth of 4.5 mm below the surface of the brain. Virus (0.1 ml of a stock of 5×10^{10} pfu/ml) were infused through the needle at a flow rate of 2 µl/ minute using a pump. The animal was then injected with antibiotic Enrofloxacin (Baytril, 10 mg/kg twice a day, subcutaneously), the hole covered with bone wax and the skin sutured into place aseptically. The rat was kept under observation until it was able to walk and administered with analgesics (Buprenorphine 0.01 mg/kg twice a day). The next day the rat was anesthetized again and the brain removed for β-galactosidase assay, or the animal's brain was infused with ^{14}C-arachidonic acid (0.25 µCi) suspended in artificial cerebrospinal fluid containing 0.1% fat free BSA (0.1 ml). After 30 minutes the animal was sacrificed and the brain removed for dissection.

1.7. Staining and sectioning the brain to monitor β-galactosidase activity

The brain was carefully cut into slices ($\sim$2 mm each) with a sharp blade. These sections were lightly fixed with PBS containing 2% paraformaldehyde and 0.025% gluteraldehyde for 5 minutes. The slices were well washed in PBS and then immersed in X-gal solution (PBS with 20 mM $K_4Fe(CN)_6$, 20 mM $K_3Fe(CN)_6$, 2 mM $MgCl_2$, 1 mg/ml of X-gal dissolved in DMSO). The samples were kept at 37 °C for 2 hours. Brains infused with control (not β-gal) virus or no virus were always included to make sure no non-specific blue color was observed. The stained tissue was washed with PBS and frozen on dry ice for sectioning. Frozen sections were cut (thickness 15 μm) and transferred onto glass slides. They were counter-stained with nuclear fast red for visualization under the microscope.

1.8. Lipid extraction from the brain

The brain was removed and cut into 0.5 cm slices with a sharp blade. Tissue from around the ventricles was dissected carefully, collected and pooled. Tissue distal to the ventricle was pooled separately. The samples were separated into 50 mg aliquots to extract lipid. Each aliquot was homogenized with 3 ml PBS acidified with 1 M formic acid to reach a pH between 3.5 and 4.0. The tissue was homogenized and extracted with one volume methanol and two volumes chloroform. The lower phase was separated after centrifugation for 5 minutes at 1500 × g in glass tubes that had been rinsed with methanol. The aqueous phase was extracted with a mixture of equal volume methanol and two volumes chloroform till it was clear and solubilized. The lower phases were collected, back extracted with water and evaporated under nitrogen. Lipid residues were dissolved in 0.5 ml of ethanol and the radioactivity in 0.1 volume determined. Extracts from the ventricle and areas distal to it, that contained equal counts were used to separate the free fatty acids from esterified lipids.

This was done using C18 Sep-Pak (purchased from Waters, # WAT054955, Milford, MA, USA). The column was pre-washed with 1 ml water, 1 ml acetonitrile followed by 1 ml water. The sample was applied to the column under a light vacuum and washed twice with 1 ml of 30% acetonitrile. The free lipids were extracted from the resin with 0.4 ml of 90% acetonitrile and dried under nitrogen. The lipid residue was resuspended in a small volume of ethanol and equal amounts of samples were used for rpHPLC analysis (see section 1.4).

2. RESULTS

2.1. Expression of Ad5/BM-3 F87V in astrocytes

Adenovirus carrying the gene for BM-3 F87V was introduced into cultures of astrocytes in increasing doses using a range of MOIs. After 24 hours, the cells were lysed and partitioned into microsomal and cytosolic fractions. Western Blotting of the proteins detected expression of the expected 130 kD band in the cytosol of cells infected with Ad5/BM-3 F87V at MOI of 6.25 and up, while the control (MOI = 0) did not show any protein (Figure 26.1). No band was detected in the microsomal

Astrocyte Cytosol

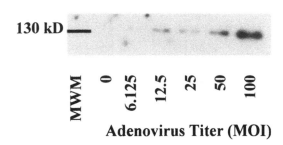

Figure 26.1 Western analysis of astrocytes infected with Ad5/BM-3 F87V. The cells were infected with increasing concentration of virus Ad5/BM-3 F87V and lysed by homogenization in hypotonic sucrose. Equal amount of cytosol from each sample was used for Western Analysis with a specific BM-3 antibody. A 130 kD band was seen in the lowest titer of viral infection, which increased with the multiplicity of infection (MOI). No BM-3 protein was seen in the lane representing an MOI of 0. Lane MWM = molecular weight marker.

fractions since the bacterial enzyme is soluble as opposed to its eukaryotic counterparts and controls using cells infected with other recombinant adenovirus did not show this band with BM-3 specific antiserum (results not shown).

The infection was repeated and the cells incubated with the substrate, ^{14}C-labeled arachidonate (3×10^{-5} M), in the absence of serum for 30 minutes. The media was removed and used for lipid extraction. The products were resolved by rpHPLC (Figure 26.2). There were three sets of prominent products seen in the media of cells infected with the Ad5/BM-3 F87V, that were not present in the media of cells infected with control virus. The tallest peak at ~ 20 minutes could not be identified by DiHETE and EET standards and may represent cycloxygenase metabolites of 14,15-EET. The second peak eluted with the DiHETE standards while the third peak (28 minutes) migrated with the early eluting EET standards that represent 14,15- and 11,12-EETs.

2.2. Growth of astrocytes carrying Ad5/BM-3 F87V

The recombinant virus was assayed for effects on growth in astrocytes. Infected cells were allowed to recover for 24 hours in serum containing media (10% FBS) before being starved to induce quiescence. Stimulation of growth by serum was then assayed by measuring thymidine incorporation in cells infected with a control virus versus Ad5/BM-3 F87V. The bacterial BM-3 F87V gene induced a three-fold greater increase in DNA synthesis over cells infected with virus carrying the bacterial lac Z gene coding for β-galactosidase, after stimulation for 18 hours with 20% FBS (Figure 26.3).

2.3. Expression of adenovirus in brain tissue

The Ad5/β-galactosidase (0.1 ml containing 5×10^9 pfu at an infusion rate of 2 μl/minute) was introduced the into the lateral ventricle of adult rats (~ 250 gm each).

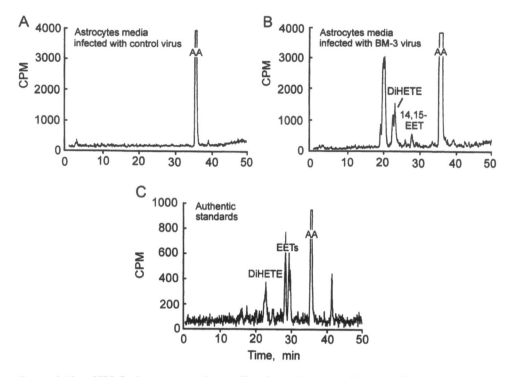

Figure 26.2 rpHPLC chromatography profile of arachidonic acid-metabolites synthesized by recombinant Ad5/BM-3 F87V. Panel A: profile of lipid extracts of media from astrocytes infected with a control recombinant adenovirus and incubated overnight with ^{14}C-labeled arachidonic acid; Panel B: profile of media from astrocytes infected with recombinant Ad5/BM-3 F87V incubated with ^{14}C-labeled arachidonic acid; Panel C: elution profile of standard mixture of epoxyeicosatrienoic acid (EETs, 14,15-, 11,12-, 8,9- and 5,6-EETs) and dihydroxyeicosatrienoic acids (DiHETEs) labeled with [14]C. Note peaks co-eluting with the DiHETE and early EET peaks present in panel B and absent in A, representing product of the bacterial epoxygense.

The animals were sacrificed after 24 hours and the brain stained for β-galactosidase activity. Care was taken to stop the color development after 2 hours to avoid nonspecific staining. No blue color was observed in brains used as controls along with the experimental samples. The tissue was frozen and thin sections (15 μm) were cut and examined for blue color in cells, after counter staining with nuclear fast red (Figure 26.4). Dark blue staining for β-galactosidase was observed in the cells which were anatomically identified from the choroid plexus (Figure 26.4).

2.4. Assay of EET production in brain after infection with Ad5/BM-3 F87V

Recombinant Ad5/BM-3 F87V was infused into the lateral ventricle of the anesthetized rat at the co-ordinates 1.2 mm lateral and 0.7 mm posterior to Bregma, at a depth of 4.5 mm below the surface of the brain. The animal was allowed to recover. The next

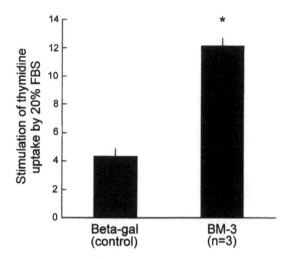

Figure 26.3 Graph showing stimulation of thymidine incorporation of astrocytes by Ad5/BM-3 F87V. Astrocytes infected with control virus and recombinant Ad5/BM-3 F87V were tested for serum stimulated growth effects by 20% fetal bovine serum for 18 hours. The cells were incubated with ^{3}H-thymidine for 3 hours after which incorporated label was counted. There was a four fold increase in DNA synthesis of cells infected with β-galactosidase while corresponding cells infected with Ad5/BM-3 F87V showed greater than twelve fold increase. The results represent the average of three independent experiments, each consisting of four samples of cells after infection with Ad5/β-galactosidase and Ad5/BM-3 F87V to cover a total of twelve samples/bar. The asterisk indicates a significant increase in the stimulation by Ad5/BM-3 F87V ($p < .05$).

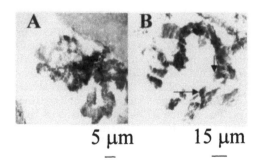

5 µm   15 µm

Figure 26.4 Staining of cells from the choroids plexus of rat infused with Ad5/β-galactosidase. Section (thickness 15 µm) of a frozen brain from a rat infused intraventricularly with Ad5/β-galactosidase (5×10^9 pfu), was stained for bacterial β-galactosidase activity for 2 hours (seen in blue) and then counterstained with nuclear fast red to display the cells. Panel B shows magnification of the choroid plexus in panel A. The arrows mark cells from the choroid plexus that stain for β-galactosidase and nuclear red, demonstrating that these cells express recombinant enzyme by viral-mediated gene transfer. (*see Color Plate 10*)

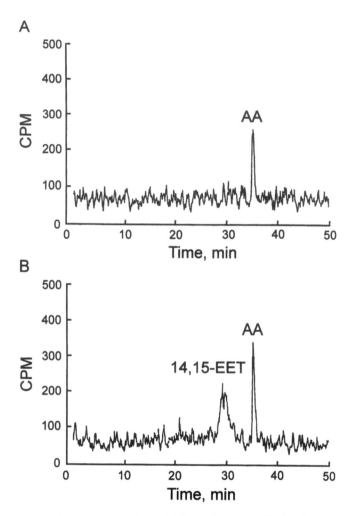

Figure 26.5 Reverse phase high performance liquid chromatography (rpHPLC) profile of arachidonic acid-metabolites formed *in vivo* by rat brain infected with Ad5/BM-3 F87V. Intraventricular infusions of recombinant Ad5/BM-3 F87V, followed by ^{14}C-labeled arachidonic acid after 24 hours, were carried out in the rat brain. Chromatographic profile of radioactive lipids are represented from A: brain tissue distal to the ventricle and B: brain tissue surrounding the ventricle. The peak at around 29 minutes in panel B has been marked as 14,15-EET and elutes with labeled standard EETs (not shown). Note the substrate arachidonic acid is present in both the samples.

day the substrate ^{14}C-arachidonic was infused at the same spot. After 30 minutes the animal was sacrificed and the brain recovered. Lipids were extracted from tissue around the ventricle as well as that obtained distal to the injection site. Analysis by rpHPLC showed 14,15-EET in the sample adjacent to the site of injection (Figure 26.5). A sample distal to this site with corresponding amounts of tissue and radioactivity did not show any EET or other metabolites, but resolved the substrate, arachidonic acid (Figure 26.5).

3. DISCUSSION

Gene delivery to the brain is a challenge that must be overcome in order to apply molecular advances for research and therapy. The epoxygenase gene is an ideal candidate because of the numerous benefits of its products and a need to investigate the mechanisms of how they function *in vivo*. The bacterial gene is especially suited for this approach as it has been engineered to metabolize arachidonic acid into a single EET, though of course these can be further metabolized by intracellular enzymes to dihydroxyeicosatrienoic acids (DiHETEs) and other products. In addition, the bacterial epoxygenase protein is immunologically distinct from epoxygenases endogenous to the mammalian brain, making it easy to follow using specific antibodies. This recombinant protein was easily detected in cultured astrocytes.

Astrocytes are an abundant cell type in the brain making them a good choice to test gene expression and function *in vitro*. They produce EETs (Alkayed *et al.*, 1996) though the amounts released in the media are considerably low. Under the conditions of the experiments there was no release of EETs in the media after 30 minutes of incubation with labeled substrate. This time was much shorter than that used in previous assays described for the production of EETs from astrocytes (Alkayed *et al.*, 1996; Medhora and Harder, 1998). Also the lipids in the previous studies were extracted from the cells and not the media (Alkayed *et al.*, 1996; Medhora and Harder, 1998). However, the recombinant Ad5/BM-3 F87V expressed the bacterial epoxygenase which was able to convert the substrate to product after 30 minutes. The levels of metabolites of the 14,15-EET were more abundant than the EET peak itself. We have obtained the same result with Cos 1 cells (Narayanan *et al.*, 2000). The abundance of distinct product formation in brain cells as compared to another mammalian epoxygenase, 2C11, prompted the use of the bacterial gene for studies *in vivo*.

First, it was determined if this recombinant virus had any adverse effect to the growth of astrocytes in culture. Next, thymidine incorporation in cells infected with bacterial β-galactosidase, which was not expected to interfere with growth, was checked. Surprisingly, quiescent cells infected with Ad5/BM-3 F87V showed significantly more stimulation by serum than the β-galactosidase controls. In fact, the thymidine incorporation was comparable to uninfected cells (results not shown), inspite of all the deleterious viral genes being coded by the vector backbone. This is in keeping with the mitogenic and growth promoting potential of BM-3 F87V and EETs in general (Chen *et al.*, 1998; Burns *et al.*, 1995).

The next part of the study was to introduce the epoxygenase gene into the mammalian brain. Delivery into the parenchyma is difficult as the densely packed cortical tissue does not accommodate injected material. Also, cortical function must be kept intact, so that multiple insertion of needles into an area of the cerebral cortex to deliver significant volumes of liquid, is undesirable. The virus was infused into the lateral ventricle since this is known to deliver recombinant genes into cells of the ependymal lining and perivascular spaces on the surface of the brain. Adenovirus has been seen to infect many cells types of the brain although *in vivo* infection of the choroid plexus has not been reported. However, if the cells of the choroid plexus that are responsible for the formation of cerebrospinal fluid were infected with Ad5/BM-3 F87V, 14,15-EET could be released into the cerebrospinal fluid from this source, in addition to levels added by release from infected ependymal cells. Once again, the bacterial epoxygenase that contained a fused P450 reductase would be advantageous, if endogenous levels of this enzyme were low in the cells lining the ventricle. Reductase must to be present for epoxygenation of arachidonic acid. The choroid plexus was closely examined after viral infection to check if the cells got infected with recombinant adenovirus (Ad5/β-gal). Therefore delivery of Ad5/BM-3 F87V into the lateral ventricle seemed a good approach to increase circulating levels of EETs in the cerebrospinal fluid.

To measure this increase the Ad5/BM-3 F87V was infused into the ventricle and the rat allowed to recover for 24 hours. This time point was chosen because longer durations would show inflammatory responses to the viral proteins and complicate the results. An aliquot of ^{14}C-labeled substrate was infused into the ventricle to facilitate detection of the EET products. However, all the substrate bound to the brain cells and too few counts from the cerebrospinal fluid were recovered to resolve by rpHPLC. Therefore, the brain tissue surrounding the ventricles was assayed for production of EET. Previous studies had showed that the virus particles were too large to diffuse into cells under the lining of the ventricles, but the arachidonic acid did permeate this layer so that it could be recovered from tissue distal to the ventricular lining. Extraction of free lipids from these two sets of tissue showed 14,15-EET only made in the cells around the ventricle. However, these conditions do not rule out the possibility that the EET detected was due to endogenous epoxygenases of the ventricle and was not coded for by Ad5/BM-3 F87V. These studies are being pursued using more sensitive fluorescent assays (Maier *et al.*, 2000) to estimate endogenous EETs in the cerebrospinal fluid.

4. SUMMARY

In summary, this study shows that the bacterial epoxygenase gene BM-3 F87V was successfully able to function in brain cells and tissue. It also highlights the need to overcome problems of gene delivery and develop more sensitive assays for measuring metabolites of arachidonic acid in tissues. By achieving this, the advantage of the P450 system can be taken in conjunction with advances in recombinant DNA technology for basic research and its applications to medicine.

ACKNOWLEDGMENTS

Thanks to Ashley Cowart for advice and Will Vandewalle in the Adenoviral Core Facility at the Medical College of Wisconsin, Milwaukee, for amplifying the Ad5/BM-3 F87V and β-galactosidase virus.

27 Identification of 11,12,15-trihydroxyeicosatrienoic acid as the mediator of acetylcholine- and arachidonic acid-induced relaxations in the rabbit aorta

Sandra L. Pfister, Nancy Spitzbarth,
Kathryn M. Gauthier and William B. Campbell

The endothelium modulates vascular tone by releasing a number of different relaxing factors, including nitric oxide (NO), prostacyclin, epoxyeicosatrienoic acids and other as yet unidentified endothelium-derived hyperpolarizing factors (EDHFs). The studies summarized in this chapter showed that in contracted rabbit aorta, arachidonic acid and acetylcholine elicited an endothelium-dependent, concentration-related relaxation that was resistant to inhibitors of both NO and cyclooxygenase. Increasing the extracellular potassium (K) concentration from 4 to 20 mM, and pretreatment with inhibitors of lipoxygenases abolished arachidonic acid- and acetylcholine-induced relaxations. In addition, arachidonic acid increased the membrane potential of rabbit aortic smooth muscle cells. Arachidonic acid had no effect on cell membrane potential in rabbit aortas without an intact endothelial layer. Rabbit aortic endothelial cells metabolized arachidonic acid to a vasodilator 15-lipoxygenase metabolite. Structural analysis of the 15-lipoxygenase products by gas chromatography/mass spectrometry indicated a trihydroxyeicosatrienoic acid (THETA) structure. Further gas chromatography/mass spectrometry analysis indicated the formation of two peaks that were the regioisomers, 11,12,15-THETA and 11,14,15-THETA. Isolation of the two products using a normal phase high pressure liquid chromatography separation found that only 11,12,15-THETA relaxed contracted aortas. The relaxation to 11,12,15-THETA was inhibited in the presence of elevated extracellular K concentrations. These studies indicate that arachidonic acid relaxes vascular smooth muscle by opening K channels and hyperpolarizing cells. They suggest that these effects are mediated by 11,12,15-THETA.

A number of endothelium-derived relaxing factors (EDRFs) have been identified including NO (Furchgott and Vanhoutte, 1989), prostacyclin (Moncada and Vane, 1979) and EDHF (Mombouli and Vanhoutte, 1997). While the chemical identity of EDHF remains controversial, its mechanism of action involves opening of K channels (Nagao and Vanhoutte, 1991). Studies from a number of laboratories have shown that EDHF is a cytochrome P450 metabolite of arachidonic acid, an epoxyeicosatrienoic acid (Campbell *et al.*, 1996). Arachidonic acid causes relaxation of blood vessels, which is dependent on the presence of the endothelium (DeMey *et al.*, 1982; Singer and Peach, 1983; Rubanyi and Vanhoutte, 1985; Pinto *et al.*, 1986). Previous work supported this observation and described an endothelium-dependent, lipoxygenase metabolite of arachidonic acid that elicits relaxation of the rabbit aorta (Pfister *et al.*, 1996). Additional studies showed that high K concentration and inhibitors of K channels blocked arachidonic acid-induced relaxations in the rabbit aorta suggesting that this metabolite may also be a arachidonic acid-derived EDHF (Pfister *et al.*, 1999). In the rabbit aorta and aortic endothelial cells, arachidonic acid is metabolized by 15-lipoxygenase to 15-HPETE which undergoes an enzymatic rearrangement to the hydroxy (H)-epoxyeicosatrienoic acids (EETA), either 11-H-14,15-EETA and/or 15-H-11,12-EETA (Pfister *et al.*, 1998). Hydrolysis of the epoxy group results in the formation of 11,12,15- and 11,14,15-THETAs. The HEETAs and THETAs relax the rabbit aorta and one or both may mediate the relaxations to arachidonic acid (Pfister *et al.*, 1998). The purpose of the present study was to determine which THETA regioisomer mediates the relaxation to arachidonic acid. Because acetylcholine-induced relaxations are reduced, but not blocked, by inhibitors of the synthesis of NO and prostaglandins, additional experiments were designed to investigate whether a HEETA and/or THETA explains the relaxations to acetylcholine not mediated by either NO or prostacyclin in the rabbit aorta. Finally, a series of experiments examined the role of K channels in arachidonic acid-induced relaxations.

1. METHODS

1.1. Vascular reactivity

Rabbits were sacrificed (pentobarbital 120 mg/kg, intravenously), the thoracic aorta removed and placed in Kreb's bicarbonate buffer (118 mM NaCl, 4 mM KCl, 3.3 mM $CaCl_2$, 24 mM $NaHCO_3$, 1.2 mM KH_2PO_4, 1.2 mM $MgSO_4$, 11 mM glucose, and 0.003 mM EDTA). The tissue was cleaned of adhering fat and connective tissue and cut into rings (3 mm thick) taking care not to damage the endothelium. Aortic rings were suspended in organ chambers containing 6 ml of Kreb's-bicarbonate buffer maintained at 37 °C and continuously bubbled with 95% O_2–5% CO_2. Isometric tension was measured with force-displacement transducers (Grass), AD Instruments ETH-400 amplifiers and recorded on a Macintosh computer using MacLab 8e software. Resting tension was adjusted to its length tension maximum of 2 grams, and vessels allowed to equilibrate for 1 hour. Increasing the KCl concentration to 40 mM produced contractions. Once the vessels reached peak contraction, the organ chambers were rinsed, and the blood vessels allowed to return to resting tension. After the aortic rings had reproducible, stable responses to KCl, the tissue was treated with indomethacin (10^{-5} M) and nitro-L-arginine (10^{-5} M) for 10 minutes prior to contraction with phenylephrine (10^{-7} M). When the contraction stabilized, cumulative concentration–response curves to acetylcholine (10^{-9}–10^{-6} M) or arachidonic acid (10^{-7}–10^{-4} M) were obtained. The responses to acetylcholine or arachidonic acid were repeated in the presence of the lipoxygenase inhibitor, cinnamyl-3,4-dihydroxy-α-cyanocinnamate (CDC) (5×10^{-5} M), or the cytochrome P450 inhibitor, miconazole (2×10^{-6} M). In other studies, responses were examined in solution containing 20 mM potassium. In an additional series of experiments, the fractions from the high pressure liquid chromatograph (HPLC) were collected, dissolved in ethanol and tested for activity in tissues contracted with phenylephrine (10^{-7} M).

1.2. Metabolism of ^{14}C-arachidonic acid by rabbit aorta

Aortas were isolated from one to two months old New Zealand White rabbits and cleaned of adhering connective tissue and fat. The vessels were rinsed in Tris buffer (0.05 M, pH 7.5), and then cut into small pieces. The blood vessel segments were homogenized in fresh buffer (500 mg of tissue/10 ml of buffer), centrifuged at 750 × g for 15 minutes and the supernatant used. Aliquots (5 mg/ml) of the supernatant were incubated for 20 minutes in Tris-HCl buffer containing indomethacin (10^{-5} M) and [^{14}C(U)]-arachidonic acid (0.05 µCi, 10^{-7} M). Reactions were stopped by adding ethanol to a final concentration of 15%. The samples were acidified (pH < 3.5) and extracted using octadecylsilyl (ODS) extraction columns (Pfister *et al.*, 1996). The extracted arachidonic acid metabolites were then resolved by HPLC (Pfister *et al.*, 1996). For reverse phase HPLC, solvent system I consisted of solvent A which was water and solvent B which was acetonitrile containing 0.1% glacial acetic acid. The program was a 40 minute linear gradient from 50% solvent B in A to 100% solvent B at a flow rate of 1 ml/minute. An aliquot of each fraction was removed and radioactivity determined by liquid scintillation spectrometry. Fractions 27–35 (5–7.5 minutes), corresponding to the THETAs were pooled, extracted with cyclohexane/ethyl acetate (50/50) and rechromatographed on reverse phase HPLC using solvent system II. Solvent system II consisted of solvent A which was water containing 0.1% glacial acetic acid and solvent B which was acetonitrile. The program consisted of a 5 minute isocratic phase with 35% B in A, followed by a 35 minute linear gradient to 85% B at a flow rate was 1 ml/minute. The column eluate was collected in 0.2 ml aliquots and radioactivity determined as described above. The fractions containing the THETAs (fractions 87–93) (17.5–18.5 minutes) were collected and extracted with cyclohexane/ethyl acetate (50/50). The THETA fraction was further purified by normal phase HPLC using a Nucleosil silica column (5 µ, 4.6 × 250 mm). Solvent system III consisted of an isocratic separation using hexane, isopropranol and glacial acetic acid (995:4:1) at a flow rate of 1 ml/minute. The column eluate was collected in 0.5 ml fractions and the radioactivity determined. The radioactive peaks were collected, dried under a stream of nitrogen and tested for biological activity on the phenylephrine-contracted aorta or derivatized and analyzed by gas chromatography/mass spectrometry (GC/MS).

1.3. Gas chromatography/mass spectrometry

The fractions isolated from solvent system III were pooled, evaporated to dryness under nitrogen and derivatized for GC–MS (Pfister *et al.*, 1988; Pfister *et al.*, 1991). The sample was dissolved in 120 µl acetonitrile and then treated with ethereal diazomethane for 6 minutes at 0 °C to form the methyl ester. The reacted sample was evaporated to dryness under nitrogen and the hydroxyl groups were then converted to the trimethylsilyl ethers by 60 minutes of incubation at 37 °C with 15 µl bis-TMS-trifluoroacetamide. GC–MS was performed with a Hewlett Packard 5989A Mass Spectrometer coupled with a 5890 Series 2 Gas Chromatograph. Ionization of the samples was done by electron impact at 65–70 eV or chemically using methane as the reagent gas. The derivatized metabolite was resolved using a 14 m capillary DB-5 column with a linear gradient from 100 ° to 300 °C. Standards were derivatized and analyzed by GC–MS using the identical methods described for the biological samples.

1.4. Membrane potential

Rabbit aortic rings were cut open laterally, and pinned, endothelial cell layer exposed, to a silastic layer on the bottom of a heated perfusion chamber (37 °C) and perfused with a physiological salt solution of the following composition: 119 mM NaCl, 4.7 mM KCl, 1.6 mM $CaCl_2$, 1.17 mM $MgSO_4$, 5.5 mM glucose, 24 mM $NaHCO_3$, 1.18 mM NaH_2PO_4, and 0.0026 mM EDTA. Perfusate solutions were equilibrated with a 21% O_2–5% CO_2–balance N_2 gas mixture to maintain a pH of 7.4 and pO_2 of 140 mmHg (Gauthier-Rein *et al.*, 1997). Indomethacin (10^{-5} M) was present in all perfusate solutions. The aortic segments were equilibrated with continual superfusion for 30 minutes before initiation of experimental protocols. Experiments were performed in preparations in which a very small section of endothelium was removed from the center of the aortic strip by gently rubbing with a small cotton swab. Impalements were performed only in the denuded area. In a subset of experiments, the entire endothelial layer was removed from the aortic strip. Intracellular membrane potential values were recorded (Harder, 1984). Briefly, glass microelectrodes were filled with 3 M KCl and had estimated tip sizes of 0.1–0.2 μm, tip resistances of 30–80 MΩ and tip potentials equal to or less than 3 mV. The electrodes were attached to a high impedance biological amplifier (Dagan Cell Explorer, Dagan Instruments, Minneapolis, MN, USA). Electrode polarization was eliminated by a Ag/AgCl half cell. Criteria for a successful impalement included an abrupt drop in potential to a new steady state value which was maintained for a minimum of 5 seconds, a cell membrane potential value greater than −20 mV) and an abrupt return to the original baseline when the electrode is pulled from the tissue. After the addition of phenylephrine (10^{-7} M) and arachidonic acid (10^{-5} M), the aortic segments were allowed to equilibrate for an additional 10 minutes before impalements were initiated.

1.5. Materials

The following drugs were used: phenylephrine, arachidonic acid (sodium salt), acetylcholine, indomethacin, nitro-L-arginine and A23187 were all from Sigma Chemical Co., St. Louis, MO, USA. CDC was from BIOMOL Research Laboratories, Plymouth Meeting, PA. [^{14}C (U)]-Arachidonic acid (specific activity 920 mCi/mmol) was obtained from New England Nuclear, Boston, MA. All solvents were HPLC grade and purchased from Burdick and Jackson, Muskegan, MI.

2. RESULTS

In isolated rings of rabbit aorta, contracted with phenylephrine, acetylcholine elicited a concentration-related, endothelium-dependent relaxation (Pfister and Campbell, 1992; Pfister *et al.*, 1996). Treatment with indomethacin, an inhibitor of cyclooxygenase, and the inhibitor of NO synthase, L-NA, reduced the relaxations to acetylcholine by approximately 40% (Figure 27.1) (Campbell *et al.*, 2000). These non-NO, non-PG-mediated relaxations to acetylcholine were abolished by pretreatment of the aorta with the lipoxygenase inhibitor, CDC (typical tracing, Figure 27.1) indicating that a metabolite of arachidonic acid produced by lipoxygenase mediates a portion of the acetylcholine-induced relaxations. The cytochrome P450 inhibitor, miconazole,

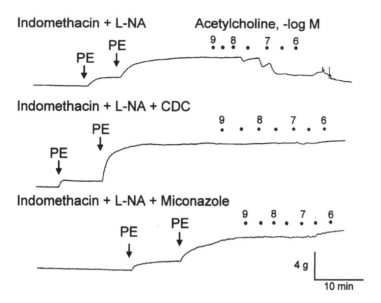

Figure 27.1 Top: Original recording showing the effect of cinnamyl-3,4-dihydroxy-α-cyanocinnamate (CDC) (middle panel) and miconazole (bottom panel) on acetylcholine (Ach)-induced relaxations of rabbit aorta. Control rings were treated with indomethacin (10^{-5} M) and nitro-L-arginine (L-NA) (10^{-5} M) for 10 minutes prior to contraction with phenylephrine (PE) (10^{-7} M). Acetylcholine was added in increasing concentrations and changes in isometric tension continuously monitored. Middle: The blood vessels were treated with indomethacin, L-NA and CDC prior to phenylephrine and acetylcholine. Bottom: The blood vessels were treated with indomethacin, L-NA and miconazole prior to phenylephrine and acetylcholine.

completely attenuated acetylcholine-induced relaxations (Figure 27.1) (Campbell *et al.*, 2000). Previous studies showed that arachidonic acid elicits endothelium-dependent relaxations of rabbit aorta (Pfister and Campbell, 1992; Pfister *et al.*, 1996). In these studies, indomethacin augmented the relaxation (Pfister and Campbell, 1992).

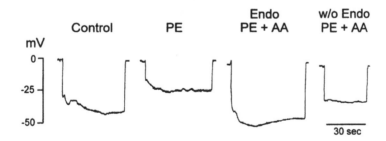

Figure 27.2 Original recordings of membrane potential of impaled rabbit aortic vascular smooth muscle cells. Membrane potential changed from a resting value of −43 mV to −25 mV with the addition of phenylephrine (PE) (10^{-7} M). In the preparations with endothelium (Endo), the subsequent addition of arachidonic acid (AA) (10^{-5} M) increased the membrane potential to −46 mV. In the preparation without endothelium (w/o Endo), the addition of arachidonic acid did not change cell membrane potential.

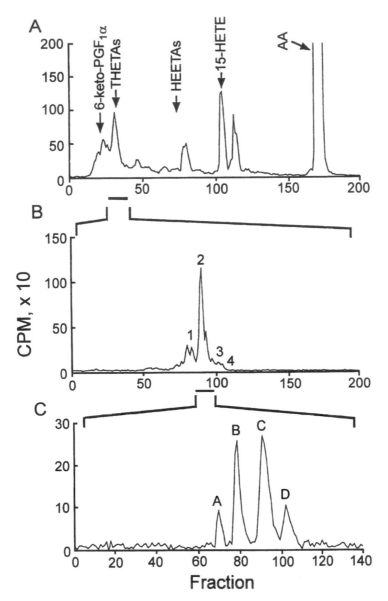

Figure 27.3 Metabolism of [^{14}C (U)]-arachidonic acid by the rabbit aorta. Aortic homogenates were incubated with indomethacin and [^{14}C (U)]-arachidonic acid for 20 minutes. The metabolites were extracted and resolved by sequential reverse phase and normal phase HPLC. (A) Separation of arachidonic acid metabolites by reverse phase HPLC using solvent system I. The migration times of known standards are shown above the chromatogram. PG = prostaglandin; THETAs = trihydroxyeicosatrienoic acids; HEETAs = hydroxyepoxyeicosatrienoic acids; HETEs = hydroxyeicosatetraenoic acids. (B) Separation of the THETA fraction (fractions 27–35, see dark bar) from panel A using reverse phase HPLC and solvent system II. (C) Separation of THETA fraction peak 2 (fractions 87–93, see dark bar) from panel B by normal phase HPLC using solvent system III. CPM = counts/min; AA = arachidonic acid.

However, treatment of vessels with CDC blocked the arachidonic acid-induced relaxations (Pfister *et al.*, 1996). Increasing the extracellular potassium concentration to 20 mM attenuated the response (Pfister *et al.*, 1999). In another set of experiments, the cell membrane potential of smooth muscle cells was measured in aortic segments. In segments with endothelium, control cell membrane potential of -42 ± 2 mV decreased to -28.5 ± 1 mV after treatment with phenylephrine (10^{-7} M). The subsequent addition of arachidonic acid increased the cell membrane potential or hyperpolarized the cells (-43.5 ± 3 mV) (Figure 27.2) (Campbell *et al.*, 2000). This hyperpolarization to arachidonic acid did not occur in blood vessels without endothelium.

When aortic homogenate was incubated with [^{14}C (U)]-arachidonic acid, extracted, and metabolites resolved by reverse-phase HPLC using solvent system I, there was the synthesis of radioactive products that migrated with the prostaglandins, the dihydroxyeicosatrienoic–dihydroxyeicosatetranoic acids and the hydroxyeicosatetraenoic acids (Pfister *et al.*, 1996; Figure 27.3). Fractions 27–35 (5–7.5 minutes) were analyzed

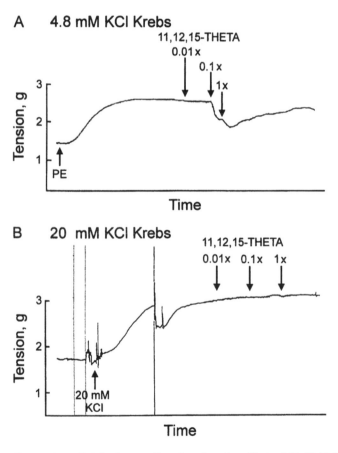

Figure 27.4 Original recording showing the effect of 11,12,15-THETA (peak B of Figure 27.3C) on isometric tension in a contracted rabbit aorta studied in Kreb's solution containing (A) 4.8 mM or (B) 20 mM KCl. The vessels were contracted with phenylephrine (PE) (10^{-7} M) when studied in 4.8 mM KCl. Dilutions of peak B of Figure 27.3C were added to the contracted vessel and isometric tension measured.

further by reverse-phase HPLC using solvent system II (Figure 27.3). A number of radioactive peaks were observed and were labeled peaks 1–4. The major peak migrated at 17.5–18.5 minutes (fractions 88–94) and was peak 2. The four peaks were isolated from aortic homogenates incubated with arachidonic acid and tested for activity on isolated rings of rabbit aorta. In contracted vessels, peak 2 elicited a concentration-dependent relaxation (Pfister *et al.*, 1996). The other peaks were inactive. The cell free incubation with arachidonic acid did not relax the rabbit aorta (data not shown). Using GC/MS analysis, additional experiments indicated that peak 2 contained two metabolites, identified as the methyl-ester trimethylsilyl ether derivatives of 11,12,15- and 11,14,15-THETA (Pfister *et al.*, 1998). When peak 2 was collected using solvent system II and rechromatographed on normal phase HPLC using solvent system III, four major products were observed (labeled A–D) (Figure 27.3). The products were collected and tested for activity in contracted rabbit aortas. Only peak B produced relaxation (Figure 27.4). The maximal relaxation was $46 \pm 13\%$ ($n = 3$). If the responses were repeated in the presence of elevated potassium, no relaxation was observed (Figure 27.4). Peak B was derivatized and analyzed by GC/MS. Mass spectra indicated that peak B was 11,12,15-THETA (data not shown) (Campbell *et al.*, 2000). Peak C, which was inactive, was identified as 11,14,15-THETA.

3. DISCUSSION

Previous studies showed that arachidonic acid caused endothelium-dependent relaxation of the rabbit aorta (Pfister *et al.*, 1996). These relaxations were blocked by inhibitors of lipoxygenase and enhanced by cycloxygenase inhibitors suggesting that the mediator of the response was a lipoxygenase metabolite. The major metabolites produced by rabbit aorta were isolated and identified (Pfister *et al.*, 1998). The results showed that arachidonic acid is metabolized by 15-lipoxygenase to HEETAs which are hydrolyzed to 11,14,15- and 11,12,15-THETAs. Both the HEETAs and THETAs relaxed rabbit aorta (Pfister *et al.*, 1998). The present study is an extension of this earlier work and provides evidence that 11,12,15-THETA is the regioisomer that elicits relaxation of the rabbit aorta. Furthermore, in the rabbit aorta, this metabolite appears to mediate the relaxations to acetylcholine that resist inhibition of NO synthase and cyclooxygenase.

In order to determine which THETA isomer was active, it was necessary to develop a HPLC system that would resolve the regioisomers. Using a normal phase HPLC with a silica column, peak 2 isolated from reverse phase HPLC using solvent system II, was resolved into four peaks with peak B being the major product. GC/MS analysis of the peaks indicated that peak B was 11,12,15-THETA and peak C was 11,14,15-THETA. Only peak B relaxed contracted rabbit aorta establishing 11,12,15-THETA as a mediator of arachidonic acid-induced relaxations. Several stereoisomers of 11,12,15-THETA are possible; however, the identity of the active stereoisomer will require additional studies. Likewise, additional experiments are needed to identify the exact structure of the HEETA or HEETAs produced by the rabbit aorta. Because the HEETAs are chemically unstable, it has been difficult to obtain structural information. Based on the ability of 11,12,15-THETA, but not 11,14,15-THETA, to relax rabbit aorta, it appears likely that 15-H-11,12-EETA should also relax rabbit aorta.

Furchgott and Zawadzki (1980) first reported that acetylcholine causes an endothelium-dependent relaxation of rabbit aorta. The substance mediating this response was called EDRF and was subsequently identified as NO (Palmer *et al.*, 1987; Ignarro *et al.*, 1987). However, NO is not the only mediator of the acetylcholine-induced relaxation in the rabbit aorta. A non-cyclooxygenase arachidonic acid metabolite may be released by acetylcholine and contribute to the observed relaxation (Rubanyi and Vanhoutte, 1985; Félétou and Vanhoutte, 1988; Hecker *et al.*, 1994; Lischke *et al.*, 1995; Campbell *et al.*, 1996). The residual relaxations in the presence of inhibitors of NO synthase and cycloxygenase are blocked by inhibitors of K channels (Cowan *et al.*, 1993) and may represent EDHF. Therefore, the studies summarized in this chapter investigated acetylcholine-induced relaxations in the rabbit aorta in vessels treated with L-NA and indomethacin. The relaxation was blocked by the lipoxygenase inhibitor, CDC or the cytochrome P450 inhibitor, miconazole. Arachidonic acid is metabolized by 15-lipoxygenase to 15-HPETE and 15-HPETE is converted by a hydroperoxide isomerase to the HEETAs (Pfister *et al.*, 1998, 2000). The HEETAs are hydrolyzed by an epoxide hydrolase to THETAs. The 15-lipoxygenase is inhibited by CDC while miconazole inhibits the hydroperoxide isomerase. The observation that both CDC and miconazole inhibit acetylcholine- and arachidonic acid-induced relaxations (Campbell *et al.*, 2000) supports the hypothesis that HEETAs and/or THETAs play a role in these relaxations.

Arachidonic acid does not increase cyclic AMP or cyclic GMP in the rabbit aorta (Pfister and Campbell, 1992). Since EDHF is thought to act by increasing the efflux of potassium from the smooth muscle cell, most likely by activating a potassium channel (Brayden and Nelson, 1992; Garland *et al.*, 1995), arachidonic acid-induced relaxations were investigated in the presence of an elevated extracellular K concentration. Under these conditions, the fatty acid failed to elicit relaxations (Pfister *et al.*, 1999). These data would suggest that arachidonic acid releases a hyperpolarizing factor that relaxes the rabbit aorta. This response was further characterized by measuring the effect of arachidonic acid on the membrane potential of vascular smooth muscle of arteries with endothelium. Under these conditions, arachidonic acid increased the membrane potential in vessels depolarized by phenylephrine. The effect of the active isomer, 11,12,15-THETA, was also tested in intact aortic segments in the presence of elevated K. Increasing extracellular K concentrations inhibited the relaxations to 11,12,15-THETA. These findings are consistent with the observation that acetylcholine causes endothelium-dependent hyperpolarization of rabbit mesenteric arteries through the activation of an apamin-sensitive K channel (Murphy and Brayden, 1995).

4. CONCLUSION

The findings summarized in this chapter support the following hypothesis (Figure 27.5). In the presence of NO synthase and cycloxygenase inhibition, various agonists such as acetylcholine stimulate the release of arachidonic acid. Arachidonic acid is metabolized by 15-lipoxygenase to 15-HPETE and further metabolized to HEETAs and THETAs. The THETAs and HEETAs act on K channels in the vascular smooth muscle to cause K efflux, membrane hyperpolarization and subsequent relaxation. While a number of these points remain to be studied, data obtained so far suggest that

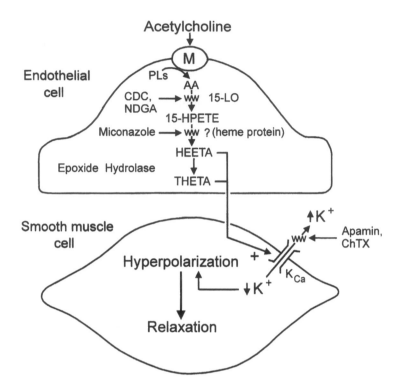

Figure 27.5 Putative role of HEETAs and THETAs on vascular tone. Agents such as acetylcholine stimulate the endothelial cell to release arachidonic acid. Arachidonic acid is metabolized by 15-lipoxygenase to 15-HPETE which is converted by a heme-containing enzyme (hydroperoxide isomerase) to the 15-H-11,12-EETA. Hydrolysis of the epoxy group of 15-H-11,12-EETA by an epoxide hydrolase produced 11,12,15-THETA. HEETAs and/or THETAs open K channels on the vascular smooth muscle to elicit hyperpolarization and relaxation; 11,12,15-THETA = 11,12,15-trihydroxyeicosatrienoic acid; 15-H-11,12-EETA = 15-hydroxy 11,12-epoxyeicosatrienoic acids; 15-LO = 15-lipoxygenase; AA = arachidonic acid; CDC = cinnamyl-3,4-dihydroxy-α-; CHTX = charybdotoxin; NDGA = nordihydroguaiaretic acid; K = potassium; PL = phospholipid.

11,12,15-THETA and/or 15-H-11,12-EETA represent new members of the EDRF family and mediate the endothelium-dependent relaxations in the rabbit aorta that cannot be explained by the release of NO or vasodilator prostaglandins.

ACKNOWLEDGMENTS

The authors thank Gretchen Barg for secretarial assistance. These studies were supported by a grant from the National Heart, Lung and Blood Institute (HL-37981).

28 Identification of hydrogen peroxide as an endothelium-derived hyperpolarizing factor in mice

Hiroaki Shimokawa, Tetsuya Matoba, Mikio Nakashima, Yoji Hirakawa, Yasushi Mukai, Katsuya Hirano, Hideo Kanaide and Akira Takeshita

The endothelium plays an important role in maintaining vascular homeostasis by synthesizing and releasing several endothelium-derived relaxing factors (EDRFs), such as prostacyclin, nitric oxide (NO), and yet unidentified endothelium-derived hyperpolarizing factor (EDHF). This study was designed to examine a hypothesis that H_2O_2 derived from endothelial NO synthase (eNOS) is an EDHF. EDHF-mediated relaxations and hyperpolarizations to acetylcholine were markedly attenuated in small mesenteric arteries from eNOS-knockout (KO) mice. In the eNOS-KO mice, vasodilating and hyperpolarizing responses of vascular smooth muscle *per se* were preserved and the increase in intracellular calcium in endothelial cells in responses to acetylcholine also was preserved. Antihypertensive treatment with hydralazine failed to improve the EDHF-mediated relaxations. Catalase, which dismutates H_2O_2 to form oxygen and water, inhibited EDHF-mediated relaxations as well as hyperpolarizations while it did not affect endothelium-independent relaxations to levcromakalim, a K^+ channel opener. Exogenous H_2O_2 elicited similar relaxations and hyperpolarizations in endo-thelium-stripped arteries. Finally, laser confocal microscopic examination with per-oxide-sensitive fluorescence dye demonstrated that the endothelium produced H_2O_2 during stimulation with acetylcholine and that the H_2O_2 production was markedly reduced in eNOS-KO mice. These results indicate that H_2O_2 is an EDHF in small mesenteric arteries of the mouse and that eNOS is a major source of the reactive oxygen species.

Since the first reports on the existence of endothelium-dependent hyperpolarization (Chen *et al.*, 1988; Félétou and Vanhoutte, 1988), several candidates for EDHF have been proposed (Mombouli and Vanhoutte, 1997; Edwards *et al.*, 1998). However, its nature still remains to be identified. While EDHF is clearly distinct from NO, these two factors share some similarities. First, both NO and EDHF are synthesized by endothelial cells in a Ca^{2+}/calmodulin-dependent manner (Nagao *et al.*, 1992a). Second, in situations where NO-mediated relaxation is reduced (e.g., hypertension and hyperlipidemia), EDHF compensates for NO to cause endothelium-dependent relaxations, while in advanced atherosclerosis, EDHF-mediated relaxations are also impaired (Shimokawa, 1999; Shimokawa *et al.*, 1999). Third, correction of the underlying risk factors improves the relaxations mediated by NO as well as those by EDHF (Shimokawa *et al.*, 1999). *In vitro*, activated eNOS can generate superoxide anions ($^\bullet O_2^-$) under conditions of depletion of L-arginine or tetrahydrobiopterin, in the presence of L-arginine analogues (Stroes *et al.*, 1998). $^\bullet O_2^-$ can be catalyzed by superoxide dismutase into H_2O_2. Vasoactive properties of reactive oxygen species were already described by Rubanyi and Vanhoutte in 1986, including H_2O_2 as a vasodilatory factor (Rubanyi and Vanhoutte, 1986a). Since H_2O_2 has been shown to elicit both hyperpolarizations and relaxations in porcine coronary arteries without endothelium (Bény and von der Weid, 1991) and a direct activation of K_{Ca} channels on vascular smooth muscle (Barlow and White, 1998; Hayabuchi et al., 1998), it could be an EDHF that is derived from eNOS.

To test this hypothesis, isometric tension recording was first performed in control and eNOS-KO mice (Huang et al., 1995). In the aorta of control mice, endothelium-dependent relaxations to acetylcholine were not affected by indomethacin, but were almost abolished by N^{ω}-L-nitroarginine (L-NNA), indicating that NO mainly mediates the relaxations to acetylcholine in the aorta (Figure 28.1). By contrast, in small mesenteric arteries, endothelium-dependent relaxations to acetylcholine were resistant to L-NNA but highly sensitive to KCl, indicating that EDHF mainly mediates the relaxations with little contribution of NO in those microvessels (Figure 28.1). Although EDHF is absent in the main trunk of the mesenteric arteries of the mouse (Chataigneau et al., 1999), EDHF-mediated relaxations and hyperpolarizations were demonstrated in the second order of the artery (200–240 μm in diameter) (Figure 28.1). The discrepancy may be due to the difference in vessel size tested since the importance of EDHF increases as the vessel size decreases in rats (Nagao et al., 1992b; Shimokawa et al., 1996) and humans (Urakami-Harasawa et al., 1997; Shimokawa et al., 1999).

In the aorta from eNOS-KO mice, endothelium-dependent relaxations to acetylcholine were absent as previously reported (Huang et al., 1995; Chataigneau et al., 1999) (Figure 28.1). In small mesenteric arteries from eNOS-KO mice, the NO-mediated component was absent, whereas indomethacin partially inhibited the acetylcholine-induced relaxations, suggesting that vasodilator prostaglandins are upregulated and partially compensate the relaxations, a finding consistent with previous reports (Godecke et al., 1998; Chataigneau et al., 1999) (Figure 28.1). EDHF-mediated relaxations, which may be enhanced by NO depletion (Olmos et al., 1995; Bauersachs et al., 1996), were also reduced in eNOS-KO mice (Figure 28.1). Electrophysiological experiments demonstrated that resting membrane potentials of smooth muscle cells from small mesenteric arteries were significantly less negative in eNOS-KO than in control mice (-60.2 ± 0.4 mV vs. -63.1 ± 0.6 mV, $p < .01$, $n = 7$ each). Treatment with L-NNA had no significant effect on the resting membrane potentials (data not shown). The extent of the hyperpolarizations to acetylcholine was markedly reduced in eNOS-KO mice (Figure 28.1). The reduced acetylcholine-induced hyperpolarizations may not be a result of the slightly depolarized resting membrane potentials because depolarized cells generally tend to hyperpolarize more upon opening of K channels. Thus, both endothelium-dependent relaxations and hyperpolarizations in response to acetylcholine are markedly reduced in eNOS-KO mice (Matoba et al., 2000).

The reduced EDHF-mediated responses in eNOS-KO mice could be caused by several mechanisms other than reduced production of the factor. First, vasodilator properties of the vascular smooth muscle might be reduced in eNOS-KO mice. However, endothelium-independent relaxations to levcromakalim, an opener of ATP-sensitive K channels, were comparable between the two strains, whereas those to sodium nitroprusside were rather enhanced in eNOS-KO mice (Figure 28.2),

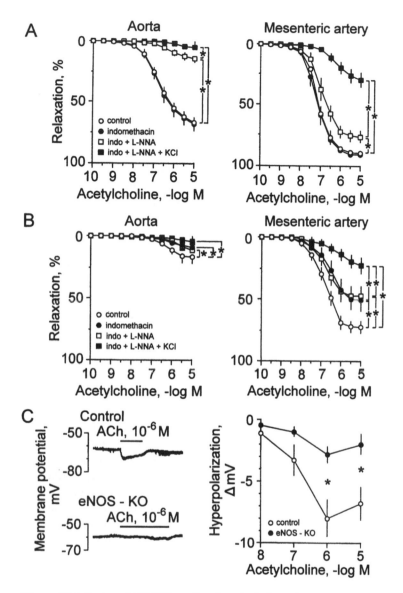

Figure 28.1 Reduced EDHF-mediated endothelium-dependent relaxations and hyperpolarizations in eNOS-KO mice. (A) Endothelium-dependent relaxations to acetylcholine of the aorta (left, $n = 11$) and of small mesenteric arteries (right, $n = 9$) in control mice. NO plays a primary role in the aorta, whereas EDHF plays a primary role in small mesenteric arteries. (B) Endothelium-dependent relaxations to acetylcholine of the aorta (left) and of small mesenteric arteries (right, $n = 10$ each) in eNOS-KO mice. The relaxations are absent in the aorta, whereas in small mesenteric arteries those responses are partially compensated by vasodilator prostaglandins with a marked reduction of EDHF-mediated responses. (C) Endothelium-dependent hyperpolarizations to acetylcholine are markedly reduced in small mesenteric arteries of eNOS-KO mice ($n = 5$–6). Data are expressed as mean ± SEM. The asterisks indicate a statistically significant difference ($p < .05$).

a consistent finding to the pervious report (Faraci *et al.*, 1998). Second, since EDHF is produced by the endothelium in a Ca^{2+}/calmodulin-dependent manner (Nagao *et al.*, 1992a; Mombouli and Vanhoutte, 1997), the acetylcholine-induced increase in intracellular Ca^{2+} levels might be reduced in eNOS-KO mice. However, the extent of the increase in intracellular Ca^{2+} levels, measured using fura-2-loaded endothelial cells on the aortic valvular leaflet (Hirano *et al.*, 1993; Aoki *et al.*, 1994), was comparable between the two strains (Figure 28.2). Third, the reduced EDHF-mediated responses in eNOS-KO mice might be the result of the mildly elevated blood pressure (Figure 28.2) (Fujii *et al.*, 1992). However, although antihypertensive treatment with oral hydralazine hydrochloride (20 mg/kg/day for six weeks) effectively lowered blood pressure in eNOS-KO mice, it failed to improve the EDHF-mediated relaxations to acetylcholine (Figure 28.2). These results indicate that the production of EDHF *per se*, which appears to be linked to the activity of eNOS, is reduced in eNOS-KO mice.

EDHF-mediated relaxations are inhibited by apamin, an inhibitor of small conductance K_{Ca} channels, or the combination of apamin plus charybdotoxin, an inhibitor of large and intermediate conductance K_{Ca} channels (Mombouli and Vanhoutte, 1997; Shimokawa *et al.*, 1999). In the present study, the combination of apamin plus charybdotoxin significantly inhibited the EDHF-mediated relaxations in small mesenteric arteries of both strains, whereas tetrabutylammonium, a non-specific inhibitor of K_{Ca} channels, was more potent to inhibit those relaxations in control mice (Table 28.1). Identical results were obtained using eNOS-KO mice (not shown). Thus, K_{Ca} channels mediate the release or action of EDHF in the arteries studied. Metabolites of arachidonic acid formed by cytochrome P450 monoxygenase, epoxy-eicosatrienoic acids, may be an EDHF (Rosolowsky and Campbell, 1993; Hecker *et al.*, 1994; Fisslthaler *et al.*, 1999). In the present study, however, 17-octadecynoic acid, an inhibitor of cytochrome P450 monoxygenase, had no inhibitory effect on the EDHF-mediated relaxations (Table 28.1). Intercellular electrical communication between endothelial cells and vascular smooth muscle cells through gap junctions could contribute to endothelium-dependent hyperpolarization (Yamamoto *et al.*, 1998). However, this mechanism does not play a role in causing hyperpolarization-mediated relaxations of mouse small mesenteric arteries, since 18β-glycyrrhetinic acid, an inhibitor of gap junctions (Yamamoto *et al.*, 1998), failed to inhibit the EDHF-mediated relaxations (Table 28.1). K^+ ions released from the endothelium also may be an EDHF in rat hepatic arteries, causing relaxations and hyperpolarizations of the smooth muscle by activating Na/K pump and inward rectifier K channels (Edwards *et al.*, 1998). However, the combination of ouabain plus barium failed to inhibit the acetylcholine-induced relaxations in the presence of indomethacin and L-NNA (Table 28.1) and cumulative addition of KCl (5–20×10^{-3} M) did not cause relaxations (not shown). Thus, this possibility may also be unlikely, at least in mouse small mesenteric arteries (Matoba *et al.*, 2000).

Then, the inhibitory effect of catalase, which dismutates H_2O_2 to form oxygen and water, on endothelium-dependent relaxations and hyperpolarizations to acetylcholine was examined in mouse small mesenteric arteries. In control mice, catalase (1250 U/ml) partially inhibited the relaxations in the presence of indomethacin alone. However, in the presence of both indomethacin and L-NNA, catalase markedly inhibited the relaxations to acetylcholine (Figure 28.3). These results suggest that in the presence of indomethacin and catalase, NO acts as the principal EDRF. However, when the generation of cycloxygenase-derived products and NO is inhibited, H_2O_2

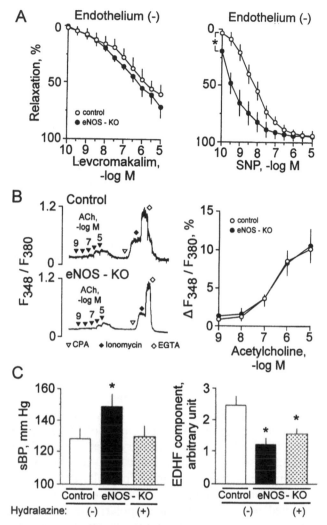

Figure 28.2 Preserved endothelium-independent relaxations and increase in intracellular Ca^{2+} levels upon stimulation by agonists and a failure of antihypertensive therapy to improve the reduced EDHF-mediated responses in eNOS-KO mice. (A) Endothelium-independent relaxations in small mesenteric arteries to levcromakalim were preserved (left, $n = 6$ each) while those to SNP were rather enhanced in eNOS-KO mice (right, $n = 5$–6). (B) Direct measurement of the changes in intracellular Ca^{2+} levels in endothelial cells, acetylcholine (10^{-9}–10^{-6} M), cyclopiazonic acid (CPA, 3×10^{-6} M) and ionomycin (2.5×10^{-5} M) caused an increase in intracellular Ca^{2+} levels as shown by F348/F380 (left). The increases in intracellular Ca^{2+} levels, when normalized to ionomycin-induced maximal F348/F380, were comparable between the two strains (right, $n = 5$ each). (C) Although the antihypertensive therapy with hydralazine normalized blood pressure in eNOS-KO mice (left), the treatment failed to improve the reduced responses mediated by EDHF (KCl-sensitive component after the blockade of cycloxygenase with 10^{-5} M indomethacin and that of eNOS with 10^{-4} M L-NNA) in eNOS-KO mice (right, $n = 8$–10). Data are expressed as mean $\pm$ SEM. The asterisks indicate $p < .05$ by ANOVA.

Table 28.1 Pharmacological characteristics of acetylcholine-induced EDHF-mediated relaxations in small mesenteric arteries of control mice. Effect of K^+ channel blockers and other inhibitors

Inhibitor(s)	Absent		Present		n
	EC_{50}	max	EC_{50}	max	
K^+ channel blockers					
Apamin (10^{-6} M) + CTx (10^{-7} M)	6.9 ± 0.2	77 ± 8	6.8 ± 0.3	$48 \pm 8^*$	7
Tetrabutylammonium (10^{-3} M)	7.1 ± 0.2	78 ± 7	ND	$18 \pm 7^*$	3
Other inhibitors					
17-octadecynoic acid (3×10^{-6} M)	7.2 ± 0.2	79 ± 6	7.6 ± 0.4	70 ± 7	4
18β-glycyrrhetinic acid (4×10^{-5} M)	7.2 ± 0.2	81 ± 5	7.3 ± 0.3	63 ± 9	4
Ouabain (10^{-3} M) + barium (3×10^{-5} M)	6.9 ± 0.2	83 ± 4	7.2 ± 0.1	77 ± 6	4

Notes
All experiments were performed in the presence of indomethacin (10^{-5} M) and L-NNA (10^{-4} M). Data are shown as mean $\pm$ SEM.
EC_{50}, negative logarithm of half-maximal effective concentration of acetylcholine; max, maximal relaxation to acetylcholine (%); ND, not determined because of abolition of the response. The asterisks indicate $p < .05$ vs. absent.

acts as the primary EDRF. Consistent with this interpretation, in eNOS-KO mice where NO cannot act as an EDRF, catalase in the presence of either indomethacin alone or both indomethacin and L-NNA almost completely blocked acetylcholine-dependent relaxation (Figure 28.3). Membrane potential recordings showed that catalase also inhibited the acetylcholine-induced endothelium-dependent hyperpolarizations of those arteries (Figure 28.3). By contrast, catalase did not affect the endothelium-independent hyperpolarizations (Figure 28.3) or relaxations (not shown) in response to levcromakalim. Deferoxamine (10^{-3} M), an inhibitor of Fenton reaction-dependent formation of hydroxyl radical, had no inhibitory effect on the EDHF-mediated relaxations (not shown). These results indicate that H_2O_2 (but not hydroxyl radical) mediates endothelium-dependent relaxations and hyperpolarizations that are attributed to EDHF in mouse small mesenteric arteries (Matoba *et al.*, 2000).

Indeed, exogenous H_2O_2 elicited relaxations and hyperpolarizations of vascular smooth muscle cells (Figure 28.3). High K^+ or tetrabutylammonium markedly inhibited H_2O_2-induced relaxations, while the combination of apamin plus charybdotoxin was relatively less effective (Figure 28.3) (Matoba *et al.*, 2000). Although the intracellular mechanism of H_2O_2-induced hyperpolarization was not determined in this study, it could be due to direct modulation of K_{Ca} channel molecules by H_2O_2 (Barlow and White, 1998; Hayabuchi *et al.*, 1998) or to a lipoxygenase-mediated mechanism (Barlow and White, 1998; Barlow *et al.*, 2000).

Finally, H_2O_2 production from endothelial cells was confirmed in the experiments using laser confocal microscopy with dichlorodihydrofluorescein diacetate (DCF), a peroxide-sensitive fluorescent dye (Ohba *et al.*, 1994). In this system, the endothelial monolayer was clearly distinguished from underlying smooth muscle cells (Figure 28.4). Acetylcholine caused an increase in the DCF fluorescence intensity in endothelial cells 3 min after the application, especially at the cell membrane (Figure 28.4). When a vascular tissue was incubated with catalase, the acetylcholine-induced increase in the fluorescence intensity was suppressed (Figure 28.4), confirming

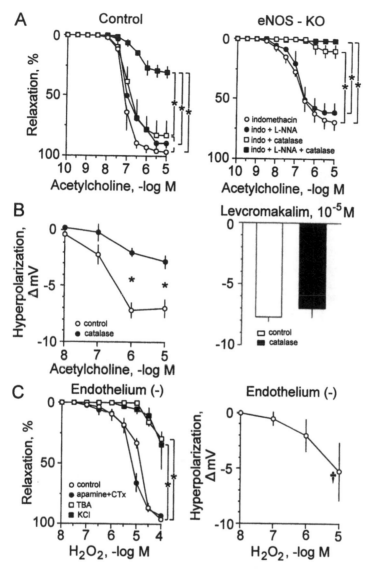

Figure 28.3 Identification of the nature of EDHF in mouse small mesenteric arteries. Experiments were performed in the presence of indomethacin (10^{-5} M) and L-NNA (10^{-4} M) (B and C). (A) Catalase (1250 U/ml) markedly inhibited the endothelium-dependent relaxations to acetylcholine in control mice (after the blockade of cycloxygenase and eNOS) (left, $n = 5$) and in eNOS-KO mice (after the blockade of cyclooxygenase) (right, $n = 4$). (B) Catalase also inhibited the acetylcholine-induced endothelium-dependent hyperpolarizations in small mesenteric arteries of control mice (left, $n = 5$), whereas it did not affect the levcromakalim (10^{-5} M)-induced hyperpolarizations (right, $n = 3$). (C) H_2O_2, when applied exogenously, caused endothelium-independent relaxations (left, $n = 5$) as well as hyperpolarizations (right, $n = 4$) in small mesenteric arteries of control mice without endothelium. Data are expressed as mean $\pm$ SEM. The asterisks indicate $p < .05$ by ANOVA. The dagger indicates $p < .05$ vs. resting membrane potentials by ANOVA.

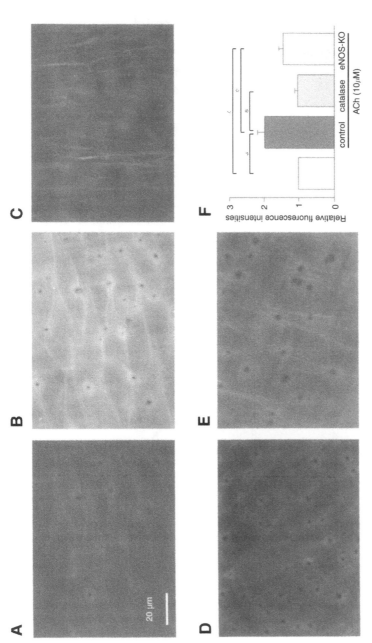

Figure 28.4 Acetylcholine-induced H$_2$O$_2$ production from the endothelium in small mesenteric artery of a control mouse were obtained before (A) and 3 min after (B) the application of acetylcholine (10^{-5} M). (C) Fluorescence image of smooth muscle layer of a control mouse obtained at the same visual field of A and B. The direction and depth of the smooth muscle layer are apparently different from those of the endothelial layer. (D) Acetylcholine-induced increase in fluorescence intensity was almost abolished by pretreatment with catalase (1250 U/ml) in a control mouse. (E) Fluorescence intensity of the endothelium in response to acetylcholine is reduced in an eNOS-KO mouse. (F) Acetylcholine-induced increase in the fluorescence intensity of the endothelium in control mice without (control) and with catalase (catalase), and in eNOS-KO mice (eNOS-KO, $n = 4$ each). The fluorescence intensity is normalized as fold increase from that under basal conditions without endothelium (before) in all three conditions. Data are expressed as mean ± SEM. The asterisks indicate $p < .05$ by ANOVA. (*see Color Plate 11*)

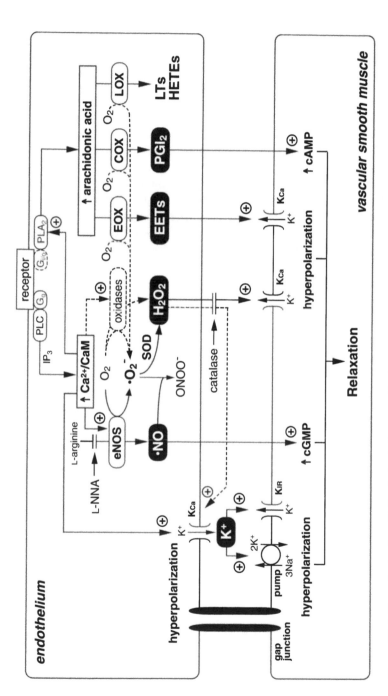

Figure 28.5 Hypothesis that H_2O_2 derived from eNOS is an EDHF in mouse small mesenteric arteries. Agonist-induced increase in intracellular calcium results in activation of eNOS in a Ca^{2+}/calmodulin (CaM) dependent manner. eNOS produces O_2^- in the presence of an L-arginine analogue, whereas several oxidases other than eNOS, including cytochrome P-450 epoxygenase (EOX), cycloxygenase (COX), and lipoxygenase (LOX), may also be sources of $\bullet O_2^-$. Subsequently, $\bullet O_2^-$ are dismutated by SOD into H_2O_2, which can freely diffuse to underlying smooth muscle, and activate K_{Ca} channels, resulting in hyperpolarizations and relaxations of vascular smooth muscle. On the other hand, H_2O_2 may also cause activation of K_{Ca} channels on the endothelium, which leads to two possible mechanism, potassium ion induced hyperpolarization of the smooth muscle, and gap junction-dependent propagation of hyperpolarization from the endothelium to the smooth muscle. (+) means stimulation.

that H_2O_2 released from endothelial cells is responsible for the oxidation of DCF. The acetylcholine-induced increase in the DCF fluorescence was markedly reduced in eNOS-KO mice (Figure 28.4), confirming the results obtained in organ chamber experiments (Matoba *et al.*, 2000).

Thus, H_2O_2 released from the endothelium was identified as an EDHF in small mesenteric arteries of mice, causing hyperpolarization and relaxation by opening K_{Ca} channels of the underlying smooth muscle. In the present study, eNOS appears to be a major source of agonist-induced H_2O_2 production since the EDHF-mediated responses and the production of H_2O_2 from the endothelium was reduced markedly in eNOS-KO mice. In eNOS-KO mice, H_2O_2 could be produced by other $^\bullet O_2^-$- or H_2O_2-producing enzymes (Figure 28.5), although not examined in this study. The decrease in the production of NO may result in an increase of $^\bullet O_2^-$ production, and thus in H_2O_2 production, which may compensate for the reduced NO-dependent endothelium-dependent relaxations by hyperpolarization-dependent mechanism. This interpretation could explain the redundancy of the endothelium-dependent relaxations caused by NO and EDHF (Mombouli and Vanhoutte, 1997; Shimokawa, 1999) and the inhibitory effect of NO on the EDHF activity (Olmos *et al.*, 1995; Bauersachs *et al.*, 1996). Superoxide dismutase appears to play an essential role in causing endothelium-dependent relaxations, not only by prolonging the half-life of NO (Rubanyi and Vanhoutte, 1986b) but also by converting vasoconstrictor $^\bullet O_2^-$ into H_2O_2, an endogenous EDHF.

29 Components of the potassium currents underlying the actions of endothelium-derived hyperpolarizing factor in arterioles

H.A. Coleman, Marianne Tare and Helena C. Parkington

The elusive nature of endothelium-derived hyperpolarizing factor (EDHF) has hampered detailed study of the underlying currents in isolated smooth muscle cells with voltage-clamp techniques. The aim of the present study was to characterize the components of current attributable to EDHF by recording from segments of intact submucosal arterioles (20–40 μm outside diameter) of guinea-pigs. These arterioles consist of a single layer of smooth muscle cells which can be voltage-clamped with single intracellular microelectrodes coupled to a switching voltage clamp amplifier. For the voltage-clamp studies, arterioles were cut into segments (100–300 μm in length), and voltage ramps were applied to determine current–voltage relationships. In the presence of nitric oxide and prostaglandin synthesis inhibitors, stimulation of the endothelium with acetylcholine evoked a hyperpolarization that was abolished by charybdotoxin plus apamin. Under voltage-clamp, acetylcholine evoked an outward current. Charybdotoxin alone reduced the amplitude of the outward current, while the presence of apamin plus charybdotoxin abolished it. Subtraction of the currents revealed charybdotoxin-sensitive and apamin-sensitive currents, and their separate current–voltage relationships were determined. Both currents reversed near the expected potassium equilibrium potential, were weakly outwardly rectifying, and displayed little, if any, time or voltage-dependent gating. The components have the biophysical and pharmacological characteristics of the intermediate conductance and small conductance calcium-activated potassium channels, respectively. Thus, the hyperpolarization attributed to endothelium-derived hyperpolarizing factor involves two current components, characteristics of which are consistent with activation of intermediate and of small conductance calcium-activated potassium channels. These channels are responsible for the prominent hyperpolarization evoked by endothelial stimulation in guinea-pig submucosal arterioles.

Endothelial cells play a central role in the regulation of vascular smooth muscle tone. The vasodilator influence of the endothelium can be mediated by a least three different "factors": nitric oxide, prostacyclin and endothelium-derived hyperpolarizing factor (EDHF) (Parkington *et al.*, 1993; Murphy and Brayden, 1995; Zygmunt *et al.*, 1998; see also Garland *et al.*, 1995; Mombouli and Vanhoutte, 1997; Edwards and Weston, 1998). The relative contribution of the three factors to vasodilatation seems to vary according to the size and location of the vessel. In general, the role of EDHF increases as vessel size decreases (Garland *et al.*, 1995). The endothelium-dependent response attributed to EDHF is that which is resistant to the combination of nitric oxide synthase and cycloxygenase inhibitors (see Mombouli and Vanhoutte, 1997; Edwards and Weston, 1998). The defining nature of this response is membrane hyperpolarization that is accompanied by relaxation.

The identity and nature of EDHF remains unresolved. Controversy surrounds whether it is actually a diffusible factor, or whether the hyperpolarization of the smooth muscle is due to electrotonic spread of activity from the endothelial cells via myoendothelial gap junctions (see Edwards and Weston, 1998). Candidates for EDHF as a diffusible factor include a metabolite of arachidonic acid produced via the cytochrome P450 enzyme (Campbell *et al.*, 1996; Popp *et al.*, 1996; Fisslthaler *et al.*, 1999), and also potassium (Edwards *et al.*, 1998). In reality, the phenomenon responsible for the EDHF response may vary between vascular beds and species.

Given the uncertainty surrounding the nature of EDHF and the possible significance of myoendothelial gap junctions (Bény, 1997, 1999; Yamamoto *et al.*, 1999), the detailed study of the currents underlying the EDHF response has remained elusive. In the present study, the use of electrically short segments of guinea-pig submucosal arterioles based on the preparation originally developed by Hirst and Neild (1980), has enabled the recording of the currents underpinning the EDHF response with the voltage-clamp technique.

1. METHODS

Guinea-pigs (190–400 g) were killed by cervical dislocation and segments of ileum were removed. The ileum was cut along the mesenteric border and the muscle layers and mucosa were removed, leaving a thin connective tissue sheet layer containing the submucosal arterioles. This sheet was then pinned to the floor of an organ bath and continuously superfused at 3 ml/min with warmed (35 °C) Krebs' solution (mM): NaCl 120, KCl 5, NaHCO$_3$ 25, KH$_2$PO$_4$ 1, MgSO$_4$ 1.2, CaCl$_2$ 2.5, glucose 11, bubbled with 95% O$_2$ and 5% CO$_2$.

Membrane potentials and currents were recorded using intracellular glass microelectrodes filled with 1 M KCl and having resistances of approximately 100 MΩ. Experiments were performed on arterioles of 20–40 μm outside diameter. For voltage-clamp experiments, short segments without branches and 100–300 μm in length, were prepared by cutting with a razor blade (Figure 29.1). For these experiments the microelectrodes were coupled to an Axoclamp-2 (Axon Instruments, Foster City, CA, USA) switching amplifier. Voltage protocols were generated using pClamp 6 software (Axon Instruments).

In these electrically short arteriole preparations membrane potential can be successfully clamped, and given that the functional endothelial/smooth muscle relationship is preserved, this enables the study of currents underlying the EDHF response (Coleman *et al.*, 2001).

For experiments where the endothelium dependence of the acetylcholine response was verified, the endothelial cells were destroyed using an antibody method (Juncos *et al.*, 1994). For this, a segment of ileum (2–3 cm in length) was placed in a chamber filled with warmed Krebs' solution. The mesenteric artery was cannulated just before it entered the ileum and perfused at 45 μl/min with the antibody solution using a syringe pump. The vasculature of the ileum was perfused for 1 h with a solution consisting of Krebs' solution containing antibody to Factor VIII (goat anti-human

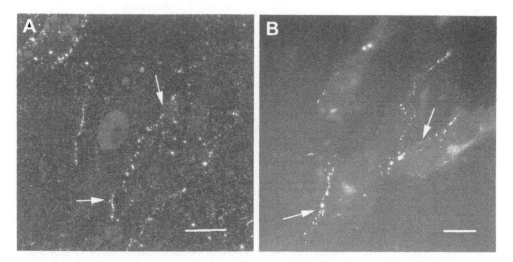

Color Plate 1 Expression of Cx43 and Cx43-GFP in A7r5 cells. A: Confluent monolayers of A7r5 cells were fixed and stained with a primary monoclonal antibody against Cx43 and secondary anti-mouse conjugated Alexa 488 secondary antibody. B: A7r5 cells were transfected with Cx43-GFP cDNA and viewed 24 hours after transfection for Cx43-GFP autofluorescence. Note the similar distribution of native Cx43 and Cx43-GFP in A and B. Arrows indicate gap junction staining. Bar = 10 μm. (*see page 44*)

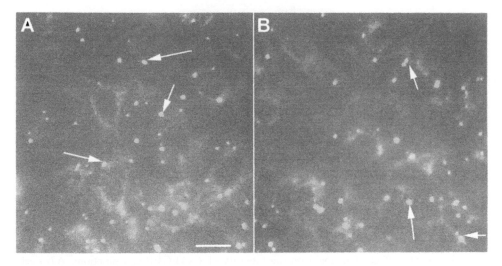

Color Plate 2 The effect of [43]Gap 27 on plaque distribution in HeLa cells expressing Cx43-GFP. Superimposed images of phase contrast and Cx43-GFP autofluorescence showing punctate gap junction locations at points of cell to cell contact in (A) non-treated cells and (B) cells treated with 5 x 10^{-4} M [43]Gap 27 peptide. Note similar distribution of staining. Arrows indicate typical Cx43-GFP gap junction plaques. Bar = 10 μm. (*see page 45*)

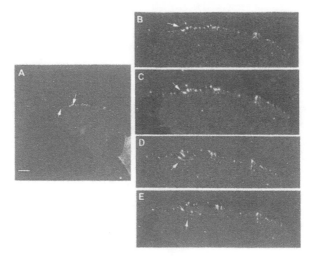

Color Plate 3 The effect of 18α-glycyrrhetinic acid on gap junction integrity in A7r5 cells. A7r5 cells were transfected with Cx43-GFP cDNA and 40 hours after transfection trafficking data was collected and analysed. A: Merged image of Cx43-GFP expression in A7r5 cells under normal conditions. B–D: Focus on the plasma membrane of the image in panel A. B: 15 to 30 minutes, C: 45 to 60 minutes before 18α-glycyrrhetinic acid treatment. At 65 minutes into the experiment 18α-glycyrrhetinic acid (2.5×10^{-5} M) was added. D and E show plaque disassembly occurring at 15–30 and 45–60 minutes after exposure to 18α-glycyrrhetinic acid. A–C: arrows indicate intact gap junctions; D and E: arrows indicate disassembled plaques. Bar = 10 μm. (*see page 48*)

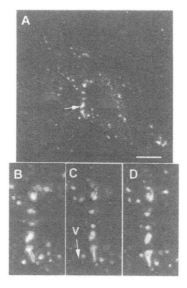

Color Plate 4 The effect of ouabain on the integrity of Cx43-GFP gap junctions. A7r5 cells were transfected with Cx43-GFP cDNA and 40 hours after transfection trafficking data was collected and analysed. A: merged image of 15–30 minutes under normal conditions. B–D focus on the plasma membrane of cells in panel A. B: 15 to 30 minutes under normal conditions. Ouabain (1×10^{-3} M) was added 30 minutes into the experiment. C: 30 to 45 minutes after exposure to ouabain: trafficking of connexons to the plasma membrane is evident as seen by movement of vesicle V (red → green → blue). D: 60 to 75 minutes after exposure to ouabain: reduced trafficking of connexons is evident as seen by the increased colocalisation of the three time points. Note that the plaques are still intact. Bar = 10 μm. (*see page 49*)

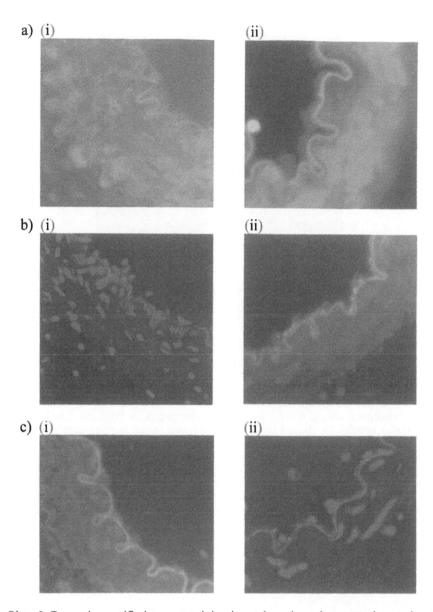

Color Plate 5 Connexin-specific immunostaining in rat hepatic and mesenteric arteries. Cx37 was abundant in both the endothelium and smooth muscle of the rat hepatic (A (i)) and mesenteric arteries (A (ii)), whereas Cx40 was restricted to the endothelium in both vessels (B (i) and (ii)). Cx43 was again evident in endothelium of both the hepatic and mesenteric arteries but also appeared at a low level in the media of these blood vessels (C (i) and (ii) respectively). (*see page 58*)

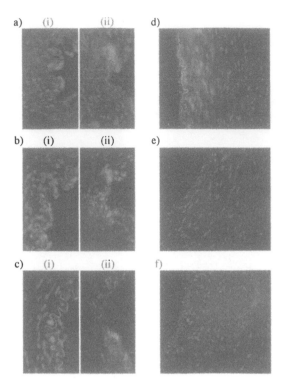

Color Plate 6 Connexin-specific immunostaining in the guinea-pig internal carotid artery and the porcine coronary artery. Cx37 staining was widespread in both the 'small' and 'large' internal carotid arteries (A (i) and (ii) respectively), and in the porcine coronary artery (D). Cx40 staining was restricted to the endothelium in the 'small' internal carotid artery (B (i)) but was evident in the media and endothelium in the 'large' internal carotid artery (B (ii)) as well as the porcine coronary artery (E). Cx43 expression was mainly endothelial in the 'small' internal carotid artery (C (i)) as was it in the porcine coronary artery (F) although there was some evidence for its expression in the smooth muscle. In the 'large' internal carotid artery, Cx43 was present in the endothelium but its expression was greatly increased in the smooth muscle (C (ii)). (*see page 59*)

Control   ß-Naphthoflavone   Nifedipine

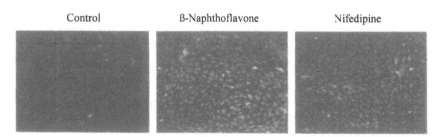

Color Plate 7 Induction of cytochrome P450 by nifedipine and β-naphthoflavone increases the generation of oxygen-derived free radicals in human endothelial cells. Endothelial cells were cultured in the presence and absence of nifedipine (10^{-7} M, 18 hours) or β-naphthoflavone (3×10^{-6} M, 48 hours) before incubation with 2',7'-dichlorodihydrofluorescein diacetate (5×10^{-6} M, 1 hour). 2',7'-Dichlorofluorescein fluorescence was monitored by confocal microscopy. Identical results were obtained using six separate cell batches. (*see page 170*)

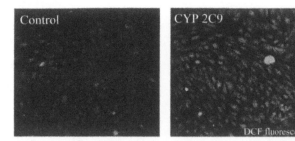

Color Plate 8 Over-expression of cytochrome P450 2C9 increases the generation of oxygen-derived free radicals in human endothelial cells. After transfection with pcDNA3.1 (control), or a cytochrome P450 2C9 expression plasmid, endothelial cells were maintained for an additional 24 hours prior to incubation with 2′,7′-dichlorodihydrofluorescein diacetate (5 x 10⁻⁶ M, 1 hour). 2′,7′-Dichlorofluorescein fluorescence was monitored by confocal microscopy. Identical results were obtained using five separate cell batches. (*see page 171*)

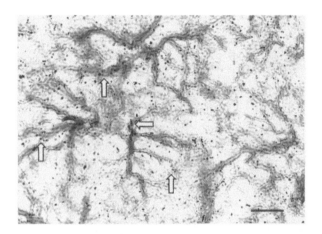

Color Plate 9 Autoradiograph showing an example of brain section that was infused with radiolabeled EET and immunohistochemically stained with glial fibrillary acidic protein (GFAP). Note the colocalization of radiolabeled EETs with GFAP-immunoreactive profiles (arrows). Scale bar, 30 μm. (*see page 225*)

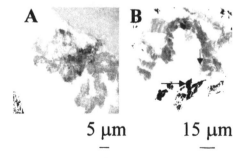

Color Plate 10 Staining of cells from the choroids plexus of rat infused with Ad5/β-galactos-idase. Section (thickness 15 μm) of a frozen brain from a rat infused intraventricularly with Ad5/β-galactosidase (5 x 10⁹ pfu), was stained for bacterial β-galactosidase activity for 2 hours (seen in blue) and then counterstained with nuclear fast red to display the cells. Panel B shows magnification of the choroid plexus in panel A. The arrows mark cells from the choroid plexus that stain for β-galactosidase and nuclear red, demonstrating that these cells express recombinant enzyme by viral-mediated gene transfer. (*see page 235*)

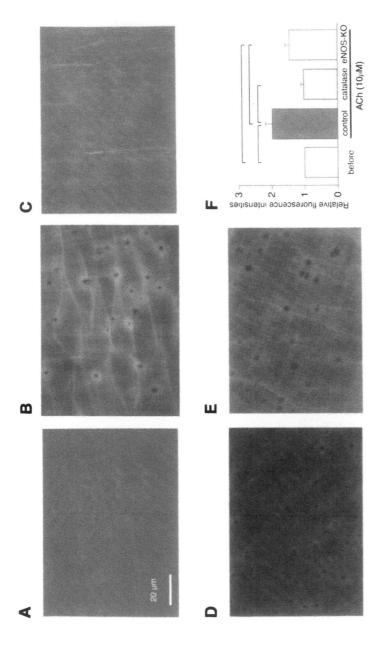

Color Plate 11 Acetylcholine-induced H_2O_2 production from the endothelium. Fluorescence images of the endothelium in small mesenteric artery of a control mouse were obtained before (A) and 3 min after (B) the application of acetylcholine (10^{-5} M). (C) Fluorescence image of smooth muscle layer of a control mouse obtained at the same visual field of A and B. The direction and depth of the smooth muscle layer are apparently different from those of the endothelial layer. (D) Acetylcholine-induced increase in fluorescence intensity was almost abolished by pretreatment with catalase (1250 U/ml) in a control mouse. (E) Fluorescence intensity of the endothelium in response to acetylcholine is reduced in an eNOS-KO mouse. (F) Acetylcholine-induced increase in the fluorescence intensity of the endothelium in control mice without (control) and with catalase (catalase), and in eNOS-KO mice (eNOS-KO, $n = 4$ each). The fluorescence intensity is normalized as fold increase from that under basal conditions without endothelium (before) in all three conditions. Data are expressed as mean ± SEM. The asterisks indicate $p < .05$ by ANOVA. (*see page 256*)

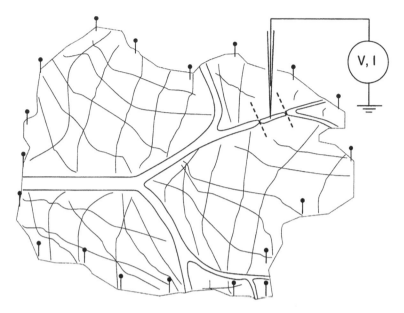

Figure 29.1 Schematic diagram of the submucosal arteriole preparation. These arterioles lie within a thin sheet of connective tissue and are accessed following the removal of the smooth muscle and mucosal layers. Segments of arterioles 20–40 μm in outside diameter were cut into electrically short lengths, typically 200 μm, which were then voltage-clamped using single intracellular microelectrodes coupled to a switching amplifier.

F8-RAg antibody, 14.29 mg/ml diluted 1:500) plus 2% complement and 5% bovine serum albumin. This was then washed out by perfusion of the vasculature with normal Krebs' solution for 20 min. Following this, the preparation was transferred to a dissecting dish and the sheet of connective tissue containing the arterioles was prepared for experiments as described above.

The following drugs were used: acetylcholine, apamin, iberiotoxin, indomethacin, N^{ω}-nitro-L-arginine methylester (L-NAME) and sodium nitroprusside (all from Sigma Chemical Co., St Louis, MO, USA), antibody to Factor VIII (goat anti-human F8-RAg antibody, Atlantic Antibodies (Incstar), Stillwater, MN, USA), bovine serum albumin (CSL Ltd, Melbourne, Vic., Australia), guinea-pig complement (Gibco BRL, Grand Island, NY, USA), nitric oxide gas (Matheson Gas Products, La Porte, TX, USA) and PCO 400 (Biomol, Plymouth Meeting, PA, USA). Iloprost was a gift from Schering (Berlin, Germany), prostaglandin E_2 was a gift from Upjohn (Kalamazoo, MI, USA), and glibenclamide was a gift from Hoechst (Melbourne, Vic., Australia). Charybdotoxin was synthesized by Auspep (Melbourne, Vic., Australia).

Nitric oxide solutions were made from nitric oxide gas (Parkington *et al.*, 1993), while nitrosocysteine was made up on a weekly basis (Field *et al.*, 1978).

Comparisons between data were made using Student's *t*-test, paired or unpaired as appropriate. Values of *p* less than .05 were considered to be statistically significant, and *n* refers to the number of tissues (animals), unless otherwise stated.

2. RESULTS

2.1. Endothelium-dependent hyperpolarization

The resting membrane potential of arteriolar smooth muscle and endothelial cells typically exceeds -70 mV (-73.7 ± 1.1 mV, $n = 13$) in normal Krebs' solution. Stimulation of the endothelium with acetylcholine under these conditions evoked only a small hyperpolarization (≤ 3 mV) (Figure 29.2). However, partial inhibition of the population of inward rectifier potassium channels with barium resulted in depolarization. When the membrane was depolarized to between -68 and -62 mV (-64.4 ± 0.6 mV, $n = 11$), endothelial stimulation now evoked hyperpolarizations of larger amplitude (7.2 ± 0.6 mV, $n = 11$) (Figure 29.2). The form of the acetylcholine-induced hyperpolarization changed with the concentration (Figure 29.2). At low concentrations ($\leq 10^{-7}$ M) the hyperpolarization was monophasic in appearance but as the concentration of acetylcholine was increased ($> 10^{-7}$ M) a second slower component emerged (Figure 29.2). The slower component was about two-fold less sensitive to acetylcholine than was the first component.

Incubation of the arterioles in N^{ω}-nitro-L-arginine methyl ester (10^{-4} M) to block nitric oxide production, or indomethacin (10^{-6} M) to prevent prostanoid synthesis, or a combination of both inhibitors, did not affect the resting membrane potential (-73 ± 1 mV, $n = 6$ tissues). Both of these inhibitors were without effect on the endothelium-dependent hyperpolarization evoked by acetylcholine. Thus, the endothelium-dependent hyperpolarization in arterioles is attributed solely to the action of EDHF. Furthermore, exogenous application of authentic nitric oxide (10^{-4} M) (Figure 29.3), sodium nitroprusside (10^{-5} M) (Figure 29.3), nitrosocysteine (8×10^{-5} M, not shown), the prostacyclin analogue, iloprost (10^{-7} M) (Figure 29.3) or prostaglandin E_2 (10^{-6} and 10^{-5} M) (not shown), all failed to evoke membrane hyperpolarization (Figure 29.3).

The endothelium-dependence of the hyperpolarization evoked by acetylcholine was determined by destroying the endothelium by treatment of the arterioles with antibody and complement. Following this treatment, the resting membrane potentials were -71 ± 1 mV ($n = 8$), which was not different from values recorded in untreated tissues. To determine the effectiveness of the antibody treatment, hyperpolarizations evoked by acetylcholine were compared between treated and untreated tissues which had been depolarized to a similar level (to between -55 and -65 mV with 2–3×10^{-5} M barium). The mean depolarized level for antibody treated tissues (-61.1 ± 0.8 mV, $n = 14$ arterioles from six tissues) was not different from the level for non-treated tissues (-60.9 ± 0.8 mV, $n = 18$ arterioles from eleven tissues). In non-treated tissues depolarized to this range, acetylcholine always evoked hyperpolarization (Figures 29.2 and 29.3). In arterioles from treated tissues, acetylcholine failed to evoke hyperpolarization (Figure 29.4).

2.2. Potassium channel blockers

The actions of potassium channel blockers were tested on the biphasic hyperpolarization evoked by 1-min applications of acetylcholine (10^{-6} M). Charybdotoxin (3×10^{-8} M), a potent but not highly specific blocker of large conductance calcium-activated potassium channels, reduced the integral of the hyperpolarization evoked by

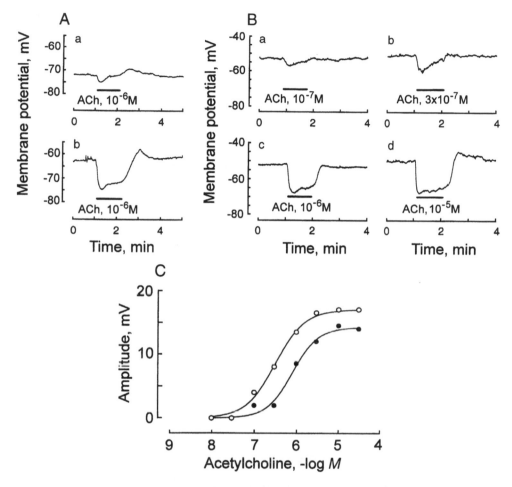

Figure 29.2 Two components of the EDHF-mediated hyperpolarization evoked by acetylcholine. (Aa) At the resting potential, in normal Krebs' solution, 1-min application of acetylcholine (ACh) (10^{-6} M) evoked only a small transient hyperpolarization. (Ab) The arteriole was subsequently depolarized with 2.5×10^{-5} M barium, and the same concentration of acetylcholine now evoked a considerably larger hyperpolarization and a second slower component was evident following the initial peak component of the hyperpolarization. (Aa,b) are from a continuous impalement. (Ba–d) Increasing concentrations of acetylcholine (10^{-7}–10^{-5} M) evoked graded hyperpolarization. At the lower concentrations the hyperpolarizations were transient in nature (Ba,b) whereas at the higher concentrations (Bc,d) the second component of the hyperpolarization became pronounced. All responses shown in (B) were from a continuous impalement. (C) Concentration–response relationships for the responses shown in B. Open circles (○) represent peak amplitude of the hyperpolarization, and filled circles (●) represent the amplitude of the hyperpolarization at the end of the 1-min application of acetylcholine. Solid lines are sigmoid curves of best fit. The EC_{50} for the initial peak component of the hyperpolarization was 3.2×10^{-7} M and the Hill slope was 1.3. The slow component of the hyperpolarization had an EC_{50} of 8.1×10^{-7} M and a Hill slope of 1.4.

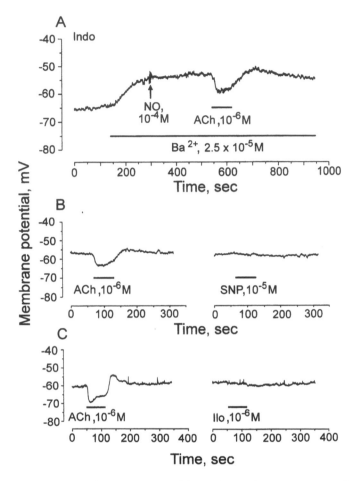

Figure 29.3 Effect of nitric oxide, sodium nitroprusside and iloprost on the membrane potential. (A) In the presence of indomethacin (10^{-6} M), the arteriole was depolarized with barium (2.5×10^{-5} M) and a 10-second application of nitric oxide (NO) (estimated final bath concentration 10^{-4} M) did not alter the membrane potential. Subsequent application of acetylcholine (10^{-6} M) for 1 min evoked membrane hyperpolarization. (B) The same arteriole as in (A), was depolarized and constricted with barium (3.5×10^{-5} M) in the presence of N^{ω}-nitro-L-arginine methylester (L-NAME, 10^{-4} M) and indomethacin (10^{-6} M). Acetylcholine evoked hyperpolarization (left panel) as before, but sodium nitroprusside (SNP, 10^{-5} M) (right panel) failed to evoke any change in the membrane potential. Continuous impalement in (B). (C) In normal Krebs' solution the arteriole was depolarized with barium (2×10^{-5} M). A 1-min application of acetylcholine (10^{-6} M) evoked substantial hyperpolarization (left panel) but the same arteriole was insensitive to iloprost (Ilo) (10^{-6} M for 1 minute). Continuous impalement in (C).

acetylcholine to $21 \pm 6\%$ ($n = 5$, paired data), with a considerable effect on the second slower component of the hyperpolarization (Figure 29.5). In contrast, the small conductance calcium-activated potassium channel blocker, apamin (2.5×10^{-7} M), had only a small and variable inhibitory effect on the hyperpolarization (Figure 29.5).

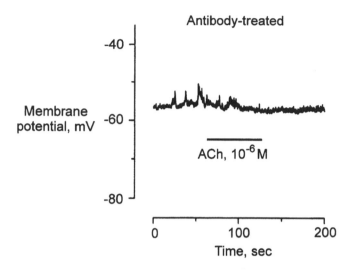

Figure 29.4 The application of acetylcholine following treatment of the arteriole with antibody. The arteriole was treated with antibody and complement (see Methods) and depolarized with 2.5×10^{-5} M barium in the presence of L-NAME (10^{-4} M) and indomethacin (10^{-6} M). Acetylcholine (10^{-6} M for 1 min) failed to evoke any hyperpolarization, indicating its endothelium-dependence.

However, the combination of both apamin plus charybdotoxin was effective in virtually abolishing the hyperpolarization, with the integral of hyperpolarization being reduced to $8 \pm 4\%$ ($n = 7$, paired data) (Figure 29.5). Iberiotoxin, a highly specific inhibitor of large conductance calcium-activated potassium channels, was without significant effect on the biphasic hyperpolarization (Figure 29.5). ATP-sensitive potassium channels were not involved in the EDHF-hyperpolarization as glibenclamide (10^{-6} M), a blocker of these channels, was without effect (Figure 29.6). Furthermore, an activator of these channels, PCO 400, failed to produce hyperpolarization when applied to the arterioles (Figure 29.6).

2.3. Currents responsible for the EDHF-mediated response

Segments of arteriole were voltage-clamped and voltage ramps were applied periodically so that current–voltage relationships could be determined. Stimulation of the endothelium evoked an outward current that appeared to consist of two components; an initial component that peaked early followed by a slower component (Figure 29.7). Charybdotoxin reduced this outward current (Figure 29.7). The charybdotoxin-sensitive current was obtained by subtraction and was large and slowly activating (Figure 29.7). Apamin also reduced the outward current evoked by acetylcholine, but to a lesser extent than charybdotoxin (Figure 29.7). The apamin-sensitive current was comparatively smaller, though it did occur over the same time course as the charybdotoxin-sensitive current (Figure 29.7). The current–voltage relationships for both charybdotoxin- and apamin-sensitive currents were outwardly rectifying (Figure 29.7) (Coleman *et al.*, 2001). The relationships for each were well described by the

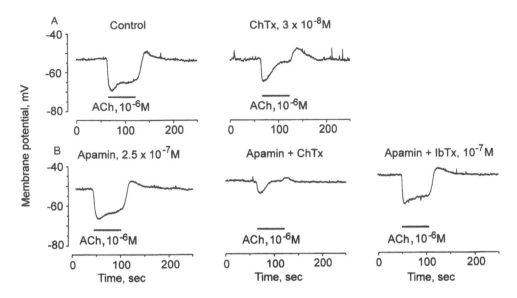

Figure 29.5 The effect of potassium channel blockers on the EDHF-induced hyperpolarization. (A) EDHF-attributed hyperpolarization evoked by acetylcholine (10^{-6} M for 1 min) before and after incubation with charybdotoxin (ChTx) (3×10^{-8} M). Although charybdotoxin reduced the initial component of the hyperpolarization, it had a greater effect on the second, slower component of the hyperpolarization. Charybdotoxin was without effect on the resting membrane potential. (B) The hyperpolarization was slightly reduced in the presence of apamin (2.5×10^{-7} M) (compare left panel of (B) with left panel of (A)). The hyperpolarization was all but abolished in the combination of apamin and charybdotoxin (3×10^{-8} M) (centre panel). In contrast, the hyperpolarization remained intact in the presence of iberiotoxin (IbTx) (10^{-7} M), even in the continuing presence of apamin (right panel). Continuous impalement in (A) and (B). All results were obtained in the presence of 4×10^{-5} M barium, L-NAME (10^{-4} M) and indomethacin (10^{-6} M).

Goldman–Hodgkin–Katz equation for a potassium conductance having reversal potentials of -85 mV, which is consistent with the likely potassium equilibrium potentials in these arterioles (see Edwards and Hirst, 1988).

3. DISCUSSION

The results from this study show that the endothelium-dependent hyperpolarization of arterioles in response to acetylcholine is mediated entirely by EDHF. The hyperpolarization was unaltered during exposure to nitric oxide synthase and cyclooxygenase inhibitors. Even if nitric oxide and prostacyclin were released from the endothelium they would not contribute to membrane hyperpolarization since exogenous application of these agents failed to elicit any membrane potential response. The endothelial origin of the response attributed to EDHF was confirmed in this study by the use of antibody to Factor VIII with complement to destroy the endothelial cells.

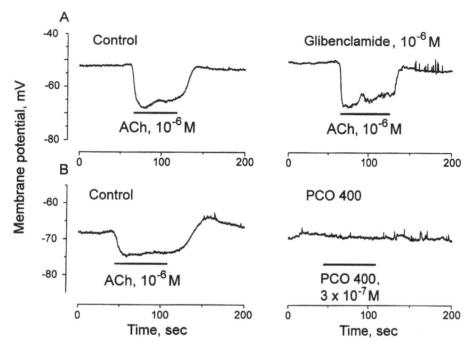

Figure 29.6 Actions of ATP-sensitive potassium channel openers and blockers. (A) The EDHF-mediated hyperpolarization evoked by 1-min application of acetylcholine (10^{-6} M) was not inhibited following incubation of the arteriole with glibenclamide (10^{-6} M). Continuous impalement, in the presence of barium (4×10^{-5} M). (B) Although acetylcholine (10^{-6} M) evoked a strong hyperpolarization the ATP-sensitive potassium channel opener PCO 400 (3×10^{-7} M) failed to evoke any change in the membrane potential. Continuous impalement, in the presence of barium (3×10^{-5} M), L-NAME (10^{-4} M) and indomethacin (10^{-6} M). Recordings in (A) and (B) are from different arterioles.

The EDHF-mediated hyperpolarization was diminished under resting conditions due to the dominance of the inward rectifier potassium conductance in these arterioles (Edwards and Hirst, 1988) which tends to make the resting membrane potential very negative. When partial blockade of the population of inward rectifier potassium channels was obtained with barium, membrane depolarization ensued, and stimulation of the endothelium under these conditions evoked robust hyperpolarization in confirmation of earlier findings (Hashitani and Suzuki, 1997). When used individually, charybdotoxin significantly reduced the hyperpolarization, while apamin had a far smaller influence. However, effective blockade of the EDHF hyperpolarization was observed when the combination of charybdotoxin and apamin was used and this is consistent with findings for responses attributed to EDHF in a variety of blood vessels (Corriu *et al.*, 1996; Zygmunt and Högestätt, 1996; Chen and Cheung, 1997; Hashitani and Suzuki, 1997; Petersson *et al.*, 1997; Plane *et al.*, 1997; Edwards *et al.*, 1998; Quignard *et al.*, 1999). The hyperpolarization was not abolished by the specific large conductance calcium-activated potassium channel blocker, iberiotoxin, alone, or in combination with apamin. ATP-sensitive potassium channels and inward

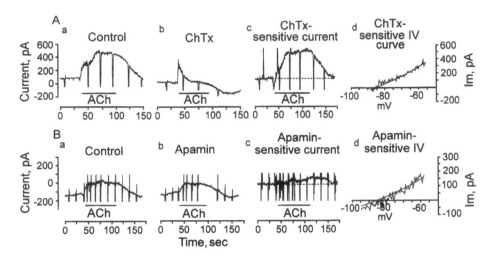

Figure 29.7 Potassium currents underlying the EDHF response and the actions of blockers. In the presence of L-NAME (10^{-4} M) and indomethacin (10^{-6} M), the
arteriole membrane potential was clamped at -55 mV for (A), and at -71 mV
for (B). Periodically the membrane potential was ramped (from -88 mV to
-55 mV (A), and -96 mV to -56 mV (B) over 1.5 seconds) as indicated by the
truncated vertical lines. (Aa, Ba) One minute applications of acetylcholine
(10^{-6} M) evoked biphasic outward currents. The outward current was
strongly inhibited by charybdotoxin (3×10^{-8} M) and only slightly reduced
by apamin (5×10^{-7} M). The current sensitive to each blocker (Ac and Bc)
was derived by subtraction (Aa minus Ab to give Ac; and Ba minus Bb to give
Bc). The current–voltage relationships for the charybdotoxin-sensitive and
apamin-sensitive currents are shown on the far right (Ad and Bd, respectively). Predicted potassium currents (smooth lines) fitted to the raw data
were calculated from the Goldman–Hodgkin–Katz equation (see Coleman
et al., 2001). Continuous impalements in each cell for (A) and (B). Recordings
in (A) and (B) are from different arterioles.

rectifier potassium channels were not involved in the EDHF response as glibenclamide
and barium, respectively, were without effect. ATP-sensitive potassium channels are
unlikely to occur in the endothelial or smooth muscle cells of these arterioles since an
activator of these channels, PCO 400, did not hyperpolarize these arterioles.

A novel aspect of the present study is the characterization of the potassium currents
underlying the EDHF response. This was made possible by the use of single electrode
voltage-clamp techniques using short segments of arterioles (Edwards and Hirst,
1988). This preparation lends itself to the clamping of membrane potential whilst at
the same time preserving the integrity of the smooth muscle and endothelial cells and
their relationship with one another. This is an important consideration in the light of
the uncertainty about the identity and nature of EDHF. Results from the present
study revealed that the hyperpolarization is underpinned by the activation of an
outward potassium current consisting of two components (see Coleman *et al.*, 2001).
As expected for potassium currents, both had reversal potentials close to the equilibrium potential for potassium ions in arterioles (see Edwards and Hirst, 1988). Both
components displayed little or no voltage sensitivity. One component was sensitive to

charybdotoxin and the other to apamin. The apamin sensitivity (Alexander and Peters, 2000) indicates that one of the currents is carried by small conductance calcium-activated potassium (SK_{Ca}) channels. The pharmacological and biophysical characteristics of the charybdotoxin-sensitive current under physiological potassium gradients are consistent with it being carried by intermediate conductance calcium-activated potassium (IK_{Ca}) channels. Cloned and native IK_{Ca} channels (conductance 18–50 pS, see Alexander and Peters, 2000) from a variety of tissues including endothelium and smooth muscle, are blocked by charybdotoxin but are insensitive to apamin and iberiotoxin (Ishii *et al.*, 1997; Cai *et al.*, 1998; Jensen *et al.*, 1998; Neylon *et al.*, 1999) and these are consistent with the observations in the present study of the effects of these blockers on EDHF hyperpolarization and the underlying currents.

Acetylcholine evoked graded hyperpolarization consisting of two components. The two components of the hyperpolarization could not be separately and selectively inhibited with either apamin or charybdotoxin. The reason for this was apparent from the voltage-clamp study, where it was revealed that the charybdotoxin-sensitive and the apamin-sensitive currents had similar temporal relationships, and each of these currents also possessed biphasic characteristics. The biphasic nature inherent to both currents is indicative of a similar origin for the triggering of the two, namely a rise in intracellular free calcium (Marchenko and Sage, 1996). Removal of external calcium abolished the second component of the hyperpolarization in guinea-pig submucosal arterioles (Yamamoto *et al.*, 1999), and although the first component was reduced it still occurred under these conditions. The persistence of the initial component of the hyperpolarization in calcium free solution indicates that calcium release from intracellular stores is important for this component (Marchenko and Sage, 1994). The second slower component of the hyperpolarization relies on calcium influx (Yamamoto *et al.*, 1999). Thus both currents appear to result from calcium release from intracellular stores, together with calcium influx.

In conclusion, the EDHF hyperpolarization in submucosal arterioles of the guinea-pig is underpinned by two calcium-activated potassium currents. The dominant current exhibits biophysical and pharmacological characteristics consistent with it being carried by intermediate conductance calcium-activated potassium channels. The second current is likely to be carried by small conductance calcium-activated potassium channels. These channels are solely responsible for carrying the currents underlying endothelium-dependent hyperpolarization in these submucosal arterioles.

ACKNOWLEDGEMENTS

This work was supported by the National Health and Medical Research Council (Australia) and the National Heart Foundation (Australia).

30 Evidence for relaxation to endothelium-derived hyperpolarizing factor (EDHF) in isolated small mesenteric arteries of the mouse

Kim A. Dora and Christopher J. Garland

Mesenteric arteries from CBA/CA mice were mounted in wire and pressure myographs. In both cases, acetylcholine evoked relaxation of the smooth muscle through an EDHF pathway, although the potency was slightly less in the wire myograph. Modest increases in extracellular potassium ion concentration also evoked smooth muscle relaxation. These data show that the mouse isolated mesenteric artery is suitable for studies on the EDHF pathway.

Attempts to demonstrate relaxation mediated by endothelium-derived hyperpolarizing factor (EDHF) in resistance arteries of the mouse have provided apparently conflicting data. In the isolated aorta, carotid, coronary and mesenteric arteries from C57BL6 mice, isometric tension recording revealed clear endothelium-dependent relaxation to acetylcholine in each case. These relaxations were abolished in all but the mesenteric artery by the presence of an inhibitor of NO synthase. In the mesenteric artery, the additional presence of indomethacin was required to abolish the relaxation. An identical profile of response was recorded in arteries taken from nitric oxide synthase knockout mice (Chataigneau *et al.*, 1999). In contrast, although relaxation in mesenteric arteries from the same strain of wild type mice was blocked by nitro-L-arginine plus indomethacin, in the knock out mice the relaxations were insensitive to this combination but inhibited in the presence of raised extracellular potassium (30 mM). A similar profile was obtained with isolated femoral arteries from these mice (Waldron *et al.*, 1999). These latter data suggested the presence of relaxation mediated by EDHF in the mesenteric and femoral arteries of the NO synthase knock out mice. The only major difference between the two studies was the fact that the mesenteric arteries studied in the latter were both pressurized and perfused.

In the present study, the involvement of EDHF in the relaxation of mouse mesenteric arteries was studied in mesenteric arteries mounted in a wire myograph and compared with the equivalent responses in pressurized and perfused vessels.

1. METHODS

Third order branches of the mesenteric artery of CBA/CA mice (30–35 g) were either normalized in a wire myograph ($D_{50} = 128 \pm 8\,\mu m$, $n = 6$) (Dora *et al.*, 2000) or pressurized to 50 mmHg and perfused intraluminally ($ID = 174 \pm 8\,\mu m$, $n = 4$) (Dora *et al.*, 1997). All experiments were performed at 37 °C in buffered Krebs solution (pH 7.4) containing indomethacin (2.8×10^{-6} M). Arteries were incubated in the presence of N^{ω}-nitro-L-arginine methyl ester (L-NAME, 100×10^{-4} M), apamin (5×10^{-8} M) and/or charybdotoxin (ChTx, 1×10^{-7} M) (synthetic forms) for 15–20 minutes prior to the addition of phenylephrine to evoke pre-contraction. All agents were added directly to the bath. Resulting data were stored at 2 Hz using a MacLab data acquisition system (Model 4e).

2. RESULTS

Acetylcholine (10^{-8} to 3×10^{-6} M) dilated the pressurized vessels by a maximum of close to 80%, and with an EC_{50} around 1×10^{-5} M ($n = 3$). Blockade of nitric oxide synthesis had no effect on the dilatation to acetylcholine, but the addition of 30 mM

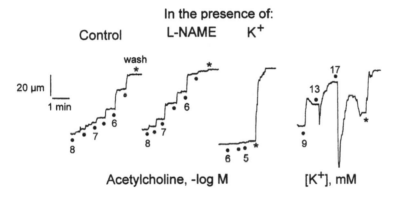

Figure 30.1 EDHF-mediated response in a mouse mesenteric artery mounted in a pressure myograph. Acetylcholine (ACh) evokes concentration dependent dilatation, which is partially due to NO release (slight rightward shift with N^{ω}-nitro-L-arginine methyl ester (L-NAME)), but predominantly due to the release of EDHF (blocked by raised extracellular potassium ion). The EDHF-mediated response evoked by acetylcholine may be due to the release of potassium ion, as small increases in the concentration of this ion (from 5 mM up to 17 mM) caused dilatation.

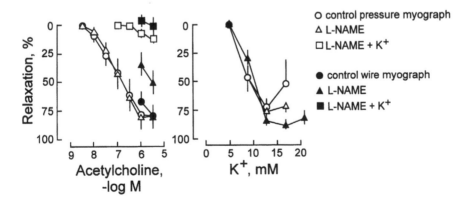

Figure 30.2 Comparison of EDHF responses in pressure- and wire-mounted mouse mesenteric arteries. Values are means ± SEM of $n = 3$–6 experiments.

K^+ abolished it (Figure 30.1). In the rat, K^+ ions released from the endothelium have been suggested to act as an EDHF (Edwards *et al.*, 1998). Pressurized mouse mesenteric arteries were dilated by increases in the concentration of K^+ ions around the outside of the vessels. The profile of dilatation was not altered in the presence of L-NAME, with K^+ causing a maximal response of close to 75%, (Figure 30.2).

In the wire myograph, cyclopiazonic acid (10^{-5} M), which evokes endothelium-dependent relaxation in arteries (Fukao *et al.*, 1995) caused a pronounced relaxation

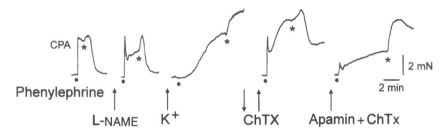

Figure 30.3 EDHF response in a mouse mesenteric artery mounted in a wire myograph. Cyclopiazonic acid (CPA) evoked concentration dependent dilatation, which was partially due to NO release (reduced in the presence of N^ω-nitro-L-arginine methyl ester (L-NAME)). The predominant mechanism for dilatation was the release of EDHF, as shown by the sensitivity to raised extracellular potassium ion and a combination of apamin (5×10^{-8} M) and charybdotoxin (ChTx, 10^{-7} M). Note that charybdotoxin reduced, but did not abolish, the EDHF response.

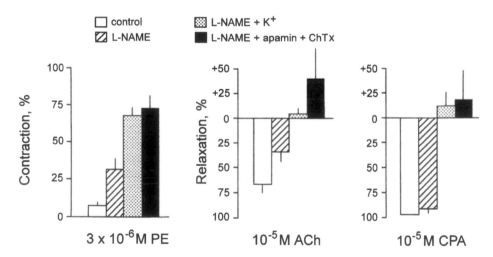

Figure 30.4 Release of EDHF during contraction and dilation of mouse mesenteric arteries mounted in a wire myograph. In each experiment, the same concentration of either phenylephrine (PE), acetylcholine (ACh) or cyclopiazonic acid (CPA), was added before and after the addition of N^ω-nitro-L-arginine methyl ester (L-NAME, 10^{-4} M) alone, or in combination with either potassium ion (K^+, 25–30 mM) or the combination of apamin (5×10^{-8} M) and charybdotoxin (ChTx, 10^{-7} M). Values are means $\pm$ SEM of $n = 3$–8 experiments.

(93 ± 4% of maximum) (Figure 30.3). Acetylcholine also relaxed mesenteric arteries contracted with phenylephrine. However, although the maximal relaxation to acetylcholine was also close to 80%, the EC_{50} was now around 3×10^{-6} M ($n = 3$). Blockade of nitric oxide synthesis had only a small effect on the relaxation to either acetylcholine or cyclopiazonic acid but raised extracellular K^+ (30 mM) almost abolished the relaxation to each agent, indicating that these responses were probably mediated by hyperpolarization ($n = 4$, Figure 30.4). Modest increases in the extracellular concentration of K^+, up to 15–20 mM, evoked a relaxation of around 90% of the contraction, followed by a secondary increase in tension with the higher concentrations. Relaxation to either acetylcholine or cyclopiazonic acid was abolished in the combined presence of the potassium channel blockers, apamin and charybdotoxin, showing that the relaxation is mediated by the EDHF pathway (Figure 30.4). In addition, the contraction mediated by phenylephrine was augmented by blockade of NO synthesis and EDHF release (Figure 30.4), underlining the importance of the endothelium in modulating contraction in this artery.

3. DISCUSSION

These data show that EDHF-mediated relaxation can be evoked in mesenteric arteries from CBA/CA mice. Furthermore, they demonstrate that increases in extracellular potassium ion concentration upto about 15 mM can evoke relaxation of the smooth muscle of these arteries. This is similar to the action of potassium in isolated rat arteries, where it has been suggested to act as an EDHF. Therefore, this possibility also exists in the mouse.

EDHF-mediated responses were demonstrated in both wire myograph mounted mesenteric arteries and arteries pressurized and perfused with physiological salt solutions. In terms of the endothelium-dependent response to acetylcholine, the only apparent difference was in the potency of the response; acetylcholine was less potent in the wire as opposed to the pressure myograph. This is consistent with previous reports in rat resistance arteries (Schubert *et al.*, 1996).

The demonstration of the similar EDHF evoked relaxations in both the wire and pressure myograph do not explain the discrepancy between these two techniques when used with mesenteric arteries from C57BL6 mice (Chataigneau *et al.*, 1999; Waldron *et al.*, 1999). The discrepancy had been suggested to be a result of the different extent of stretch applied by the two different techniques. Based on the present data, this appears not to be a satisfactory explanation (Waldron *et al.*, 1999).

The contraction to phenylephrine was augmented in mouse mesenteric arteries after inhibition of NO synthase, and more so after preventing endothelial cell hyperpolarization and the release of EDHF (Figure 30.4). This finding is a direct parallel to observations in the rat mesenteric artery (Dora *et al.*, 2000), and is consistent with the activation of heterocellular calcium signalling during contraction (Dora *et al.*, 1997). Indeed, the possibility that calcium or another signal travels down the concentration gradient from activated smooth muscle cells to adjacent endothelial cells is made possible by the presence of myoendothelial gap junctions in mesenteric arteries of both the rat (Sandow and Hill, 2000) and mouse (Sandow and Hill, personal communication). The importance of homocellular and heterocellular calcium signalling and current spread in the mouse mesenteric artery is unknown.

31 Pharmacological characterization of potassium channels in intact mesenteric arteries and single smooth muscle cells from eNOS −/− and +/+ mice

Hong Ding and Chris Triggle

Acetylcholine-mediated relaxation of blood vessels from endothelial nitric oxide synthase "knockout" mice (eNOS −/−) was insensitive to a combination of cyclo-oxygenase, nitric oxide synthase, and soluble guanylyl cyclase inhibitors and possessed the characteristics of being mediated by an endothelium-dependent hyperpolarizing factor (EDHF). The release and/or cellular action of this putative EDHF was inhibited by a combination of apamin and charybdotoxin and thus assumed to involve calcium-activated charybdotoxin- and apamin-sensitive potassium channels. Patch clamp studies of myocytes from the small mesenteric arteries revealed differences in whole cell current density between myocytes obtained from eNOS −/− versus eNOS +/+ mice that may reflect differences in potassium channel subtype and thus contribute to the alterations in endothelium-dependent relaxation that have previously been reported in eNOS −/− mice. Four components of outward current were identified: (a) a 4-aminopyridine-sensitive transient outward current; (b) a 4-aminopyridine-sensitive delayed rectifier current; (c) a 4-aminopyridine-resistant delayed rectifier current; and (d) a tetraethylammonium-sensitive calcium-activated and delayed rectifier potassium (K_{Ca} and K_{DR}) currents. An apamin and charybdotoxin-sensitive current could not be detected in the myocytes. These data indicate that the apamin and charybdotoxin-sensitive component of the EDHF-mediated response observed in the mesenteric artery does not reflect the cellular action of EDHF at the level of the vascular smooth muscle cell and that, most likely, the site of action of apamin and charybdotoxin is on the endothelium.

Studies of endothelial cell function in the vasculature from mice that do not express eNOS provide a tool to investigate the contributions of non-nitric oxide endothelium-derived vasodilators. The thoracic aorta from eNOS knockout (eNOS −/−) mice does not relax when challenged with acetylcholine suggesting that, at least in this artery, there is no compensatory increase in the production of endothelium-derived hyperpolarizing factor (EDRF) (Huang *et al.* 1995). In contrast, the acetylcholine-mediated dilatation of pial vessels from eNOS −/− is partially sensitive to tetrodotoxin and reduced by N^G-nitro-L-arginine indicating that neuronal NOS (nNOS)-dependent mechanism may compensate for the loss of eNOS-derived nitric oxide (Meng *et al.*, 1996). The pharmacological identity of the non-nitric oxide endothelium-derived relaxing factor (EDRF) in the pial vessels was not determined. In the aorta, carotid, coronary and mesenteric arteries from eNOS −/− mice neither a nitric oxide-dependent relaxation, nor a relaxation attributable to EDHF, could be evoked by acetylcholine (Chataigneau *et al.*, 1999). Thus, endothelium-dependent hyperpolarization of smooth muscle appeared to be absent in blood vessels from eNOS −/− mice. Only in the mesenteric vessels from the eNOS −/− an indomethacin-sensitive EDRF partially compensated for the loss of eNOS-derived nitric oxide (Chataigneau *et al.*, 1999).

In the absence of endothelium-derived nitric oxide there is an apparent upregulation of the contribution by EDHF to acetylcholine-mediated relaxation in the resistance arterioles from the mesenteric bed of eNOS −/− mice (Waldron *et al.*, 1999). Indeed, acetylcholine relaxations of pressurized arterioles of gracilis muscle from eNOS −/− mice is inhibited by cytochrome P450 inhibitors and high K^+ or iberiotoxin, suggesting a contribution of an EDHF that may be derived from, or depend on the presence, of a cytochrome P450 product (Huang *et al.*, 2000). Thus, the data from studies of endothelium-dependent relaxation of vessels from eNOS −/− mice indicate a considerable heterogeneity suggesting that the chronic loss of eNOS-derived NO has varying effects on the response to acetylcholine relaxation in different blood vessels.

The present study investigated the pharmacological properties of the K^+ channels that are involved in mediating endothelium-dependent hyperpolarization, to examine the hypothesis that the chronic lack of eNOS may lead to changes in the identity, contributions and density of both endothelial and vascular potassium channels. Acetylcholine increases the probability of opening of K_{Ca} channels in native endothelial cells (Rusko *et al.*, 1992) and the target on vascular smooth muscle cells of the putative EDHF is a K^+ channel(s) and/or the Na^+/K^+-ATPase (Figure 31.1) (Edwards *et al.*, 1998, 1999). Hence, the properties of K^+ channels were investigated in freshly dispersed mouse myocytes from second order mesenteric arterioles and the obtained results correlated with data obtained from studies of the effects of a variety of K^+ channel blockers on endothelium-dependent relaxations in the same vascular preparation.

1. METHODS

1.1. Materials

Mice (20–24 weeks of age) were stunned and killed by cervical dislocation following a protocol approved by the Canadian Council of Animal Care.

1.2. Myograph studies

Mesenteric arteries were removed and kept in Krebs' solution. Arteries were cut into rings (2 mm) and mounted on a Mulvany–Halpern myograph (Mulvany and Halpern, 1977). Tension studies were performed using a wire myograph. All experiments were performed at 37 °C.

1.3. Single cell studies

Second order mesenteric arteries from eNOS +/+ and −/− were incubated in a nominally calcium-free medium for 30 min to facilitate dispersion by disruption of desmosones connecting adjacent cells. To improve the yield and calcium tolerance of the myocytes, ethyleneglycol-bis-(β-amino-ethylether) n,n-tetra-acetic acid (EGTA)

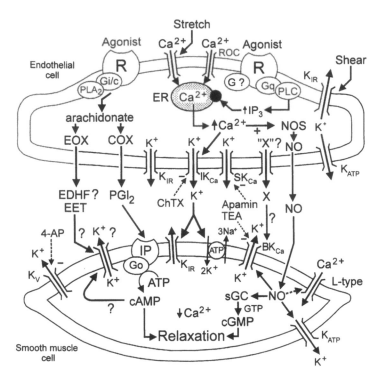

Figure 31.1 Relationship between an endothelial cell and vascular smooth muscle cell, and the regulation of the synthesis/release of nitric oxide (NO), prostacyclin (PGI$_2$), epoxyeicosandoids (EET), as well as the release of K$^+$ and a hypothesized endothelium-dependent hyperpolarization factor, "X", from the endothelial cell. Depicted on the endothelial cell is a G protein (Gi/o or Ga) coupled receptor (R) that regulates phospholipase A$_2$ (PLA$_2$) or phospholipase C (PLC). PLA$_2$ regulates the mobilization of arachidonate (arachidonic acid) from phospholipids, and epoxygenase (EOX) and cycloxygenase (COX) regulate the production of EETs and PGI$_2$ respectively. Ca^{2+} influx into the endothelial cell may be regulated via stretch-activated and/or receptor-operated (ROC) cation channels, as well as a store-operated influx mechanism linked with the superficial endoplasmic reticulum (ER). Intracellular Ca^{2+} release may also be regulated by inositol trisphosphate (IP$_3$). The putative role of K$^+$ channels (K$_{ir}$-inward rectifying; IK$_{Ca}$-intermediate conductance Ca^{2+}-activated; SK$_{Ca}$-small conductance Ca^{2+}-activated) in regulation of shear and chemical-mediated endothelial cell activation of EDRF/EDHF synthesis is also illustrated. NO and PGI$_2$ are depicted as acting via the soluble guanylyl cyclase and adenylate cyclase systems respectively, with PGI$_2$ activating adenylate cyclase via the IP prostanoid receptor. However, possible direct effects of NO on calcium-activated K$^+$ (K$_{Ca}$) and L-type voltage-gated Ca^{2+} (L-type Ca^{2+}) channels are also illustrated. EDHF, which may reflect a small increase (5 mM) in extracellular K$^+$, is assumed to mediate VSMC hyperpolarization via the activation of K$_{ir}$ and/or K$_{Ca}$ as well as the Na$^+$/K$^+$-ATPase. The SK$_{Ca}$ inhibitor, apamin, and the IK$_{Ca}$ inhibitor, charybdotoxin (ChTX), inhibit the synthesis/release of EDHF via their action on K$^+$ channels on the endothelium. 4-aminopyridine (4-AP) and tetraethylammonium (TEA) inhibit vascular smooth muscle cell hyperpolarization by an action on voltage dependent (K$_V$) and large conductance Ca^{2+}-activated K$^+$ channels (BK$_{Ca}$) respectively. A broken arrow, -----▶, reflects an inhibitory action (i.e, apamin inhibits the SK$_{Ca}$ channel) and a solid arrow, ——▶, indicates a pathway.

(10^{-4} M) was added to the solution. Single smooth muscle cells were dissociated enzymatically with 1 mg/ml collagenase IV and 0.2–0.5 μ/ml elastase III in 10 μM Ca^{2+} medium for 12 min. After digestion, the arteries were rinsed three times in fresh 10 μM Ca^{2+}-containing medium and triturated to harvest the cells. Cells were kept in the ice-cold solution. Single cells were voltage clamped using the whole cell configuration. Pipette potential and capacitance were nulled. Voltage clamp protocols were applied using pCLAMP 6.0 software. Whole cell current records were displayed and analysed using pCLAMP. A 10 mV junction potential was employed to correct all whole cell voltage clamp protocols. Macroscopic current values were normalized in pA/pF. Current–voltage (I–V) relation for end-pulse current amplitude was measured at the end of 250 ms command pulses to voltages between −65 and +45 mV. The standard bath solution contained the following (mM): 120 NaCl, 3 $NaHCO_3$, 4.2 KCl, 1.2 KH_2PO_4, 0.5 $MgCl_2$, 10 glucose, 1.8 $CaCl_2$ and 10 N-(2-hydroxyethyl)piperazine-N'-(2-ethanesulfonic acid (HEPES), pH 7.4. The pipette solution contained the following (mM): 30 KCl, 0.5 $MgCl_2$, 10 HEPES, 5 Na_2ATP, 1 GTP and 10 1,2-bis(2-amino-phenoxyl)-ethane-N,N,N',N'-tetraacetic acid (BAPTA).

1.4. Data analysis

Relaxation is expressed as percentage of phenylephrine-induced tone. Data are shown as means ± SEM. The significance of differences between mean values was calculated by Student's t-test for paired data. Statistical significance of differences between the means of data groups was estimated using ANOVA. Significance was assumed if p was less than .05.

1.5. Drugs

Acetylcholine, Na_2ATP – adenosine 5′-triphosphate (ATP), 4-aminopyridine(4-AP), apamin, charybdotoxin, 1,2-bis(2-aminophenoxyl)-ethane-N,N,N',N'-tetraacetic acid (BAPTA), ethyleneglycol-bis-(β-amino-ethylether)N,N-tetra-acetic acid (EGTA), N-(2-hydroxyethyl)piperazine-N'-(2-ethanesulfonic acid (HEPES), GTP (guanosine 5′-triphosphate), iberiotoxin, indomethacin, N^{ω}-nitro-L-arginine, (L-NA), 1H-(1,2,4) oxadiazolo(4,3-a)quinoxalin-1-one, (ODQ), phenylephrine, tetraethylammonium (TEA).

All drugs were obtained from Sigma (St. Louis, MO, USA). All drugs were dissolved in distilled water except for indomethacin and ODQ which were dissolved in 95% ethanol and dimethyl sulfoxide, respectively.

2. RESULTS

2.1. Mesenteric arterioles

The relaxation to acetylcholine in mesenteric vessels from eNOS −/− mice contracted with phenylephrine (10^{-5} M) was endothelium-dependent and insensitive to nitric oxide synthase and cycloxygenase inhibition, as well as combined inhibition of nitric oxide synthase, cycloxygenase and soluble guanylyl cyclase (Figure 31.2). In contrast, in arterioles from eNOS +/+ mice inhibition of nitric oxide synthase and

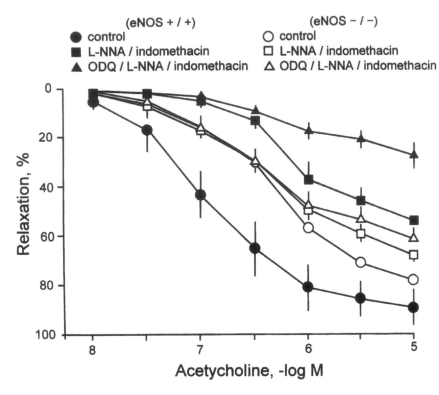

Figure 31.2 Concentration–relaxation curves to acetylcholine (ACh) in second order mesenteric arteries with endothelium from eNOS –/– and +/+ mice in the absence or presence (in combination) of inhibitors of either nitric oxide synthase (N^ω-nitro-L-arginine; L-NA, 10^{-4} M) plus cyclooxygenase (indomethacin, 10^{-5} M) or nitric oxide synthase, cyclooxygenase and soluble guanylyl cyclase (1H-(1,2,4)oxadiazolo(4,3-a)quinoxalin-1-one; ODQ, 10^{-5} M) inhibitors. The preparations were contracted with phenylephrine (10^{-6} M). Data are shown as means ± SEM ($n = 6–7$). The asterisk(s) indicate a statistically significant difference between the two strains ($p < .05$).

cyclooxygenase, as well as a combination of inhibitors of nitric oxide synthase, cyclooxygenase, and soluble guanylyl cyclase significantly reduced acetylcholine-induced relaxations.

In mesenteric arteries with endothelium from eNOS +/+ mice during contractions to phenylephrine (10^{-6} M), acetylcholine induced a concentration-dependent relaxation response (Figure 31.2). In the presence of the cycloxygenase inhibitor, indomethacin, (10^{-5} M) and the nitric oxide synthase inhibitor, N^ω-nitro-L-arginine, (L-NA, 10^{-4} M) the relaxation was attenuated significantly. The relaxation was significantly inhibited by the combination of the putatively specific soluble guanylyl cyclase inhibitor, ODQ, (10^{-5} M), indomethacin plus L-NA (Figure 31.2). In arteries from eNOS –/– mice the maximal relaxation induced by acetylcholine was significantly smaller than in those from wild type animals. However, the combination of L-NA and indomethacin or L-NA, indomethacin plus ODQ did not affect significantly the acetylcholine-induced relaxation (Figure 31.2).

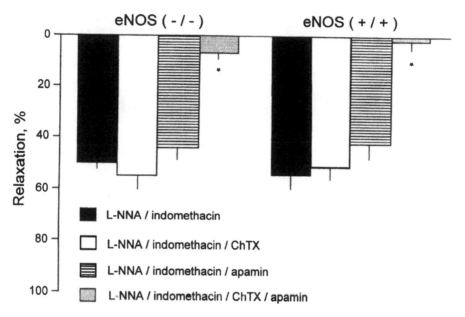

Figure 31.3 Effects of apamin (10^{-6} M), charybdotoxin (ChTX, 10^{-7} M) or a combination of apamin and charybdotoxin on acetylcholine-induced relaxations in second order mesenteric arteries from eNOS $-/-$ and $+/+$ mice. All studies were performed in the presence of N^ω-nitro-L-arginine (L-NA, 10^{-4} M) and indomethacin (10^{-5} M). Data are shown as means $\pm$ SEM ($n = 6$–7). The asterisks indicate a statistically significant difference between the drug treatments ($p < .05$).

The acetylcholine-induced relaxation was determined also in the presence of the calcium-activated potassium channel (K_{Ca}) inhibitors charybdotoxin and apamin. Neither charybdotoxin (10^{-7} M) nor apamin (10^{-6} M) alone significantly affected the relaxation to (Figure 31.3). The combination of apamin plus charybdotoxin completely abolished the acetylcholine-induced relaxation in both eNOS $+/+$ and $-/-$ mice. Substitution of charybdotoxin with iberiotoxin, or the combination of iberiotoxin and apamin could not completely inhibit acetylcholine-induced relaxation (data not shown).

2.2. Dispersed mesenteric myocytes

Whole cell currents were recorded during 250 ms pulses between -65 and $+65$ mV in 10 mV steps from myocytes in eNOS $+/+$ and $-/-$ mice (Figure 31.4). Activation of current during the depolarizing steps to $+65$ mV revealed significantly smaller whole-cell outward current densities in myocytes from eNOS $-/-$ (55.6 ± 6.3; $n = 12$) than in those from eNOS $+/+$ mouse myocytes (75.6 ± 10.9 pA/pF; $n = 7$. The half activation voltage was not significantly different, -10.3 ± 1.2 mV and -9.9 ± 1.7 mV, respectively. In the range from -65 mV to $+45$ mV there was no significant difference between the two strains.

Whole cell currents (Figure 31.5) were recorded from a single myocyte before and after treatment with tetraethylammonium at 10^{-3} M. At 10^{-3} M tetraethylammonium significantly reduced currents; at 10^{-2} M it almost totally eliminated whole cell currents

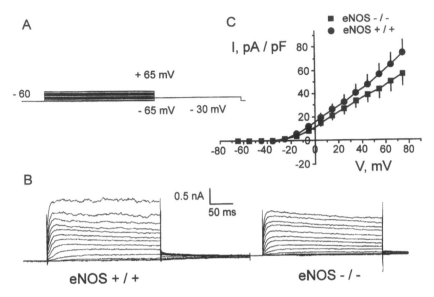

Figure 31.4 Whole cell currents recorded, during 250 ms pulses between −65 and +75 mV in 10 mV steps with holding potential of −60 mV, in myocytes from eNOS +/+ and −/− mice ($n = 10$–12). (A) Protocol of voltage step. (B) Original recordings of whole cell current. (C) Current (I)–Voltage (V) relationship of the end-pulse current.

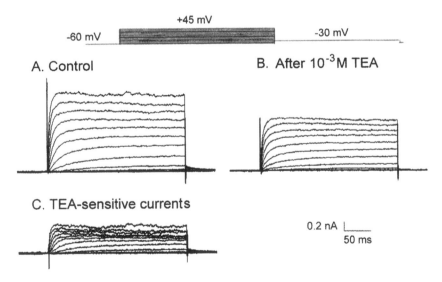

Figure 31.5 Whole cell currents recorded, during 250 ms pulses between −65 and +45 mV in 10 mV steps with holding potential of −60 mV, in myocytes from eNOS −/− mice. Currents were recorded from a single myocyte before (A), and after treatment with (10^{-3} M) tetraethylammonium (TEA) (B); in the presence of tetraethylammonium (10^{-3} M), the tetraethylammonium-sensitive (TEA-sensitive) current, C, is depicted as A minus that shown in B, (C).

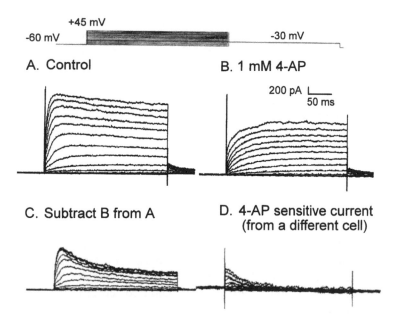

Figure 31.6 Whole cell currents recorded, during 250 ms pulses between −65 and +45 mV in 10 mV steps with holding potential of −60 mV in myocytes from eNOS −/− mice. Original recordings of whole cell currents were obtained in a single myocyte before (A), and after treatment with 4-aminopyridine (4-AP, 10^{-3} M) (B); C illustrates data from panel B subtracted from that presented in panel A; D represents similar data as in panel C but obtained from a different cell.

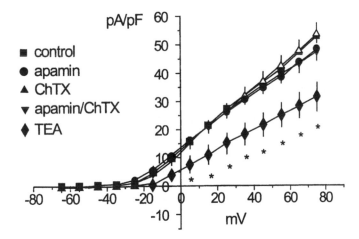

Figure 31.7 Current (I)–Voltage (V) relationship of the end-pulse current depolarizing step to +75 mV. Whole cell currents recorded during 250 ms pulses between −65 and +75 mV in 10 mV steps with holding potential of −60 mV in myocytes from eNOS −/− mice in the absence and presence of the K_{Ca} channel blockers apamin (10^{-6} M), or charybdotoxin (ChTX, 10^{-7} M) either alone or in combination, or in the presence of tetraethylammonium (TEA, 10^{-3} M). Data are shown as means ± SEM ($n = 6$). The asterisks indicate a statistically significant difference with the respective from control ($p < .05$).

(data not shown). 4-Aminopyridine (10^{-3} M) also significantly attenuated whole cell currents (Figure 31.6). The recordings indicate that there are both transient and sustained outward currents sensitive to 4-aminopyridine. Activation of current during the depolarizing steps to $+75$ mV revealed a whole-cell outward current density in eNOS $-/-$ mouse myocytes of 52.8 ± 4.7 pA/pF (Figure 31.7). The presence of the K_{Ca} channel blockers apamin (10^{-6} M) or charybdotoxin (10^{-7} M) singularly or in combination, had no significant effect on the outward whole cell current, and current densities of 48.3 ± 3.9, and 53.4 ± 3.5 pA/pF were recorded, respectively. The combination of apamin (10^{-6} M), plus charybdotoxin (10^{-7} M) had no significant inhibitory action on the current with a current density 47.5 ± 2.9 pA/pF. Tetraethylammonium (10^{-3} M) significantly inhibited the outward current density to 31.5 ± 5.1 pA/pF.

3. DISCUSSION

The present study demonstrates that in mesenteric arterioles from eNOS $+/+$ mice the relaxation mediated by acetylcholine is almost totally abolished by the combination of inhibitors of cyclooxygenase, nitric oxide synthase and soluble guanylyl cyclase. This observation leads to the conclusion that acetylcholine-induced relaxation is mediated mainly by nitric oxide and prostacyclin in eNOS $+/+$ mice. In contrast, in mesenteric vessels from the eNOS $-/-$ mice a mediator(s) other than nitric oxide and prostacyclin is responsible for the acetylcholine-induced endothelium-dependent relaxation. Neither apamin nor charybdotoxin alone inhibit the acetylcholine-mediated endothelium-dependent relaxation (and presumably the hyperpolarization), relaxation of mesenteric arterioles from eNOS $-/-$ mice. However, the combination of these K_{Ca} channel blockers completely inhibited the response to acetylcholine. Analysis of whole cell K^+ currents in freshly dispersed myocytes from the mouse mesenteric resistance vessels failed to demonstrate an apamin/charbdotoxin current suggesting that these K_{Ca} channels most likely are associated with the endothelial cells. Tetraethylammonium reduced and eventually abolished whole cell outward currents, indicating the contribution of K_{Ca} channels in the mouse myocyte. 4-Aminopyridine also significantly reduced the whole cell outward currents, suggesting the contribution of a K_V channel(s). Charybdotoxin can inhibit not only the large conductance, BK_{Ca}, and intermediate conductance, IK_{Ca}, K^+ channels, but also K_V channels (Nelson and Quayle, 1995). Thus, one could expect some inhibitory effect of charybdotoxin alone on whole cell currents in the mouse myocytes. The present data does not permit further speculation and such an inhibitory effect of charybdotoxin was not detected. In contrast, the lack of sensitivity of mesenteric myocytes to apamin was predictable. Indeed, although intestinal smooth muscle contains SK_{Ca} (Vogalis and Goyal, 1997), this is not the case in native vascular smooth muscle cells (Marchenko and Sage, 1996; Muraki *et al.*, 1997; Wang *et al.*, personal communication). Thus, the sensitivity of the nitric oxide and prostacyclin-independent relaxation of the eNOS $-/-$ mouse mesenteric arteriole to the combination of apamin and charybdotoxin probably results from an action of the toxins on the endothelial cell that leads to inhibition of the release of EDHF and/or inhibition of endothelial-smooth muscle cell communication via myo-endothelial cell gap junctions (Figure 31.1).

Two possible explanations can be offered for the requirement for both apamin and charybdotoxin to inhibit the EDHF-mediated relaxation of eNOS $-/-$ mouse mesenteric arterioles. First, the target for these two toxins may be a novel K_{Ca} channel that, perhaps through the heteromultimeric assembly of α-subunits derived from SK_{Ca} and IK_{Ca} posseses the binding sites for both toxins (Zygmunt *et al.*, 1997). Second, two EDHFs may be released; the release of one being sensitive to apamin and the second sensitive to charybdotoxin and thus, in the presence of only one toxin, the ratio of the EDHFs released would change and only a partial inhibition of endothelium-dependent hyperpolarization would be achieved (Edwards and Weston, 1998). In studies of the nitric oxide- and prostacyclin-independent relaxation of mesenteric arterioles from eNOS $-/-$ mice, iberiotoxin, that is selective for BK_{Ca} (Galvez *et al.*, 1990), does not substitute for charybdotoxin (unpublished data). This indicates that the putative novel potassium channel, or the release mechanism for EDHF(s), does not involve a BK_{Ca} channel. Since it is unlikely that BK_{Ca} channels are expressed in native endothelial cells (Triggle, 2000, unpublished data) the present data indicate that the apamin- and charybdotoxin-sensitive K^+ channel(s) cannot be part of the vascular smooth muscle cells. In the rat hepatic artery the IK_{Ca} channel opener, 1-ethyl-2-benzenimidazolinone (1-EBIO) (Jensen *et al.*, 1998), causes a charybdotoxin-sensitive, iberiotoxin-insensitive hyperpolarization that is absent in preparations without endothelium. Furthermore, 1-EBIO induced a charybdotoxin-sensitive, and iberiotoxin-insensitive, current in cell cultures of bovine aortic endothelial cells and had no effect in rat hepatic myocytes (Edwards *et al.*, 1999). In rabbit aortic endothelial cells acetylcholine causes a hyperpolarization that has two components; the transient component is inhibited by charybdotoxin and the sustained one by apamin- and charybdotoxin. These data support the hypothesis that the apamin- and charybdotoxin-sensitive channel(s), that are critical for the mediation of endothelium-dependent hyperpolarization reside on the endothelial cells (Figure 31.1). During depolarization, the whole cell current density was lower in the mouse myocytes from eNOS $-/-$ mice suggesting that the chronic lack of eNOS-derived nitric oxide leads to changes in expression of K^+ channels. However, under hyperpolarizing and resting conditions whole cell current density was not different in myocytes from eNOS $-/-$ versus $+/+$ mice. Thus, the physiological significance of the differences under depolarizing conditions is uncertain.

The data on endothelium-dependent relaxations of blood vessels from eNOS $-/-$ mice indicate a considerable heterogeneity suggesting that the chronic loss of eNOS-derived nitric oxide has different effects on the response to acetylcholine depending on the origin and/or the size of the preparations studied. This may reflect the different role and contribution or chemical nature of EDHFs in these blood vessels (Meng *et al.*, 1996; Waldron *et al.*, 1999; Ding *et al.*, 2000; Huang *et al.*, 2000). For example the endothelium-dependent relaxation (and presumably the hyperpolarization) to acetylcholine of saphenous arteries from eNOS $-/-$ and $+/+$ mice cannot be mimicked by elevating extracellular K^+. However, an elevation in the concentration of extracellular K^+ may be a contributor to the endothelium-dependent hyperpolarization in mouse mesenteric arterioles (Ding *et al.*, 2000).

ACKNOWLEDGEMENTS

Dr John McGuire for his critical reading of the manuscript and Dr William C. Cole for his help with the analysis of the data from the electrophysiology studies.

32 EDHF, which is not NO, is a major endothelium-dependent vasodilator in mice

Ralf P. Brandes, Michel Félétou,
Friedrich-Hubertus Schmitz-Winnenthal,
Paul M. Vanhoutte, Ingrid Fleming
and Rudi Busse

Endothelial control of vascular tone is mediated mainly by nitric oxide and the endothelium-derived hyperpolarizing factor (EDHF). The properties of EDHF and the contribution of EDHF to endothelium-dependent relaxation were determined by studying vasodilator responses to endothelial agonists in wild-type and endothelial NO synthase knockout mice (eNOS −/−).

Vasodilator responses to bradykinin were determined *in vivo* by recording changes in mean arterial pressure. *In vitro* vasodilator responses were determined as changes in perfusion pressure in the saline perfused heart and hindlimb under constant flow conditions. Bradykinin induced a pronounced, dose-dependent decrease in mean arterial pressure which did not differ between wild-type and eNOS −/− mice, and was unaffected in both strains by treatment with N^{ω}-nitro-L-arginine methylester and diclofenac. In the perfused hindlimb and heart of wild-type and eNOS −/− mice, vasodilator responses to acetylcholine were unaffected by N^{ω}-nitro-L-arginine (L-NA) and diclofenac. The acetylcholine-induced vasodilatation in the hindlimb of wild-type was not attenuated by L-NA. In the presence, but not the absence of L-NA, the vasodilator response to acetylcholine was sensitive to KCl, and to the combination of apamin plus charybdotoxin. In addition, gap junction inhibitors (18α-glycyrrhetinic acid, octanol, heptanol) but not inhibition of cytochrome P450 enzymes impaired the EDHF-mediated vasodilator response. These results demonstrate that in murine resistance vessels the predominant agonist-induced endothelium-dependent vasodilator principle *in vivo* and *in vitro*, is a non-NO, non-prostacyclin metabolite, which displays the classical characteristics of EDHF and requires functional gap junctions.

Endothelium-derived NO is an important determinant of local vascular tone and resistance and plays a predominant role in agonist-induced, endothelium-dependent relaxations both *in vivo* and *in vitro*. In contrast, the contribution of endothelium-derived hyperpolarizing factor (EDHF) to relaxation and vasodilatation is still poorly understood as the chemical nature of the different EDHFs generated in different vascular beds and species is uncertain (Campbell and Harder, 1999; Cohen and Vanhoutte, 1995; Edwards and Weston, 1998; Furchgott and Vanhoutte, 1989; Quilley *et al.*, 1997; Waldron and Cole, 1999).

The present experiments were designed to determine the contribution of EDHF to agonist-induced vasodilator responses in resistance vessels of mice. By including endothelial synthase knockout (eNOS −/−) mice in this study, the question was addressed of whether or not EDHF might be identical to NO released from an incompletely inhibited NO-synthase.

1. MATERIALS AND METHODS

1.1. Animals and drugs

Wild-type control mice and homozygote eNOS −/− mice were obtained from Iffa Credo/Charles Rivers. The colony was founded on eNOS −/− breeders kindly supplied by P.L. Huang, Boston, MA, USA.

Iberiotoxin and charybdotoxin were purchased from Bachem, Heidelberg. Germany. All other drugs were obtained from Sigma, Deisenhofen, Germany.

1.2. *In vivo*

Vasodilator responses were recorded in sodium pentobarbital (90 mg/kg, intra-peritoneal, 0.2 ml) anesthetized mice as changes in mean arterial pressure following the bolus application of bradykinin (1, 10, 30 µg/kg). Bradykinin was applied via a catheter inserted into the jugular vein. Blood pressure was recorded using a pressure transducer in one carotid artery. Studies were performed in wild-type and eNOS −/− mice in the presence and absence of the inhibitor of the NO synthase N^{ω}-nitro-L-arginine methylester (L-NAME, 30 mg/kg) and the inhibitor of the cycloxygenase diclofenac (10 mg/kg), both applied intra-peritoneally at least 30 min prior to the study.

1.3. *In vitro*

Conduit arteries were studied in a conventional organ chamber. Arterial segments were mounted on tungsten wire triangles and studied under isometric conditions (passive tension 10 N). Relaxations to increasing concentrations of acetylcholine were recorded in the continuous presence of diclofenac (10^{-5} M) in modified Krebs–Henseleit buffer (concentrations in mM: NaCl 118.3, KCl 4.7, $CaCl_2$ 1.8, $MgSO_4$ 1.2, KH_2PO_4 1.2, $NaHCO_3$ 25, EDTA 0.026, glucose 11.1, pH 7.40 aerated with 95% O_2–5% CO_2) in the presence or absence of N^{ω}-nitro-L-arginine (L-NA, 3×10^{-4} M).

Resistance vessels of the isolated heart and the hindlimb were studied in a perfusion system: For recordings in the hindlimb a catheter was inserted into one of the common iliac arteries via the abdominal aorta. The isolated heart was studied under non-working conditions by retrograde perfusion via the aortic arch through a blunt steel cannula. Vasodilator responses to bolus applications (0.1 ml) of endothelial agonists (bradykinin, acetylcholine and substance P) or the NO-donor sodium nitroprusside were determined as changes in perfusion pressure since flow rate was maintained constant during the experiment. To facilitate comparison of the response to endothelium-dependent agonists in the absence and presence of a given inhibitor, control responses were obtained in each animal and after an equilibration period of 20 min, inhibitors were added to the perfusate and the response to the endothelial agonist was assessed again.

1.4. Statistics

Data presented are mean ± SEM. Statistical analysis was performed using analysis of variance for multiple measurements. Differences were considered to be statistically significant when *p* was less than .05.

2. RESULTS

2.1. *In vivo*

Bradykinin elicited a dose-dependent and transient decrease in mean arterial pressure. At doses higher than 1 μg/kg the effect of bradykinin was significant. No difference in bradykinin-induced changes in mean arterial pressure were observed between wild-type and eNOS −/− mice. Moreover, neither diclofenac, nor L-NAME significantly affected the changes in blood pressure induced by bradykinin in either mouse strain (Figure 32.1, Table 32.1).

2.2. *In vitro*

Endothelium-dependent relaxations to acetylcholine were observed in aortic rings of wild-type mice in the absence of eNOS inhibitors. In contrast, acetylcholine failed to elicit relaxations of aortas from wild-type mice treated with L-NA, or from eNOS −/− mice. Neither bradykinin nor substance P induced relaxations of the mouse aorta.

In the perfused hindlimb and perfused heart, acetylcholine and bradykinin induced dose-dependent vasodilator responses, which were similar in wild-type and eNOS −/− mice and were unaffected by L-NA. Chemical removal of the endothelium using Triton X-100, significantly attenuated vasodilatation to acetylcholine (Figures 32.2 and 32.3).

Table 32.1 Baseline characteristics of the anesthetized mice

	Mean arterial pressure (mmHg)	Heart rate (BPM)	n
Wild-type			
Control	$68.0 \pm 2.7^{\dagger}$	$428 \pm 8^{\dagger}$	22
Diclofenac	$60.1 \pm 1.9^{\dagger}$	$396 \pm 6^{\dagger}$	30
L-NAME	$78.0 \pm 2.9^{\dagger}$	$388 \pm 9^{*,\dagger}$	26
L-NAME + Diclofenac	$78.3 \pm 3.8^{\dagger}$	$377 \pm 5^{*,\dagger}$	28
eNOS(−/−) mice			
Control	$114.8 \pm 13.8^{\dagger}$	$489 \pm 18^{\dagger}$	16
Diclofenac	$87.0 \pm 6.4^{\dagger}$	$477 \pm 16^{\dagger}$	22
L-NAME	$94.2 \pm 6.9^{\dagger}$	$474 \pm 16^{\dagger}$	22
L-NAME + Diclofenac	$98.0 \pm 10.1^{\dagger}$	$472 \pm 9^{\dagger}$	26

Notes
BPM = Beats per minute; L-NAME = N$^{\omega}$-nitro-L-arginine methylester.
The asterisks (*) indicate statistical significant differences ($p < .05$) with the respective control, and the daggers ($\dagger$) between wild-type and eNOS −/− mice.

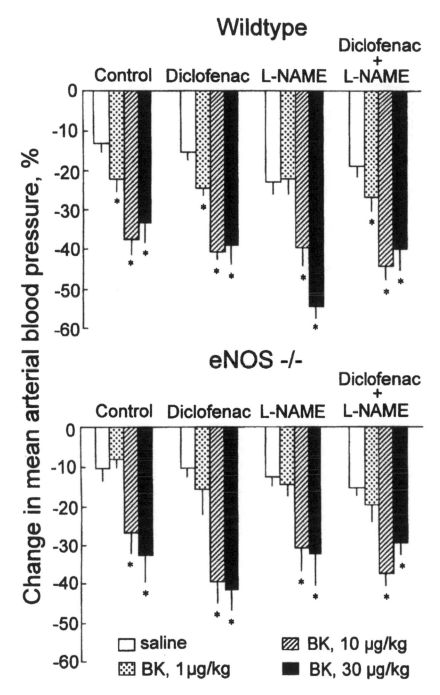

Figure 32.1 Effect of bolus application of saline or bradykinin (BK) on mean arterial pressure (MAP) (A) in anesthetized wild-type, or (B) in eNOS −/− mice in the presence or absence of diclofenac and N^{ω}-nitro-L-arginine methylester (L-NAME). The asterisks (∗) indicate statistically significant differences ($p < .05$) with the respective control. Data shown are mean ± SEM ($n \geq 5$).

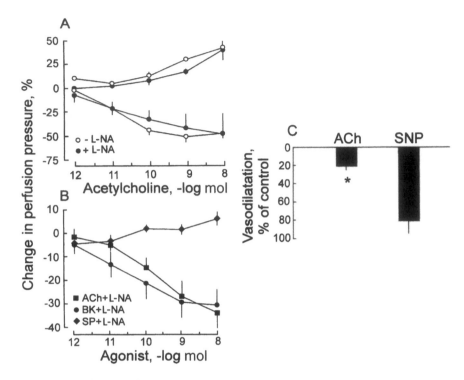

Figure 32.2 (A) Vasodilator responses to acetylcholine (ACh, 100 μl bolus) in the isolated perfused heart, in the presence of diclofenac (10^{-5} M) and presence or absence of N^{ω}-nitro-L-arginine (L-NA, 3×10^{-4} M). Acetylcholine elicited a biphasic response with initial increase in pressure and subsequent drop. (B) Vasodilator responses to bolus applications (100 μl) of acetylcholine (ACh), bradykinin (BK) and substance P (SP) in the presence of diclofenac (10^{-5} M). (C) Effect of removal of the endothelium using Triton X-100. Responses to either the endothelial agonist acetylcholine (ACh, 10^{-5} mol) or to the NO-donor sodium nitroprusside (SNP, 10^{-5} mol) as percent of vasodilator response prior to the infusion of Triton X-100. Data expressed are percent reduction in perfusion (Perf.) pressure, and are expressed as means $\pm$ SEM ($n \geq 5$). The asterisk ($*$) indicates a statistically significant difference ($p < .05$) with the control.

Although L-NA had only a negligible effect on agonist-induced vasodilatation, it significantly increased resistance in the perfused hindlimb of wild-type mice ($43.7 \pm 7\%$, $n = 7$). In contrast, L-NA had no effect on resistance in the hindlimb of eNOS $-/-$ mice ($2.3 \pm 1.7\%$, $n = 7$).

2.3. Characterization of the L-NA-resistant vasodilatation

In the perfused hindlimb of the wild-type mice, in the presence of L-NA, $K^+ (4 \times 10^{-2}$ M), as well as the combination of the K^+-channel blockers charybdotoxin (10^{-7} M) plus apamin (10^{-7} M), inhibited acetylcholine-induced vasodilatation. Charybdotoxin alone only slightly impaired the responses to acetylcholine. Apamin or the combination of iberiotoxin (10^{-7} M), apamin, glibenclamide (10^{-6} M), and 4-aminopyridine (5×10^{-3} M), did not significantly inhibit the vasodilatation

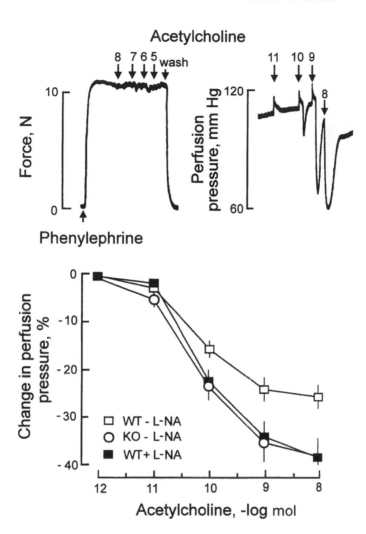

Figure 32.3 (Top) Original recordings showing the effect of acetylcholine on the tone of isolated aortic rings contracted with phenylephrine (PE, 10^{-7} M, numbers above the arrows indicate the concentration in 10^{-x} M of the agonist applied, left panel) and on perfusion pressure in the perfused hindlimb of eNOS −/− mice (numbers above the arrows indicate the amount of the agonist applied with the bolus in 10^{-x} mol, right panel). (Lower) Vasodilator responses to bolus applications (100 µl) of acetylcholine (ACh) on the perfusion pressure of the hindlimb of wild-type (WT; □) and eNOS −/− mice (KO; ○) in the absence (open symbols) and presence (closed symbols) of N^{ω}-nitro-L-arginine (L-NA, 3×10^{-4} M). Data are expressed as percent of the maximal response to sodium nitroprusside and shown as means ± SEM ($n \geq 8$).

elicited by acetylcholine. In the absence of L-NA, only the combination of charybdotoxin plus apamin exerted a small inhibitory effect on acetylcholine-induced vasodilatation (Figure 32.4). In the presence of L-NA, the acetylcholine-induced vasodilatation of the hindlimb vasculature was inhibited by 18α-glycyrrhetinic acid (10^{-4} M), octanol (10^{-3} M), and heptanol (10^{-3} M). These substances had no significant effect on

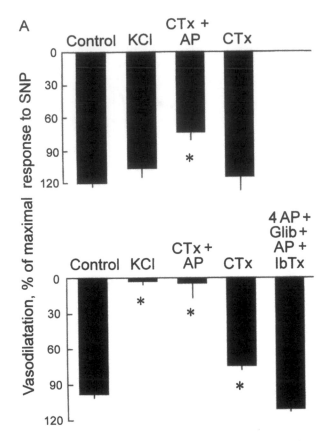

Figure 32.4 Vasodilator responses to acetylcholine in the hindlimb of wild-type mice. Experiments were performed in the presence of diclofenac (10^{-5} M) and in the absence (A) and presence (B) of N^{ω}-nitro-L-arginine (3×10^{-4} M). CTL = control, potassium channel blockade with charybdotoxin (CTX, 10^{-7} M), apamin (APA, 10^{-7} M), 4-aminopyridine, (4 AP, 5×10^{-3} M), glibenclamide, (Glib, 10^{-6} M) and iberiotoxin (IbTX, 10^{-7} M). Data expressed as percent of the maximal response to sodium nitroprusside (SNP) and shown as means $\pm$ SEM ($n \geq 3$). The asterisks (∗) indicate statistically significant differences ($p < .05$) with the respective control.

vasodilatation in the absence of L-NA (Figure 32.5). 8-cyclopentyl-1,3-dipropylxanthine (10^{-6} M) and 17-octadecynoid acid (10^{-5} M), miconazole (5×10^{-6} M) and sulfaphenazole (10^{-5} M) had no significant effect on acetylcholine-induced vasodilatation (data not shown).

Similar results were obtained in the perfused hindlimb of eNOS $-/-$ mice (data not shown).

3. DISCUSSION

The present study determined the role of EDHF in mediating agonist-induced vasodilatation in resistance vessels of mice both *in vivo* and *in vitro*. The results obtained

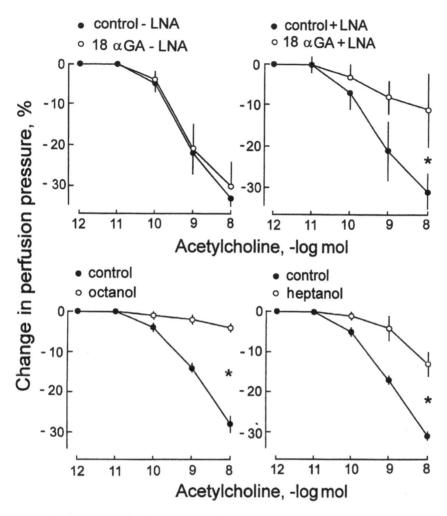

Figure 32.5 Effects of the gap junction uncoupler 18α-glycyrrhetinic acid (18αGA, 3×10^{-5} M) on the decrease in perfusion pressure caused by acetylcholine in the hindlimb of wild-type mice in the presence (+L-NA) or absence (−L-NA) of N^{ω}-nitro-L-arginine (3×10^{-4} M), and of heptanol (10^{-3} M) and octanol (10^{-3} M) in the presence of N^{ω}-nitro-L-arginine (3×10^{-4} M). Diclofenac (10^{-5} M) was continuously present during the experiment. Data are expressed as means $\pm$ SEM ($n \geq 5$). The asterisks (∗) indicate statistically significant differences ($p < .05$) with the respective control.

demonstrate that a factor exhibiting the characteristic profile of EDHF is a, if not the, major determinant of endothelium-dependent vasodilatation to bradykinin or acetylcholine in both wild-type and eNOS −/− mice. These data highlight the crucial role played by EDHF in the regulation of vascular tone and demonstrate that EDHF is not NO in the mouse.

The term "EDHF", as used in the present study, implies that the NO- and prostacyclin-independent vasodilator response occurs as a consequence of the opening of K^{+} channels, and of the hyperpolarization of vascular smooth muscle cells (Cohen and Vanhoutte, 1995; Félétou and Vanhoutte, 1999). However, since hyperpolarization of smooth muscle was not measured in the present study, the contribution of EDHF-mediated vasodilatation has to be infered from the pharmacological profile of the response. The sensitivity of the L-NA/diclofenac-resistant vasodilatation to depolarizing concentrations of K^+, as well as to the combination of the K^+ channel blocker charybdotoxin plus apamin is a characteristic of EDHF-mediated responses (Cohen and Vanhoutte, 1995; Corriu et al., 1996; Félétou and Vanhoutte, 1999; Waldron and Cole, 1999). The EDHF-mediated relaxation of mesenteric arteries from wild-type and eNOS $-/-$ mice is sensitive to charybdotoxin plus apamin (Ding et al., 2000). However, in the gracilis artery of mice, iberiotoxin alone inhibits the NO- and prostacyclin-independent acetylcholine-induced relaxation (Huang et al., 2000). Different experimental conditions may help to explain the apparent discrepancy in these results. For example, in the present study, vasodilatation was recorded under conditions of constant flow. Therefore, the luminal surface of the endothelium was exposed continuously to shear stress, which activates multiple signal transduction pathways in endothelial cells (Davies, 1995). In addition, acetylcholine was applied as a bolus and, as a consequence of the perfusion, washed out immediately. This very transient stimulus may elicit responses which differ from those elicited by the prolonged application of the muscarinic agonist.

Studies addressing the contribution of EDHF to endothelium-dependent vasodilatation are usually limited by the fact that the involvement of the various endothelium-derived mediators can only be estimated by the inclusion of pharmacological inhibitors. This approach is usually complicated by unwanted side effects of the inhibitors (Amezcua et al., 1989; Lamontage et al., 1991), and by the fact that some of the inhibitors used do not fully inhibit the activity of the enzyme system targeted (Cohen et al., 1997). In this regard, EDHF has been proposed to be NO generated by an incompletely inhibited nitric oxide synthase (Cohen et al., 1997). This latter point is of particular relevance since, at high concentrations, NO can cause hyperpolarization (Archer et al., 1994; Bolotina et al., 1994), although by activating a different K^+ channel (Chataigneau et al., 1998). Thus, an aim of the present study was to demonstrate that EDHF is not NO. By demonstrating agonist-induced vasodilatation in eNOS $-/-$ mice, endothelium-derived NO can be completely excluded from the list of candidate EDHFs in mice. In addition, the inclusion of a NOS inhibitor even in the eNOS $-/-$ mouse group makes it unlikely that NO, generated by other NO synthase isoforms (Meng et al., 1996), can contribute to the observed effects (Meng et al., 1998).

In some arterial beds EDHF may be a CYP-epoxygenase metabolite (Fisslthaler et al., 1999; Quilley and McGiff, 2000). In the present study, no evidence was found to suggest that this is the case in the mouse hindlimb. In contrast, EDHF-mediated vasodilator responses in the mouse hindlimb were sensitive to gap junction uncouplers. These agents, which attenuate EDHF-mediated relaxation in some rabbit arteries (Chaytor et al., 1998; Taylor et al., 1998), usually have no effect in vascular beds, in which EDHF has been characterized as a CYP metabolite see chapters 14 and 21. Nevertheless, the factor transmitted through gap junctions and the exact chemical nature of the EDHF generated in mouse resistance vessels remains elusive.

K^+ ions may be an EDHF in some blood vessels (Edwards et al., 1998). However, since the inhibitors which can be employed to test this hypothesis (oubain and barium) exert severe side effects on myogenic tone in the mouse hindlimb, the role of K^+ could not be determined in the present study. However, the evident contribution of gap junctions renders the potential role of K^+ less likely, as K^+ ions would be expected to leave endothelial cells readily and accumulate in the subendothelial space, without the need for functional myoendothelial gap junctions.

4. CONCLUSION

The present study demonstrates a significant role for EDHF in mediating endothelium-dependent, agonist-induced vasodilatation, both *in vivo* and *in vitro*. Moreover, the use of eNOS −/− mice excludes endothelium-derived NO as candidate EDHF. The experimental observations made however, highlight the role of charybdotoxin plus apamin-sensitive K^+ channels and of gap junctions in EDHF-mediated vasodilator responses in the mouse.

33 Prostacyclin and iloprost in the isolated carotid artery of the guinea-pig

Catherine Corriu, Paul M. Vanhoutte and Michel Félétou

The purpose of the present study was to characterize the changes in membrane potential produced by prostacyclin or its stable analog iloprost in vascular smooth muscle cells. The membrane potential was measured in isolated guinea-pig carotid arteries with intracellular microelectrodes in the presence of inhibitors of cycloxygenase and nitric oxide synthase.

In the presence of endothelial cells, prostacyclin and iloprost induced a concentration-dependent hyperpolarization of the smooth muscle cells. The hyperpolarization produced by iloprost was significantly larger than the one produced by prostacyclin. In presence of Bay U3405, the responses to iloprost were unaffected while those to prostacyclin were increased significantly with a shift to the left of the concentration–response curve. The metabolite of prostacyclin, 6-ketoPGF$_{1\alpha}$ did not affect the membrane potential of the smooth muscle cells while U46619 and prostaglandin F$_{2\alpha}$ produced a significant, sustained and stable depolarization. Glibenclamide abolished the hyperpolarization induced by iloprost. In contrast, the response to prostacyclin was either unaffected, converted to depolarization or converted to slow wave activity with firing of action potentials. In the presence of the association of glibenclamide, charybdotoxin and apamin, prostacyclin produced only depolarization. The electrical changes induced by prostacyclin, in the presence of glibenclamide were abolished by Bay U3405. After removal of the endothelium, iloprost and prostacyclin produced hyperpolarizations that were not significantly different from those observed in controls. The concentration–response curve to prostacyclin was still significantly enhanced and shifted in the presence of Bay U3405. However, in the presence of glibenclamide, prostacyclin produced only a depolarization that was abolished by Bay U3405. These results indicate that in the carotid artery of the guinea-pig, iloprost activate IP receptor on the smooth muscle cells and produce hyperpolarization by the opening of ATP-sensitive potassium channels. In contrast, prostacyclin (or one of its metabolite different from 6-ketoPGF$_{1\alpha}$) can produce additional endothelium-dependent and independent effects that are sensitive to Bay U3405. In the absence of the endothelium, the activation of TP-receptors produces depolarization and partially antagonizes the hyperpolarization mediated by IP receptors. In the presence of the endothelial lining, the changes in membrane potential produced by prostacyclin involve the activation of calcium-activated potassium channels. Whether or not this endothelial effect involves the release of an unidentified factor or myo-endothelial gap junctions remains uncertain.

Prostacyclin is the principal metabolite of arachidonic acid produced by cyclooxygenase in most blood vessels (Moncada *et al.*, 1976) and the endothelium is the major site of its synthesis (Moncada *et al.*, 1977). Prostacyclin usually causes vasodilation (Kadowitz *et al.*, 1978) that involve the stimulation of specific cell surface receptors (IP receptors) and are associated with the activation of the adenylate cyclase. This leads to an elevation of intracellular cyclic-AMP (Gryglewski *et al.*, 1991; Wise and Jones, 1996), and in some instances the hyperpolarization of the vascular smooth muscle cells (Jackson *et al.*, 1993; Parkington *et al.*, 1995). At high concentration, prostacyclin can evoke contractions or biphasic responses in the rabbit and rat aorta (Borda *et al.*, 1983; Williams *et al.*, 1994), human coronary and umbilical arteries (Davis *et al.*, 1980; Pomerantz *et al.*, 1978) and rabbit pulmonary blood vessels (Kaapa *et al.*, 1991). These contractions are linked either to the direct activation of TP-receptors (Zhao *et al.*, 1996) or to the release of endothelium-derived contracting factors (Rapoport and Williams, 1996; Adeagbo and Malik, 1990).

The purpose of the present study was to compare, in smooth muscle cells of the guinea-pig carotid artery, the changes in membrane potential produced by various concentrations of prostacyclin and of its stable analogue iloprost.

1. METHODS

Male Hartley guinea-pigs (300–400 g, Charles River, France) were anaesthetized with pentobarbitone (250 mg/Kg i.p.) and the carotid arteries were dissected, cleaned of adherent connective tissue and pinned down to the bottom of an organ chamber (1 ml). They were superfused continuously with modified Krebs–Ringer bicarbonate solution (37 °C, aerated with a 95% O_2, 5% CO_2 gas mixture, pH 7.4) of the following composition (mM): NaCl 118.3, KCl 4.7, $CaCl_2$ 2.5, $MgSO_4$ 1.2, KH_2PO_4 1.2, $NaHCO_3$ 25, calcium disodium EDTA 0.026 and glucose 11.1.

In most experiments, care was taken to preserve the endothelium as intact as possible; in some preparations, the endothelium was removed with a rapid infusion of saponin (1 mg/ml) in the lumen of the blood vessel (Corriu *et al.*, 1996b). Trans-membrane potentials were recorded with glass microelectrodes filled with KCl (3 M), with a tip resistance of 30–90 MΩ. The microelectrode was mounted on a sliding micromanipulator (Leitz, St Gallen, Switzerland). The potential recorded was amplified by means of a recording preamplifier (WPI (intra767), New Haven, CT, USA) with capacitance-neutralization. Impalements were not accepted as valid unless they were signaled by a sudden change in voltage, and were maintained for at least 3 minutes; at that point the membrane potential had stabilized. The impalements were performed from the adventitial side. In order to prevent endogenous release of endothelial factors, indomethacin (5×10^{-6} M) and N^ω-nitro-L-arginine (L-NA, 10^{-4} M) were present throughout the experiments.

1.1. Drugs

Indomethacin; N^ω-L-nitro-Arginine (L-NA); prostacyclin, PGE_2, $PGF_{2\alpha}$, 6-keto$PGF_{1\alpha}$, U46619 (Sigma, La Verpillère, France); charybdotoxin, apamin (Latoxan, Rosans, France); glibenclamide (Boeringer, Manheim, Germany); iloprost (Schering, Berlin, Germany); Bay U3405 was synthetized in the Institut de Recherches Servier (Suresnes, France). Prostacyclin was dissolved in Tris(hydroxymethyl)-aminomethan (5×10^{-2} M, pH 9.4). Stock solutions of glibenclamide, and 6-keto$PGF_{1\alpha}$ (10^{-3} M) were prepared in dimethyl sulfoxide (DMSO), prostaglandin E_2 and U46619 (10^{-3} M) in ethanol (70%) and indomethacin (5×10^{-6} M) in $NaHCO_3$ 5%. The other drugs were dissolved in distilled water.

1.2. Statistics

Data are shown as mean $\pm$ SEM; n indicates the number of cells in which membrane potential was recorded. Statistical analysis was performed with unpaired Student's t-test for unpaired observations. Differences were considered to be statistically significant when p was less than .05.

2. RESULTS

2.1. Guinea-pig carotid artery without endothelium

In the absence of endothelial cells, the membrane potential of the smooth muscle was -51.9 ± 1.1 mV ($n = 29$). Iloprost (10^{-7} M) produced a sustained hyperpolarization (-16.6 ± 1.9 mV, $n = 6$). Prostacyclin (10^{-5} M) produced a hyperpolarization that was biphasic with an initial transient phase followed by a sustained second phase that persisted even after wash out. In the presence of Bay U3405 (10^{-6} M), a statistically significant increase of the maximal hyperpolarization to prostacyclin was observed, especially during the sustained second phase (Figure 33.1). In the presence of glibenclamide (10^{-6} M), prostacyclin (10^{-5} M) produced a depolarization that was abolished by Bay U3405 (10^{-6} M; Figure 33.1).

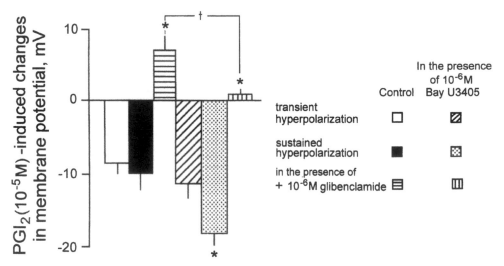

Figure 33.1 Prostacyclin (PGI$_2$, 10^{-5} M)-induced changes in membrane potential of the smooth muscle cells of isolated guinea-pig carotid arteries without endothelium (in the presence of indomethacin: 5×10^{-6} M plus L-nitro-arginine: 10^{-4} M). Effects of glibenclamide (10^{-6} M), Bay U3405 (10^{-6} M) and glibenclamide plus Bay U3405. Data are shown as means $\pm$ SEM of n experiments ($n = 3-8$). The asterisk indicates a statistically significant difference between the sustained hyperpolarization induced by prostacyclin in the absence and presence of Bay U3405. The dagger indicates a statistically significant difference between the effect of prostacyclin in the presence of glibenclamide only and that observed in presence of glibenclamide plus Bay U3405.

2.2. Guinea-pig carotid artery with endothelium

In the presence of the endothelium, the cell membrane potential of the smooth muscle cells was significantly more hyperpolarized than in absence and averaged -55.8 ± 0.7 mV ($n = 72$). Iloprost induced concentration-dependent sustained hyperpolarizations that were significantly larger than those produced by prostacyclin (Figure 33.2). Prostacyclin, at the highest concentration tested (10^{-5} M), induced also a biphasic hyperpolarization with a first transient hyperpolarization (-7.6 ± 1.1 mV, $n = 10$) followed by a sustained hyperpolarization (-12.3 ± 2.5 mV, $n = 4$).

The membrane potential of smooth muscle cells was not influenced by the presence of the antagonist of TP receptors Bay U3405 (10^{-6} M, $- 55.2 \pm 1.0$ mV, $n = 47$). In the presence of this antagonist, the hyperpolarization induced by iloprost was not affected significantly (Figure 33.2). In contrast, the concentration–response curve to prostacyclin was shifted to the left and the amplitude of the hyperpolarization was enhanced. In the presence of Bay U3405, the effects of iloprost were no longer significantly different from those of prostacyclin (Figure 33.2). At the highest concentration tested, prostacyclin (10^{-5} M) produced a biphasic effect. The transient hyperpolarization was not significantly affected by Bay U3405, but the sustained hyperpolarization was significantly enhanced (presence of Bay U3405: -7.8 ± 1.2 and 15.3 ± 1.6 mV, $n = 6$, transient and sustained hyperpolarization, respectively).

The metabolite of prostacyclin, 6-ketoPGF$_{1\alpha}$ (10^{-5} M; Figure 33.3), did not significantly influence the cell membrane potential while prostaglandin E$_2$ (PGE$_2$, 10^{-6} M; Figure 33.3) and the agonists at the TP-receptors, U46619 (10^{-8} M) and PGF$_{2\alpha}$ (10^{-6} M) produced a depolarization (Figure 33.4). The effects of U46619 and PGF$_{2\alpha}$ were abolished in presence of Bay U3405 (Figure 33.4). Glibenclamide (10^{-6} M), did not significantly affect the membrane potential of the smooth muscle cells (-53.3 ± 1.2 mV, $n = 38$). The hyperpolarization induced by iloprost (10^{-7} M) was

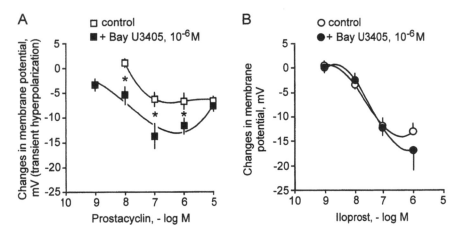

Figure 33.2 Effect of Bay U3405 (10^{-6} M) on the concentration–hyperolarization curves to prostacyclin (A: transient hyperpolarization) and to iloprost (B) in smooth muscle cells of the isolated guinea-pig carotid arteries with endothelium in the presence of indomethacin (5×10^{-6} M) and L-nitro-arginine (10^{-4} M). Data are shown as means $\pm$ SEM ($n = 3-10$). The asterisk indicates a statistically significant difference between control and Bay U3405.

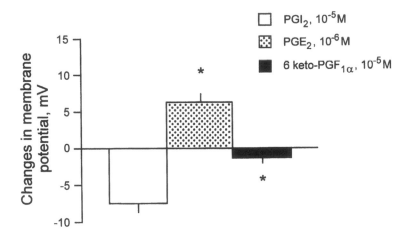

Figure 33.3 Effects of prostacyclin, prostaglandin E_2 (PGE$_2$) and 6-keto prostaglandin
$F_{1\alpha}$ (6-ketoPGF$_{1\alpha}$), on the membrane potential of smooth muscle cells from
isolated guinea-pig carotid arteries with endothelium in the presence of indomethacin (5×10^{-6} M) plus L-nitro-arginine (10^{-4} M). Data shown as
means $\pm$ SEM ($n = 3$–10).

blocked by glibenclamide (Figure 33.5). In contrast, in the presence of glibenclamide,
prostacyclin (10^{-5} M) depolarized 39% of the cells ($+7.4 \pm 1.4$ mV, $n = 9$), hyperpolarized 30% of the cells studied (-11.7 ± 3.5 mV, $n = 7$), or induced spontaneous
electrical activity in the remaining 30% of the cells ($n = 7$; Figure 33.6). In the presence
of glibenclamide, and after the addition of the combination of charybdotoxin (10^{-7} M)
plus apamin (5×10^{-7} M), prostacyclin depolarized all the cells studied (Figure 33.7). In
the presence of glibenclamide and after the addition of Bay U3405 (10^{-6} M), prostacyclin (10^{-5} M) no longer influenced the membrane potential (Figure 33.7).

3. DISCUSSION

These results of the present study suggest that in guinea-pig carotid artery, iloprost
activates IP receptors on the smooth muscle cells and produces hyperpolarization by
opening ATP-sensitive potassium channels. In contrast, prostacyclin (or a metabolite
different from 6-ketoPGF$_{1\alpha}$) produces additional endothelium-dependent and independent effects that are prevented by a TP receptor antagonist.

In the present study, prostacyclin and its stable analogue iloprost induced
hyperpolarization of guinea-pig vascular smooth muscle cells, confirming earlier results
obtained in various species (Siegel *et al.*, 1987; Parkington *et al.*, 1993, 1995; Murphy
and Brayden, 1995; Corriu *et al.*, 1996a). These hyperpolarizations were observed in
the presence of inhibitors of nitric oxide synthase and cycloxygenase and in the presence or absence of endothelium, indicating a direct effect on the smooth muscle.
Iloprost has a high affinity for IP receptors but also for EP$_1$ and EP$_3$ receptors
(Narumiya *et al.*, 1999). The receptor involved in the hyperpolarization induced by
prostacyclin and iloprost is most likely the IP receptor as prostaglandin E$_2$, an agonist
of the EP$_1$ and EP$_3$ receptors did not hyperpolarize the smooth muscle cells of the

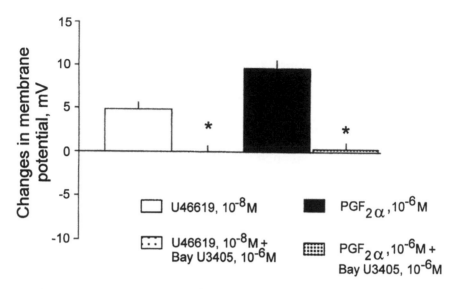

Figure 33.4 Effects of U46619 (10^{-8} M) and prostaglandin $F_{2\alpha}$ ($PGF_{2\alpha}$, 10^{-6} M) on the membrane potential of smooth muscle cells from isolated guinea-pig carotid arteries with endothelium, in the presence of indomethacin (5×10^{-6} M) plus L-nitro-arginine (10^{-4} M). Experiments were performed in the presence and the absence of Bay U3405 (10^{-6} M). Data are shown as means ± SEM ($n = 3-6$). The asterisks indicate statistically significant effects of Bay U3405 (10^{-6} M).

guinea-pig carotid artery (Narumiya *et al.*, 1999). Under the present experimental conditions, the hyperpolarizations produced by iloprost were similar in arteries with and without endothelium. They were abolished by glibenclamide, indicating that the prostacyclin analogue activated exclusively IP receptors on the smooth muscle, resulting in the opening of ATP-sensitive potassium channels. In most of the blood vessels studied so far, the hyperpolarizations produced by prostacyclin and its various analogues involve the opening of ATP-sensitive potassium channels that are blocked by sulfonylureas such as glibenclamide (Siegel *et al.*, 1987; Jackson *et al.*, 1993; Parkington *et al.*, 1993, 1995; Murphy and Brayden, 1995; Corriu *et al.*, 1996a). However, in the guinea-pig carotid artery, prostacyclin shows an additional effect when compared to iloprost. In arteries without endothelium, the hyperpolarization induced by prostacyclin was enhanced by Bay U3405, an antagonist of TP receptors (Rosentreter *et al.*, 1989), suggesting that prostacyclin activates simultaneously IP and TP receptors on the smooth muscle with opposite effects on the cell membrane potential. This interpretation is confirmed further by the observations that in the presence of glibenclamide, prostacyclin produces a depolarization blocked by Bay U3405 and that TP receptor agonists $PGF_{2\alpha}$ and U 46619 produce depolarizations also sensitive to Bay U3405. Whether or not the activation of the TP-receptors is due directly to prostacyclin or to one of its metabolites is unknown at present. However, 6-ketoPGF$_{1\alpha}$, the stable metabolite of prostacyclin (Moncada and Vane, 1979), is inactive in this preparation.

A   Control

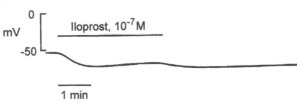

B   In the presence of glibenclamide, 10^{-6} M

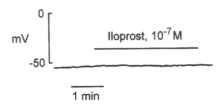

C   Changes in membrane potential

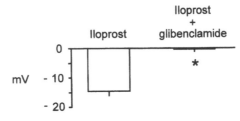

Figure 33.5 Effects of glibenclamide on iloprost (10^{-7} M)-induced hyperpolarizations of smooth muscle cells of the isolated guinea-pig carotid arteries with endothelium in the presence of indomethacin (5×10^{-6} M) plus L-nitro-arginine (10^{-4} M). (A) Control. (B) Presence of glibenclamide (10^{-6} M). (C) Summary graph. Data are shown as means $\pm$ SEM ($n = 4$–6). The asterisks indicate a statistically significant effect of glibenclamide.

In blood vessels with endothelium, the concentration–response curve to prostacyclin was shifted to the left by Bay U3405, confirming that prostacyclin activates simultaneously IP and TP receptors. In 30% of the vessels studied, the results obtained were consistent with what was observed in vessels without endothelium, i.e., in presence of glibenclamide, prostacyclin produced a depolarization sensitive to Bay U3405. However, in the other blood vessels, and in contrast to what is observed with iloprost, glibenclamide either did not affect the hyperpolarization produced by prostacyclin or unmasked a spike-like repetitive electrical activity. These endothelium-dependent effects of prostacyclin unmasked by glibenclamide were inhibited by the combination of charybdotoxin and apamin. Indeed, in the presence of these two potassium channel blockers the effects of prostacyclin were similar to those observed in carotid arteries without endothelium. Furthermore, in the presence of the TP receptor antagonist, all the effects of prostacyclin unmasked by glibenclamide were abolished. Sulfonyureas, such as glibenclamide and to a lesser extent tolbutamide, at high concentrations

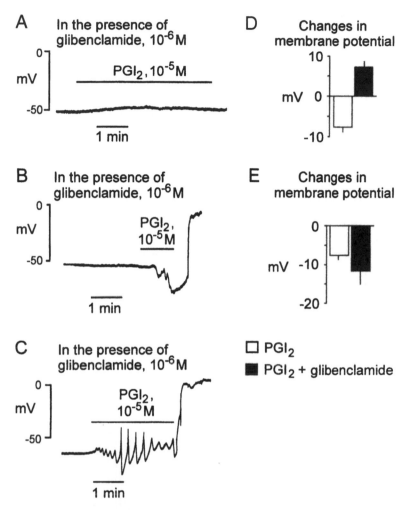

Figure 33.6 Effects of glibenclamide on prostacyclin (10^{-5} M)-induced hyperpolarizations of smooth muscle cells of the isolated guinea-pig carotid arteries with endothelium in the presence of indomethacin (5×10^{-6} M) plus L-nitro-arginine (10^{-4} M). (A) and (D) Original traces of prostacyclin (10^{-5} M)-induced depolarization as observed in 39% of the cells studied ($n = 9$) and summary bar graph. (B) and (E) Original traces of prostacyclin (10^{-5} M)-induced hyperpolarization as observed in 30% of the cells studied ($n = 7$) and summary bar graph. (C) Original traces of prostacyclin (10^{-5} M)-induced spike-like rhythmic activity as observed in 30% of the cells studied ($n = 7$). (D) and (E) Data are shown as means $\pm$ SEM ($n = 7-9$).

inhibit thromboxane receptors (Cocks *et al.*, 1990; Zhang *et al.*, 1991). This could have explained the complex observations performed in presence of glibenclamide and prostacyclin as both substances may interact with TP receptors. However, the addition of Bay U3405 produced clear-cut inhibition of the responses, suggesting that this unspecific action of glibenclamide is unlikely to explain the effects of prostacyclin. These results suggest that prostacyclin (or a metabolite different from 6-ketoPGF$_{1\alpha}$)

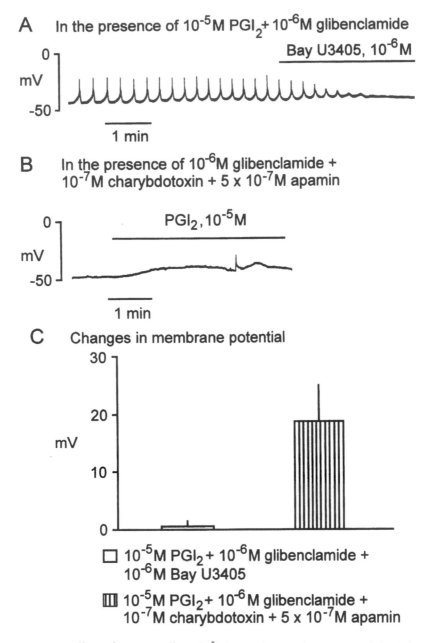

Figure 33.7 Effect of prostacyclin (10^{-5} M) on the membrane potential of the smooth muscle cells of isolated guinea-pig carotid arteries with endothelium in the presence of glibenclamide (10^{-6} M) plus indomethacin (5×10^{-6} M) plus L-nitro-arginine (10^{-4} M). (A) Original trace showing the effect of Bay U3405 (10^{-6} M) on prostacyclin (10^{-5} M) induced spike-like rhythmic activity. (B) Original trace showing the effect prostacyclin (10^{-5} M) in the presence of charybdotoxin (10^{-7} M) plus apamin (5×10^{-7} M). (C) Summary bar graph. Data shown as means $\pm$ SEM ($n = 3-10$).

activates calcium-sensitive potassium channels. Whether or not this endothelial effect involves the release of an unidentified factor or myo-endothelial gap junctions remains to be determined (Figure 33.8).

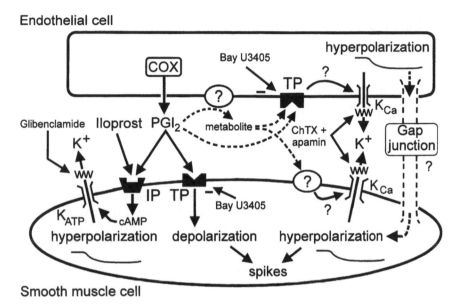

Figure 33.8 Effects of prostacyclin and iloprost on the membrane potential of the smooth muscle cells of the isolated guinea-pig carotid artery. COX = cyclooxygenase; cAMP = cyclic adenosine mono-phosphate; IP = prostaglandin IP receptor; K_{ATP} = adenosinc tris-phosphate-sensitive potasium channel; K_{Ca} = calcium-activated potassium channel. Iloprost activate IP receptor on the smooth muscle cells and produce hyperpolarization by the opening of ATP-sensitive potassium channels. In contrast, prostacyclin (or one of its metabolite different from 6-ketoPGF$_{1\alpha}$) can produce additional endothelium-dependent and independent effects that are sensitive to Bay U3405. In the absence of the endothelium, the activation of TP-receptors produces depolarization and partially antagonizes the hyperpolarization mediated by IP receptors. In the presence of the endothelial lining, the changes in membrane potential produced by prostacyclin involve the activation of calcium-activated potassium channels. Whether or not this endothelial effect involves the release of an unidentified factor or myo-endothelial gap junctions remains uncertain.

34 Role of charybdotoxin/apamin sensitive K^+_{Ca} channels in pulsatile perfusion-mediated coronary vasodilatation *in vivo*

*Nazareno Paolocci, Takayoshi Isoda,
Walter F. Saavedra, Pasquale Pagliaro
and David A. Kass*

In vivo, coronary flow increases when the perfusion pulsatility is enhanced, and nitric oxide is responsible for about half of this response. The role of K^+_{Ca} channels to a nitric oxide/cyclooxygenase-independent pulsatility-response was studied, and the channel subtypes involved in the response were identified. The canine left descending coronary artery was perfused with whole blood at constant mean pressure, and perfusion pulsatility set to 40 or 100 mmHg by a computer-servo-pump. Cyclooxygenase was inhibited by indomethacin. Mean flow increased with enhanced pulsatility. This response declined by half with blockade of nitric oxide synthase with N^ω-monomethyl-L-arginine (L-NMMA) or K^+_{Ca} (charybdotoxin plus apamin). While inhibiting either or both pathways did not alter basal coronary flow, the combined blockade of nitric oxide synthase plus K^+_{Ca} eliminated the pulsatility-induced as well as bradykinin-stimulated increases in flow. Bradykinin-induced vasodilatation was more sensitive to charybdotoxin plus apamin than L-NMMA whereas the response to acetylcholine was blunted more by L-NMMA than charybdotoxin plus apamin, and not eliminated by combined blockade. Iberiotoxin plus apamin was minimally effective in inhibiting either pulsatility or agonist-evoked flow responses (with or without nitric oxide synthase inhibition), and not different from apamin alone in this regard. This supports a more prominent role of small and intermediate conductance channels, but a minimal role of iberiotoxin-sensitive large-conductance K^+_{Ca} channels. Low-dose bradykinin, which activates K^+_{Ca} channels enhanced pulsatility-triggered increases in flow, whereas this was not observed with acetylcholine. Hence, K^+_{Ca} activation and nitric oxide modulate pulsatility-stimulated increases in coronary flow in an additive fashion *in vivo*. These data support an important role of hyperpolarization in mechano-vascular signaling, and highlight the prominence of small and intermediate-conductance K^+_{Ca} channels in this response.

Nitric oxide can modulate coronary arterial tone *in vivo* as it is the mediator of shear stress signaling (Rubanyi *et al.*, 1986; Ohno *et al.*, 1993), perfusion pulsatility (Recchia *et al.*, 1996; Pagliaro *et al.*, 1999) and endothelium-dependent relaxations to agonists such as acetylcholine and bradykinin. In a variety of arteries, however, a component of endothelium-dependent dilatations are resistant to inhibition of nitric oxide synthase and cyclooxygenase. The mechanism underlying this pathway is relaxation of vascular smooth cells mediated by an endothelium-derived hyperpolarizing factor (EDHF) (Quilley *et al.*, 1997) whose nature remains controversial

(Cohen *et al.*, 1997; Edwards *et al.*, 1998; Fisslthaler *et al.*, 1999). A common footprint of EDHF-mediated relaxation is the activation of calcium-dependent potassium (K_{Ca}^+) channels inhibitable by charybdotoxin plus apamin (Félétou and Vanhoutte, 1999). These channels may also be activated by nitric oxide and cyclicGMP (Robertson *et al.*, 1993; Bolotina *et al.*, 1994) suggesting a role of K_{Ca}^+ channels conductance to nitric oxide (Archer *et al.*, 1994) and shear stress signaling as well (Takamura *et al.*, 1999).

Endothelium-dependent hyperpolarization has also been evoked *in vitro* by increased shear stress (Takamura *et al.*, 1999) or pulsatile stretch (Popp *et al.*, 1998). However, *in vivo* evidence supporting a role for EDHF remains scant, and has mostly focused on agonist-stimulated responses. Furthermore, while *in vitro* blockade of K_{Ca}^+, nitric oxide synthase and/or cycloxygenase blockade produces vasoconstriction, in intact hearts basal coronary tone is unaltered by these treatments (Nishikawa *et al.*, 1999; Jones *et al.*, 1995). Since intact blood vessels are always exposed to mechanical stimuli, K_{Ca}^+ activation might play a greater role when stress is enhanced, as with higher pulsatility for example during exertion. Indeed, *in vivo* pulsatility raises mean coronary flow without altering regional metabolism or function (Gregg effect), and this response can be only partially explained by the enhanced release of nitric oxide (Recchia *et al.*, 1996; Pagliaro *et al.*, 1999).

The present study tested the hypothesis that K_{Ca}^+ channels prominently contribute to the *in vivo* modulation of coronary flow due to enhanced perfusion pulsatility. The channel sub-types underlying this modulation, contrasting it to that for bradykinin and acetylcholine, were determined.

1. METHODS

1.1. Animal preparation

The protocol was approved by the Animal Care and Use Committee of the Johns Hopkins University, following guidelines established by the National Institutes of Health. Coronary pulsatile perfusion was modified selectively using a custom designed computer-controlled servo-system (Recchia *et al.*, 1996; Pagliaro *et al.*, 1999) (Figure 34.1). Adult mongrel dogs (25–30 kg, $n = 28$) were anesthetized with pentobarbital (30 mg/kg intravenous) and fentanyl (50 mg/kg intravenous), and ventilated using enhanced inspired oxygen to maintain physiological arterial PO_2, PCO_2, and pH. Animals were administered indomethacin (5.0 mg/kg intramuscular) to inhibit cycloxygenase activity, and heparin (8000 IU bolus, 1000 IU/h). Arterial blood was withdrawn by means of a flow pump from a femoral artery, pressurized to a constant 100 mmHg pressure, passed through a heat-exchanger and filter, and then into a 30 ml chamber with a movable floor coupled to a linear motor (Ling Apparatus, CT, USA) (Figure 34.1). The position of the chamber floor was controlled by digital real-time feedback to generate a given desired pulse-pressure waveform. Blood exiting the chamber perfused a rigid cannula inserted into the proximal left anterior descending artery. Perfusate pressure was measured with a micromanometer (SPC 350, Millar Inst., TX, USA) to provide the feedback signal to the computer-servo-system. The central aortic pressure was digitally recorded, modified in memory to generate a waveform with the desired pulse amplitude, and then played back in real-time as the command signal to the servo-pump.

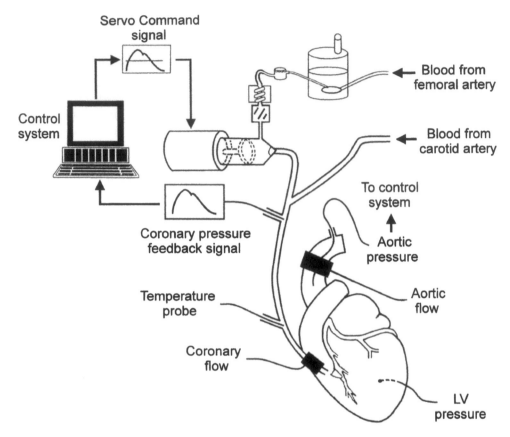

Figure 34.1 Schematic of the servo-perfusion system used to study effects of varying pulse pressure. Blood is withdrawn from the femoral artery of the dog and passed through a pressurized reservoir to establish a mean 100 mmHg pressure. It then passed through a filter and heat exchanger (B) to enter a chamber with a movable floor (C) that is coupled with a linear motor (D). This motor is computer-controlled to generate the desired pressure waveform. Blood exits the chamber via a rigid tube (E), past an indwelling micromanometer (F) and inline flow meter to perfuse the left anterior descending artery. Central aortic pressure is recorded by a second micromanometer, and this is used to generate the command signal controlling the servomotor. This system can thereby generate any desired mean and pulse pressure in the isolated left anterior descending artery bed, while maintaining ventricular loading constant. LV = left ventricle.

1.2. Drugs

The following drugs were used: acetylcholine (ACh) (Sigma, St Louis, MO, USA); adenosine (Fujisawa USA, Deerfield, IL); apamin (AP) (Sigma, St Louis, MO); bradykinin (BK) (Sigma, St Louis, MO); charybdotoxin (CbTX) (Sigma, St Louis, MO); diethylamine/NO complex (DEA/NO) from Dr D.A. Wink (Radiation Biology Branch, National Health Institute, Bethesda, MD); iberiotoxin (IbTX) (Sigma, St Louis, MO); N^{ω}-monomethyl-L-arginine (L-NMMA) (CalBiochem, LaJolla, CA); sodium nitroprusside (Sigma, St Louis, MO).

1.3. Experimental protocols

Perfusion pulsatility was set to 40 mmHg, and the preparation stabilized for at least 15–20 min. Data were subsequently obtained with the servo-pump generating a pulsatility of either 40 or 100 mmHg, at the same mean pressure. Data were measured at steady-state, occurring after 2 min following a change in perfusion pulsatility, and average values measured over the ensuing 1–2 min period. Perfusion pulsatility was switched several times to confirm the reproducibility for each condition, and mean results derived at each pulse pressure. Basal flow, pulse pressure-altered flow, and agonist-altered flow (acetylcholine: 150 µg/30 sec intracoronary and bradykinin: 100 µg/30 sec intracoronary) were assessed under the following conditions: (a) baseline ($n = 28$); (b) 5 min treatment and continued infusion of apamin (15 nmol/min, intracoronary; mean concentration of 417×10^{-9} M at 36 ml/min average coronary blood flow) and charybdotoxin (1.5 nmol/min, intracoronary, 42×10^{-9} M) to block K_{Ca}^+-channels ($n = 20$); (c) new controls after charybdotoxin plus apamin washout, (10–15 min after discontinuing both agents); (d) L-NMMA ($n = 20$) (0.5 mg/kg/min, intracoronary) administered for 20 min prior to and continuing during pulse pressure and agonist testing; and (e) combined charybdotoxin plus apamin and L-NMMA ($n = 11$). In seven studies, the protocol was conducted substituting iberiotoxin (4.7 nmol/min, 131×10^{-9} M) for charybdotoxin. Lastly, to test the involvement of apamin-sensitive K_{Ca}^+ channels, apamin alone was infused ($n = 6$) and pulse pressure and agonist tests performed.

Each drug was dissolved in isotonic saline at 37 °C immediately before use. All the drugs were administered intracoronary through a side-port in the servo-perfusion cannula at flow rates equal to/or less than 2 ml/min. Given the nature of the servo-perfusion, coronary flow was unaltered by saline infusion alone at such rates.

1.4. Data analysis and statistics

Hemodynamic data were digitized at 200 Hz and analyzed off-line by custom software. Mean and pulsatile coronary flow and pressure, left ventricular pressure, and aortic flow, were measured in each study. Data were analyzed using repeated measures ANOVA, using a Tukey test for multiple comparisons. All data are presented as mean ± SEM. Differences were considered to be statistically significant when p was less than .05.

2. RESULTS

2.1. Basal coronary tone

Basal flow at a constant 100 mmHg mean- and 40 mmHg pulse-pressure in the servo-perfused left anterior descending coronary artery territory was 36.7 ± 17.7 ml/min ($n = 28$), similar to the baseline flow prior to servo-pump regulation. Inhibition of K_{Ca}^+ by charybdotoxin plus apamin, iberiotoxin plus apamin, or apamin alone did not significantly alter the basal flow. However there was a small, but significant decline in mean flow following L-NMMA (Figure 34.2). Subsequent addition of the K_{Ca}^+-channel blockers did not significantly further reduce flow, although the combination of charybdotoxin plus apamin and L-NMMA also reduced basal flow below untreated control hearts.

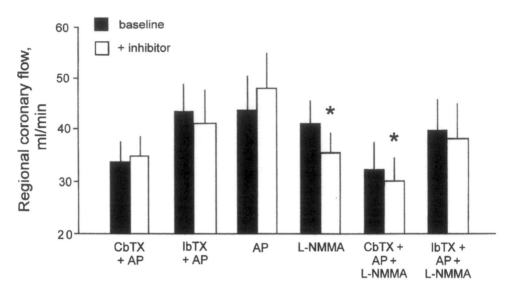

Figure 34.2 Effects of various nitric oxide synthase and $K_{Ca^{2+}}^{+}$ inhibitors and combinations of inhibitors on basal coronary flow at a mean pressure of 100 mmHg and pulse pressure of 40 mmHg. Only N^{ω}-monomethyl-L-arginine (L-NMMA) had a slight effect on lowering basal flow, and this was also observed with the addition of charybdotoxin plus apamin and L-NMMA. Data shown are means ± SEM. The asterisks indicate statistically significant differences from baseline ($p < .05$). CbTX = charybdotoxin, AP = apamin, and IbTX = iberiotoxin.

2.2. Pulsatility

Elevating perfusion pulsatility resulted in a significant sustained rise in mean flow (averaging 36.0 ± 4.5–41.8 ± 4.9 ml/min, $n = 20$) (Figure 34.3). Charybdotoxin plus apamin significantly blunted this flow augmentation by $35 \pm 3\%$. It was fully restored to baseline 10–20 min after discontinuing drug infusion, and it again declined following L-NMMA by a similar magnitude. Combining inhibition of nitric oxide synthase and K_{Ca}^{+} inhibition eliminated pulse pressure–flow responses (31.1 ± 4.4 versus 31.9 ± 4.2, $n = 11$) (Figure 34.3C). However, this did not prevent direct nitric relaxation to both sodium nitroprusside and diethylamine/NO complex still induced vasodilatation ($+140 \pm 9\%$ and $+110 \pm 11\%$ after and before the blockade, respectively).

2.3. Bradykinin and acetylcholine

Both acetylcholine and bradykinin were infused to achieve near-maximal flow responses (acetylcholine: $+274.6 \pm 22.7\%$; bradykinin: $+274.5 \pm 24.6\%$) (Figure 34.4). Charybdotoxin plus apamin blunted responses to bradykinin by $-66.3 \pm 5.2\%$ (residual flow rise $+89 \pm 20\%$, $n = 13$), whereas the acetylcholine response declined less ($-44.5 \pm 7.2\%$, $n = 11$). Inhibition of nitric oxide synthase reduced the acetylcholine- significantly more than the bradykinin-induced elevation (bradykinin: $-45.8 \pm 7.0\%$, acetylcholine: $-70.6 \pm 3.1\%$). Disparities were also observed when these agents were combined, revealing full inhibition of bradykinin-induced dilata-

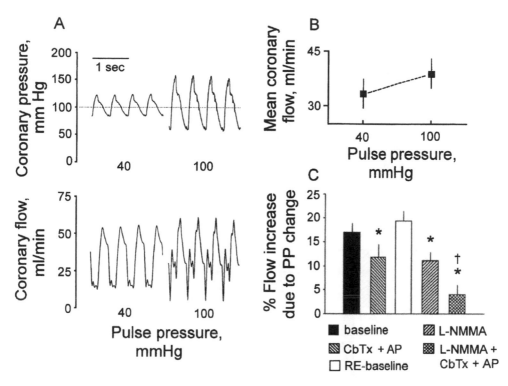

Figure 34.3 Influence of increasing *in vivo* perfusion pulse pressure on mean coronary flow. (A) Tracings for coronary artery pressure and flow at normal (40 mmHg) and elevated (100 mmHg) pulse pressure. With higher pulsatility, the coronary flow during the systolic period increases, while the diastolic flow is maintained despite the fall in mean diastolic pressure. (B) Mean ($n = 28$) elevation in coronary flow at higher perfusion pulsatility. (C) Influence of $K_{Ca^{2+}}^{+}$ and/or nitric oxide synthase inhibition on pulsatile perfusion-dependent coronary flow augmentation. Data shown are means $\pm$ SEM. The asterisks indicate statistically significant differences from baseline ($p < .05$). The dagger indicate statistically significant differences from N^{ω}-monomethyl-L-arginine (L-NMMA) alone ($p < .05$). CbTX = charybdotoxin, AP = apamin.

tions, similar to the response to pulse pressure, whereas a residual acetylcholine-induced increase in flow ($+41.3 \pm 8.1\%$) persisted.

2.4. Sub-types of K_{Ca}^{+} channels

Iberiotoxin plus apamin blunted responses to pulse pressure and bradykinin by less than half the extent observed with charybdotoxin plus apamin, both with or without concomitant nitric oxide synthase inhibition (Figure 34.4). Furthermore, iberiotoxin plus apamin had no appreciable effect on the acetylcholine-mediated response, and yielded a similar inhibition to that with L-NMMA alone when combined with the latter. Further studies were performed employing only apamin. The absolute reduction in response to enhanced pulse pressure or bradykinin with apamin alone was not significantly different from that with iberiotoxin plus apamin (Figure 34.4).

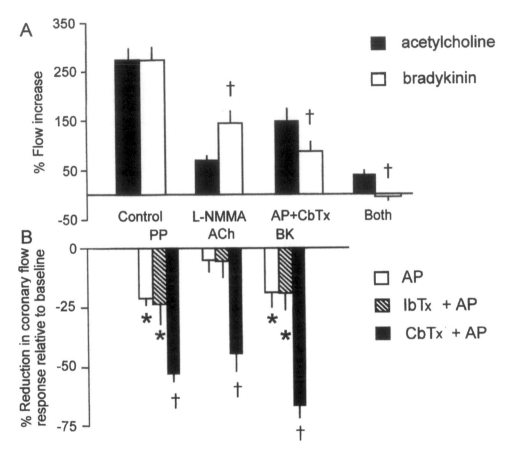

Figure 34.4 (A) Effect of $K_{Ca^{2+}}^+$ and/or nitric oxide synthase inhibition on the percent rise in mean coronary flow in response to maximal-dilator doses of acetylcholine and bradykinin. There were differential effects on each dilator depending upon the pathway blocked, and combined inhibition fully eliminated bradykinin but not acetylcholine dilation. (B) Comparison of iberiotoxin plus apamin versus charybdotoxin plus apamin and apamin alone in modulating pulse perfusion, acetylcholine, and bradykinin dilator responses. See text for details. Asterisks indicate statistically significant differences ($p < .05$) versus pre-inhibitor response. Daggers indicate statistically significant differences versus apamin or iberiotoxin plus apamin ($p < .05$). CbTX = charybdotoxin, AP = apamin, and IbTX = iberiotoxin.

2.5. Low-dose acetylcholine or bradykinin with pulse pressure

In eleven dogs, pulse pressure effects were assessed after infusion of low doses of acetylcholine or bradykinin, sufficient to raise basal coronary flow by 40–50%. With acetylcholine, subsequent flow associated with increasing pulse perfusion was not significantly different from that observed under control conditions (8.1 ± 2.1 and $11 \pm 1.8\%$) respectively. Enhancing perfusion pulsatility during bradykinin infusion amplified the flow augmentation compared to control (20.3 ± 1.8 and $15.1 \pm 2.7\%$, respectively).

3. DISCUSSION

This study demonstrates *in vivo* that in the presence of blockade of nitric oxide synthase and cyclooxygenase, K_{Ca}^+ channels inhibitable by charybdotoxin plus apamin play a major role in modulating coronary flow due to enhanced perfusion pulsatility. This pathway appears additive to nitric oxide-dependent dilatation, and resembles that underlying bradykinin-induced vasodilatation. This interpretation is supported by the facts that: combined blockade of nitric oxide synthase and cycloxygenase was sufficient to prevent responses to both pulse pressure and bradykinin responses; and that bradykinin, but not acetylcholine infused with higher pulse pressure was synergistic in elevating mean coronary flow. Furthermore, these data provide *in vivo* evidence that these signaling pathways do not involve large-conductance K_{Ca}^+ channels inhibitable by iberiotoxin, but rather highlight the importance of small and intermediate conductance channels sensitive to apamin plus charybdotoxin-sensitive. These data support the physiological role of K_{Ca}^+ channels *in vivo*, and by extension, that of an EDHF-dependent pathway.

In vivo K_{Ca}^+ channels play a role in nitric oxide synthase/cyclooxygenase independent acetylcholine-induced dilatations (Nishikawa *et al.*, 1999). In the present study, residual dilatation of distal arterioles (less than 100 µm in diameter) was inhibited by suffusion with K^+ buffer or by K_{Ca}^+ blockade. Furthermore, inhibition of nitric oxide synthase and cycloxygenase inhibition alone was effective in blocking the acetylcholine- induced dilatation in larger less distal arterioles, supporting a more prominent role of nitric oxide in such vessels (Jones *et al.*, 1995). Charybdotoxin or iberiotoxin combined with N^G-Nitro-L-arginine methyl ester prevent bradykinin-dependent dilatation *in vivo*, and this pathway plays a role in post-ischemic dilatation (Node *et al.*, 1997). This suggests that K_{Ca}^+ channel activation, like K_{ATP}^+-channel activation (Ishibashi *et al.*, 1998), can modify the impact of the imbalance between coronary supply and demand. The present data extend these observations by showing a role for K_{Ca}^+ activation in pulse pressure signaling. As such, these results can help explain beneficial effects of exercise (which is accompanied by enhanced pulse pressure) on flow reserve (Griffin *et al.*, 1999). Furthermore, given the fact that bradykinin stimulation triggers release of factors other than nitric oxide, the observed synergy between bradykinin and pulse pressure in elevating mean coronary flow could explain nitric oxide-independent coronary vasodilatation during exercise (Traverse *et al.*, 2000).

The present data are consistent with the proposed role of EDHF to pulse-stretch (Popp *et al.*, 1998) and shear (Takamura *et al.*, 1999) mediated vascular signaling. Nonetheless, alternative hypotheses should be considered. One is that nitric oxide synthase inhibition was incomplete, and that residual pulse pressure and/or agonist-induced dilatation was due to the persistent production of nitric oxide (Cohen *et al.*, 1997; Simonsen *et al.*, 1999). In larger conductance vessels, direct correlation exists between residual acetylcholine-responses and persistent nitric oxide release despite inhibition of nitric oxide synthase (Cohen *et al.*, 1997; Simonsen *et al.*, 1999). However, if this were true in the present study, any residual nitric oxide would have to preferentially act via opening of K_{Ca}^+ channels. While potentially possible (Robertson *et al.*, 1993; Bolotina *et al.*, 1994; Archer *et al.*, 1994), nitric oxide and cyclicGMP activation of K_{Ca}^+ channels has thus far only been reported in large-conductance channels, whereas these did not play a dominant role in the response to pulse pressure or bradykinin. Also, the extent of inhibition of the pulse pressure response by nitric oxide or K_{Ca}^+ inhibition were similar and additive, and this would not be expected if substantial crosstalk was present between these pathways. A second mechanism is mechanically mediated vascular distension and decline in resistance due to the wider pulse pressure (Kuo *et al.*, 1991; Goto *et al.*, 1996; Recchia *et al.*, 1999). However, mean and pulse pressures were identical in all protocols despite near-complete inhibition of pulse pressure–flow responses with charybdotoxin plus apamin and L-NMMA. This is not likely due to reduced distensibility of the smooth muscle, as the basal coronary flow was altered little, and relaxation to nitric oxide donors was preserved. Furthermore, intravascular charybdotoxin employed at similar doses to those in the present study, acts principally on the endothelium rather than vascular smooth muscle (Edwards *et al.*, 1998; Doughty *et al.*, 1999) making direct effects on smooth muscle less likely.

The sensitivities of the pulse pressure-mediated flow changes to pharmacological inhibitors closely matched those observed with bradykinin, identifying small and intermediate conductance channels as the dominant subtypes involved. Unlike acetylcholine, both responses to pulse pressure and bradykinin were very near or blocked by combined charybdotoxin plus apamin and L-NMMA, and diminished by apamin alone. Iberiotoxin altered none of these responses. Bradykinin, which plays an important role in the coronary vasculature under normal and pathological conditions, induces microvascular relaxation by hyperpolarization of the cell membrane (Kemp and Cocks, 1997; Miura *et al.*, 1999). Combined nitric oxide synthase inhibition and charybdotoxin plus apamin consistently inhibited this, whereas far less blockade was observed with iberiotoxin (Frieden *et al.*, 1999). Charybdotoxin blocks both intermediate and large conductance channels, whereas iberitotoxin selectively inhibits the latter (Brugnara *et al.*, 1995; Neylon *et al.*, 1999). At concentrations above those employed in the present study, charybdotoxin also inhibits voltage gated K^+ channels. However, these channels are not thought to play a prominent role in the coronary endothelium. Apamin is relatively selective for small-conductance channels, and these may interact with nitric oxide synthase signaling to mediate vasodilatation (Adeagbo and Triggle, 1993). The lack of sensitivity to iberiotoxin in agonist or pulse pressure response in the present study is supported by several studies performed in renal vessels (Rapacon *et al.*, 1996). However, there are discrepancies between data reported in coronary arteries. For example, iberiotoxin inhibited nitric oxide synthase/cyclooxygenase-independent acetylcholine-induced (Nishikawa *et al.*, 1999) and bradykinin-induced dilatations in canine coronary arteries (Node *et al.*, 1997). In both cases, a lower dose of agonist and/or nitric oxide synthase inhibitors could have played a role in this disparity. The present data suggests greater involvement of iberiotoxin-insensitive channels at higher bradykinin doses, showing a similar selectivity for pulse pressure. Residual acetylcholine-mediated dilatation *in vivo* despite full inhibition of bradykinin (or pulse pressure) signaling with charybdotoxin plus apamin and L-NMMA has not been previously reported, but suggests a further pathway. This would be consistent with the induction of a hyperpolarizing K^+ current different from that resulting from the opening of K_{Ca}^+ channels by acetylcholine (Edwards *et al.*, 1998).

ACKNOWLEDGMENTS

This study was funded by a grant from the National Institutes of Health (HL-47511). The authors also thank Dr David A. Wink for his helpful insights.

35 Essential role of estrogen in the EDHF-mediated responses of mesenteric arteries from middle-aged female rats: possible contribution of gap junctional protein connexin43

Mitsuhiro Fukao, Ichiro Sakuma, Atsushi Sato, Ming-Yue Liu, Satoshi Nawate, Satoko Watanuki, Yasuhiro Akaishi, Hiroko Takano, Satoshi Watanabe, Kazuhiro Abe, Akira Kitabatake and Morio Kanno

Experiments were designed to examine whether or not responses mediated by endothelium-derived hyperpolarizing factor (EDHF) and the gap junctional protein connexin43 are altered after ovariectomy in the middle-aged female rat mesenteric arteries. Female rats were divided into three groups: sham-operated (control), ovariectomized and estrogen-replacement (17β-estradiol 10 µg/day). Four weeks later, the mesenteric arteries were excised and used for the experiments. Prostaglandin-dependent arterial relaxation was minimal or none in the rat mesenteric arteries. NO-induced endothelium-dependent relaxation was not different among the arteries from the three groups. However, EDHF-mediated relaxation was significantly reduced in the ovariectomized group. The resting membrane potential in vascular smooth muscle from ovariectomized rats was shallower. The EDHF-mediated membrane hyperpolarization by acetylcholine was reduced in the ovariectomized group, but the endothelium-independent hyperpolarization by pinacidil was not different. Estrogen replacement therapy prevented the impaired EDHF-mediated arterial relaxation and membrane hyperpolarization in the mesenteric arteries from ovariectomized rats. Estrogen *per se* had no effect on the resting membrane potential and the EDHF-induced membrane hyperpolarization when added acutely. The gap junctional protein inhibitor, 18β-glycyrrhetinic acid, almost completely inhibited EDHF-mediated responses in both control and ovariectomized rats. Western blot analysis showed that the expression of the connexin43 is reduced in the aorta and mesenteric artery from ovariectomized rats. Immunohistochemical staining demonstrated that the connexin43 protein is expressed in both arterial endothelial and smooth muscle cells. These results suggest that estrogen may upregulate EDHF-mediated responses at least in part through the expression of gap junctional protein connexin43. The increase of EDHF-mediated responses by estrogen may partly account for the protecting effect of the hormone against atherosclerosis.

The incidence of cardiovascular disorders of premenopausal women is significantly lower than that of men of a similar age. After the menopause, however, the incidence of cardiovascular diseases becomes comparable in both genders. Hormone replacement therapy decreases the ischemic cardiac event leading to the suggestion that estrogen plays an essential role in preventing the development of coronary athero-sclerosis and ischemic heart disease in postmenopausal women (Grodstein *et al.*, 1997). Estrogen has been shown to have a number of beneficial effects on the cardio-vascular system. Orally administered estrogen raises the level of HDL cholesterol and lowers that of total cholesterol, LDL cholesterol and lipoprotein(a) in serum (Walsh *et al.*, 1991). Other mechanisms underlying the beneficial effect of estrogen include protection of LDL from oxidation, potentiation of fibrinolysis, and improvement in endothelium-dependent vasodilator function (Gisclard *et al.*, 1988; Sack *et al.*, 1994; Koh *et al.*, 1997).

Estrogen induces arterial relaxation in the various vascular beds both *in vivo* (Gilligan *et al.*, 1994) and *in vitro* (Shan *et al.*, 1994). An acute and direct effect of estrogens on the vascular wall is consistent with the finding that the vascular wall contains specific estrogen receptors (Green *et al.*, 1986). Several hypotheses exist as to the mechanisms by which 17β-estradiol induces vasodilatation: release of nitric oxide; prostaglandin release; activation of potassium channels, or calcium channel anta-gonism (Gisclard *et al.*, 1988; Williams *et al.*, 1988; Weiner *et al.*, 1994). In addition to the acute effects of estrogen on the vascular wall, estrogen exerts additional chronic effects through the regulation of the expressional levels of various proteins, which affect arterial tone, including ion channels, contractile apparatus, gap junctional proteins and relaxing factors. However, the acute and chronic effects of estrogen on EDHF-mediated responses have not yet been examined.

Gap junctional communication between and among the endothelial and the vas-cular smooth muscle cells may mediate the relaxing effect of EDHF in rabbit, guinea-pig and rat mesenteric arteries (Chaytor *et al.*, 1998; Yamamoto *et al.*, 1998; Edwards *et al.*, 1999). Gap junctional proteins are membrane-localized channels, facilitating intercellular communication and coordination of cellular activities (Christ *et al.*, 1996). A hexamer of individual connexin proteins constitutes the gap junction. The family of connexins contains at least twenty-two identified members in mammals. Three of the characterized connexins, connexin43 (Cx43), connexin40 and con-nexin37, occur in cells of the vascular system, and Cx43 may play a major role in mediating the relaxing effect of EDHF (Little *et al.*, 1995; Chaytor *et al.*, 1998). The expression of the myometrial Cx43 increases dramatically with the onset of labor, in association with an increase in the level of estrogen in the plasma. Thus, estrogen may exert its beneficial effect on the cardiovascular system by up-regulating the EDHF-mediated responses through regulation of the expressional level of Cx43. This study examined the acute and chronic effects of estrogen on EDHF-mediated relaxation and membrane hyperpolarization by acetylcholine in mesenteric arteries of middle-aged female rats. It also assessed whether or not the expression of Cx43 is altered by ovariectomy in the aorta and mesenteric arteries using western blot analysis and immunohistochemistry.

1. METHODS

Fifty-week-old female Wistar rats were studied. The female rats (at normal cycling) were divided into three groups: control (sham-operated), ovariectomized and estro-gen-replacement in which an osmotic pump (Alza Corporation, 2ML4, Palo Alto, CA, USA) delivering 10 µg/day of water soluble estradiol was implanted at ovariectomy. Four weeks after the operation, the rats were anaesthetized with diethyl ether, and the main branch of the superior mesenteric arteries were removed carefully and cleaned of surrounding fat and connective tissues in oxygenated physiological salt solution at room temperature. The arteries were cut into rings (3 mm in length). Care was taken to ensure that the endothelial layer was not damaged during preparation.

1.1. Membrane potential

The main branch of the superior mesenteric artery was placed on a plate and opened longitudinally. Where indicated, the endothelial cells were removed by gently rubbing the intimal surface of the blood vessel with a moistened cotton ball. The tissue was pinned down, intimal side upward, on the bottom of an organ chamber (capacity 3 ml), and superfused at a constant flow rate (7 ml/min) with physiological salt solution aerated with 95% O_2 and 5% CO_2. The temperature of perfusate was kept constant at 37 °C. The composition of the physiological salt solution was as follows (in mM): NaCl 118.2; KCl 4.7; $CaCl_2$ 2.5; $MgCl_2$ 1.2; KH_2PO_4 1.2; $NaHCO_3$ 25.0; and glucose 10.0. After the preparations were allowed to equilibrate for 60 min, glass microelectrodes filled with 3 M KCl (tip resistance 40–80 MΩ) were inserted into the smooth muscle cells from the intimal side. After a stable recording of membrane potential for at least 2 min was obtained, changes in membrane potential produced by acetylcholine and pinacidil were registered using a high-impedance amplifier (Nihon Kohden MEZ-8201, Tokyo, Japan) in continuous recording. Electrical signals were continuously monitored on an oscilloscope (Nihon Kohden VC-10, Tokyo, Japan) and recorded on a chart recorder (Watanabe Sokki WR3101, Tokyo, Japan).

1.2. Relaxation

Rings of rat mesenteric artery were suspended by a pair of stainless steel pins in a water-jacketed chamber filled with 6 ml of normal physiological salt solution. The solution in the bath was gassed with 95% O_2 and 5% CO_2 (pH 7.4) and its temperature was maintained at 37 °C. The rings were stretched until an optimal resting tension of 1.0 g was obtained and then allowed to equilibrate for at least 60 min. Force generation was monitored using an isometric transducer (Unique Medical UMTB-1, Tokyo, Japan) and a carrier amplifier (Nihon Kohden AP-621G, Tokyo, Japan). The output of the force transducer was registered on a pen recorder (Rikadenki R-64, Tokyo, Japan). After the equilibration period, the rings were exposed several times to solution with high K^+ (80 mM $[K^+]_o$) until reproducible contractile responses were obtained. High K^+ solution was prepared by substituting NaCl with equimolar KCl. The vessels were contracted with 10^{-6} M [in the absence of N^ω-nitro-L-arginine (L-NA)] or 10^{-7} M (in the presence of L-NA) phenylephrine. Indomethacin (10^{-5} M), L-NA (10^{-4} M) and 18β-glycyrrhetinic acid (3×10^{-5} M) were added to the organ chamber 15 min before the application of phenylephrine. After the contraction had reached a plateau level, acetylcholine was applied in a cumulative manner. The responses to acetylcholine in the presence of L-NA plus indomethacin were regarded as EDHF-mediated relaxations, since preliminary experiments showed that L-NA- and indomethacin-resistant relaxations were reduced in 20 mM K^+ solution and abolished either by 30 mM K^+ solution or by charybdotoxin (10^{-7} M) plus apamin

$(5 \times 10^{-7} \text{ M})$ (Fukao *et al.*, 1997a). Relaxations were expressed as a percentage of the contraction induced by phenylephrine.

1.3. Western blot

Aortas and mesenteric arteries were excised. The blood vessels were minced and homogenized in ice-cold tris buffered saline (pH 7.4) (Tris-HCl 75 mM, $MgCl_2$ 25 mM, EDTA 5 mM, EGTA 1 mM). Protein extracts were obtained by centrifugation at $1000\,g$ for 10 min at 4 °C. Sodium dodecyl sulfate polyacrylamide gel electrophoresis was performed on 10% laemmli gel. Electrophoresis and transfer to polyvinylidene difluoride membranes (Bio-Rad, Hercules, CA, USA) was carried out using a Bio-Rad Mini-Protean II apparatus. Cx43 protein was detected using Cx43 monoclonal antibody (1:250 dilution; Zymed Laboratories, San Francisco, CA, USA) and a horseradish peroxidase-linked secondary anti-mouse antibody (1:4000 dilution; Bio-Rad) was used for the experiment. The band of Cx43 was visualized on the X-ray film using a chemiluminescence kit (ECL + plus, Amersham, Buckinghamshire, UK), according to the manufacturer's protocols.

1.4. Immunohistochemistry

For immunohistochemical analysis of Cx43, rabbit anti-Cx43 antibodies were used (Zymed Laboratories). Aortas and mesenteric arteries were fixed in 2% paraformaldehyde, embedded in paraffin, and cut in slices (5-μm thick). After deparaffinization, the sections were immersed in 3% hydrogen peroxide for 15 min was used for blocking. The nonspecific binding of protein was blocked with 5% skim milk (15 min). Anti-Cx43 antibody was applied at a dilution of 1:500 and incubated overnight at 4 °C in a humidified environment. After the sections were washed in phosphate-buffered saline, rabbit anti-mouse IgG was applied for 60 min at room temperature. Staining was visualized with diaminobenzidine at room temperature for 10 min. The immunoreactive level of Cx43 was evaluated with light microscopy.

1.5. Drugs

The following drugs were used: acetylcholine chloride (Wako, Osaka, Japan), pinacidil (Shionogi, Osaka, Japan), L-NA, indomethacin, sodium nitroprusside, 17β-estradiol, 18β-glycyrrhetinic acid, charybdotoxin, apamin, tetrabutylammonium, tetraethylammonium and glibenclamide (Sigma Chemical, St. Louis, MO, USA). Pinacidil and L-NA were prepared in 0.2 N HCl, and glibenclamide in 0.05 N NaOH. 18β-glycyrrhetinic acid was dissolved in dimethyl sulfoxide. Other drugs were dissolved in distilled water. Physiological salt solution was used for further dilution to the proper concentrations. Solvents used to dissolve drugs did not, themselves, affect electrical and mechanical responses at their final concentrations in the organ chamber.

1.6. Statistical analysis

All values are expressed as means ± SE. Two-way analysis of variance (ANOVA) was used to compare concentration–response curves of hyperpolarization and relaxation.

Other variables were compared using Student's *t*-test for paired and unpaired observations. Differences were considered to be statistically significant when $p < .05$.

2. RESULTS

2.1. General characteristics

Four weeks after the operation, body weight was not different among the three groups of rats. The serum estrogen levels in ovariectomized rats were significantly decreased compared with those in sham-operated controls. Estrogen-replacement therapy normalized the estrogen levels. The serum levels of total cholesterol, HDL cholesterol, LDL cholesterol, and triglycerides were not affected by ovariectomy or estrogen supplementation.

2.2. EDHF-mediated relaxation

Acetylcholine elicited endothelium-dependent relaxations in the arteries contracted with phenylephrine in the three groups. Treatment with indomethacin (10^{-5} M) had no significant effect on the relaxations to acetylcholine. In the presence of L-NA (10^{-4} M), the concentration–response curves for the peak amplitude of arterial relaxation by acetylcholine were shifted to the right, and the peak amplitudes of relaxation were reduced significantly in the three groups. In the absence of indomethacin and L-NA, acetylcholine-induced relaxations were not different among the three groups. Endothelium-dependent relaxations by acetylcholine in the presence of indomethacin or in the combination of indomethacin, charybdotoxin plus apamin were also not different among the groups. However, acetylcholine-induced endothelium-dependent relaxations of arteries from ovariectomized rats in the presence of indomethacin plus L-NA was significantly reduced compared with controls. The concentration–response curves for the peak amplitude of arterial relaxation by acetylcholine in ovariectomized group in the presence of indomethacin and L-NA was shifted to the right and the peak amplitude of relaxation significantly reduced compared with controls. For example, the peak amplitudes of relaxation at the concentration of 10^{-6} M acetylcholine in the presence of indomethacin and L-NA were $66.0 \pm 1.9\%$ in the control and $24.5 \pm 10.9\%$ in the ovariectomized group. Estrogen replacement therapy restored the reduced EDHF-mediated relaxation in the ovariectomized group. The concentration–relaxation curve by acetylcholine in estrogen supplemented group in the presence of indomethacin and L-NA was not significantly different from that of the control group.

2.3. Membrane hyperpolarization

Acetylcholine produced sustained hyperpolarization of the smooth muscle cells in control rats. When the endothelium was removed, acetylcholine no longer produced significant changes in resting membrane potential. The hyperpolarizing response to acetylcholine was reduced in 20 mM K^+ solution and enhanced in 1 mM K^+ solution. Tetrabutylammonium (5×10^{-4} M), a non-specific K^+ channel blocker, markedly inhibited the acetylcholine-induced hyperpolarization. A combination of apamin

(5×10^{-7} M; a specific blocker of small conductance Ca^{2+}-activated K^+ channel) plus charybdotoxin (10^{-7} M; a blocker of large conductance Ca^{2+}-activated K^+ channels and voltage dependent K^+ channels) almost completely inhibited the hyperpolarization by acetylcholine. Tetraethylammonium, a relatively specific blocker of large conductance Ca^{2+}-activated K^+ channels, inhibited acetylcholine-induced hyperpolarization only at high concentration (10^{-2} M). However, glibenclamide (10^{-5} M; an ATP-sensitive K^+ channel blocker) and ouabain (10^{-5} M; a Na/K-ATPase inhibitor) were without effect on the hyperpolarization caused by acetylcholine.

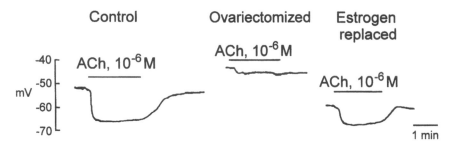

Figure 35.1 Original recordings of cell membrane potential, and effects of acetylcholine (ACh, 10^{-6} M) in the mesenteric arteries from middle-aged female rats with intact endothelium. ACh was applied during the period indicated by horizontal bars.

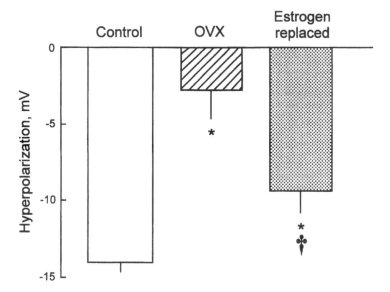

Figure 35.2 Summary data of acetylcholine (10^{-6} M)-induced hyperpolarizations in mesenteric arteries from control, ovariectomized (OVX) and estrogen-replaced rats. Data are shown as mean ± SE of three experiments. Membrane hyperpolarization by acetylcholine in ovariectomized rat was significantly reduced ($p < .05$) compared with controls. Estrogen replacement therapy significantlly restored the reduced EDHF-mediated response in ovariectomized rats. The asterisk denotes a statistically significant difference from control; the dagger indicates a statistically significant difference between ovariectomy and replacement therapy ($p < .05$).

The resting membrane potential of the mesenteric arterial smooth muscle cells was significantly shallower in arteries from the ovariectomized group (-41.7 ± 2.4 mV, $n = 3$) compared to controls (-49.0 ± 2.0 mV, $n = 3$) and the estrogen-replacement group (-49.5 ± 3.7 mV, $n = 3$). The acetylcholine-induced hyperpolarization in the mesenteric artery with endothelium was significantly depressed in the artery from the ovariectomized group in comparison with the control group (Figures 35.1 and 35.2). The decrease in endothelium-dependent membrane hyperpolarization by acetylcholine was partially restored in the estrogen-replacement group (Figures 35.1 and 35.2).

Pinacidil, an ATP-sensitive K^+ channel opener, elicited endothelium-independent hyperpolarization in the rat mesenteric artery. Membrane hyperpolarizations by pinacidil were not different among arteries from the three groups. Estrogen *per se* had no effect on the resting membrane potential. Estrogen also did not modify the hyperpolarization caused by acetylcholine when added acutely (15–60 min before the application of acetylcholine).

2.4. 18β-glycyrrhetinic acid

At 5×10^{-5} M, 18β-glycyrrhetinic acid significantly inhibited the contraction to phenylephrine in the rat mesenteric artery. Therefore, a lower concentration (3×10^{-5} M) was used. 18β-glycyrrhetinic acid (3×10^{-5} M) had not significant effect on phenylephrine-induced contractions in arteries from the control and ovariectomized groups. It slightly inhibited acetylcholine-induced relaxations in control solution, and nearly abolished the response to acetylcholine in the presence of indomethacin and L-NA in both groups (Figure 35.3). 18β-glycyrrhetinic acid also

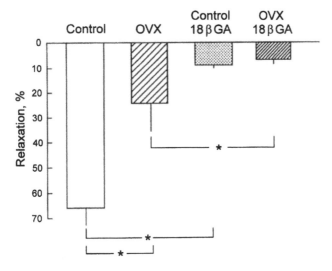

Figure 35.3 Effect of 18β-glycyrrhetinic acid (18β-GA) on endothelium-dependent relaxations induced by acetylcholine (10^{-6} M) in the presence of indomethacin (10^{-5} M) and L-NA (10^{-4} M) in mesenteric arteries from control and ovariectomized (OVX) rats. Data are shown as mean $\pm$ SE ($n = 6$). The asterisk indicates statistically significant differences between groups ($p < .05$).

inhibited the endothelium-dependent membrane hyperpolarization caused by acetylcholine in the rat mesenteric artery.

2.5. Western blot analysis

Anti-Cx43 antibody recognized a single band of 43 kDa in the homogenates of rat aorta and mesenteric artery. The densities of immunoreactive bands of Cx43 were reduced in preparations from the ovariectomized group compared with controls.

2.6. Immunohistochemical analysis

The aorta and mesenteric artery from control and ovariectomized rats were examined for expression of Cx43 protein by immunohistochemistry. Positive staining for Cx43 protein was observed in the endothelium and smooth muscle cells in both arteries. The stainings of Cx43 were decreased in preparations from the ovariectomized group.

3. DISCUSSION

The protective role of sex hormones in the cardiovascular system has been established in numerous clinical trials. Estrogen is largely responsible for the decreased incidence of cardiovascular diseases in premenopausal women compared to men. The present study demonstrates that EDHF-mediated membrane hyperpolarizations and relaxations are impaired in mesenteric arteries from ovariectomized rats and that estrogen replacement restores the reduced EDHF-mediated responses. These results suggest that estrogens may exert their beneficial effect, in part, through the upregulation of the EDHF pathway.

The resting membrane potential of the smooth muscle of rat mesenteric arteries became shallower following ovariectomy and was normalized by estrogen-replacement. These observations suggest that estrogens function physiologically to increase the cell membrane potential, and that deprivation of these hormones renders vascular smooth muscle prone to constriction. Possible mechanisms underlying these estrogen effects include a direct effect on potassium channels of the vascular smooth muscle cell membrane, which regulate the resting membrane potential, or an indirect effect through activation of the release or the action of EDHF.

The endothelium-dependent relaxation to acetylcholine was not affected by indomethacin, indicating that prostaglandins contribute little to the response in the rat mesenteric artery. The acetylcholine-induced relaxation in the presence of the combination of indomethacin, charybdotoxin and apamin, which block both the prostaglandin- and EDHF-mediated relaxations, was not significantly reduced in the ovariectomized group. This result suggests that NO-mediated arterial relaxation is not impaired by ovariectomy. The effect of chronic treatment with estrogen on NO-mediated relaxations is controversial. Long-term treatment with estrogens in ovariectomized rat increases endothelium-dependent relaxations in the rat aorta (Andersen *et al.*, 1999). However, estrogens do not increase the production or release of endothelium-derived nitric oxide in the same preparation (Vedernikov *et al.*, 1997). The present study demonstrates that, in contrast to the effect of estrogens on NO-mediated response, the EDHF-mediated relaxation to acetylcholine (in the presence of L-NA)

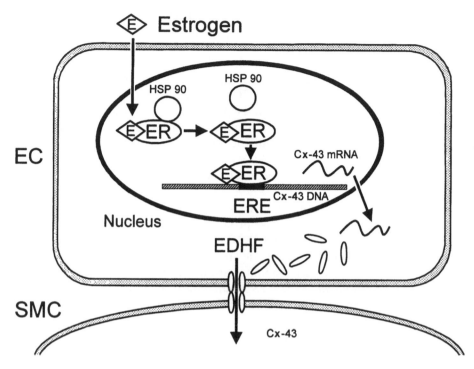

Figure 35.4 Proposed upregulation of EDHF-mediated responses by estrogen through the expression of connexin43 (Cx43). Estrogen receptors in the nucleus usually are bound to the heat shock protein 90 (HSP90) and are inactivated. Binding of estrogens to the estrogen receptors in the nucleus dissociates HSP90 and activates signal transduction. Estrogen-receptor complexes stimulate transcription of the Cx43 gene by binding to the specific promoter DNA elements, estrogen responsive element.

was reduced in the rat mesenteric artery after ovariectomy. These results suggest that EDHF-mediated relaxation is specifically impaired by ovariectomy. In other words, estrogens may play an important role in the maintenance of EDHF-mediated responses in the rat mesenteric artery.

Estrogen exerts its effect through binding to specific receptors, ERα and ERβ (Green *et al.*, 1986; Mosselman *et al.*, 1996) (Figure 35.4). These receptors are mainly expressed in the nucleus, although a small percentage are expressed in the plasma membrane. The latter couple to Gqα and Gsα coupling proteins, which mediate the acute effect of estrogens. In the present experiments, estrogens *per se* had no effect on resting membrane potential and the hyperpolarization to acetylcholine, suggesting that the effect of estrogen on EDHF-responses is not due to its acute but rather to its chronic effect, through the activation of estrogen receptors in the nucleus. Estrogen receptors in the nucleus usually are bound to heat shock protein 90 and inactivated. Binding of estrogens to the estrogen receptor in the nucleus dissociates heat shock protein 90 and activates the estrogen receptor. The estrogen-receptor complexes stimulate transcription of estrogen-regulated genes by binding to the specific promoter DNA elements, referred to as estrogen responsive elements. Such elements in estrogen responsive genes exhibit the properties of hormone-inducible enhancers (Yamamoto, 1985). A structural and functional analysis of the promoter region of various estrogen regulated genes revealed a common 13 bp-palindromic estrogen responsive element with the consensus sequence 5′-GGTCANNNTGACC-3′ (Klein-Hitpass et al., 1986). In the present study, western blot analysis and immunohistochemical study showed that the expression of Cx43 protein is decreased in the aorta and mesenteric arteries of ovariectomized rats. From the analysis of Cx43 gene reported in GenBank, there is no complete estrogen responsive element in the promoter region of Cx43 DNA. However, interestingly, 5′ upstream of Cx43 DNA have six half estrogen responsive elements. These half-palindromic elements are sufficient to activate gene transcription of the rat Cx43 gene expressed in HeLa cells (Yu et al., 1994). These data support the present finding that estrogens enhance the expression of Cx43 protein in the rat mesenteric artery.

The nature of EDHF is still unclear. In some arteries, especially in the coronary and renal small vessels, a P450 epoxygenase product, such as an epoxyeicosatrienoic acid, may be an essential component of EDHF-mediated responses. However, in other blood vessels, including the rat mesenteric artery, this is obviously not the case. Indeed P450-derived arachidonic acid metabolites are not EDHF in the rat mesenteric and hepatic arteries (Fukao et al., 1997b; Zygmunt et al., 1996). K^+ has been proposed as an EDHF in the rat hepatic and mesenteric arteries (Edwards et al., 1998). However, in the present experimental conditions, K^+ reduced rather than increased the resting membrane potential, and Ba^{2+}, ouabain or the combination of Ba^{2+} plus ouabain had little or no effect on the acetylcholine-induced hyperpolarization. Thus, an unidentified factor different from P450 metabolites or K^+ must be responsible for the EDHF-mediated responses in the rat mesenteric artery.

Myoendothelial gap junctions play a central role in the EDHF-mediated hyperpolarization and relaxation in some smooth muscle cells (Chaytor et al., 1998). 18β-glycyrrhetinic acid has been recently considered as a potential tool for studying the role of gap junctions in electrical coupling between endothelial and smooth muscle cells in the mesenteric artery (Yamamoto et al., 1998). EDHF-mediated relaxations and hyperpolarizations of the rat mesenteric artery were almost completely inhibited by the gap junctional inhibitor 18β-glycyrrhetinic acid. Although nonspecific actions of 18β-glycyrrhetinic cannot be excluded, a more specific inhibitor, the synthetic gap junctional protein inhibitor Gap 27, which is identical in sequence to a portion of an extracellular loop of a Cx43, inhibits EDHF-mediated responses in rabbit and rat mesenteric arteries (Chaytor et al., 1998; Edwards et al., 1998). Therefore, in the rat mesenteric artery, EDHF-mediated responses almost depend on myoendothelial gap junctions. The expressional level of connexin may play a key role in controlling the EDHF-mediated responses.

4. CONCLUSION

Estrogens may exert their effect by increasing the EDHF-mediated responses through upregulation of the expression of the gap junctional protein Cx43. This effect may partly account for the antiatherogenic effect of estrogens in the arterial wall.

36 Endothelium-derived hyperpolarizing factor (EDHF) and utero-feto-placental circulation in the rat

Y.P. Vedernikov, E.E. Fulep, G.R. Saade and R.E. Garfield

The objective of this study was to find out whether or not endothelium-derived hyper-polarizing factor (EDHF) plays a role in the rat utero-feto-placental circulation. In the rat utero-feto-placental units from non-pregnant, mid and late pregnant rats perfused with Krebs buffer containing dextran and indomethacin, N^{ω}-nitro-L-arginine methyl ester (L-NAME) did not significantly influence perfusion pressure. Phenylephrine-induced increases in perfusion pressure did not differ in the utero-feto-placental units from the all three groups. L-NAME after phenylephrine further increased perfusion pressure that was greater at late gestation. Acetylcholine and bradykinin decreased perfusion pressure independently of the gestational age or the presence of L-NAME. Decreases in perfusion pressure caused by the nitric oxide (NO) donor diethylamine/NO were greater in the utero-feto-placental units from late pregnant animals and were not influenced by L-NAME. The decreases in perfusion pressure induced by acetylcholine in the presence of indomethacin and L-NAME in the utero-feto-placental units from late pregnant rats were abolished by potassium chloride, attenuated by miconazole, but not by linolcyl hydroxamic acid. The data suggest that basal, but not the stimulated production and/or release of nitric oxide as well as the sensitivity to NO are increased in the utero-feto-placental circulation at late gestation. EDHF is acting via activation of delayed rectifier type of voltage-sensitive potassium channels and seems not to be NO or a metabolite of arachidonic acid produced by either lipoxygenase or cytochrome p450 monooxygenase. The factor may control fetal perfusion during pregnancy.

Pregnancy is accompanied by increases in blood and plasma volumes, blood flow and cardiac output, while total peripheral resistance and arterial blood pressure decrease (Gant *et al.*, 1980). These changes are thought to be due in part to uteroplacental circulation acting as a low resistance shunt (Ferris, 1983). Another characteristic of the cardiovascular adaptations during pregnancy is decreased responsiveness to some vasoconstrictors (Abdul-Karim and Assali, 1961; Ferris *et al.*, 1983; Davidge and McLauphlin, 1992), which may result from changes in number and function of adrenoceptors (Smiley and Finster, 1996), in baroreflex control of the sympathetic outflow because of an increased level of some metabolites (Heesh and Rohger, 1995), and in pre- and post-junctional nerve endings (Ravelic and Burnstock, 1996).

Nitric oxide (NO) may also be implicated in the adaptive responses to pregnancy (Sladek *et al.*, 1997). The myogenic tone in resistance mesenteric arteries of late pregnant rats is reduced (Meyer *et al.*, 1993) or unchanged (Cockell and Poston, 1996), although flow-induced NO-mediated dilatation may operate (Cockell, 1996). Basally released

NO does not modify myogenic tone, at least under no-flow condition, although acetyl-choline-induced relaxation is greater in myometrial versus omental arteries from term pregnant women (Kublickiene *et al.*, 1997). However, bradykinin-induced endo-thelium-dependent relaxation of human omental versus myometrial arteries is not influenced by pregnancy (Ashworth *et al.*, 1996). The release of NO is enhanced in pressurized uterine arteries from pregnant rats (Ni *et al.*, 1997), while the low vascular tone and arterial pressure is not mediated by NO in pregnant rabbits (Losoncky *et al.*, 1996) or in the rat mesenteric artery bed (Ravelick and Burnstock, 1996).

The role of endothelium-derived hyperpolarizing factor (EDHF) in blood vessels at pregnancy has been demonstrated in aorta (Bobadilla *et al.*, 1997) and the mesenteric artery of the rat (Gerber *et al.*, 1998), and in human omental arteries (Vedernikov *et al.*, 1996, 1999). The data regarding utero-placental vascular physiology, obtained in isolated vessels, do not provide information about the responses of the utero-feto-placental circulation and negates the effect on the downstream resistance vessels, although most of the vasodilatation in microvessels are achieved by EDHF (Urakami-Harasawa *et al.*, 1997).

The objective of this study was to compare the role of EDHF and NO, and the role and probable nature of the former in the utero-feto-placental circulation.

1. METHODS

1.1. Animals

Timed pregnant Sprague-Dawley rats obtained from Charles River Laboratories (Houston, TX, USA) were housed separately in temperature- and humidity-controlled quarters and provided with food and water *ad libitum*. The pregnant rats used in this study were at day 14 (considered mid gestation) and day 21 (considered late gestation). Day 1 was the day when the sperm plug was observed. Nonpregnant female rats of the same age were used as controls.

The animals were euthanized by the inhalation of carbon dioxide. A middle incision of abdomen was made and the aorta close to the iliac bifurcation or the iliac artery was cannulated. All other vessels were ligated to enable perfusion of the right uterine horn through the uterine artery (Langer *et al.*, 1993). The utero-feto-placental units were perfused either in an organ chamber or *in situ* with Krebs buffer (in mmol/l): NaCl 119, KCl 4.7, $MgSO_4$ 1.2, KH_2PO_4 1.2, $CaCl_2$ 2.5, $NaHCO_3$ 25, dextrose 11.1, sodium EDTA 0.03 containing 2% dextran and indomethacin, 10^{-5} M, bubbled with 5% CO_2 in air (37 °C, pH $\sim$ 7.4) a peristaltic pump (Minipuls 3, Gilson Inc., Middleton, WI, USA). Agents were applied by addition to the Krebs buffer, by bolus injection into the perfusion line, or by constant infusion in the perfusion line by means of a syringe pump (kd scientific, model 100, KD Scientific Inc., Boston, MA, USA). The intraluminal pressure was monitored using a pressure transducer (Kent Scientific Corp., Litchfield, CT, USA) connected to an on-line computer.

1.2. Experimental protocol

Flow-rate was gradually adjusted to achieve 50 mmHg of perfusion pressure for the preparations, which was maintained throughout the experiment. Under these conditions, any changes in perfusion pressure reflect changes in the resistance of the downstream vasculature. Phenylephrine (10^{-6} M) was added to the perfusate to increase perfusion pressure. After stabilization of the pressure, acetylcholine (10^{-6} M), bradykinin (10^{-7} M) or substance P (10^{-7} M) were infused in sequence for five minutes with 15-min intervals. This was followed by a bolus injection of 10 μl of 10^{-4} M of diethylamine/NO complex (DEA/NO). The experiment was repeated after 30-min perfusion with N^{ω}-nitro-L-arginine methyl ester (L-NAME, 10^{-4} M). Finaly, inhibitors of ATP-dependent (K_{ATP}), Ca-dependent (K_{Ca}) and delayed rectifier type (K_V) potassium channels as well as some agents supposed to inhibit the effect of EDHF had been studied in the utero-feto-placental units from late pregnant rats. Vascular bed was exposed to the inhibitors for 30 min.

1.3. Drugs used

Concentrations are given as final molar concentrations in the perfusion solution. Phenylephrine, acetylcholine, bradykinin, substance P, indomethacin, N^{ω}-nitro-L-arginine methyl ester (L-NAME), N^{ω}-nitro-L-arginine (L-NA), 2 Phenyl-4,4,5,5-tetra-methyl-imidazoline-1-oxyl-3-oxide (PTIO), miconazole, glibenclamide, 4-aminopyridine, tetraethylammonium chloride (Sigma Chemical Co., St. Louis, MO, USA), linoleyl hydroxamic acid [octa-9,12-dienehydroxamic acid (z,z-)] (Penn Bio-Organics, Inc., State College, PA, USA), 17-octadecynoic acid, diethylamine/nitric oxide complex sodium (DEA/NO) /NO (RBI, Natick, MO, USA).

1.4. Data analysis

The data were collected, stored and analyzed using a DI-220 data acquisition system and Windaq/200 software (DataQ Instruments Inc., Akron, OH, USA). They are presented as means ± SEM of percent changes from the perfusion pressure during administration of phenylephrine in the presence of inhibitors of cycloxygenase and NO-synthase. Independent Student's *t*-test and one way analysis of variance (ANOVA) with post hoc Newman–Keuls test were used when two or more means were compared, respectively (GraphPad Prism; GraphPad Software Inc., San Diego, CA, USA). A *p*-values less than .05 were considered to be statistically significant.

2. RESULTS

Infusion for 30 min of N^{ω}-nitro-L-arginine methyl ester (L-NAME, 10^{-4} M) into the utero-feto-placental units from mid ($n = 4$) or term ($n = 4$) pregnant rats, did not significantly increase perefusion pressure ($+3.3 \pm 1.5$ mmHg and $+5.0 \pm 3.5$ mmHg, respectively). Infusion of phenylephrine (10^{-6} M) into the utero-feto-placental units from non-pregnant, mid pregnant and term pregnant rats, increased intraluminal pressure by 27.9 ± 2.7 mmHg ($58.9 \pm 5.4\%$) ($n = 5$), 36.8 ± 6.4 mmHg ($73.5 \pm 12.7\%$) ($n = 7$) and 32.2 ± 4.7 mmHg ($74.4 \pm 9.5\%$) ($n = 8$), respectively. The increase was not significantly different between the three groups (Figure 36.1). Infusion of L-NAME in the presence of phenylephrine, significantly increased perfusion pressure in the utero-feto-placental units of the three groups of animals which was greater in the units from late pregnant animals (Figure 36.1). Infusion of L-arginine or L-citrulline

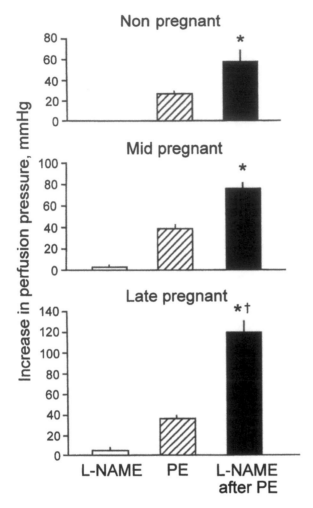

Figure 36.1 Increases in perfusion pressure caused by N^{ω}-nitro-L-arginine methyl ester (L-NAME, 10^{-4} M, $n = 4$), phenylephrine (PE, 10^{-6} M) and L-NAME in the presence of phenylephrine in rat utero-feto-placental units from non-pregnant ($n = 5$), mid ($n = 7$) and late pregnant $n = 8$ rats. Data shown as means $\pm$ SEM. The asterisks indicate statistically significant effect of L-NAME plus phenylephrine versus phenylephrine and L-NAME alone ($p < .05$). The dagger indicates a statistically significant difference versus non-pregnant and mid pregnant groups ($p < .05$).

(both at 10^{-3} M for 30 min) did not significantly affect the perfusion pressure increased by L-NAME in the presence of phenylephrine (data not shown).

Decreases in perfusion pressure induced by acetylcholine (10^{-6} M) were not significantly different in the utero-feto-placental units from non-pregnant, mid pregnant and late pregnant animals. L-NAME did not significantly inhibit acetylcholine-induced decreases in perfusion pressure in the three groups (Figure 36.2). Decreases in perfusion pressure induced by bradykinin (10^{-7} M) were not significantly different in the utero-feto-placental units from non-pregnant, mid pregnant and late pregnant animals. Infusion of L-NAME attenuated the bradykinin-evoked decreases in perfusion pressure the pregnant rat utero-feto-placental units. However the decrease did not reach statistically significant levels (Figure 36.2). Substance P (10^{-7} M) did not significantly affect perfusion pressure in the utero-feto-placental units of any group (data not shown).

Decreases in perfusion pressure induced by bolus injection of the NO-donor, DEA/NO were significantly higher in the utero-feto-placental units from late pregnant versus non-pregnant rats either in the absence or presence of L-NAME (Figure 36.2).

Decreases in perfusion pressure induced by acetylcholine (10^{-5} M) in the presence of indomethacin (10^{-5} M) and L-NAME were not significantly affected by glibenclamide (3×10^{-6} M), tetraethylammonium (10^{-3} M), but were significantly inhibited

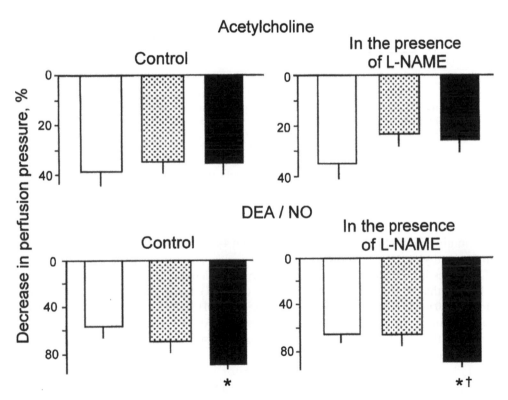

Figure 36.2 Infusion of N^{ω}-nitro-L-arginine methyl ester (L-NAME, 10^{-4} M, right panel) into utero-feto-placental units from non pregnant (open bars), pregnant (hatched bars) and late pregnant (closed bars) rats tends to decrease the dilatation induced by acetylcholine (10^{-6} M). Decreases in perfusion pressure induced by bolus (10 µl of 10^{-4} M solution) injection of nitric oxide donor diethylamine/NO (DEA/NO) are more pronounced in utero-feto-placental units from late pregnant rats, and were not significantly influenced by L-NAME. Data shown as means ± SEM. The asterisks indicate a statistically significant difference versus non-pregnant animals ($p < .05$). The dagger indicates a statistically significant difference versus mid pregnant animals ($p < .05$).

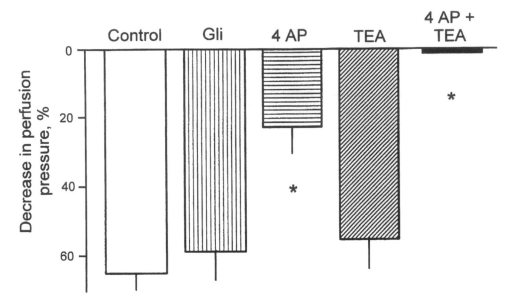

Figure 36.3 Decrease in perfusion pressure caused by acetylcholine (10^{-5} M) in the presence of indomethacin (10^{-5} M) and N^{ω}-nitro-L-arginine methyl ester (10^{-4} M) during constrictions to phenylephrine (10^{-6} M). The response before (control, pooled, $n = 14$, open bars) and after infusion of glibenclamide (3×10^{-6} M, $n = 4$, vertical lined bar), 4-amionopyridine, 10^{-3} M, $n = 5$, horizontal lined bar) and 4-amiono-pyridine plus tetraethylammonium ($n = 6$, closed bar). Data shown as means ± SEM. The asterisks indicate a statistically significant effect of the treatment ($p < .05$).

by 4-aminipyridine (10^{-3} M) and abolished when 4-aminopyridine was infused together with tetraethylammonium (Figure 36.3).

Decreases in perfusion pressure induced by acetylcholine (10^{-5} M) in the presence of indomethacin (10^{-5} M) and L-NAME (10^{-4} M) were abolished by potassium chloride (30 mM) (Figure 36.4). Miconazole (10^{-6} M) significantly attenuated acetyl-choline-induced decreases in perfusion pressure. At 10^{-5} M, however, miconazole abolished the increases in perfusion pressure caused by phenylephrine (data not shown). Neither linoleyl hydroxamic acid (10^{-6} M, an inhibitor of lipoxygenase) or 17-octadecynoic acid (3×10^{-6} M, an inhibitor of P450) significantly influenced the decrease in perfusion pressure induced by acetylcholine (Figure 36.4). Finally, experiments were performed to find out whether EDHF may be nitric oxide still formed and released in spite of the presence of the NO-synthase inhibitor used. After the response to acetylcholine in the presence of indomethacin and L-NAME was obtained, utero-feto-placental units from late pregnant rats were perfused for 30 min with Krebs solution containing additionally N^{ω}-nitro-L-arginine (10^{-4} M, L-NA), followed by addition of 2 Phenyl-4,4,5,5-tetramethyl-imidazoline-1-oxyl-3-oxide (PTIO, 10^{-5} M), a scavenger of nitric oxide. Neither addition of L-NA or L-NA plus PTIO significantly affected decreases in perfusion pressure induced by acetylcholine (10^{-5} M) (Figure 36.5).

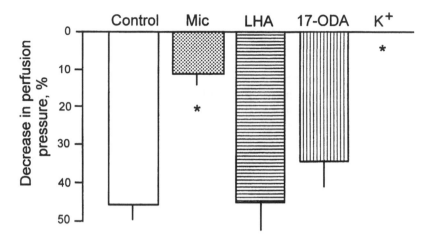

Figure 36.4 Decrease in perfusion pressure caused by of acetylcholine (10^{-5} M) in the presence of indomethacin (10^{-5} M) and N^{ω}-nitro-L-arginine methyl ester (10^{-4} M) during constrictions to phenylephrine (10^{-6} M). The response before (control, pooled, $n = 18$, open bar) and after infusion of miconazole (10^{-6} M, $n = 4$, dotted bar), linoleyl hydroxamic acid (10^{-6} M, $n = 5$, horizontal lined bar), 17-octadecynoic acid (3×10^{-6} M, $n = 5$, vertical lined bar) and potassium chloride (30 mM, $n = 4$, closed bar). Data shown as means $\pm$ SEM. The asterisks indicate a statistically significant effects of the treatment ($p < .05$).

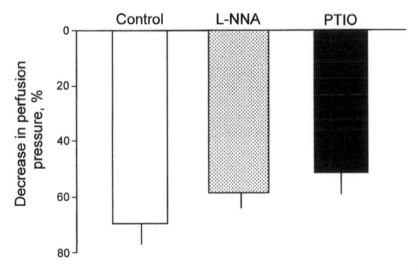

Figure 36.5 Decrease in perfusion pressure caused by of acetylcholine (10^{-5} M) in the presence of indomethacin (10^{-5} M) and N^{ω}-nitro-L-arginine methyl ester (L-NAME, 10^{-4} M) during constrictions to phenylephrine (10^{-6} M) in utero-feto-placental units from late pregnant rats ($n = 4$). The response in control (open bar) and after infusion of N^{ω}-nitro-L-arginine (L-NA, 10^{-4} M, hatched bar) and 2 Phenyl-4,4,5,5-tetramethyl-imidazoline-1-oxyl-3-oxide (PTIO, 10^{-5} M, closed bar). Data shown as means $\pm$ SEM.

3. DISCUSSION

The data of this study demonstrate that in the utero-feto-placental units from non-pregnant, mid and late pregnant rats, equilibrated at perfusion pressure of 50 mmHg, the increase in perfusion pressure induced by phenylephrine does not differ significantly. The infusion of the inhibitor of NO-synthase L-NAME did not induce changes in perfusion pressure in the utero-feto-placental units from the three groups of animals. However, after treatment with phenylephrine, the basal release of endothelium-derived relaxing factor/NO, estimated by the increase in perfusion pressure after infusion of L-NAME, was larger in utero-feto-placental units from late pregnant animals than those from mid pregnant and non-pregnant rats. Thus, in the utero-feto-placental circulation, the basal release of NO is revealed during stimulation of α_1-adrenoceptors, and it is larger at term, despite a comparable responses to phenylephrine.

The observed increase in the basal release of endothelial NO in the utero-feto-placental units at pregnancy is in line with earlier findings (Sladek *et al.*, 1997). The responses to the endothelium-dependent vasodilator acetylcholine and bradykinin, were similar in the utero-feto-placental units from non-pregnant, mid and late pregnant rats and were not significantly inhibited by L-NAME. The finding of a non-dependency on gestational age and on NO is at variance with data obtained in isolated uterine arteries (Ni *et al.*, 1997) and suggests that in perfused utero-feto-placental units non-prostanoid non NO factor(s) may be released to modulate vascular tone.

The decreases in perfusion pressure of the utero-feto-placental units in response to NO, released from the NO donor diethylamine/NO, was larger at late pregnancy and was not influenced by the presence of basal release of endothelium-derived NO, demonstrating that the responsiveness of the utero-feto-placental unit smooth muscle to NO at this stage of gestation is higher versus those in non-pregnant and mid pregnant rats. Since in the perfused utero-feto-placental units the resistance is largely determined by small resistance arteries the data may indicate the particular sensitivity of their smooth muscle to NO at late pregnancy.

All experiments were performed in the presence of indomethacin. Thus, the present experiments do not allow to speculate further on the role of cycloxygenase products in modulating the responses of the utero-feto-placental circulation.

The ability of the endothelial dilators to decrease perfusion pressure in the presence of inhibitors of cycloxygenase and NO synthase suggests that EDHF may be involved in the response in the utero-feto-placental circulation. Indeed, the decrease in perfusion pressure caused by acetylcholine was inhibited by 30 mM potassium chloride, which depolarizes the cell membrane and prevents the action of factor (Nagao and Vanhoutte, 1992).

The data demonstrate that relaxation induced by EDHF in the utero-feto-placental units from late pregnant rats at least, results from preferential activation of delayed rectified type (K_V), but not ATP-dependent potassium channels. Calcium-dependent potassium channels (K_{Ca}) may also be involved in the effect of EDHF since tetraethylammonium, having no effect when applied alone, potentiated the effect of 4-aminopyridine.

In the utero-feto-placental circulation 17-octadecynoic acid or an inhibitor of lipoxygenase did not influence the decreases in perfusion pressure induced by acetylcholine. Miconazole inhibited the acetylcholine-induced decrease in perfusion pressure. However, at higher concentration (10^{-5} M) miconazole abolished the tone induced by phenylephrine. This suggests that the inhibition may be due to nonspecific interference with the activation of contractile apparatus. Thus, the present experiments do not allow firm conclusions as to the chemical nature of the EDHF involved. They do not confirm, at least in the utero-feto-placental unit the suggestion that NO still produced and released in the presence of NO-synthase inhibition may serve as an EDHF (Cohen *et al.*, 1997). Indeed, in the presence of two inhibitors of nitric oxide synthase, L-NAME plus L-NA, or in the presence of the two inhibitors plus NO scavenger PTIO, acetylcholine still decreased perfusion pressure in the rat utero-feto-placental units.

4. CONCLUSION

In the perfused rat utero-feto-placental units the response to endothelium-dependent dilators does not depend on the gestational age. It is not prevented by inhibitors of cycloxygenase and NO-synthase. The basal release and direct effect of nitric oxide are larger at late gestation. EDHF-mediated responses to acetylcholine are inhibited by potassium-chloride depolarization and by inhibition of delayed rectifier type of voltage sensitive potassium channels. It appears that both EDHF and NO are important in the regulation of the utero-feto-placental circulation.

37 Endothelium-derived hyperpolarizing factor maintains a normal relaxation to bradykinin despite impairment of the nitric oxide pathway in porcine coronary arteries with regenerated endothelium

C. Thollon, M.-P. Fournet-Bourguignon,
L. Lesage, D. Saboureau, C. Cambarrat,
H. Reure, Paul M. Vanhoutte and
J.-P. Vilaine

Four weeks after balloon denudation, porcine coronary arteries with regenerated endothelium selectively lose endothelium-dependent relaxations to agonists such as serotonin while those to bradykinin or adenosine diphosphate (ADP) are maintained. The aim of the present study was to investigate the relative contribution of endothelium-derived hyperpolarizing factor (EDHF) to the relaxation induced by bradykinin in arteries with regenerated endothelium.

Transmembrane potential, isometric tension and levels of cyclic-Guanosine Monophosphate and cyclic-Adenosine Monophosphate (cyclic GMP and cyclic AMP) were measured simultaneously in each strip with regenerated endothelium and compared with those of the corresponding control coronary artery. Under basal conditions, in coronary arteries with regenerated endothelium, a depolarization of vascular smooth muscle cells was associated with a decreased level of cyclic GMP without alteration in that of cyclic AMP. Exogenous nitric oxide (NO) was added in order to compensate for the reduced level of cyclic GMP. The resulting repolarization of the injured coronary arteries demonstrated the involvement of the NO pathway in the control of resting membrane potential. This effect was cyclic GMP-dependent, as it was blocked by an inhibitor of soluble guanylate cyclase, oxadiazoloquinoxalin (ODQ). When contracted with prostaglandin F2α, arteries with normal or regenerated endothelium depolarized whatever the conditions studied (control, inhibition of cycloxygenase with or without that of nitric oxide synthase). In the presence of regenerated endothelium, spikes and phasic contraction were observed. In all blood vessels, both in the presence or the absence of indomethacin, bradykinin evoked nearly maximal relaxations suggesting no involvement of prostacyclin in the response. Additional blockade of nitric oxide synthase by N^{ω}-nitro-L-arginine, reduced the relaxation, demonstrating a small contribution of NO. In both coronary arteries, the relaxation induced by bradykinin was mediated essentially by EDHF. The membrane potential reached during exposure to bradykinin was always less negative in the presence of regenerated endothelium, suggesting that the NO pathway participated to the hyperpolarization in repolarizing the blood vessel. Thus, the unaltered relaxation to bradykinin despite the reduced production of NO, suggests that the endothelium-dependent hyperpolarization is sufficient to maintain a normal relaxation in coronary arteries with regenerated endothelium.

Abnormal endothelium-dependent relaxation is an early event in the development of vascular disease both in animal models (Yamamoto *et al.*, 1987; Shimokawa *et al.*, 1987; Cohen *et al.*, 1988) and in humans (Förstermann *et al.*, 1988; Creager *et al.*, 1990).

In porcine coronary arteries with regenerated endothelium after balloon denudation, endothelium-dependent relaxations are normalized 8 days after the procedure (Shimokawa *et al.*, 1987). However, 4 weeks after such denudation, the pertussis-toxin sensitive G-protein coupled relaxation to serotonin is reduced while that induced by bradykinin is normal (Shimokawa *et al.*, 1987, 1989; Borg-Capra *et al.*, 1997). In the porcine coronary artery, it is unlikely that NO fully explains the endothelium-dependent relaxations induced by bradykinin (Richard *et al.*, 1990; Cowan and Cohen, 1991; Nagao and Vanhoutte, 1992), suggesting an important contribution of endothelium-derived hyperpolarizing factor (EDHF) in the response (Bény and Haefliger, 1999). Four weeks after balloon denudation, in porcine coronary arteries with regenerated endothelium, the smooth muscle cells are depolarized and the hyperpolarization induced by bradykinin, in the presence of inhibitors of nitric oxide synthase and cyclooxygenase, is correlated with the value of membrane potential before the administration of the kinin. As a result, an increase in the hyperpolarization in response to bradykinin occurs in the most depolarized cells, suggesting a greater contribution of EDHF in these coronary arteries (Thollon *et al.*, 1999a). During contractions to prostaglandin $F_{2\alpha}$, in the presence of a blocker of cyclooxygenase, the hyperpolarization induced by bradykinin was normal in previously denuded coronary arteries (Thollon *et al.*, 1999b), suggesting that nitric oxide may curtail the EDHF-mediated component (Olmos *et al.*, 1995). Thus the aim of the present study was to measure the endothelium-dependent hyperpolarization in response to bradykinin in porcine coronary ateries with regenerated endothelium contracted with prostaglandin $F_{2\alpha}$ and to investigate its relative contribution in the relaxation evoked by the peptide.

1. MATERIALS AND METHODS

1.1. Endothelial denudation

Thirty-two Large White pigs (8 weeks, 19–25 kg), were anesthetized with an intramuscular injection of Tiletamine plus Zolazepam (20 mg/kg). Additional doses of anesthetic (sodium thiopental) were given intravenously, as needed. Animals were intubated and ventilated with a respirator. Heparin (250 I.U./kg) and lysine acetyl-salicylate (10 mg/kg) were administrated. Using a percutaneous transluminal coronary angioplasty (PTCA) guide catheter, a balloon (3.5 mm diameter × 20 mm length) was introduced via the femoral artery and advanced under fluoroscopic guidance into the coronary artery. The endothelium was removed locally by inflating the balloon three times. The pressure of inflation was adjusted so that the blood vessel was not over-stretched (2–8 atm). The animals were sacrified 28 days after the endothelial denudation.

1.2. Simultaneous recording of membrane potential and tension

The coronary arteries were dissected free, cleaned of adherent fat and connective tissue and maintained in oxygenated Krebs–Ringer solution at room temperature. Each coronary artery with regenerated endothelium was compared with a coronary artery with native endothelium from the same heart. Rings of coronary arteries (approximately 4 mm long) were cut open along the longitudinal axis and installed for simultaneous recording of tension and membrane potential (Thollon *et al.*, 1999b). One end of the segment was pinned down to the bottom of an experimental chamber, the endothelial side upward. At the other end three ligatures with micro-surgical silk thread (8/0) were performed to attach the tissue to a wire connected to a force transducer in order to measure contraction. The strips were superfused continuously at 5 ml/min with oxygenated, modified Krebs–Ringer solution of the following composition (mmol/L): NaCl 118, KCl 4.7, MgSO$_4$ 1.2, KH$_2$PO$_4$ 1.2, CaCl$_2$ 2.5, NaHCO$_3$ 25, EDTA 0.026 and glucose 11. The preparations were allowed to equilibrate for 30–45 min. During this period a basal tension of about 5 g was applied progressively.

For some experiments the strips were opened and fixed to the bottom of the experimental chamber without application of a determined resting tension. In all experiments, the membrane potential was measured with conventional glass micro-electrodes (30–40 MΩ), filled with 3 M KCl.

1.3. Measurement of cyclic nucleotides

The tissue segments were frozen rapidly in liquid nitrogen at the end of the experiments and stored at $-80\,^{\circ}$C. At the time of assay, frozen tissue was placed in medium containing acetate buffer (0.05 M, pH 5.8) and a phosphodiesterase inhibitor, 3-isobutyl-1-1-methylxanthine (IBMX, 10^{-4} M). The coronary segment then was homogenized rapidly and sonicated. The total protein content was determined in each homogenate using the Biorad method. The homogenate was centrifugated at 2000g for 20 min at 4 $^{\circ}$C. The cyclic GMP and cyclic AMP levels were determined in the supernatant by radioimmunoassay using the Amerlex method. The results are expressed in pmol per mg of total protein content.

1.4. Drugs

The following drugs were used: bradykinin, indomethacin, IBMX, N$^{\omega}$-nitro-L-arginine, 1H-(1,2,4)oxadiazolo(4,3-a)quinoxalin-1-one (ODQ), prostaglandin F$_{2\alpha}$, and sodium nitroprusside (all from Sigma Chemical Co.). Indomethacin (10^{-2} M, in ethanol), prostaglandin F$_{2\alpha}$ (3×10^{-3} M, in ethanol) and bradykinin (10^{-3} M, in H$_2$O) were prepared as stock solutions ($-20\,^{\circ}$C) and diluted in Krebs–Ringer solution to reach the final concentrations reported.

1.5. Statistical analysis

Data are expressed as the mean $\pm$ SEM from n experiments. Student's t-test for paired observations was used. Differences were considered to be statistically significant when p was less than .05.

2. RESULTS

Twenty-eight days after surgery, the smooth muscle cells of coronary arteries with regenerated endothelium were polarized significantly less than the corresponding control arteries (Figure 37.1). This depolarization was associated with a decrease in cyclic GMP levels (-79.7%) while the cyclic AMP contents were not changed (Figure 37.2). Prostaglandin $F_{2\alpha}$ $(6 \times 10^{-6}\,M)$ induced similar contractions in both types of coronary arteries, associated with a depolarization of vascular smooth muscle cells only for coronary arteries with native endothelium (Figure 37.1). Addition of

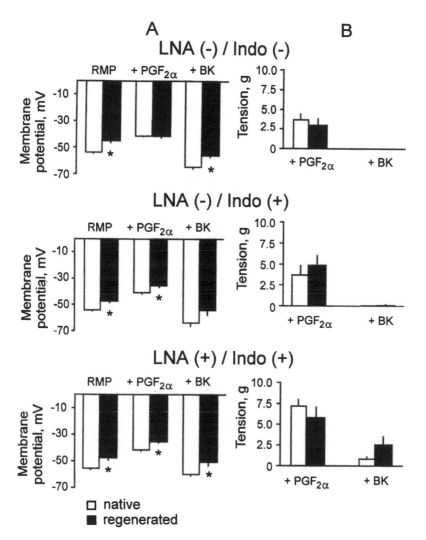

Figure 37.1 Changes in membrane potential of smooth muscle cells (A) and tension (B) during contractions to prostaglandin $F_{2\alpha}$ $(2-6 \times 10^{-6}\,M)$ $(+PGF_{2\alpha})$ and relaxations to bradykinin $(3 \times 10^{-8}\,M)$ $(+BK)$ in porcine coronary arteries with native or regenerated endothelium. RMP represent the resting membrane potential under resting tension, before the addition of drugs. The tension is expressed as changes from the basal values of resting tension. Data are mean $\pm$ SEM from seven experiments for each group. The experiments were performed in the absence $(-)$ or in the presence $(+)$ of indomethacin $(10^{-5}\,M)$ (Indo) alone or in addition to N^{ω}-nitro-L-arginine $(3 \times 10^{-5}\,M)$ (L-NA). The asterisks indicate statistically significant differences from the corresponding control coronary arteries with native endothelium $(p < .05)$.

bradykinin $(3 \times 10^{-8}\,\mathrm{M})$ produced a total change in cell membrane potential (repolarization plus hyperpolarization) which was more important in arteries with native $(-23.0 \pm 1.6\,\mathrm{mV})$ than with regenerated endothelium $(-14.3 \pm 1.4\,\mathrm{mV})$ (Figure 37.1). In both blood vessels, bradykinin induced a complete endothelium-dependent relaxation (Figure 37.1). Bradykinin induced an increase in cyclic GMP and AMP in both preparations, but the levels of cyclic GMP were significantly lower in coronary arteries with regenerated endothelium (Figure 37.2).

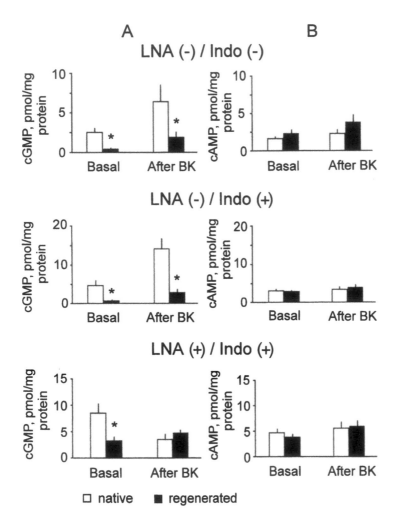

Figure 37.2 Levels of cyclic GMP (A) and cyclic AMP (B) in porcine coronary arteries with native or regenerated endothelium: under basal conditions ("Basal") and at the maximal level of relaxation with bradykinin (BK, $3 \times 10^{-8}\,\mathrm{M}$) ("After BK", same segments as those tested in the experiments of Figure 37.1). Both vascular segments are frozen at the same time and correspond to the same vascular tissue. Data are mean $\pm$ SEM from seven experiments for each group. Some experiments were performed in the presence of indomethacin (Indo, $10^{-5}\,\mathrm{M}$) or indomethacin plus N^{ω}-nitro-L-arginine (L-NA, $3 \times 10^{-5}\,\mathrm{M}$). The asterisks indicate statistically significant differences from the corresponding control coronary arteries with native endothelium ($p < .05$).

Under basal conditions, control preparations and arteries incubated with indomethacin only presented similar alterations of resting membrane potential and cyclic GMP content (Figures 37.1 and 37.2). The presence of indomethacin (10^{-5} M) did not significantly change the contractions induced by prostaglandin $F_{2\alpha}$ (3×10^{-6} M) (Figure 37.1). This contraction was associated with a depolarization of similar amplitude for coronary arteries with native (13.7 ± 1.2 mV) and regenerated (12.1 ± 1.6 mV) endothelium (Figure 37.1). The membrane potential in coronary arteries with regenerated endothelium was polarized significantly less than in those with native endothelium, both before and during contraction (Figure 37.1). The endothelium-dependent hyperpolarization in response to the addition of bradykinin was not different in both types of preparations: -22.9 ± 3.01 mV in coronary arteries with native endothelium vs -18.4 ± 3.5 mV in those with regenerated endothelium. The membrane potential reached during exposure to bradykinin was reduced

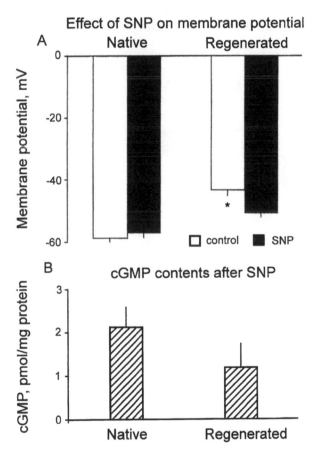

Figure 37.3 Changes in membrane potential of smooth muscle cells (A) and levels of cyclic GMP (B) in porcine coronary arteries with regenerated endothelium during exposure to a NO donor, sodium nitroprusside (SNP, 10^{-6} M). Both vascular segments are frozen at the end of exposure to SNP (17 min). Data are mean $\pm$ SEM from five experiments for each group. The asterisks indicate statistically significant differences from the corresponding control coronary arteries with native endothelium ($p < .05$).

in the presence of regenerated endothelium (Figure 37.1). Bradykinin induced maximal relaxations (99.3 ± 0.6% and 95.4 ± 3.0% for coronary arteries with native and regenerated endothelium, respectively) (Figure 37.1). The production of cyclic AMP in response to bradykinin was inhibited by indomethacin. As observed in the control group, the content of cyclic GMP after bradykinin stimulation was reduced by 63% in the previously denuded blood vessels (Figure 37.2).

In the presence of inhibitors of both nitric oxide synthase and cyclooxygenase, the electrophysiological parameters were not different from those obtained in preparations incubated with indomethacin only (Figure 37.1). The difference in the basal levels of the two nucleotides between the two types of blood vessels was similar to those observed in the two other experimental groups (Figure 37.2). During comparable contractions induced by prostaglandin $F_{2\alpha}$ (2×10^{-6} M), the relaxation of coronary arteries with regenerated endothelium in response to bradykinin (64.7 ± 9.9%) was reduced in comparison to the corrresponding control coronary arteries (87.9 ± 4.7%) (Figure 37.1). Under such conditions, the production of cyclic nucleotides was inhibited by the combination of indomethacin plus N^{ω}-nitro-L-arginine (Figure 37.2).

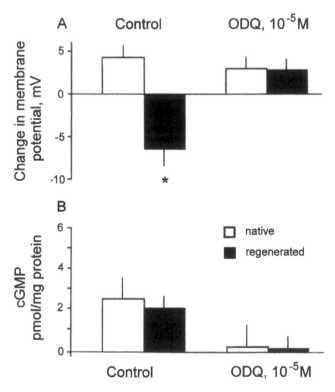

Figure 37.4 Changes in membrane potential of smooth muscle cells (A) and levels of cyclic GMP (B) in porcine coronary arteries with native or regenerated endothelium after exposure to a NO donor, sodium nitroprusside (SNP, 10^{-6} M) in the presence or absence of an inhibitor of soluble guanylate cyclase, ODQ (10^{-5} M). Data are mean ± SEM from six experiments for each group. The asterisks indicate statistically significant differences from the corresponding control coronary arteries with native endothelium ($p < .05$).

Addition of the donor of nitric oxide, sodium nitroprusside (10^{-6} M), repolarized the smooth muscle cells of coronary arteries with regenerated endothelium without affecting the membrane potential in the control arteries (Figure 37.3). As a result, the difference in the resting membrane potential between the two types of blood vessels was corrected by the exposure to nitric oxide. This repolarization was associated with an increase in the level of cyclic GMP (Figure 37.3). ODQ (10^{-5} M) inhibited the change in resting membrane potential induced by nitric oxide (Figure 37.4).

3. DISCUSSION

As previously demonstrated, the smooth muscle cells from porcine coronary arteries with regenerated endothelium were depolarized in comparison to those from corresponding control arteries (Thollon *et al.*, 1999a,b). This depolarization was associated with spontaneous electrical activity inducing phasic contractions in some arteries with regenerated endothelium while such membrane potential instability was never observed in the corresponding control arteries. Rhythmic spontaneous activity has been observed in coronary arteries from patients with cardiovascular diseases (e.g., Ross *et al.*, 1980; Kalsner, 1985). In the model of angioplasty used in the present study, the electrophysiological modifications were associated with a decrease in the levels of cyclic GMP and unchanged levels of cyclic AMP in the injured blood vessels. This decrease in cyclic GMP levels (Thollon *et al.*, 1999b) is the result of a reduced cellular production of nitric oxide by the regenerated endothelium (Fournet-Bourguignon *et al.*, 2000). In order to study if the change in membrane potential is related to the alteration of nitric oxide pathway, the injured blood vessels were exposed to sodium nitroprusside as a donor of nitric oxide. Sodium nitroprusside repolarized the vascular smooth muscle cells from coronary arteries with regenerated endothelium, normalizing the resting membrane potential. By contrast, sodium nitroprusside did not hyperpolarize coronary arteries with native endothelium, as previously demonstrated (Bény and Brunet, 1988). This repolarizing effect is cyclic GMP-dependent, as it is blocked by an inhibitor of soluble guanylate cyclase. These results suggest that nitric oxide via the production of cyclic GMP can inhibit an inward depolarizing current and/or activate an outward potassium current, both possibly altered in the injured blood vessels.

Four weeks after balloon denudation, porcine coronary arteries with regenerated endothelium selectively lose endothelium-dependent relaxations to some agonists such as serotonin while that to bradykinin is maintained (Shimokawa *et al.*, 1987, 1989; Borg-Capra *et al.*, 1997). The present study investigated the relative contribution of EDHF, prostacyclin and nitric oxide to the relaxation induced by bradykinin in arteries with regenerated endothelium. The hyperpolarization and relaxation were measured simultaneously and the evaluation of cyclic nucleotides contents was performed in the same vascular segments.

The contraction induced by prostaglandin $F_{2\alpha}$ was always associated with a depolarization of smooth muscle cells from coronary arteries with normal and regenerated endothelium. Under control conditions, the concentration of bradykinin used in these experiments induced a complete relaxation of both types of blood vessels. Under these conditions, the three pathways of endothelium-dependent relaxation are supposed to participate: prostacyclin, nitric oxide and EDHF. Contribution of the cycloxygenase pathway was evaluated by change in the levels of its second messenger, cyclic AMP. A modest increase in cyclic AMP contents was observed after application of bradykinin with no difference between coronary arteries with native or regenerated endothelium. Furthermore, the inhibition of cycloxygenase did not affect the amplitude of this relaxation. These results show the minor contribution of prostacyclin in the endothelium-dependent relaxation in response to bradykinin in both preparations.

The levels of cyclic GMP after exposure to bradykinin were lower in the previously denuded arteries than in the controls. When nitric oxide synthase was blocked additionally, as shown by the absence of increase in cyclic GMP levels after exposure to bradykinin, the relaxation was reduced, demonstrating a contribution of nitric oxide in both types of blood vessels.

The present study points EDHF as the major factor contributing to the relaxation induced by bradykinin in porcine coronary arteries both with native and regenerated endothelium. The hyperpolarization was not modified by the inhibition of nitric oxide synthase and cycloxygenase indicating the absence of regulation of the EDHF production by nitric oxide and prostacyclin in this preparation. Moreover, the hyperpolarization involved a participation of repolarization as demonstrated by similar hyperpolarizations in both types of preparations except when the depolarization during contraction was different. Nevertheless, for identical relative hyperpolarizations, in the presence of blockers of the production of prostacyclin and nitric oxide, the relaxation in response to bradykinin was smaller in arteries with regenerated endothelium in comparison to those with native endothelium. These findings suggest a possible reduction of the efficiency of EDHF in relaxing the injured blood vessels that could involve endogenous contracting agents.

4. CONCLUSIONS

Four weeks after balloon denudation, in porcine coronary arteries with regenerated endothelium, a major finding was the selective reduction of the production of nitric oxide. Under basal conditions, this alteration is associated with a depolarization of the smooth muscle cells. Exogenous nitric oxide could restore resting membrane potential and counteract abnormal spontaneous electrical activities in these previously denuded blood vessels.

In control vessels contracted with prostaglandin $F_{2\alpha}$, both nitric oxide and EDHF contribute to the relaxing effect of bradykinin, with a greater contribution of the latter.

In the coronary arteries with regenerated endothelium, the production of nitric oxide in response to bradykinin was reduced while the EDHF component was not changed. In contrast to the augmented endothelium-dependent hyperpolarization observed previously under basal conditions in the more depolarized previously denuded blood vessels (Thollon *et al.*, 1999a), this did not occur in the present experiments probably as a result of the further depolarization induced by the contracting agent. Nevertheless, EDHF remains the main contributor to the relaxing effect of bradykinin in coronary arteries with regenerated endothelium and this explains the maintained relaxation to this agent despite the reduced production of nitric oxide.

38 Mechanisms underlying the vasodilatation caused by bradykinin in essential hypertensive patients

Stefano Taddei, Lorenzo Ghiadoni,
Agostino Virdis, Simona Buralli
and Antonio Salvetti

In essential hypertension endothelium-dependent vasodilatation is impaired because of reduced availability of nitric oxide (NO), mainly caused by oxidative stress. The present study was designed to identify the mechanism(s) responsible for NO-independent vaso-dilatation to bradykinin in essential hypertensive patients. In healthy subjects and essential hypertensive patients modifications in forearm blood flow (strain-gauge plethysmography) were measured during the intrabrachial infusion of bradykinin in the presence of saline, N^ω-monomethyl-L-arginine (L-NMMA, to inhibit NO-synthase), and ouabain (to block Na^+K^+/ATPase and prevent hyperpolarization). In healthy subjects, the vasodilatation to bradykinin was blunted by L-NMMA and unaffected by ouabain. In essential hypertensive patients, the response to bradykinin was not modified by L-NMMA, but reduced by ouabain. When, in a further group of hypertensive patients the response to bradykinin was repeated during intrabrachial infusion of vitamin C (a scavenger for oxygen-derived free radicals), the L-NMMA-induced inhibition of the vaso-dilatation to bradykinin was restored while ouabain was no longer effective. In a final group of normotensive controls, the vasodilatation to bradykinin which resisted to L-NMMA was inhibited further by the simultaneous infusion of ouabain. These findings suggest that the vasodilatation to bradykinin is impaired in essential hypertensive patients because the production of NO is altered by oxidative stress, and that it is mediated by an alternative pathway possibly involving endothelium-dependent hyperpolarization.

After the original report by Furchgott and Zawadzki (1980) demonstrating that the endothelium releases a vasodilator substance in response to acetylcholine, it soon became clear that various relaxing and contracting factors play a role in endothelium-dependent responses (Lüscher and Vanhoutte, 1990). Probably the most important endothelium-derived relaxing factor is nitric oxide (NO), which is released from endothelial cells in response to shear stress or stimulation of different receptors on the endothelial cell surface. These stimuli increase the activity of a constitutive enzyme, NO synthase, which converts L-arginine into NO and citrulline (Moncada *et al.*, 1991). However, this substance does not universally explain endothelium-dependent relaxations. Thus in isolated blood vessels and the intact circulation, the action of endothelial vasodilators is, at least in part, resistant to inhibitors of NO synthase (Cowan and Cohen, 1991; Mügge *et al.*, 1991). An alternative mechanism is an endothelial factor that causes hyperpolarization of smooth muscle cells (Cohen and Vanhoutte, 1995), possibly mediated by an increase in conductance to potassium ions (Standen *et al.*, 1989; Edwards *et al.*, 1998), activation of the Na^+K^+/ATPase (Fèlètou and Vanhoutte, 1998; Edwards *et al.*, 1998) or inactivation of chloride channels (Fèlètou and Vanhoutte, 1998).

In healthy human subjects several agonists including acetylcholine and bradykinin, when directly injected into the brachial or coronary circulation, cause vasodilatation (Vallance *et al.*, 1989; Vita *et al.*, 1990; Kuga *et al.*, 1995) which is mainly NO-mediated and presumably endothelium-dependent since it can be inhibited by specific inhibitors of NO synthase, such as N^{ω}-monomethyl-L-arginine (L-NMMA) (Rees *et al.*, 1989). In essential hypertensive patients the response to endothelium-dependent agonists, mainly acetylcholine or bradykinin, is blunted in different vascular beds (Linder *et al.*, 1990; Panza *et al.*, 1990; Taddei *et al.*, 1993; Panza *et al.*, 1995). This diminished dilator response to acetylcholine or bradykinin is resistant to L-NMMA, indicating the presence of compromised NO-availability caused, at least for acetylcholine (Taddei *et al.*, 1998), by oxidative stress. Therefore some other mediator(s) account(s) for the dilator effects of these agents in the presence of an impaired availability of NO.

The aim of the present study was to explore the mechanisms responsible for the dilator response to bradykinin in the peripheral circulation of essential hypertensive patients.

1. METHODS

1.1. Subjects

Twenty-two healthy subjects and twenty-four matched essential hypertensive patients participated in the study (Table 38.1). Subjects with smoking history (more than five cigarettes per day), ethanol consumption (more than 60 g per day), hypercholesterolemia (total cholesterol greater than 200 mg/dl), diabetes mellitus, cardiac and/or cerebrovascular ischaemic vascular disease, impaired renal function and other major pathologies were excluded. In accordance with institutional guidelines, all patients were aware of the investigational nature of the study and gave written consent to it.

Subjects were defined as normal according to the absence of familial history of essential hypertension and blood pressure values below 140/90 mmHg (Table 38.1). Essential hypertensive patients were recruited from among newly diagnosed cases when they reported the presence of positive family history of essential hypertension and if supine arterial blood pressure (after 10 min of rest), measured by mercury sphygmomanometer three times at 1-week intervals, was consistently found to be greater than 140/90 mmHg (Table 38.1). Secondary forms of hypertension were excluded by routine diagnostic procedures. Patients were enrolled if never-treated ($n = 18$) or reporting a history of discontinued or ineffective pharmacological antihypertensive treatment ($n = 6$).

1.2. Experimental model

Vascular reactivity was assessed by the perfused forearm technique. Briefly, the brachial artery was cannulated for drug infusion at systemically ineffective rates, intraarterial blood pressure and heart rate monitoring. Forearm blood flow was measured in both forearms (experimental and contralateral forearm) by strain-gauge venous plethysmography (Whitney, 1953). Circulation to the hand was excluded 1 min before forearm blood flow measurement by inflating a pediatric cuff around the wrist

Table 38.1 Characteristics of subjects

Parameter	Normotensive subjects ($n = 22$)	Essential hypertensive patients ($n = 24$)
Age (years)	47.7 ± 5.6	48.8 ± 4.9
Sex (male/female)	17/5	18/6
Smoking (yes/no)	No	No
Body Mass Index (Kg/m^2)	21.3 ± 2.6	21.7 ± 2.9
Systolic blood pressure (mmHg)	116.9 ± 3.1	$155.3 \pm 5.1^*$
Diastolic blood pressure (mmHg)	79.1 ± 2.6	$103.4 \pm 3.6^*$
Heart rate (beats/min)	69.2 ± 5.1	71.4 ± 6.2
Plasma glucose (mg/dl)	88.5 ± 3.9	91.2 ± 5.5
Plasma total cholesterol (mg/dl)	181.7 ± 13.4	189.7 ± 10.4
Plasma HDL cholesterol (mg/dl)	44.3 ± 4.1	41.9 ± 5.3
Plasma LDL cholesterol (mg/dl)	106.3 ± 7.2	110.4 ± 8.6

Notes
HDL: High Density Lipoprotein; LDL: Low Density Lipoprotein.
The asterisks indicate statistical, significant ($p < .05$) difference between the two groups.
Data are shown as mean $\pm$ SD.

at suprasystolic blood pressure. Forearm volume was measured according to the water displacement method (Taddei *et al.*, 1993).

1.3. Study design

In eight normotensive subjects and eight essential hypertensive patients, endothelium-dependent forearm vasodilatation was evaluated by obtaining a dose–response curve to intraarterial bradykinin (cumulative increase in infusion rates: 5, 15, 50 ng/100 ml of forearm tissue/min for 5 min at each dose). Endothelium-independent vasodilatation was assessed with sodium nitroprusside (1,2 and 4 µg/100 ml of forearm tissue/min for 5 min at each dose), which acts directly on the smooth muscle cells (Schultz *et al.*, 1997).

To identify the mediator responsible for bradykinin-induced vasodilatation, the dose–response curve to the peptide was repeated in the presence of intra-arterial L-NMMA (100 µg/100 ml forearm tissue/min, an inhibitor of NO-synthase), and in the presence of intraarterial ouabain (0.7 µg/100 ml forearm tissue/min, to block $Na^+K^+/ATPase$ and thereby prevent EDHF effects on smooth muscle) (Cohen and Vanhoutte, 1995; Edwards *et al.*, 1998; Tonomura, 1986). In essential hypertensive patients, the response to sodium nitroprusside was also repeated in the presence of ouabain.

To assess whether the production of oxygen-derived free radicals can impair NO-mediated endothelium-dependent vasodilatation, thereby activating a compensatory pathway, the dose–response curve to bradykinin was performed in eight normotensive subjects and eight hypertensive patients during saline (0.2 ml/min), in the presence of L-NMMA (100 µg/100 ml forearm tissue/min) or ouabain (0.7 µg/100 ml forearm tissue/min). These three infusions were then repeated during the intra-arterial administration of vitamin C (8 mg/100 ml forearm tissue/min), an antioxidant (Frei *et al.*, 1989).

Finally, to further assess the possibility that in presence of a reduced NO-availability, a NO-independent compensatory pathway is activated, in six normotensive subjects bradykinin was infused during saline (0.2 ml/min), in the presence of L-NMMA (100 μg/100 ml forearm tissue/min) or ouabain (0.7 μg/100 ml forearm tissue/min) and in the presence of simultaneous infusion of L-NMMA and ouabain.

L-NMMA, ouabain and vitamin C were started 10 min before bradykinin and continued throughout. The sequence of L-NMMA and ouabain infusion was randomized. Thirty minutes of washout were allowed between each dose–response curve, while a 60 min period was allowed when L-NMMA was infused. These periods of time were validated in preliminary studies (data not shown).

1.4. Data analysis

Data were analyzed in terms of changes in forearm blood flow. Because arterial blood pressure did not change significantly during the study, increments in forearm blood flow were taken as evidence of local vasodilatation. The results are expressed as mean ± SD, except for the figures, where results are described as mean ± SEM. Differences between two means were compared by Student's t-test for paired or unpaired observations, as appropriate. Responses to bradykinin and sodium nitroprusside were analyzed by ANOVA for repeated measures and Scheffè's test was applied for multiple comparison testing. Differences were considered to be statistically significant when $p < .05$.

1.5. Drugs

Bradykinin HCl (Clinalfa AG, Läufelfingen, Switzerland), N^G-monomethyl-L-arginine (Clinalfa AG, Läufelfingen, Switzerland), ouabain (Ouabaine Arnaud), vitamin C (Bracco, Milan, Italy) and sodium-nitroprusside (Malesci, Milan, Italy) were obtained from commercially available sources and diluted freshly to the desired concentration by adding normal saline. Sodium nitroprusside was dissolved in glucosate solution and protected from light by aluminum foil.

2. RESULTS

Age, sex, plasma cholesterol, glycemia and smoking history were similar, and within a normal range, between the two study groups, which differed significantly only as regards arterial blood pressure (Table 38.1).

2.1. Bradykinin and sodium nitroprusside in essential hypertensive patients

The forearm blood flow increase induced by bradykinin was significantly reduced in essential hypertensive patients (from 3.0 ± 0.3 to a maximum of 14.6 ± 2.9 ml/100 ml/min) as compared to normotensive subjects (from 3.1 ± 0.3 to a maximum of 22.3 ± 3.7 ml/100 ml/min) (Figure 38.1). In contrast, vasodilatations to sodium nitroprusside were similar in normotensive subjects (from 3.1 ± 0.3 to 21.4 ± 4.8 ml/100 ml/min) and hypertensive patients (from 3.1 ± 0.3 to 21.9 ± 4.9 ml/100 ml/min) (Figure 38.1).

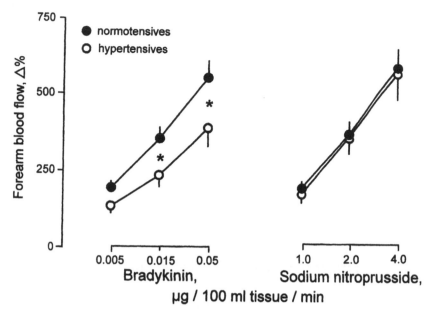

Figure 38.1 Increases in forearm blood flow (FBF) above basal induced by bradykinin and sodium nitroprusside infused at cumulative increasing rates into the brachial artery of normotensive subjects (●) and essential hypertensive patients (○). Data are shown as means ± SEM ($n = 8$) and expressed as percent increases in forearm blood flow above basal. The asterisks denote significant differences ($p < .05$) between infusion in normotensive subjects and essential hypertensive patients.

2.2. L-NMMA and ouabain and vasodilatation to bradykinin

In normotensive subjects, the L-NMMA infusion decreased basal forearm blood flow (from 3.3 ± 0.4 to 2.0 ± 0.2 ml/100 ml forearm tissue/min) and significantly blunted the vasodilator effect of bradykinin (from 2.0 ± 0.2 to 7.0 ± 1.8 ml/100 ml forearm tissue/min) while ouabain decreased basal forearm blood flow (from 3.4 ± 0.4 to 2.4 ± 0.2 ml/100 ml forearm tissue/min), but did not change the response to the agonist (from 2.4 ± 0.2 to 16.8 ± 1.8 ml/100 ml forearm tissue/min) (Figure 38.2). In essential hypertensive patients, L-NMMA, which caused a lesser decrease in forearm blood flow (from 3.2 ± 0.5 to 2.4 ± 0.2 ml/100 ml forearm tissue/min) as compared to controls (per cent decrease: 40% vs 25%, respectively), did not change the response to bradykinin (from 2.4 ± 0.2 to 12.3 ± 2.9 ml/100 ml forearm tissue/min) (Figure 38.2). In contrast, ouabain caused a decrease in forearm blood flow comparable to that with L-NMMA (from 3.0 ± 0.4 to 2.2 ± 0.2 ml/100 ml forearm tissue/min), significantly and blunted the response to bradykinin (from 2.2 ± 0.3 to 8.3 ± 1.6 ml/100 ml forearm tissue/min) (Figure 38.2). Ouabain did not alter the response to sodium nitroprusside (data not shown).

2.3. Vitamin C

In the second group of normotensive subjects, L-NMMA blunted the vasodilator effect of bradykinin (saline: from 3.6 ± 0.5 to 22.7 ± 3.7 ml/100 ml forearm tissue/min;

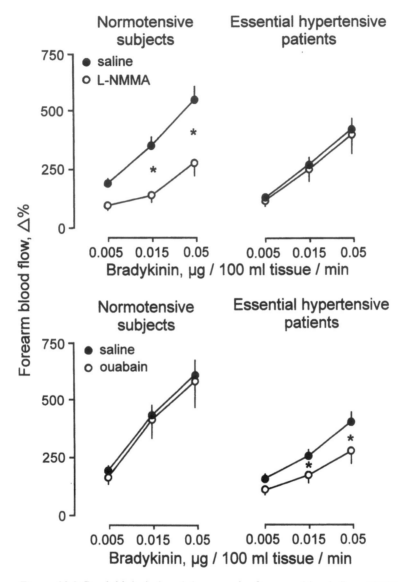

Figure 38.2 Bradykinin-induced increase in forearm blood flow (FBF) under control conditions (saline at 0.2 ml/min), in the presence of N^ω-monomethyl-L-arginine (L-NMMA, 100 μg/100 ml forearm tissue/min) or ouabain (0.7 μg/100 ml forearm tissue/min) in normotensive subjects and essential hypertensive patients. Data are shown as means ± SEM ($n = 8$) and expressed as per cent increases in forearm blood flow above basal. The asterisks denote significant differences between infusion with and without N^ω-monomethyl-L-arginine or ouabain ($p < .05$).

L-NMMA: from 2.2 ± 0.2 to 9.0 ± 1.8 ml/100 ml forearm tissue/min; per cent increase: 531 ± 58 and 309 ± 38, respectively), while ouabain was ineffective. Vitamin C infusion did not alter basal forearm blood flow or change either the response to bradykinin (from 3.7 ± 0.5 to 23.1 ± 3.2 ml/100 ml forearm tissue/min) or the

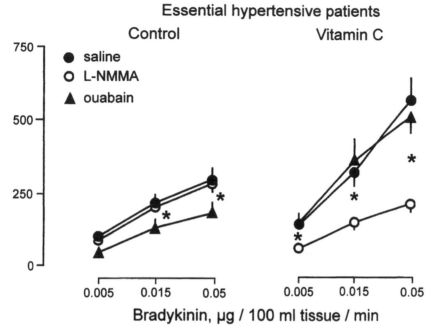

Figure 38.3 Bradykinin-induced increase in forearm blood flow (FBF) under control conditions (saline at 0.2 ml/min) (●) and in the presence of N$^{\omega}$-monomethyl-L-arginine (L-NMMA, 100 µg/100 ml forearm tissue/min) (○) or ouabain (0.7 µg/100 ml forearm tissue/min) (▲) in essential hypertensive patients before and after intra-arterial infusion of vitamin C (8 mg/100 ml tissue/min). Data are shown as means ± SEM ($n = 8$) and expressed as per cent increase above basal. The asterisks denote significant differences between infusion with and without N$^{\omega}$-monomethyl-L-arginine or ouabain ($p < .05$).

inhibiting effect of L-NMMA on vasodilatation to bradykinin (from 2.2 ± 1.0 to 10.9 ± 2.1 ml/ 100 ml forearm tissue/min). Under vitamin C, ouabain did not alter the vasodilatation to bradykinin. In the final group of hypertensive patients, L-NMMA did not change the response to bradykinin (saline: from 3.0 ± 0.5 to 11.9 ± 2.3 ml/ 100 ml forearm tissue/min; L-NMMA: from 2.3 ± 0.2 to 9.1 ± 2.2 ml/100 ml forearm tissue/min) (Figure 38.3). In contrast ouabain inhibited the response to the endothelial agonist (from 2.1 ± 0.2 to 5.9 ± 0.9 ml/100 ml forearm tissue/min) (Figure 38.3). Vitamin C increased the response to bradykinin (from 3.2 ± 0.4 to 21.5 ± 4.6 ml/100 ml forearm tissue/min) (Figure 38.3). Moreover L-NMMA, when tested again under vitamin C, significantly blunted the vasodilating effect of bradykinin (from 2.2 ± 0.2 to 7.1 ± 0.8 ml/100 ml forearm tissue/min) (Figure 38.3). During infusion of vitamin C, ouabain no longer inhibited the response to the agonist (from 2.1 ± 0.2 to 12.9 ± 2.8 ml/100 ml forearm tissue/min) (Figure 38.3).

2.4. L-NMMA plus ouabain

As in the previous series, ouabain did not change the response to bradykinin (saline: from 2.8 ± 0.4 to 18.5 ± 2.1 ml/100 ml forearm tissue/min; ouabain: from 1.9 ± 0.1 to

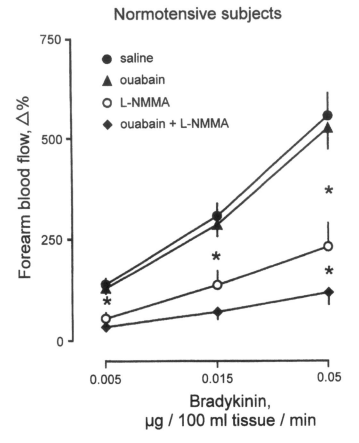

Figure 38.4 Bradykinin-induced increase in forearm blood flow (FBF) under control conditions (saline at 0.2 ml/min) (●) and in the presence of N^ω-monomethyl-L-arginine (L-NMMA, 100 μg/100 ml forearm tissue/min) (○), ouabain (0.7 μg/100 ml forearm tissue/min) (▲) or ouabain plus N^ω-monomethyl-L-arginine (◆) in normotensive subjects. Data are shown as means ± SEM ($n = 6$) and expressed as per cent increase above basal. The asterisks denote significant differences between infusion with and without N^ω-monomethyl-L-arginine or ouabain or N^ω-monomethyl-L-arginine plus ouabain ($p < .05$).

12.5 ± 1.6 ml/100 ml forearm tissue/min) while L-NMMA infusion significantly blunted the vasodilator effect of the agonist (from 1.7 ± 0.2 to 5.6 ± 0.9 ml/100 ml forearm tissue/min) (Figure 38.4). However, when the dose–response curve to bradykinin was repeated during of simultaneous administration of ouabain and L-NMMA, the vasodilatation to bradykinin was reduced (from 1.3 ± 0.2 to 2.8 ± 0.4 ml/100 ml forearm tissue/min) (Figure 38.4) to a significantly greater extent than with L-NMMA alone.

2.5. Contralateral forearm

In both normotensive subjects and essential hypertensive patients the contralateral forearm blood flow did not significantly change throughout the study (data not shown).

3. DISCUSSION

In agreement with previous evidence, the vasodilator effect of bradykinin, an endothelial agonist, but not of sodium nitroprusside, a dilator acting directly on smooth muscle cells, was blunted in hypertensive patients compared to controls (Panza *et al.*, 1995), confirming the presence of impaired endothelium-dependent vasodilatation to bradykinin in the peripheral circulation of essential hypertensive patients (Panza *et al.*, 1995). These observations further reinforce the concept of endothelial dysfunction is present in essential hypertension (Linder *et al.*, 1990; Panza *et al.*, 1990; Taddei *et al.*, 1993; Panza *et al.*, 1995; Taddei *et al.*, 1998).

In healthy subjects the vasodilator response to bradykinin was blunted by L-NMMA, an inhibitor of NO-synthase, in confirmation of earlier observations (Panza *et al.*, 1995). This finding indicates that the relaxing activity of this agonist must be predominantly mediated by activation of the L-arginine-NO pathway. This interpretation is supported by the present evidence that in normotensives ouabain, a Na^+K^+/ATPase inhibitor, did not change the response to bradykinin. In contrast in essential hypertensive patients the vasodilatation to bradykinin was resistant to L-NMMA, indicating the presence of an alteration in the L-arginine-NO pathway, leading to impaired availability of NO. On the other hand, the response to bradykinin was reduced by ouabain, at a dose that did not change the vasodilator effect of sodium nitroprusside. Taken together these results indicate that while under healthy conditions endothelium-dependent vasodilatation to bradykinin seems to be mainly dependent on NO-production, in essential hypertensive patients it is not dependent on the NO-system, but rather is related to activation of a ouabain-sensitive pathway (Figure 38.5).

Finally, when the response to bradykinin was tested in the presence of vitamin C, which probably blocks oxidative stress by a scavenger activity (Frei *et al.*, 1989), vasodilatation to the endothelial agonist and the inhibiting effect of L-NMMA was not changed in normotensive subjects, indicating that oxidative stress plays no major role in affecting endothelial responses under healthy conditions (Taddei *et al.*, 1998). In contrast, in essential hypertensive patients the response to bradykinin was significantly increased, suggesting that, in line with the results observed with acetyl-choline (Taddei *et al.*, 1998; Solzbach *et al.*, 1997), oxidative stress may be the main mechanism leading to impaired vasodilatation to bradykinin in essential hypertension. During administration of vitamin C the inhibitor effect of L-NMMA was restored while ouabain proved no longer effective in blunting the response to bradykinin. These results indicate that in essential hypertensive patients the vasodilatation to bradykinin depends mainly on an ouabain-dependent pathway when NO activity is impaired because of the presence of oxidative stress (Figure 38.5).

This possibility is further reinforced by the study evaluating the effect of ouabain on the vasodilatation to bradikynin resistant to L-NMMA blockade in healthy subjects. In this situation of decreased NO availability, ouabain, although ineffective when tested under control conditions, produced a further decrease in the response to bradykinin. Therefore, these findings suggest that in the peripheral human circulation an ouabain-sensitive pathway may operate as a rapid compensatory mechanism for a decreased NO activity.

Although the present study does not allow identification of the exact nature of the ouabain-sensitive pathway, the following line of evidence supports the hypothesis that this compensatory pathway could be related to hyperpolarization. Thus, in animal

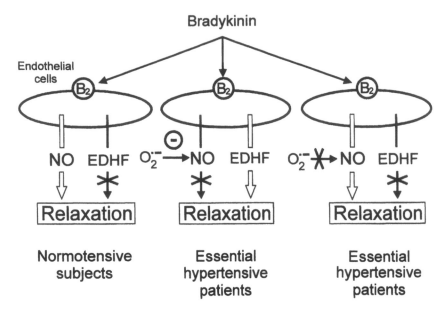

Figure 38.5 Mechanisms involved in the response to bradykinin in the human peripheral circulation. In healthy subjects NO almost completely accounts for endothelium-dependent vasodilatation to bradykinin. In essential hypertensive patients oxidative stress impairs the availability of NO. Thus an ouabain-sensitive pathway (EDHF?) is activated as a compensatory mechanism. When oxidative stress is blocked, the availability of NO is restored and, as a consequence, the ouabain-sensitive pathway is inhibited. B_2: B_2-kinin receptor; EDHF: endothelium-derived hyperpolarizing factor.

isolated blood vessels and the intact circulation, when the action of endothelium-dependent vasodilators is, at least in part, resistant to inhibitors of NO-synthase (Cohen and Vanhoutte, 1995), as was the case in the hypertensive population, hyperpolarization accounts for endothelium-dependent relaxation (Vanhoutte *et al.*, 1996). Moreover bradykinin-dependent EDHF production has been demonstrated in human coronary arteries from transplant hearts (Nakashima *et al.*, 1993). Finally, *in vitro* studies suggest that NO can inhibit the release of EDHF evoked by bradykinin (Olmos and Vanhoutte, 1995; Bauersachs *et al.*, 1996). These findings are in agreement with our present results in humans indicating that the ouabain-sensitive pathway can be detected in both normotensive subjects and hypertensive patients only when the NO system is not active.

Ouabain blocks $Na^+K^+/ATPase$ (Schultz *et al.*, 1997), but it is uncertain whether or not EDHF acts through activation of this pump (Cohen and Vanhoutte, 1995; Vanhoutte *et al.*, 1996). It is more likely that ouabain, by depolarizing the cell membrane, non-specifically inhibits the smooth muscle to EDHF (Cohen and Vanhoutte, 1995; Edwards *et al.*, 1998).

4. CONCLUSIONS

The present results indicate that in human peripheral circulation vasodilatation to bradykinin is mediated mainly by NO, since it can be blocked by L-NMMA.

In essential hypertensive patients, the availability of NO is impaired since the vaso-dilatation to bradykinin is resistant to L-NMMA. In these patients an alternative compensatory pathway sensitive to ouabain is activated acutely. The possibility exists that this compensatory mechanism could be related to the production of EDHF.

39 Influence of diabetes on endothelium-dependent responses in mesenteric and femoral arteries of rats

Susan J. Wigg, Marianne Tare, Richard C. O'Brien and Helena C. Parkington

The impact of diabetes on endothelium-dependent hyperpolarization and relaxation was compared in mesenteric and femoral arteries of rats in which the functional complement of endothelial vasodilators is different. Arteries, 200–300 μm in diameter, obtained from rats following eight weeks of streptozotocin-induced diabetes and from their age-matched euglycaemic controls, were mounted on a Mulvany-style myograph. Using conventional intracellular glass microelectrodes, the cell membrane potential was measured, simultaneously with isometric tension, in arteries depolarized and constricted with phenylephrine. Acetylcholine evoked relaxation in mesenteric and femoral arteries of control rats and the hyperpolarization was ten-fold larger in the mesenteric than in the femoral arteries. N^ω-nitro-L-arginine methylester (L-NAME) abolished the responses in the femoral artery and shifted the concentration–response curves to the right in mesenteric artery, although maximal hyperpolarization and relaxation were still achieved. Indomethacin had no effect in either artery. Diabetes was without effect on the responses in the femoral artery. Although the maximal relaxation was unaltered in the mesenteric artery, the pD_2 for acetylcholine was shifted significantly to the right in the diabetics and the maximal hyperpolarization was reduced by half. The shift in the relaxation curve to the right by L-NAME was the same as in the controls and the maximal amplitudes of the hyperpolarization and relaxation were reduced to 19 and 58%, respectively. Vitamin E for 8 weeks preserved the nitric oxide-dependent relaxations in both control and diabetic mesenteric arteries but impaired the EDHF-dependent responses, particularly in the arteries from euglycaemic animals.

Endothelium-dependent vasodilatation is impaired in diabetes. Both human and animal studies suggest that the impact of diabetes on endothelial function varies significantly according to the vascular bed studied.

Most studies of vessels from rats in which diabetes mellitus had been induced by streptozotocin have focussed on the mesenteric arterial bed where endothelium-dependent relaxation to acetylcholine is impaired. Evidence to elucidate the contributions of the different endothelium-dependent vasodilators, namely nitric oxide, prostanoid and endothelium-derived hyperpolarizing factor (EDHF), to this impairment of endothelial function in diabetes is still evolving.

The increased risk of vascular disease in diabetes is not fully explained by known cardiovascular risk factors. There is accumulating evidence that advanced glycation of proteins and oxidation and glycation of circulating lipoproteins are important in the pathogenesis of diabetic vasculopathy.

1. VASODILATOR ABNORMALITIES IN DIABETES

1.1. The relative contributions of nitric oxide, prostanoid and EDHF in endothelial impairment in diabetes

1.1.1. Variability between vascular beds

Early animal studies of the impact of diabetes on endothelial vasodilator function mostly examined conduit arteries such as the aorta and yielded conflicting results, with some demonstrating impairment of endothelium-dependent relaxation (Kamata *et al.*, 1989; Cameron and Cotter, 1992) and others finding no change (Ralevic *et al.*, 1993). This inconsistency suggests that the effect of diabetes on endothelial vasodilator function may vary with the vascular preparation used, the animal model and the duration of diabetes.

Human studies also revealed variability between vascular beds. *In vitro* studies have demonstrated vasodilator impairment in the corpora cavernosa of impotent men (deTejada *et al.*, 1989) and in isolated subcutaneous arteries (McNally *et al.*, 1994). However, the results of *in vivo* studies vary, with some showing impaired vasodilatation in the forearm resistance circulation of patients with type 1 and type 2 diabetes (Williams *et al.*, 1996; Ting *et al.*, 1996), while others have reported preserved endothelial function (Calver *et al.*, 1992; Elliott *et al.*, 1993).

In non-diabetic animals, different arteries may rely on different suites of vasodilators for relaxation, and different agonists stimulate the release of different vasodilators from endothelial cells. For example, endothelium-dependent relaxations evoked by acetylcholine in the femoral artery of rats is almost entirely dependent on nitric oxide whereas the mesenteric artery in that species relies on both nitric oxide and EDHF (Zygmunt *et al.*, 1995; Fukao *et al.*, 1997). Furthermore, bradykinin stimulates the release of predominantly nitric oxide in mesenteric arteries (Taylor *et al.*, 1995).

1.1.2. Resistance arteries

Studies of resistance arteries in animal models of diabetes, such as mesenteric arteries in streptozotocin-induced diabetic rats, generally demonstrate impaired endothelium-dependent vasodilatation in response to acetylcholine. While some suggest that a reduction of nitric oxide bioavailability is responsible for this impairment (Taylor *et al.*, 1992; Abiru *et al.*, 1993), other studies demonstrate that nitric oxide bioavailability is unchanged or may even be increased in this arterial bed (Diederich *et al.*, 1994; Heygate *et al.*, 1996). Nitric oxide may mediate the increases in regional blood flow and vascular permeability seen early in diabetic complications. A decrease in EDHF may be the most significant vasodilator abnormality in diabetes (Fukao *et al.*, 1997; Wigg *et al.*, 2000; Makino *et al.*, 2000). Prostacyclin is generally regarded as playing no significant role in relaxation of mesenteric arteries (Taylor *et al.*, 1992; Diederich *et al.*, 1994; Fukao *et al.*, 1997).

Direct comparison of mesenteric and femoral arteries of streptozotocin-induced diabetic rats (8 weeks) demonstrates the role of EDHF in diabetic endothelium-dependent vasodilator dysfunction. While the relaxation evoked by acetylcholine in the mesenteric artery, which involves both nitric oxide and EDHF, is impaired, the

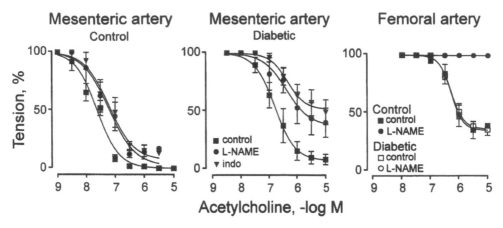

Figure 39.1 In mesenteric and femoral arteries constricted with phenylephrine, discrete 2-min applications of acetylcholine induced endothelium-dependent relaxation. In mesenteric arteries: The curve was shifted to the right in tissues obtained from diabetic rats, compared with euglycaemic controls. N^ω-nitro-L-arginine methylester (L-NAME, 10^{-4} M) caused a greater rightward shift in the curves from diabetic compared with control tissues. Indomethacin (10^{-6} M plus L-NAME) was without significant effect. In femoral arteries: The concentration–relaxation curves from diabetic and control tissues were superimposed. Relaxations were abolished by L-NAME.

response in the femoral artery, which relies on nitric oxide alone, is not (Figure 39.1 and Table 39.1). When bradykinin, which releases predominantly nitric oxide (Taylor *et al.*, 1992), is used to stimulate the endothelium of the mesenteric artery, there is no difference in endothelium-dependent relaxations between mesenteric arteries of diabetic and control rats. This suggests that, in these arteries, in this rat model at least, the endothelial impairment in diabetes is most pronounced in situations in which EDHF contributes substantially to endothelium-dependent responses (e.g., acetylcholine-induced stimulation of mesenteric artery). Nitric

Table 39.1

	Control	*Diabetic*
Mesenteric artery		
Control	7.61 ± 0.06	6.81 ± 0.12
L-NAME	7.21 ± 0.10	6.40 ± 0.32
L-NAME + indomethacin	7.20 ± 0.08	6.36 ± 0.20
Femoral artery		
Control	6.28 ± 0.09	6.27 ± 0.05
L-NAME		

Notes
The values of pD_2 ($-\log EC_{50}$) for acetylcholine-induced relaxation of phenylephrine-constricted mesenteric and femoral arteries ($n = 5$ in each group) obtained from euglycaemic control and diabetic rats. Data shown as means $\pm$ SEM. L-NAME: N^ω-nitro-L-arginine methylester.

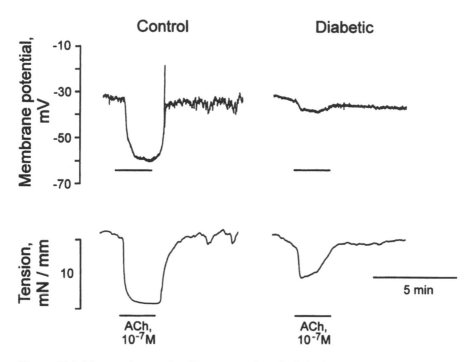

Figure 39.2 Mesenteric arteries from control and diabetic rats were depolarized and constricted with phenylephrine. Acetylcholine evoked a pronounced (up to 30 mV) hyperpolarization and relaxation in the control tissue and these responses were severely impaired in the tissue from the diabetic animal. (The responses shown were recorded in the presence of N^{ω}-nitro-L-arginine methylester (L-NAME, 10^{-4} M) plus indomethacin (10^{-6} M)).

oxide-dependent relaxation (e.g., acetylcholine-induced responses in the femoral artery and bradykinin-induced relaxation in the mesenteric artery) appears to resist the effects of diabetes.

Hyperpolarization to acetylcholine, attributed to EDHF when measured in the presence of L-NAME and indomethacin to block nitric oxide and prostacyclin production, respectively, was reduced significantly (Figure 39.2). The maximal amplitude of hyperpolarization in mesenteric arteries of diabetic animals was only 19% of the response observed in tissues of control rats. These electrophysiological data support the role of reduced EDHF in the endothelial dysfunction associated with diabetes.

2. MECHANISMS OF IMPAIRED ENDOTHELIUM-DEPENDENT VASODILATOR FUNCTION IN DIABETES

2.1. Glucose dependent metabolic processes

A number of mechanisms have been proposed to explain the abnormal endothelial function in diabetes, in terms of hyperglycemia *per se*. Glucose-dependent biochemical processes such as the polyol pathway (which converts glucose to sorbitol via aldose reductase), oxygen derived free radicals, increased protein kinase C, reduced sodium–potassium ATPase activity and advanced glycation of proteins have all been implicated in the pathogenesis of diabetic vasodilator dysfunction.

2.2. Advanced glycation

2.2.1. *Advanced glycation end products*

Glucose reacts non-enzymatically with amino groups of amino or nucleic acids in a process known as non-enzymatic glycosylation. The initial products of this reaction (Schiff bases) are rearranged to form early glycation products (Amidori products such as haemoglobin A1c). These are in equilibrium with their precursors, and the levels therefore tend to rise and fall depending on the ambient glucose concentration. Amidori products are gradually degraded into reactive carbonyl compounds, which can further react with free amino groups to form irreversible glucose-derived cross-links that accumulate. These advanced glycation end products accumulate on long-lived proteins, such as collagen and elastin, during normal aging and this process is accelerated in diabetes. Advanced glycation end products are increased in a variety of tissues in experimentally induced diabetes in rats (Soulis-Liparota *et al.*, 1991) and in human diabetes (Monnier *et al.*, 1986). Advanced glycation causes marked changes in the structure and function of proteins, and tissue concentrations of advanced glycation end products have been shown to correlate with the severity of diabetic microvascular complications (Monnier *et al.*, 1986).

The principal means through which advanced glycation end products exert their cellular effects is via specific cellular receptors, one of which, advanced glycation end product receptor (RAGE) is expressed in endothelium. Blockade of RAGE inhibits the impairment of endothelial barrier function induced by advanced glycation end products and largely reverses the early vascular hyperpermeability observed in streptozotocin-induced diabetic rats (Wautier *et al.*, 1996). In addition, advanced glycated collagen covalently traps low-density lipoproteins, which are then susceptible to oxidative modification. Oxidized low-density lipoproteins are chemo-attractant to circulating monocytes and are cytotoxic, with the potential to damage endothelial cells. Furthermore, the cross-links between advanced glycation end products and arterial collagen decrease arterial elasticity and may therefore contribute to the structural abnormality of arteries in diabetes (O'Brien and Timmins, 1994).

2.2.2. *Aminoguanidine*

Aminoguanidine is a phenylhydrazine derivative that inhibits advanced glycosylation and reduces the excessive accumulation of advanced glycation end products in diabetes (Soulis-Liparota *et al.*, 1991). Aminoguanidine also selectively inactivates the inducible isoform of nitric oxide synthase (Wolff *et al.*, 1995) and furthermore inhibits aldose reductase (Kumari *et al.*, 1991) and diamine oxidase, and reduces the uptake by macrophages of oxidatively damaged low-density lipoproteins (Picard *et al.*, 1992). Aminoguanidine may prevent or ameliorate many of the functional complications of diabetes, such as diabetes-induced vascular dysfunction in the retina (Tilton *et al.*, 1990), peripheral nerves (Cameron and Cotter, 1992), the aorta (Bucala *et al.*, 1991) and the kidneys (Ido *et al.*, 1990). Other functional complications of diabetes reduced by aminoguanidine include albuminuria (Soulis-Liparota *et al.*, 1991), early structural changes in the arterial wall (Tilton *et al.*, 1992), and electrophysiological changes in peripheral nerves (Kihara *et al.*, 1991). The prevention of diabetic complications by aminoguanidine appears to relate to the duration of treatment. (Soulis *et al.*, 1996). There is also evidence that aminoguanidine may reverse experimental diabetic nephropathy (Soulis *et al.*, 1996).

Despite this variety of evidence demonstrating the beneficial effects of aminoguanidine in the prevention of diabetic vascular complications, treatment of streptozotocin-induced diabetic rats with aminoguanidine for 8 or 32 weeks did not prevent the impairment of endothelium-dependent relaxation to acetylcholine in mesenteric arteries. However, treatment of control rats did prevent the age-related impairment in endothelium-dependent vasodilatation.

2.3. Oxidative Stress

2.3.1. Oxidant stress in diabetes

Diabetes is a state of increased oxidant stress resulting from increased free radical generation, decreased circulating antioxidant concentrations, and probably also impaired regeneration of the reduced forms of antioxidants. Free radicals can cause cellular damage directly via effects on DNA, and indirectly via oxidation of lipids in the arterial wall and also via advanced glycation of long-lived proteins. Inhibition of the hyperpermeability induced by advanced glycation end products and diabetes by antioxidants suggests the central role of advanced glycation end products in RAGE induced oxidant stress in the development of diabetic complications (Wautier *et al.*, 1996). Oxidized low-density lipoproteins can impair endothelium-dependent relaxation of arteries and decrease the expression of endothelial nitric oxide synthase. Several studies suggest that antioxidants such as vitamins E, C and β-carotene reduce the susceptibility of low-density lipoproteins to oxidative modification (Reavan *et al.*, 1993).

2.3.2. Antioxidant supplementation and vascular disease

Antioxidant supplementation may be of benefit to vascular function. Large, randomized, placebo controlled clinical trials demonstrate benefit from vitamin E (Stephens *et al.*, 1996) and β-carotene (Gaziano *et al.*, 1990) in preventing cardiovascular events in patients with previous cardiovascular disease. However, the HOPE trial, a large study of almost 10,000 patients (approximately 40% with diabetes) with cardiovascular disease, showed no significant benefit from vitamin E supplementation (400 IU daily) in the secondary prevention of cardiovascular events (Yusuf *et al.*, 2000). A much smaller study demonstrated that vitamin E supplementation (1000 IU daily for 3 months) normalized impaired endothelium-dependent vasodilatation in patients with insulin-dependent diabetes, as measured by the flow-dependent dilatation of the brachial artery evoked by acetylcholine (Skyrme-Jones *et al.*, 2000).

In the streptozotocin-induced diabetic rat, antioxidant supplementation may improve endothelium-dependent vasodilatation in conduit arteries (Keegan *et al.*, 1995) and endoneurial blood flow (Cotter *et al.*, 1995). Incubation of diabetic rat mesenteric arteries with the free radical scavengers superoxide dismutase and

1,3-dimethyl-2-thiourea significantly improved the relaxation evoked by acetylcholine, whereas pretreatment with an inhibitor of protein kinase C did not (Diederich *et al.*, 1994).

In mesenteric arteries of streptozotocin-induced diabetic rats, studies examining the effect of vitamin E on endothelium-dependent vasodilatation show conflicting results, which may be due to differences in the dose used and/or the duration of the treatment. Vitamin E supplementation at a dose of 250 mg/kg for 4 weeks made no difference to the impairment of endothelium-dependent relaxation to acetylcholine, while 500 mg/kg for 4 weeks significantly increased this impairment when compared with arteries of

Table 39.2

	Control	Diabetic
No treatment		
Control	7.63 ± 0.29	7.10 ± 0.06
L-NAME + indomethacin	7.36 ± 0.20	6.50 ± 0.14
Vitamin E (1 g/kg/day)		
Control	7.38 ± 0.03	7.05 ± 0.11
L-NAME + indomethacin	6.68 ± 0.06	5.82 ± 0.21

Notes
The values of pD_2 ($- \log EC_{50}$) for acetylcholine-induced relaxations of phenylephrine-constricted mesenteric arteries ($n = 4-6$ in each group) obtained from euglycaemic control and diabetic rats, with and without treatment with vitamin E. Data shown as means $\pm$ SEM. L-NAME: N^{ω}-nitro-L-arginine methylester.

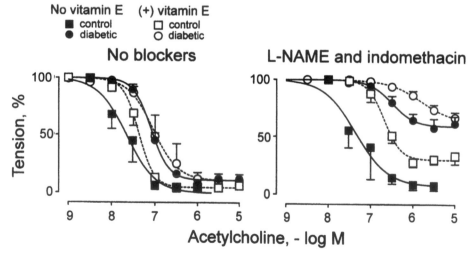

Figure 39.3 In mesenteric arteries constricted with phenylephrine, discrete 2-min applications of acetylcholine induced endothelium-dependent relaxation. In tissues from both diabetic and control rats, vitamin E treatment was without effect on the concentration–relaxation curves in the absence of blockers. The curves attributed to EDHF (obtained in the presence of N^{ω}-nitro-L-arginine methylester (L-NAME, 10^{-4} M) plus indomethacin (10^{-6} M) were shifted to the right by vitamin E treatment.

diabetic rats fed a standard chow (Palmer *et al.*, 1998). Combination of vitamin E (250 mg/kg) and vitamin C (250 mg/kg) in that study did not improve the endothelium-dependent vasodilator response to acetylcholine but did worsen endothelium-independent responses to sodium nitroprusside. A higher dose of vitamin E (1 g/kg rat daily) for 8 weeks did not change the endothelium-dependent relaxation to acetylcholine in mesenteric arteries of diabetic rats (Figure 39.3 and Table 39.2). This study suggested that treatment with vitamin E preserves nitric oxide-dependent relaxation but impairs EDHF responses in mesenteric arteries. Vitamin E supplementation made no significant difference to endothelium-dependent relaxations in femoral arteries. Thus, intervention studies may be deleterious to selected components of endothelium-dependent relaxation.

3. CONCLUSION

Variability between arterial beds, between species and in the suite of relaxants released from endothelial cells by different stimulants contribute to the uncertainty in the understanding of endothelial dysfunction in diabetes. It appears that reduced nitric oxide bioavailability may not be the only, or even the major reason for endothelial impairment in diabetes. A reduced effectiveness of EDHF is evident, at least in the mesenteric artery of rats in which diabetes has been induced with streptozotocin. The continued uncertainty regarding the nature of EDHF complicates a resolution of endothelial dysfunction in diabetes. In addition, it would appear that interventions such as vitamin administration must be approached with caution, since observations with vitamin E suggest that, while it may preserve one component of endothelium-dependent vasodilator function, it may be deleterious to others.

ACKNOWLEDGEMENTS

The authors thank Ms M.A. Tonta for technical assistance. This work was supported by the National Health & Medical Research Council and the National Heart Foundation of Australia.

40 Folate restores the NO synthase- and cyclooxygenase-resistant renal vasodilator response to acetylcholine in diabetes

A.S. De Vriese, Johan Van de Voorde, Paul M. Vanhoutte and N.H. Lameire

Impaired endothelium-dependent relaxations have been reported in different types of blood vessels of different animal models of diabetes. The majority of the studies were performed *in vitro* in conduit arteries, and endothelial dysfunction was generally attributed to a reduced bioavailability of endothelium-derived nitric oxide (EDNO). Little attention has been paid to endothelium-dependent responses in the microcirculation in diabetes and in particular to the role of endothelium-derived hyperpolarizing factor (EDHF). The present study investigates endothelium-dependent vasodilator responses *in vivo* in the renal microcirculation of rats with streptozotocin-induced diabetes. Total renal blood flow was measured with an electromagnetic flow probe placed on the renal artery and the segmental responses of the renal microcirculation were evaluated with videomicroscopy, using the split hydronephrotic kidney technique. The N^G-nitro-L-arginine methyl ester (L-NAME)- and indomethacin-resistant rise in renal blood flow to intrarenal acetylcholine was significantly reduced in the diabetic versus control rats, suggesting impaired EDHF-mediated vasodilatation. The vasodilatations to the NO donor detaNONOate and to the K^+-channel opener pinacidil were similar in diabetic and control animals, indicating intact endothelium-independent vasodilator mechanisms. In the hydronephrotic kidney, the L-NAME- and indomethacin-resistant component of the vasodilatation to acetylcholine increased as vessel size decreased. In diabetic rats, the impairment of the response to acetylcholine was most pronounced in the smallest vessels. Administration of 5-methyltetrahydrofolate, the active form of folate, normalized the L-NAME- and indomethacin-resistant vasodilatation in diabetes, suggesting a potential role for folate in the prevention of diabetic microvascular disease.

Worldwide, the prevalence of diabetes has been rising over the past few decades. Currently, about 4% of the population in Europe and in the United States have diabetes. Macro- and microvascular disease, including diabetic nephropathy, are the principal causes of morbidity and mortality in these patients and account for more than 80% of the health budget spent on diabetes (Ismail *et al.*, 1999). Despite intensive research, the possibilities for prevention and treatment of diabetic vascular complications are limited.

Loss of the modulatory role of the endothelium may be a critical and initiating factor in the development of diabetic vascular disease. The presence of endothelial dysfunction, in the absence of obstructive vascular disease, is associated with an increased incidence of cardiac events (Suwaidi *et al.*, 2000).

Endothelial integrity is generally assessed by evaluating the vasodilator response of a blood vessel or a vascular bed to an endothelium-dependent agonist (Nagao *et al.*, 1992). Impaired endothelium-dependent relaxations have been reported in different types of blood vessels of different animal models of diabetes (De Vriese *et al.*, 2000a). The majority of the studies were performed in large conduit arteries such as the aorta, and the endothelial dysfunction was generally attributed to a reduced production or increased inactivation of endothelium-derived NO, or to an overproduction of endothelium-derived vasoconstrictors. Information concerning endothelial cell dysfunction in the diabetic microvasculature is more limited. In particular, little attention has been paid to the potential role of an impaired release or action of endothelium-derived hyperpolarizing factor (EDHF) in diabetes.

A better understanding of the pathophysiology of diabetic endothelial dysfunction may enable the development of therapies to modify the natural history of diabetic vascular disease. Although strict glycemic control (The Diabetes Control and Complications Trial Research Group, 2000) and rigorous antihypertensive treatment (UK Prospective Diabetes Study Group, 1998) prevent or delay the occurrence of microvascular complications, these measures may not be sufficient in some patients. There is, therefore, a need for additional preventive and therapeutic measures.

Administration of folate improves impaired endothelial function associated with hypercholesterolemia (Verhaar *et al.*, 1998, 1999) and with hyperhomocysteinemia (Usui *et al.*, 1999), two conditions characterized by increased oxidative stress. The beneficial effects of folate were independent of its homocysteine-lowering properties. Folate may reduce the generation of superoxide anions (Verhaar *et al.*, 1998). These observations raise the possibility that the beneficial effect of folate might be extended to other pathologies associated with endothelial dysfunction and increased oxidative stress, including diabetes.

Against this background, the present *in vivo* study examined the different components of the endothelium-dependent vasodilator response in the renal microcirculation of streptozotocin-induced diabetic rats. The influence of acute administration of 5-methyltetrahydrofolate (5-MTHF), the active form of folate, on endothelium-dependent vasodilatation was investigated.

1. MATERIALS AND METHODS

1.1. Laboratory animals

The studies were performed in female Wistar rats (Iffa Credo, Brussels, Belgium) receiving care in accordance with NIH and national guidelines for animal protection. Diabetes was induced by the intravenous injection of streptozotocin 65 mg/kg. Slow release insulin pellets with a release rate of 1 U/24 h were implanted. Experiments were performed 6 weeks later. In the rats with a hydronephrotic kidney, diabetes was induced 8 weeks after the ligature to the ureter. During each experiment, plasma samples were drawn for analysis of glucose, fructosamine, total protein, cholesterol and total homocysteine levels.

1.2. Measurement of total renal blood flow

The rats were anesthetized with thiobutabarbital 100 mg/kg intraperitoneally. The trachea was intubated. The right jugular vein was cannulated for the continuous infusion of isotonic saline (3 ml/h) and administration of drugs, and the right carotid artery was cannulated for the continuous monitoring of mean arterial blood pressure. The right suprarenal artery was cannulated for the intrarenal administration of drugs. A blood flow sensor with an inner diameter of 0.6–0.8 mm was placed on the right renal artery, allowing continuous renal blood flow monitoring by an electromagnetic square wave flow meter (Skalar Medical, Delft, The Netherlands) (Verbeke et al., 1999).

The renal blood flow response to intrarenal acetylcholine (0.1–50 ng, in bolus) was examined in diabetic ($n = 8$) and age-matched control rats ($n = 8$), before and after the intravenous administration of N^G-nitro-L-arginine methyl ester (L-NAME 10 mg/ kg in bolus, followed by 20 mg/kg/h) plus indomethacin (4 mg/kg in bolus, followed by 8 mg/kg/h). Before administration of the next dose of acetylcholine, renal blood flow was allowed to return to baseline values. The renal blood flow response to intrarenal detaNONOate (16–112 µg, in bolus) and pinacidil (25–175 µg, in bolus) was examined in diabetic ($n = 8$) and control rats ($n = 8$), before and after intravenous administration of L-NAME plus indomethacin. The renal blood flow response to intrarenal acetylcholine after intravenous administration of L-NAME plus indomethacin was examined before and 15 min after an intravenous bolus of 5-MTHF (200 µg in 0.5 ml saline) in diabetic ($n = 8$) and control rats ($n = 8$), and before and after a bolus of 0.5 ml saline without 5-MTHF in diabetic rats ($n = 8$).

1.3. Intravital microscopy of the hydronephrotic kidney

After anesthesia with halothane (Fluothane; Zeneca, Destelbergen, Belgium) a unilateral hydronephrosis was induced by a permanent ligation of the left ureter (Steinhausen et al., 1983; De Vriese et al., 1999). About 8 to 10 weeks following the induction of hydronephrosis, the renal parenchyma has become a thin translucent tissue sheet due to tubular atrophy. The microcirculation remains, however, intact (Steinhausen and Endlich, 1993; Nobiling et al., 1986) and is accessible for study by intravital microscopy. For the final experiments, the rats were anesthetized with thiobutabarbital. The hydronephrotic kidney was exposed by a left flank incision and split with a thermal cautery along its greater curvature. The ventral half of the kidney was sutured to a semicircular frame and attached to the bottom of an organ chamber in plexiglass. The entry of the renal hilus into the chamber was sealed with silicone grease. The chamber was filled with an isotonic, isocolloidal solution maintained at 37°C. Glomeruli and renal vessels were visualized by transillumination microscopy (Axiotech Vario 100 HD; Zeiss, Jena, Germany) using water immersion objectives (Achroplan 10×, 40×, 63×). The resulting image was recorded by a high-speed video camera (Kodak Motioncorder Analyser; Eastman Kodak Company, San Diego, CA, USA) and forwarded to the videorecorder (S-VHS Panasonic AG-7355), either on-line or from the memory of the camera. Luminal diameters and red blood cell velocities were analysed off-line, with image analysis software (Cap-Image; Ingenieurbüro Zeintl, Heidelberg, Germany). For red blood cell velocity measurements, sequences were recorded with the high-speed camera at a rate of 600 fps and forwarded to the videorecorder at a rate of 25 fps. The sequences were thus slowed with a factor of 24, allowing analysis of the red blood cell velocities with the line-shift-diagram method (De Vriese et al., 2000b). The luminal diameters of the following vascular segments were measured: proximal arcuate artery (45–55 µm), distal arcuate artery (35–45 µm), proximal interlobular artery (20–25 µm), distal interlobular artery

(10–15 μm), proximal afferent arteriole (8–12 μm), distal afferent arteriole (6–9 μm), proximal efferent arteriole (8–12 μm), distal efferent arteriole (15–25 μm). Red blood cell velocity (V_{RBC}) was measured in the efferent arteriole, and glomerular blood flow (GBF) was calculated from the equation: GBF = $V_{RBC} \times \pi D^2/4$, where D = luminal diameter. Acetylcholine (10^{-5} M) was added to the organ chamber before and after administration of L-NAME (10^{-4} M) plus indomethacin (10^{-3} M) in diabetic ($n = 6$) and control rats ($n = 6$).

1.4. Drugs

Acetylcholine (Sigma Chemical Co, St. Louis, MO, USA)
DetaNONOate (Alexis, Grünberg, Germany)
Indomethacin (Sigma)
5-methyltetrahydrofolate (5-MTHF, Sigma)
N^G-nitro-L-arginine methyl ester (L-NAME, Sigma)
Pinacidil (Sigma)
Slow release insulin pellets (Linshin, Scarborough, Canada)
Streptozotocin (Pfanstiel, Davenham, UK)
Thiobutabarbital (Inactin, RBI, Natick, USA).

1.5. Statistical analysis

The data are presented as mean ± SEM. The renal blood flow response to the different agonists is expressed as the area under the curve of the change in renal blood flow (ml/min × min). The changes of vascular diameters and of glomerular blood flow are expressed as percentage changes from control values. Analysis of variance or Student's t-tests of paired and unpaired observations were used as appropriate. When p was less than .05, differences were considered to be statistically significant.

2. RESULTS

As compared to the age-matched control rats, diabetic animals had significantly lower body weights (242 ± 4 and 270 ± 4 g, respectively) and higher plasma glucose (455.1 ± 28.9 and 164.3 ± 8.3 mg/dl, respectively) and fructosamine levels (3.36 ± 0.18 and 1.78 ± 0.08 μmol/g total protein, respectively). Mean arterial blood pressure (119.1 ± 2.2 and 121.4 ± 4.0 mmHg, respectively) and plasma cholesterol (74.6 ± 3.4 and 70.3 ± 2.8 mg/dl, respectively) were not significantly different between diabetic and control rats. Plasma total homocysteine was significantly lower in diabetic than in control animals (6.0 ± 0.4 and 8.3 ± 0.5 μmol/l, respectively). Homocysteine levels were not significantly different before and after the administration of 5-MTHF, whether in control (8.9 ± 0.6 and 9.3 ± 0.6 μmol/l, respectively) or in diabetic rats (6.0 ± 0.2 and 6.3 ± 0.9 μmol/l, respectively).

2.1. Total renal blood flow

The infusion of L-NAME plus indomethacin increased blood pressure with significantly more in control rats (28.7 ± 2.9%, $n = 24$) than in diabetic rats

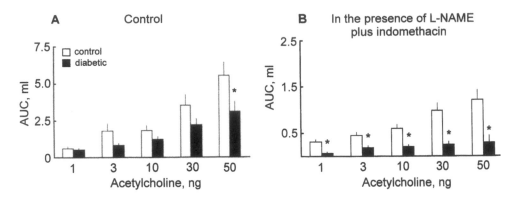

Figure 40.1 The renal blood flow response to intrarenally administered acetylcholine in control (open bars) and diabetic rats (full bars) before (A) and after (B) administration of L-NAME (10 mg/kg in bolus, followed by 20 mg/kg/h) plus indomethacin (4 mg/kg in bolus, followed by 8 mg/kg/h). The area under the curve (AUC) of the change from baseline values was calculated for each bolus acetylcholine. Data are shown as mean ± SEM. The asterisks indicate statistically significant differences.

($20.2 \pm 1.6\%$, $n = 32$). Basal renal blood flow was significantly higher in diabetic than in control rats (4.21 ± 0.14 ml/min and 3.79 ± 0.09 ml/min, respectively). After systemic administration of L-NAME plus indomethacin, renal blood flow was not different in diabetic and control animals (2.73 ± 0.14 ml/min and 2.70 ± 0.08 ml/min, respectively).

In diabetic animals, the global renal blood flow response to acetylcholine was not significantly different from that in control rats, except at the highest acetylcholine dose (Figure 40.1A). The residual L-NAME- and indomethacin-resistant responses to all doses of acetylcholine were significantly lower in diabetic than in control rats (Figure 40.1B).

2.2. Intravital microscopy

The local application of acetylcholine, L-NAME and indomethacin in the organ chamber had no significant effects on arterial blood pressure. The basal vascular diameters and glomerular blood flow were higher in diabetic rats as compared to control rats. After the local administration of L-NAME plus indomethacin, the vascular diameters and the glomerular blood flow were not different in diabetic and control animals (data not shown). In control rats, the vasodilatation to acetylcholine was most pronounced in the smallest preglomerular arterioles, whereas the larger preglomerular vessels and the distal efferent arterioles dilated only moderately in response to acetylcholine (Figure 40.2A). The vasodilatation to acetylcholine was impaired in the diabetic kidneys, with the most pronounced deficit in the smallest preglomerular vessels (Figure 40.2A). The increase in glomerular blood flow in response to acetylcholine was less pronounced in the diabetic animals as compared to control rats ($73.9 \pm 6.9\%$ and $106.0 \pm 9.6\%$, respectively). The local administration of L-NAME plus indomethacin decreased the response to acetylcholine especially in the larger preglomerular vessels, whereas an important residual response was apparent in the distal interlobular, proximal afferent and distal afferent arterioles (Figure 40.2B). In

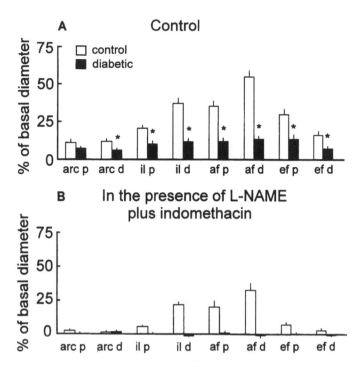

Figure 40.2 Percentage changes of basal vascular diameters in the hydronephrotic kidney of control (open bars) and diabetic rats (full bars) in response to local application of acetylcholine 10^{-5} M in the tissue bath before (A) and after (B) local application of L-NAME 10^{-4} M plus indomethacin 10^{-3} M. arc p = proximal arcuate artery; arc d = distal arcuate artery; il p = proximal interlobular artery; il d = distal interlobular artery; af p = proximal afferent arteriole; af d = distal afferent arteriole; ef p = proximal efferent arteriole; ef d = distal efferent arteriole. Data are shown as mean ± SEM. The asterisks indicate statistically significant differences.

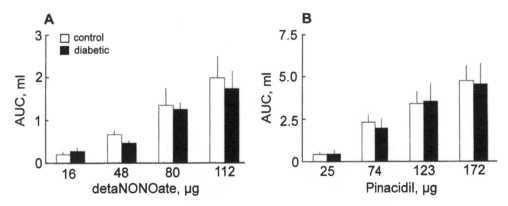

Figure 40.3 The renal blood flow response to intrarenally administered detaNONOate (A) and pinacidil (B) in control (open bars) and in diabetic rats (full bars). The area under the curve (AUC) of the change from baseline values was calculated for each bolus detaNONOate and pinacidil. Data are shown as mean ± SEM.

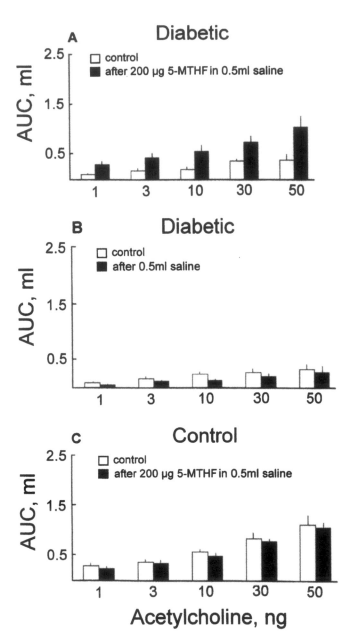

Figure 40.4 The renal blood flow response to intrarenally administered acetylcholine (A) in diabetic rats before (full bars) and 15 min after (hatched bars) an intravenous bolus of 200 μg 5-MTHF dissolved in 0.5 ml saline; (B) in diabetic rats before (full bars) and 15 min after (hatched bars) an intravenous bolus of 0.5 ml saline without 5-MTHF; (C) in control rats before (open bars) and 15 min after (hatched bars) an intravenous bolus of 200 μg 5-MTHF dissolved in 0.5 ml saline. The experiments were performed under systemic NO synthase and cycloxygenase blockade. The area under the curve (AUC) of the change from baseline values was calculated for each bolus acetylcholine. Data are shown as mean ± SEM. The asterisks indicate statistically significant differences.

the diabetic rats, L-NAME plus indomethacin reduced the vasodilator response to acetylcholine in all blood vessels (Figure 40.2B). The L-NAME- and indomethacin-resistant rise in glomerular blood flow was significantly lower in diabetic than in control kidneys ($53.4 \pm 6.0\%$ and $8.6 \pm 2.1\%$, respectively).

2.3. Endothelium-independent responses

The renal blood flow responses to detaNONOate and to pinacidil were not significantly different in diabetic and control rats (Figure 40.3). The systemic administration of L-NAME plus indomethacin did not significantly influence the increase in renal blood flow to detaNONOate and to pinacidil, whether in control or in diabetic animals (data not shown).

2.4. 5-MTHF

The administration of a bolus of 5-MTHF in the diabetic rats restored the impaired L-NAME- and indomethacin-resistant response to acetylcholine, to values that were not significantly different from the response in control rats (Figure 40.4A). A bolus injection of saline did not significantly affect the L-NAME- and indomethacin-resistant response to acetylcholine in the diabetic rats (Figure 40.4B). The administration of 5-MTHF did not alter the L-NAME- and indomethacin-resistant response to acetylcholine in control rats (Figure 40.4C).

3. DISCUSSION

The present study aimed to analyse the influence of diabetes on the different components of the endothelium-mediated vasodilatation in the renal microcirculation of the rat *in vivo*. Two complementary techniques were used, providing information both on the variations in total renal blood flow as well as on the intrarenal distribution of the changes in vascular reactivity. Acetylcholine was used as an endothelium-dependent agonist and its effects were compared with those of the endothelium-independent agonists detaNONOate and pinacidil. A considerable part of the acetylcholine-induced increase in total renal blood flow is resistant to inhibition with L-NAME and indomethacin. The NO synthase- and cyclooxygenase-independent component of the vasodilatation to an endothelium-dependent agonist can be attributed to EDHF (Cohen and Vanhoutte, 1995). The contribution of EDHF to relaxation is dependent on vessel size, being most prominent in small arteries (Nagao *et al.*, 1992; Shimokawa *et al.*, 1996). Therefore, additional experiments were performed using the split hydronephrotic kidney model, an intravital microscopy technique that offers the possibility to examine the different segments of the renal microcirculation *in vivo*. There was a clear gradient in the overall response to acetylcholine. It increased progressively from the proximal arcuate arteries to the afferent arterioles and decreased again in the postglomerular vessels. The pronounced vasodilatation to acetylcholine in the smallest arterioles was in large part insensitive to inhibition of NO and prostaglandin synthesis, suggesting the involvement of EDHF.

In the diabetic animals, the global renal blood flow response to acetylcholine tended to be lower, but the difference was significant only for the highest acetylcholine dose. However, the L-NAME- and indomethacin-resistant component of the response to acetylcholine was impaired at all doses. These results suggest a decreased EDHF-mediated component in the diabetic kidneys. In the experiments with the hydronephrotic kidney in diabetic animals, the vasodilator response to acetylcholine was impaired more as the vessel caliber became smaller. Administration of L-NAME and indomethacin almost abolished the response to acetylcholine in the smallest preglomerular arterioles. Taken together, the present results suggest an increasing importance of the EDHF-mediated component of the acetylcholine-induced vasodilatation towards the most distal arterioles and a severe impairment of this EDHF-mediated vasodilatation in the diabetic kidney.

This decreased response cannot be explained by a decreased general responsiveness of the vascular smooth muscle cells, since vasodilatation in response to pinacidil and detaNONOate was not altered under the same conditions. Neither can the results be attributed to the differential effects of L-NAME on systemic blood pressure in diabetic and control rats, since the renal blood flow results were parallelled closely by the intravital microscopy findings, where L-NAME was administered locally and no systemic blood pressure changes were observed.

So far, only a few studies addressed the role of EDHF in diabetes and none of these were performed *in vivo*. Endothelium-dependent hyperpolarization and the NO synthase and cyclooxygenase-independent component of the relaxation to acetylcholine are decreased in isolated mesenteric arteries from diabetic rats (Fukao *et al.*, 1997). The NO synthase- and cyclooxygenase-resistant vasodilatation to bradykinin or acetylcholine is impaired in the Langendorff perfused heart (Quilley *et al.*, 1996) and in the isolated perfused kidney (Fulton *et al.*, 1996) of diabetic animals. Another study, performed in the isolated aorta, found no evidence for an impaired EDHF release in diabetes (Endo *et al.*, 1995), which may illustrate the difference in relative contribution of NO and EDHF to endothelium-dependent relaxations in the aorta, as compared with distal arterioles. *In vivo*, hyperpolarization cannot be measured directly. Nevertheless, such studies yield valid information, since they are performed under physiological flow conditions. Indeed, the experimental conditions may determine the magnitude of the contribution of EDHF to endothelium-dependent vasodilatation, by setting the resting membrane potential. In particular, depolarization of the vessel by pressurization may enhance the EDHF response (Campbell and Harder, 1999). The controversy on the identity of EDHF and the absence of specific inhibitors of EDHF hampers the establishment of its physiological role. EDHF may provide a mechanism to induce a rapid dilatation, followed by a relatively slow NO-mediated response (Bakker and Sipkema, 1997). Rhythmic alterations in intraluminal pressure induce the synthesis of EDHF (Popp *et al.*, 1998). Pulsatile pressure may thus be the physiological stimulus for EDHF release, whereas shear stress is a major stimulus for NO release (Cohen and Vanhoutte, 1995). Blockade of EDHF reduced vascular compliance (Popp *et al.*, 1998). Elevated blood pressure is injurious to glomeruli and accelerates the development of diabetic glomerulosclerosis (Ismail *et al.*, 1999). The present results may therefore have implications for the pathophysiology of diabetic nephropathy. A decreased action of EDHF in the small resistance vessels of the diabetic kidney may lead to a failure to protect the glomeruli from the deleterious effects of high blood pressure and thus contribute to the development of glomerulosclerosis.

The impaired NO synthase- and cyclooxygenase-independent renal vasodilator response in diabetic rats was restored to normal by acute systemic administration of 5-MTHF, which is the active and circulating form of folic acid. The effect was specific for the pathological vessels, since 5-MTHF did not augment the response to acetylcholine in control kidneys. The mechanisms underlying the beneficial effects of folate on endothelial function was not related to the lowering of homocysteine levels. Folate is the primary therapy in patients with hyperhomocysteinemia, since it is the cosubstrate for the homocysteine-metabolizing enzyme methionine synthase. However, in the present study, plasma homocysteine levels were lower in the diabetic than in the control rats, as described previously (Jacobs *et al.*, 1998), and were not influenced by the acute administration of 5-MTHF. Folate restores endothelial dysfunction during a methionine load test in healthy volunteers without affecting the rise in plasma homocysteine levels (Usui *et al.*, 1999). Other data also support vascular effects of folate independent of the lowering of homocysteine levels. A single intravenous bolus of 5-MTHF (Verhaar *et al.*, 1998) and 4 weeks of treatment with oral folate (Verhaar *et al.*, 1999) normalized impaired endothelium-dependent vasodilatation in the forearm circulation of patients with familial hypercholesterolemia. 5-MTHF reduced the generation of superoxide by both xanthine oxidase and recombinant endothelial NO synthase *in vitro* (Verhaar *et al.*, 1998). Folate may thus exert its beneficial effects on endothelium-dependent vasodilatation by preventing the oxidative breakdown of endothelium-derived NO (Verhaar *et al.*, 1998). The present results were obtained under systemic NO synthase blockade and, therefore, the effects of folate cannot be explained by an improved availability of endothelium-derived NO. Increased oxidative stress could, however, also have adverse effects on the production and/or the availability of EDHF. While the precise mechanism underlying the beneficial effect of folate remains to be determined, the present results and these of others (Verhaar *et al.*, 1998, 1999; Usui *et al.*, 2000) suggest a potential role for folate in the prevention or treatment of cardiovascular complications.

ACKNOWLEDGMENTS

The authors thank Dirk Degruytere, Tommy Dheuvaert, Julien Dupont and Cyriel Mabilde for their expert technical assistance.

41 Resistance of EDHF-mediated relaxations to oxidative stress in human radial arteries

C.A. Hamilton, G.A. Berg, V. Pathi,
J.L. Reid and A.F. Dominiczak

Nitric oxide-dependent relaxation is decreased by atherosclerosis disease in both man and animal models of disease. Increased superoxide levels may contribute by decreasing the bioavailability of nitric oxide. The effects of oxidative stress and increased production of superoxide anions on endothelium-dependent hyperpolarizing factor is less clear. The present experiments were designed to compare the effects of superoxide anions and another potentially harmful species, hydrogen peroxide, on endothelium-dependent relaxations in human arteries used in coronary artery bypass graft surgery. Relaxation of isolated rings of artery to carbachol was studied in organ chambers before and after addition of superoxide dismutase and catalase. Superoxide anions levels in the arteries were measured using lucigenin chemiluminescence. The endogenous levels of superoxide anions were similar in internal mammary and radial arteries. In internal mammary artery no relaxation to carbachol was observed in the presence of the inhibitor of nitric oxide synthase N^G-nitro-L-arginine methyl ester (L-NAME). The nitric oxide-dependent relaxation was enhanced in the presence of superoxide dismutase. In radial arteries, both nitric oxide-dependent and independent relaxations to carbachol were observed. Superoxide dismutase and the polyethylene glycolated form of the enzyme both enhanced the nitric oxide-dependent but not the nitric oxide independent relaxation. Catalase had no effect on relaxations to carbachol either in the presence or absence of L-NAME. These results suggest that nitric oxide dependent relaxation to carbachol is attenuated by superoxide in internal mammary and radial arteries. In radial arteries, nitric oxide-independent relaxation to carbachol is also observed which appears not to be modified by superoxide or hydrogen peroxide. Resistance to oxidative stress could contribute to long term patency of radial arteries used in revascularization surgery.

Nitric oxide, prostanoids and endothelium-dependent hyperpolarizing factors (EDHFs) are the main endothelium-derived vasodilators in human arteries. Nitric oxide plays the major role in most human conduit arteries (Joannides *et al.*, 1995). The bioavailability of nitric oxide is reduced in many forms of cardiovascular disease (Yang and Lüscher, 1991; Woodman, 1995). There is increasing evidence that this may be related to increased levels of reactive oxygen species, particularly superoxide anions (Munzel and Harrison, 1999; McIntyre *et al.*, 1999). EDHFs may be less susceptible to degradation by superoxide anions and other products of oxidative stress (Kaw and Hecker, 1999). Due to the uncertainties as to the nature of EDHFs in different vascular beds the effects of oxidative stress on EDHF-mediated vasodilatation, particularly in human arteries, is unclear.

A response with the pharmacological characteristics of EDHF, is responsible for around 50% of relaxation to acetylcholine and bradykinin in human radial arteries

(Hamilton *et al.*, 1999). Mammary arteries and saphenous veins are the two blood vessels most frequently used for coronary artery bypass graft surgery. However long term patency of venous grafts is poor and radial arteries may be used in preference to saphenous veins for revascularization in some patients. Patients undergoing this type of surgery are likely to have one or more risk factors for cardiovascular disease and higher than normal plasma levels of reactive oxygen species. The susceptibility of endogenous vasodilators produced by the grafted vessels to oxidative degradation may influence long term patency and survival of the graft. The present study compares superoxide anions levels and the effects of superoxide dismutase, polyethylene glycolated superoxide dismutase and catalase, on nitric oxide-dependent and independent relaxations of human internal mammary and radial arteries.

1. METHODS

Human internal mammary and radial arteries were obtained from patients undergoing coronary artery bypass graft surgery. Approval to use discarded tissues was granted by the Western Infirmary Ethical Committee, Glasgow, UK. The blood vessels were surgically prepared (Hamilton *et al.*, 1999) and transferred to the laboratory in physiological salt solution. They were cleaned of muscle and connective tissue and cut into rings (2–3 mm) for organ chamber experiments or for measurement of superoxide anions (3–4 mm).

Superoxide anions were measured by lucigenin chemiluminescence (Berry *et al.*, 2000). Rings were suspended in organ chambers for tension measurement (Hamilton *et al.*, 1999). After an appropriate equilibrium period rings were contracted with phenylephrine (3×10^{-6} M), which causes 50–70% of maximal constriction. Relaxation to carbachol ($10^{-8} - 10^{-5}$ M) was then examined. The organ chambers were washed out, the tissues allowed to recover and vehicle or scavengers of reactive oxygen species added. After 20 min, the vessels were constricted again with phenylephrine and relaxation to carbachol studied.

Superoxide dismutase (SOD 50–200 U/ml) or polyethylene glycolated superoxide dismutase (PEG SOD 50 U/ml) were used to dismutase superoxide anions and catalase (1000 U/ml) to scavenge hydrogen peroxide.

In another series of experiments relaxation to carbachol was studied first in the absence of L-NAME, again in the presence of L-NAME (2×10^{-4} M) and in radial arteries for a third time in the presence of L-NAME and scavengers of reactive oxygen species, or vehicle.

1.1. Analysis of results

The maximal relaxation to carbachol (E max) and the concentration of agonist required to produce 50% relaxation (EC_{50}) were calculated for each individual ring using Microsoft Excel (R). Values obtained before and after treatment with scavengers of reactive oxygen species or L-NAME were compared using students *t*-tests for paired observations. Superoxide anion levels in radial and internal mammary arteries were compared using the students *t*-test for unpaired observations. Differences were considered to be statistically significant when *p* was less than .05.

2. RESULTS

2.1. Tissue levels of superoxide anions

Superoxide anions levels were similar in internal mammary and radial arteries (0.91 ± 0.09 and 0.96 ± 0.30 n moles/min/mg respectively).

2.2. Organ chamber studies

2.2.1. *Superoxide dismutase*

In internal mammary artery treatment with superoxide dismutase (50 U/ml) caused a significant increase in relaxation fom $58 \pm 4\%$ before treatment to $77 \pm 5\%$ in the presence of superoxide dismutase ($n = 14$) as calculated form the fitted dose response curves. The EC_{50} was decreased significantly from 10.9 ± 2.5 to $4.6 \pm 0.7 \times 10^{-7}$ M in the presence of superoxide dismutase. Vehicle treatment had no significant effect on relaxation. Data from individual points on the dose response curve is shown in Figure 41.1. Increasing the concentration of superoxide dismutase to 200 U/ml had no additional effect on the relaxations.

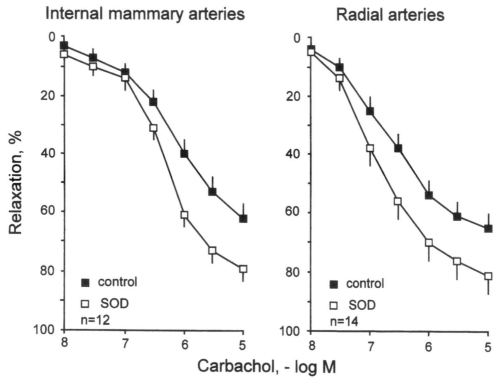

Figure 41.1 Effect of treatment with superoxide dismutase on relaxation to carbachol in internal mammary arteries. Relaxations to carbachol were studied before and after treatment with superoxide dismutase 50 U/ml (left hand panel). Before treatment ■. In the presence of superoxide dismutase or vehicle □. Results are mean ± SEM ($n = 12$).

In radial arteries superoxide dismutase also enhanced relaxations to carbachol. The maximal relaxation was $68 \pm 5\%$ before treatment and $81 \pm 6\%$ in the presence of superoxide dismutase (50 U/ml) ($n = 14$). The mean EC_{50} was lower after superoxide dismutase treatment (2.18 ± 0.65 vs $3.13 \pm 0.76 \times 10^{-7}$ M) but the difference was not statistically significant. In vehicle treated samples maximal relaxation was $68 \pm 6\%$ and $69 \pm 7\%$ before and after treatment respectively ($n = 16$).

2.3. L-NAME

No significant relaxation to carbachol was observed in internal mammary arteries after incubation with L-NAME. In radial arteries L-NAME did not abolish relaxation but reduced it from $83 \pm 4\%$ to $58 \pm 4\%$ ($n = 18$). In radial arteries treated with L-NAME neither superoxide dismutase nor vehicle significantly modified the relaxation to carbachol. Maximal relaxation was $64 \pm 7\%$ before and $63 \pm 8\%$ after superoxide dismutase treatment ($n = 10$) and $60 \pm 5\%$ and $58 \pm 5\%$ after vehicle treatment ($n = 11$).

2.4. PEG-Superoxide dismutase

In radial arteries PEG-Superoxide dismutase had no additional effects above those of normal superoxide dismutase. In the absence of L-NAME, the relaxation was increased from $79 \pm 8\%$ to $90 \pm 9\%$ ($n = 5$). In blood vessels treated with L-NAME, the maximal relaxation was $60 \pm 8\%$ and $55 \pm 4\%$, in the absence and presence of PEG-Superoxide dismutase (50 U/ml), respectively ($n = 10$).

2.5. Catalase

Incubation with catalase (1000 U/ml) had no effect on the relaxation to carbachol either in the absence or presence of L-NAME. In the absence of L-NAME, the maximal relaxation was 63 ± 13 and $58 \pm 11\%$ ($n = 5$), while in rings of radial artery treated with L-NAME it averaged $61 \pm 11\%$ before and $63 \pm 9\%$ after addition of catalase to the organ chambers ($n = 4$). The combination of catalase and PEG-Superoxide dismutase also failed to modify relaxations to carbachol in L-NAME-treated preparations. The maximal relaxation was $45 \pm 8\%$ in the absence, and $41 \pm 9\%$ in the presence of PEG-Superoxide dismutase plus catalase ($n = 4$).

3. DISCUSSION

These results show the scavenger of superoxide anions, superoxide dismutase improves nitric oxide-dependent dilation to the acetylcholine analogue carbachol in internal mammary and radial arteries. In contrast nitric oxide-independent dilation was not improved by scavenging superoxide anions.

Superoxide anions are generated by both internal mammary and radial arteries. The rate constant for the interaction of superoxide anions with nitric oxide is high. Thus the radical produced in vascular tissue may react rapidly with nitric oxide synthesized in endothelial cells reducing its bioavailability (Thompson *et al.*, 1995).

Less is known about the potential interactions of superoxide with non-nitric oxide vasodilators. As indomethacin was present in the buffer throughout the present studies the nitric oxide-independent dilatation observed in radial arteries was unlikely to be due to prostanoids. Previous studies have shown that this nitric oxide/prostanoid independent relaxation has the characteristics of EDHF (Hamilton *et al.*, 1999). The lack of an effect of superoxide dismutase on this nitric oxide/prostanoid-independent relaxation in radial arteries might suggest that in this preparation superoxide does not react with EDHF(s).

Superoxide dismutase is relatively tissue impermeable. Radial arteries are muscular vessels and poor penetration of superoxide dismutase into the tissue could, at least in part, explain the absence on effect of superoxide dismutase on the nitric oxide/prostanoid-independent relaxation. However PEG-Superoxide dismutase, which fully penetrates the vascular wall, also failed to modify the nitric oxide/prostanoid independent relaxations.

Superoxide anions are not the only reactive oxygen species found in the vasculature. *In vivo* superoxide anions are dismutated to hydrogen peroxide by superoxide dismutase. Hydrogen peroxide is a toxic species and can interfere with endothelial function and attenuate relaxation (Dowell *et al.*, 1993; Mian and Martin, 1997). Thus although superoxide dismutase may decrease the concentration of one harmful species it could increase the concentration of another. However catalase, when added alone or in the presence of PEG-Superoxide dismutase, had no effect on the response to carbachol. Catalase is a high capacity system for removal of hydrogen peroxide (Halliwell, 1982). It is possible that the concentration of endogenous catalase in the arteries is sufficient to convert hydrogen peroxide generated in the tissue to water before it can impair relaxation. Alternatively hydrogen peroxide may not react directly with nitric oxide or EDHF(s) in radial arteries.

Overall these results suggest that the nitric oxide/prostanoid independent relaxations in radial arteries are not attenuated by interaction with superoxide anions or hydrogen peroxide. Studies in other tissues also suggest that EDHF-mediated relaxation may be resistant to oxidative stress. Scavenging of superoxide does not influence the release of EDHF in the isolated rat heart (Fulton *et al.*, 1997). The EDHF-mediated relaxations of bovine coronary arteries is unchanged in the presence of superoxide dismutase or catalase, and is unaffected by incubation with menadione or pyrogallol both of which can generate superoxide anions (Kaw and Hecker, 1999).

Superoxide anion levels are elevated in animal models of hypercholesterolemia (Mugge *et al.*, 1994), hypertension (Kerr *et al.*, 1999) and diabetes (Hattori *et al.*, 1991), all of which are risk factors for coronary artery disease. The relative importance of nitric oxide-independent relaxation is increased in pulmonary hypertension in sheep (Kemp *et al.*, 1995). In carotid arteries from hypercholesterolemic rabbits the contribution of nitric oxide-cyclic GMP to acetylcholine induced relaxation is reduced while that mediated by an hyperpolarizing factor remains unchanged (Najibi *et al.*, 1994). In a rat model of congestive heart failure, nitric oxide-mediated dilatation is decreased, while EDHF-dependent dilatation is upregulated (Malmsjo *et al.*, 1999). Taken together these results suggest that while the levels of superoxide anions increase and that of nitric oxide decrease in atherosclerotic disease, EDHF-mediated relaxation may remain unchanged or become upregulated. Its contribution to endothelium-dependent relaxations increase. Thus there may be advantages in using blood vessels in which EDHF makes a substantial contribution to endothelium-dependent relaxations for revascularization surgery. Long term survival of venous grafts in coronary artery bypass surgery is poor. Radial arteries are being used in preference to saphenous veins for revascularization in selected patients. Short to medium term survival of these grafts appears good (Acar *et al.*, 1992; Manasse *et al.*, 1996). EDHF-dependent relaxations which are resistant to oxidative stress may contribute to the long term patency of radial arteries used in revascularization surgery.

42 Critical limb ischemia results in different types of endothelial dysfunction depending on the vascular bed studied

Paul Coats, Yagna P. Jarajapu and Chris Hillier

Critical limb ischemia is a state of advanced peripheral vascular disease resulting in paraesthesia, pain, tissue breakdown, gangrene and necrosis of the distal portion of the affected limb. The effects of chronic ischemia on resistance artery function have yet to be fully determined. Endothelial function in isolated arteries from patients with critical limb ischemia were investigated. Immediately following amputation, arteries were isolated from proximal and distal sites from both subcutaneous and skeletal muscle vascular beds. The distal arteries were harvested from the ischemic portion of the leg. Whereas the proximal arteries were harvested from a non-ischaemic site and served as internal controls. Isolated resistance-sized arteries were studied on a pressure myograph. Endothelium-dependent relaxation were significantly impaired in both subcutaneous and skeletal muscle arteries from the distal ischaemic sites when compared with the proximal, non-ischaemic arteries. In subcutaneous resistance arteries, chronic ischemia specifically attenuated the component of relaxation that was insensitive to N^G-nitro-L-arginine (L-NOARG) and indomethacin. The response was sensitive to high potassium saline solution and therefore, presumably mediated by endothelium-derived hyperpolarizing factor. The opposite was observed in the skeletal muscle resistance arteries where ischemia attenuated the endothelium-dependent relaxation sensitive to L-NOARG and indomethacin. In this vascular bed, the component sensitive to high potassium saline solution was unaffected by chronic ischemia. Therefore, the mechanisms underlying endothelium-dependent relaxations are altered differentially in the two main vascular beds in the ischemic limb of patients with advanced peripheral vascular disease.

Critical limb ischemia is a state of advanced peripheral vascular disease, where limb function and survival are endangered. It is caused by the development of diffuse atherosclerotic plaques in the large communicating arteries resisting blood flow and reducing perfusion pressure (Haq *et al.*, 1997). The resulting ischemia and metabolic insufficiency produces clinical symptoms of paraesthesia, pain, tissue breakdown, gangrene and necrosis of the distal portion of the affected limb (McEwan and Ledingham, 1971; Fagrell, 1977).

Advances in diagnostic techniques such as capillary microscopy, laser doppler fluxmetry, fluorescein angiography and transcutaneous oxygen measurement have allowed analysis of local haemodynamics at a superficial subcutaneous level (Franzeck, 1982; Fagrell and Lundberg, 1984; Seifert *et al.*, 1988). However, these techniques give no information on vascular function in the important resistance-sized arteries nor are they able to provide information on the deep skeletal muscle resistance bed. *In vitro* techniques (small vessel wire myography) have been adopted to identify general abnormalities in the endothelial function of subcutaneous resistance arteries from patients undergoing bypass surgery for critical limb ischemia (Hillier *et al.*, 1999).

Peripheral resistance is, in part, modulated via vasodilator stimuli mediated by the three endothelium-derived relaxing factors: prostacyclin, nitric oxide, and endothelium-derived hyperpolarizing factor (EDHF) (Moncada and Vane, 1979; Furchgott and Zawadzki, 1980; Komori *et al.*, 1988; Taylor and Weston, 1988). However, it is not clear to what extent each of these endothelium-derived factors contributes to a single response or under what circumstances their relative contribution changes.

The aim of the present study was to investigate endothelial function in skeletal muscle and subcutaneous resistance arteries, to identify the relative importance of nitric oxide, prostacyclin and EDHF in both vascular beds and to examine the degree of endothelial dysfunction in the chronically ischemic limb.

1. METHODS

1.1. Patients and biopsy preparation

This study has been performed according to the Declaration of Helsinki (Declaration of Helsinki, 1997). Biopsies were obtained from thirty-two patients (Table 42.1) undergoing amputation for critical limb ischemia. Each patient fulfilled the criteria for critical limb ischemia defined in the European Consensus Document as follows (European Consensus Document, 1991).

1.2. Biopsy procedure

Immediately following leg amputation, biopsies ($1\,cm^3$) were removed from four anatomical sites: proximal and distal subcutaneous and proximal and distal skeletal muscle (Figure 42.1). Proximal tissue represents an internal control as it is harvested

Table 42.1 Clinical details of patients involved in this study

Number	32
Sex	15 male, 17 female
Age	male 67 ± 2, female 68 ± 3
Systolic BP	$132 \pm 5\,mmHg$
Diastolic BP	$75 \pm 4\,mmHg$
Diabetic	14 (NIDDM 8, IDDM 6)
Hypertension	9
Drug therapy	
Ace inhibitor	6
Ca^{2+} channel antagonist	3
Diuretic	7
Digoxin	6
Nitrates	7
Aspirin	12
HMG CoA reductase inhibitor	5

BP = blood pressure; HMG CoA = hydroxy-3-methylglutaryl coenzyme A; IDDM = insulin-dependent diabetes mellitus; NIDDM = non-insulin-dependent diabetes mellitus. Values are means $\pm$ SEM.

from a non-ischemic region and distal tissue is taken from an ischemic diseased region. Proximal subcutaneous and skeletal muscle biopsies were isolated approximately 2 cm below the level of amputation. The distal subcutaneous biopsies were isolated from the subcutaneous tissue directly inferior to the medial malleolus. Distal skeletal muscle biopsies were isolated from the distal portion of the soleus muscle. Each biopsy was transferred to the laboratory in cold saline solution. Resistance size arteries (diameter less than 200 µm) were isolated from each biopsy and cleaned of any adherent tissue under a dissection microscope (Zeiss Stemi 2000, Mag 6X–45X).

1.3. Apparatus and data acquisition

All the experiments in this study were performed on a Danish Myo Tech P100 pressure myograph system. Real time images of the artery (752 × 582 pixels) were

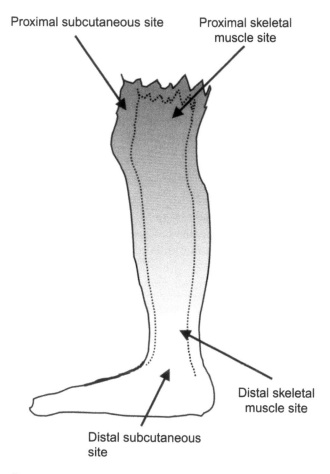

Figure 42.1 Schematic representation of an amputated leg identifying the site of biopsies. Proximal biopsies are taken from the non-ischaemic part of the amputated leg represented by deep shading. Conversely, the distal biopsies are taken from the ischaemic part of the amputated leg represented by the white area. Relative blood perfusion of the limb is represented by the intensity of the shading. The broken line represents the subcutaneous-skeletal muscle border.

taken with the myograph block placed on the stage of an inverted microscope (Zeiss axiovert 25C) above a high-resolution 16-bit CCD video camera (Sony XC-73CE monochrome). A Data Translation's digital DT3157 Mach frame grabber processed the digital image. The final viewed magnification of the prepared artery was 100×. Dedicated data acquisition software (Vessel View, Danish Myo Tech, Denmark) integrated edge detection image analysis, measuring vessel morphology (external and internal diameter, wall thickness, lumen), recording of time, luminal pressure, longitudinal force, temperature and manual intervention. Data were acquired at 1-second intervals.

1.4. Experimental methodology

Following isolation the arteries were cannulated and secured with two fine nylon sutures to a size-matched micro-cannula (80 μm). The lumen was flushed gently with saline solution to remove any blood or debris, following which the second end of the artery was cannulated and secured. During all experiments the saline solution was gassed with 95% O_2/5% CO_2 maintaining pH 7.4 at 37 °C. Following pressurization to 40 mmHg all arteries were equilibrated for 60 minutes in a no-flow state. To ensure functional viability, arteries were activated with 60 mM K^+ saline solution three times. Arteries not developing tone in response to 60 mM K^+ saline solution were disregarded. Additionally, all arteries were exposed to $1-10^{-5}$ M norepinephrine; arteries that did not respond to norepinephrine were similarly disregarded.

Endothelium-dependent relaxation was assessed by constructing cumulative dose response curves ($10^{-9}-3 \times 10^{-4}$ M) to acetylcholine alone or following cumulative incubation with: (a) L-NOARG (10^{-3} M for 1 hour); (b) indomethacin (3×10^{-5} M for 30 minutes in the presence of L-NOARG); and (c) 25 mM K^+ solution (in the presence of both L-NOARG and indomethacin). To obtain a level of constriction (diameter) similar to that used for cumulative concentration responses to acetylcholine the concentration of norepinephrine was reduced in the presence of 25 mM K^+ solution.

1.5. Drugs and solutions

All drugs and solutions were prepared on the day of the experiment. Acetylcholine, indomethacin, L-NOARG and norepinephrine were purchased from Sigma (Poole, Dorset, UK). All were dissolved in distilled water with the exception of indomethacin. A stock solution of indomethacin (10^{-1} M) was dissolved in dimethyl sulphoxide (DMSO) and subsequent dilutions were made in physiological saline solution. The final bath concentration of DMSO never exceeded 0.03%. The control physiological saline solution had the following composition (mM): NaCl 119, KCl 4.5, NaHCO$_3$ 25, KH$_2$PO$_4$ 1.0, MgSO$_4$7H$_2$O 1.0, Glucose 6.0 and CaCl$_2$ 2.5. To obtain solutions containing 25 mM and 60 mM potassium an equimolar substitution of NaCl with KCl was performed.

1.6. Data and statistical analysis

All arteries were constricted with norepinephrine to approximately 80% of their maximal constriction diameter. Relaxations are represented relative to the constricted

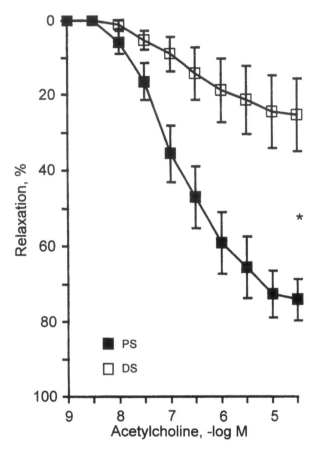

Figure 42.2 Relaxation to cumulative addition of acetylcholine (ACh) in proximal subcutaneous (PS) and distal subcutaneous (DS) arteries. Data shown as
means ± SEM ($n = 12$ pairs, $*p < .05$, one way ANOVA for repeated measures).

diameter of the artery. Values are shown as means ± standard error of the mean
(SEM). Statistical comparisons of sensitivity (pD_2, negative log of the concentration of
acetylcholine required to produced 50% of the maximum response) and maximal
responses (R_{MAX}) between proximal and distal arteries were performed using Student's
t-test for paired observations. Comparisons of concentration response curves were by
one-way ANOVA for repeated measures. Statistical significance was assumed if p was
less than .05.

2. RESULTS

2.1.

Endothelium-dependent relaxations to the cumulative addition of acetylcholine were
significantly reduced in distal subcutaneous arteries when compared to the proximal

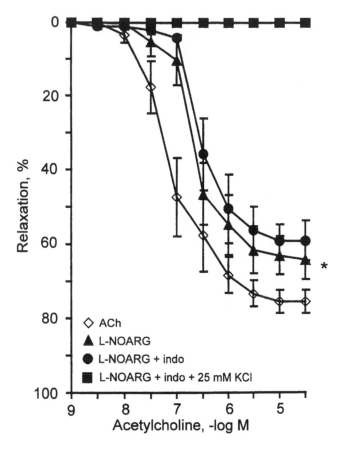

Figure 42.3 Relaxation to acetylcholine (ACh) in proximal subcutaneous arteries before and after cumulative incubation with N^G-nitro-L-arginine (L-NOARG), indomethacin (INDO) and $25\,mM$ K^+. Data shown as means $\pm$ SEM ($n = 9$, $^*p < .05$, one way ANOVA for repeated measures).

arteries (Figure 42.2). Both the sensitivity and the maximal relaxation in response to acetylcholine were significantly impaired when compared with the proximal arteries from the same leg.

In a separate set of arteries, incubation with L-NOARG significantly reduced the maximal relaxation and the sensitivity to acetylcholine in proximal subcutaneous arteries when compared with the control response (Figure 42.3; 6.4 ± 0.2 vs. 7.5 ± 0.2). Subsequent incubation with indomethacin, (in the presence of L-NOARG), failed to modify this response. Introduction of a $25\,mM$ K^+ solution, (in the presence of L-NOARG and indomethacin) abolished the relaxation to acetylcholine in these arteries (Figure 42.3). In distal subcutaneous arteries incubation with L-NOARG and subsequently indomethacin (in the presence of L-NOARG) failed to significantly modify the response to acetylcholine (Figure 42.4). However, replacement of the superfusate/perfusate with $25\,mM$ K^+ solution in the presence of L-NOARG and indomethacin, resulted in abolition of the relaxation to acetylcholine (Figure 42.4).

The comparison of the proximal subcutaneous and distal subcutaneous artery maximal values indicates that the L-NOARG/indomethacin-sensitive component of the response to acetylcholine is relatively preserved in the distal ischaemic region ($16 \pm 5\%$ and $18 \pm 4\%$, respectively). However, the L-NOARG/indomethacin-insensitive, K^+-sensitive component was significantly reduced in the distal subcutaneous arteries when compared with that observed in the proximal preparation ($59 \pm 5\%$ and $15 \pm 8\%$ respectively, $p < .05$).

2.2.

The relaxation to acetylcholine was also significantly impaired in the arteries isolated from distal skeletal muscle biopsies (Figure 42.5). The maximal response to acetylcholine observed in distal skeletal muscle arteries was significantly reduced when compared with that in the proximal preparation. However, there was no significant difference in the sensitivity to acetylcholine. In a separate set of arteries, following a concentration response to acetylcholine, incubation with L-NOARG, resulted in a significant reduction in the sensitivity to acetylcholine (6.1 ± 0.3 vs. 6.9 ± 0.1) and

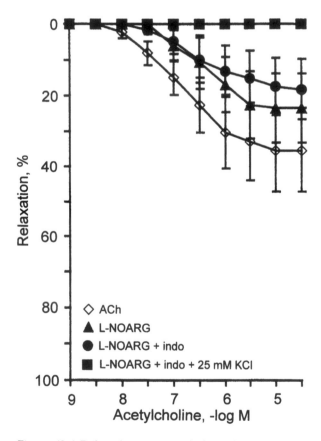

Figure 42.4 Relaxation to cumulative addition of acetylcholine (ACh) in distal subcutaneous arteries before and after cumulative incubation with N^G-nitro-L-arginine (L-NOARG), indomethacin (INDO) and 25 mM K^+ ($n = 10$).

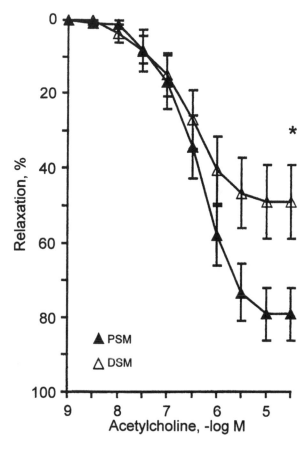

Figure 42.5 Results of cumulative addition of acetylcholine (ACh) in proximal skeletal muscle (PSM) and distal skeletal muscle (DSM) arteries, Data shown as means ± SEM ($n = 12$ pairs, $^*p < .05$, Student's t-test comparison of the maximal responses).

maximal relaxation when compared with the control response (Figure 42.6). The combination of L-NOARG plus indomethacin had no significant further effect on the sensitivity or maximal response to acetylcholine. In the presence of L-NOARG and indomethacin 25 mM K^+ abolished the acetylcholine-induced relaxation in proximal skeletal muscle arteries. In distal skeletal muscle arteries, incubation with L-NOARG and L-NOARG plus indomethacin produced only marginal effects (Figure 42.7). Replacement of the physiological saline with 25 mM K^+ in the presence of L-NOARG and indomethacin eliminated the response to acetylcholine. In the distal skeletal muscle arteries reveals that, in contrast to subcutaneous arteries, the L-NOARG/indomethacin-insensitive component of the relaxation response to acetylcholine was relatively preserved compared to the proximal preparations (42 ± 5% and 35 ± 10%, respectively). However, there was a significant reduction in the L-NOARG/indomethacin-sensitive component (39 ± 7% and 9 ± 5% respectively).

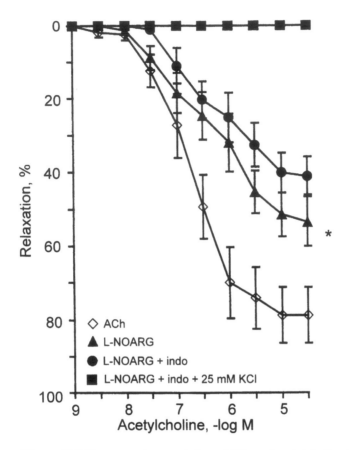

Figure 42.6 Responses to cumulative addition of acetylcholine (ACh) in proximal skeletal muscle arteries before and after cumulative incubation with N^G-nitro-L-arginine (L-NOARG), indomethacin (INDO) and 25 mM K^+. Data shown as means $\pm$ SEM ($n = 9$, $^*p < .05$, one way ANOVA for repeated measures).

3. DISCUSSION

The present study shows that endothelium-dependent relaxations are abnormal in the ischemic part of the limb of patients with advanced peripheral vascular disease known as critical limb ischemia. Moreover, the specific mechanisms underlying the dysfunction in endothelium-dependent relaxation are differentially altered depending on the vascular bed examined. In subcutaneous resistance arteries, ischemia specifically attenuates the L-NOARG/indomethacin-insensitive, K^+-sensitive component of the relaxation response, which is presumably mediated via EDHF (Adeagbo and Triggle, 1993; Petersson *et al.*, 1995). However, in the skeletal muscle resistance arteries the contribution of this component is preserved while the L-NOARG/indomethacin-sensitive component is significantly reduced.

Generalized endothelial dysfunction in the chronically ischemic limb has been suggested by *in vivo* measurement techniques of skin perfusion (McEwan and Ledingham, 1971; de Gaetano, 1992). This dysfunction has also been recently confirmed

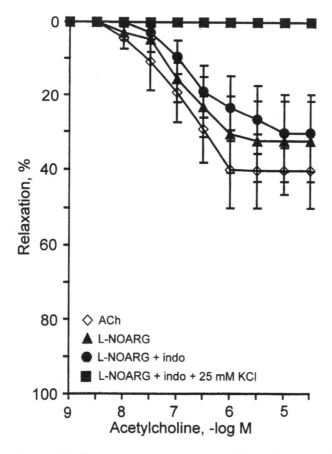

Figure 42.7 Responses to cumulative addition of acetylcholine (ACh) in distal skeletal muscle arteries before and after cumulative incubation with N^G-nitro-L-arginine (L-NOARG), indomethacin (INDO) and 25 mM K^+. Data shown as means $\pm$ SEM ($n = 9$).

in subcutaneous resistance arteries isolated from ischaemic limbs using small vessel wire myography (Hillier *et al.*, 1999).

The importance of the endothelium-derived factor known as EDHF has become apparent. Both potassium ions and a P450 enzyme product have been proposed as EDHF, although the identity and mechanisms through which EDHF acts remain controversial (Chataigneau *et al.*, 1998; Edwards *et al.*, 1998; Doughty and Langton, 1999; Fisslthaler *et al.*, 1999; Quignard *et al.*, 1999; Boltz *et al.*, 2000). EDHF is of primary importance in the resistance-sized arteries whereas nitric oxide appears to be more important in larger conduit arteries (Nagao and Vanhoutte, 1993; Garland *et al.*, 1995; McCulloch *et al.*, 1997). The present study confirms the relative importance of a non-nitric oxide, non-prostanoid component, presumably mediated by an EDHF, to the endothelium-dependent responses in both the subcutaneous (about 75%) and skeletal muscle (about 50%) vascular beds. In skeletal muscle arteries this of the relaxation response to acetylcholine is unaffected by ischemic conditions. However, the opposite was observed in the subcutaneous resistance arteries isolated from the distal ischemic part of the amputated leg.

In vivo and *ex vivo* studies show a deficiency in vasodilator response in subcutaneous small arteries of patients with peripheral vascular disease (Conrad, 1968; Fagrell, 1977; Hillier *et al.*, 1999). This correlates with the clinical observation of ulceration, gangrene and necrosis of the subcutaneous tissue while the skeletal muscle tissue is relatively intact. This has led to suggestions that there is a redistribution of blood in the ischemic limb from skin to protect the deep skeletal muscle tissue (Diamantopoulos and Grigoriadou, 1997). The 'redistribution hypothesis' has derived from clinical observations in critical limb ischemia patients presenting with ischemic lesions on an affected limb(s) who are asymptomatic in terms of limb pain and paraesthesia (Criqui *et al.*, 1985). In the present study, comparison of the endothelium-dependent relaxations from the distal portion of the ischemic limb shows that the response in the subcutaneous arteries is relatively poor when compared to the skeletal muscle arteries. If representative of *in vivo* conditions, a greater resistance to blood flow may be present in the subcutaneous vascular bed as a direct consequence of attenuated release of endothelial-derived relaxing factors offering a potential rationale for redistribution of blood to the skeletal muscle tissue.

The present data demonstrates that the importance of prostacyclin in the endothelium-dependent modulation of tone in both skeletal muscle and subcutaneous resistance arteries *ex vivo* is marginal. This supports similar findings in earlier studies of the role of prostacyclin in endothelium-dependent relaxation of human subcutaneous resistance arteries (Buus *et al.*, 1998, 2000; Hillier *et al.*, 1998).

Limitations to the interpretation of this study involve the heterogeneity of the patient group in terms of underlying pathology and treatment. The subcutaneous resistance bed of hypertensive patients is structurally altered and exhibits endothelial dysfunction. The subcutaneous vessels from diabetics show no structural differences at the level of resistance vessels but also show endothelial dysfunction (Bucala *et al.*, 1991; McNally *et al.*, 1994). The present study revealed both structural atrophy (data not shown) and endothelial dysfunction in arteries from ischaemic limbs. The endothelial dysfunction may be affected by the underlying pathologies. However, *post hoc* analysis revealed no specific subgroup effect of the pathology on these results. However, the reduction in group sizes necessitated by these analyses increased the risk of a type II statistical error.

The present study did not use a separate cohort of patients as controls but has used proximal tissue from the same limb as an internal non-ischemic control tissue. This means that any observed differences between proximal and distal sites must be due to an intrinsic difference between sites or due to the level of ischemia since other variables such as drug interactions, anaesthetic and underlying pathologies are identical. Previous studies comparing subcutaneous tissue from ischemic patients with control tissue from non-ischemic patients have shown that there is no intrinsic difference in either structure or function (endothelium-dependent and independent vasodilatation) between small arteries from proximal ischemic limbs and those from proximal or distal non-ischemic limbs (Hillier *et al.*, 1999). No similar studies have been carried out on human skeletal muscle because of the difficulty in obtaining control tissue. It is possible that the skeletal muscle bed is unlike the subcutaneous bed and possesses intrinsic differences in structural and functional responses between proximal and distal sites.

4. CONCLUSION

Impaired endothelium-dependent relaxation were observed in both subcutaneous and skeletal muscle of arteries from the chronically ischemic limb. Furthermore, we have provided mechanistic insight into the specific components of endothelial function affected by chronic ischemia and intriguingly have identified differences between the responses of skeletal muscle and subcutaneous resistance arteries to chronic ischemia.

ACKNOWLEDGEMENTS

This study was supported by Barnwood House Trust. The authors wish to thank the vascular surgical teams at Glasgow Gartnavel Hospital and Glasgow Royal Infirmary for their assistance in this study.

43 Potentiated EDHF-mediated dilatations in the rat middle cerebral artery following ischemia/reperfusion

*Sean P. Marrelli, William F. Childres,
Jan Goddard-Finegold and
Robert M. Bryan Jr.*

EDHF-mediated dilatations were studied in the rat middle cerebral artery following ischemia/reperfusion. The ischemia/reperfusion model consisted of 2 hours of unilateral focal ischemia followed by 24 hours of reperfusion. Controls or sham-injured rats underwent brief vessel occlusion followed by 24 hours of reperfusion. Following the ischemia/reperfusion or sham-injury protocols, middle cerebral arteries were isolated, pressurized to 85 mmHg, and luminally perfused. EDHF-mediated responses were evaluated using luminal applications of uridine triphosphate (UTP), a P2Y$_2$ selective agonist, or A23187, a Ca^{2+} ionophore, following the inhibition of nitric oxide synthase. Middle cerebral arteries from both sham and ischemia/reperfusion rats dilated maximally to the luminal application of UTP or A23187 in the presence of N$^{\omega}$-nitro-L-arginine methyl ester (L-NAME, 10^{-5} M). However, UTP was seven times more potent and A23187 was three times more potent in middle cerebral arteries from ischemia/reperfusion rats compared to shams. Indomethacin (10^{-5} M), an inhibitor of cyclooxygenase, did not alter the L-NAME insensitive component of the UTP-mediated dilatation in reperfused arteries. In the presence of L-NAME, dilatations to UTP were accompanied by smooth muscle hyperpolarization. Dilatations to UTP and A23187 in the presence of L-NAME were blocked by charybdotoxin (10^{-7} M), an inhibitor of the calcium activated potassium channels. Thus, ischemia/reperfusion potentiates EDHF-mediated dilatations in the rat middle cerebral artery. The upregulation of the EDHF-mediated response may offer cerebral protection during pathological conditions.

Following inhibition of nitric oxide synthase, isolated cerebral arteries and arterioles from normal rats dilate through a mechanism involving EDHF when P2Y$_2$-like purinoceptors on the endothelium are stimulated by either adenosine triphosphate (ATP) or UTP (You *et al.*, 1997; You *et al.*, 1998; Marrelli *et al.*, 1999; You *et al.*, 1999). In these studies, EDHF was identified by the following criteria: (a) endothelium-derived; (b) not NO; (c) not a metabolite of cycloxygenase such as prostacyclin; (d) hyperpolarized the vascular smooth muscle; and (e) blocked by charybdotoxin, an inhibitor of calcium activated potassium channels (K$_{Ca}$).

The EDHF pathway may be upregulated during some pathological conditions where the NO/cyclic GMP pathway is suppressed (Olmos *et al.*, 1995; Hecker, 2000). Thus, EDHF could have a crucial, if not vital, role for the maintenance of blood flow when the nitric oxide pathway has been compromised. The purpose of the present study was to extend this hypothesis to the cerebrovascular circulation and to determine whether or not the EDHF pathway is upregulated following ischemia/

reperfusion in the brain. UTP, a $P2Y_2$ selective agonist, and A23187, a calcium ionophore, were used to elicit EDHF-mediated responses.

1. METHODS

1.1. Surgery

Studies were conducted on male Long-Evans rats (275–325 g) following approval of the Animal Protocol Review committee at Baylor College of Medicine. For surgical procedures, rats were anesthetized with isoflurane (3%). Rectal temperature was maintained at 37 °C with a temperature controller coupled to a heat lamp. A nylon occluder (approximately 240 µm diameter) was inserted into the right internal carotid artery and advanced into the circle of Willis past the ostium of the middle cerebral artery (Longa *et al.*, 1989) (Figure 43.1). The occluder fit snugly into the circle of Willis and, thus, occluded blood flow to the middle cerebral artery without actually entering it. Heparin (50 units) was administered prior to and 1 hour after placement of the occluder to reduce blood clot formation. After 2 hours of placement, the occluder was removed to restore blood flow. Rats were allowed to recover for 24 hours before

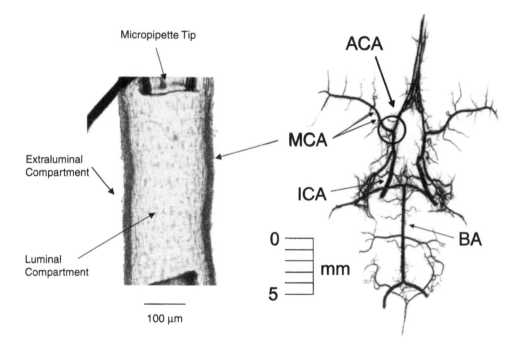

Figure 43.1 (Left) Image of a pressurized perfused rat middle cerebral artery. Note the micropipette tips at the top and bottom of the vessel and the two compartments consisting of the luminal compartment (endothelial side) and extraluminal compartment (vascular smooth muscle side). (Right) A resin cast of the cerebrovascular system of the Long-Evans rat. The circle shows the origin of the middle cerebral artery (MCA) and the approximate location of occlusion in the ACA. ACA = anterior cerebral artery; ICA = internal carotid artery; BA = basilar artery.

middle cerebral arteries were harvested. Sham operated animals underwent the same procedure, except that the occluder was removed immediately after placement.

1.2. Isolated middle cerebral arteries

Following 24 hours of reperfusion, rats were anesthetized with isoflurane and decapitated. The brain was removed from the cranium and placed in cold Krebs solution. A segment of the right middle cerebral artery approximately 3 mm from the circle of Willis was dissected from the brain and mounted on two glass micropipettes. Each vessel was bathed in physiological saline solution (37 °C) which was equilibrated with 20% O_2 and 5% CO_2 with a balance of N_2 (Bryan Jr. *et al.*, 1995; Bryan Jr. *et al.*, 1996). The pH of the bath solution was approximately 7.40, the P_{CO_2} approximately 35 mmHg and the P_{O_2} approximately 130 mmHg. The vessels were pressurized to 85 mmHg and a flow of 200 µl/min was established through the lumen. Pressure transducers on either side of the vessel provided a measurement of perfusion pressure. The isolated arteries had two compartments, a luminal compartment and an extraluminal compartment (Figure 43.1). Drugs could be selectively delivered to the vascular smooth muscle by adding them to the extraluminal compartment. Conversely, drugs could be selectively delivered to the endothelium by adding them to the luminal compartment.

After the artery was mounted, the chamber was placed on the stage of an inverted microscope (Nikon) equipped with a video camera and video monitor (final magnification of 600×). Outer diameters were measured continuously (1.1 Hz) using an image analysis system (Optimas Corporation, Bothell, WA, USA).

Dilatations were elicited by the luminal application of UTP, a $P2Y_2$-selective agonist, or the luminal application of A23187. UTP dilates the rat middle cerebral artery through the release of NO and/or EDHF (You *et al.*, 1998; Marrelli *et al.*, 1999). Only one concentration–response curve was obtained for each preparation to avoid the risk of tachyphylaxis (You *et al.*, 1997). Concentration–response curves were obtained in the absence or presence of L-NAME ($10^{-5}, 5 \times 10^{-5}$ or 10^{-3} M), N^{ω}-nitro-L-arginine (L-NA, 5×10^{-5} M), indomethacin (10^{-5} M), or after removal of the endothelium by perfusing the lumen with air (Bryan, Jr. *et al.*, 1996; You *et al.*, 1997).

In one group of arteries, membrane potential was measured in individual vascular smooth muscle cells using glass microelectrodes filled with 3 M KCl (impedance from 55 to 75 MΩ). The measurements of membrane potential were made in pressurized/perfused arteries so that diameters could be recorded simultaneously (You *et al.*, 1998; Marrelli *et al.*, 1999; You *et al.*, 1999). The potential difference between the glass microelectrode and a reference electrode, placed in the bathing solution of the arteriograph, was measured using a Dagan 8700 Cell Explorer (Dagan Corporation, Minneapolis, MN, USA) with the output being displayed on a Tektronix 5223 Digitizing Oscilloscope (Beaverton, OR, USA). Micropipettes were made by pulling capillary tubing to a rapid taper (tip diameter approximately 0.1 µm) using a model P-87 Brown–Flaming micropipette puller (Sutter, San Francisco, CA, USA). Primary criteria for a successful impalement included a sharp drop in voltage from baseline upon entry of the microelectrode tip into the cell and no change in microelectrode resistance after exiting the cell. Membrane potentials from several different smooth muscle cells were averaged to obtain a single value for a given condition in a given artery.

1.3. Histology

Following removal of the right middle cerebral artery (ipsilateral to the injury), the brains were placed in a rat brain matrix (Braintree Scientific Inc., Braintree, MA, USA) and cut into coronal sections (2 mm). The sections were incubated in a 2% Triphenyltetrazolium chloride solution for 30 minutes and placed in a formalin solution for at least 24 hours (Marrelli *et al.*, 1999). Viable tissue stained deep red while the lesion area due to the occlusion remained white. Lesion volumes were evaluated using image analysis (MCID, Imaging Research, St. Catharines, Ontario, Canada). Confirmation of lesion by Triphenyltetrazolium chloride was a prerequisite for all "ischemia/reperfusion" vessels.

1.4. Transmission electron microscopy

Following ischemia/reperfusion or sham injury, rats were anesthetized with Nembutal sodium (60 mg/kg). Brains were fixed with 3% glutaraldehyde/phosphate buffer for 24 hours and sectioned for transmission electron microscopy. Sections of the middle cerebral artery were magnified to 3300 and 6600×.

1.5. Drugs and reagents

Indomethacin, N^ω-nitro-L-arginine methyl ester, N^ω-nitro-L-arginine (L-NA), Triphenyltetrazolium chloride, and UTP were purchased from Sigma Chemical Co. (St. Louis, MO, USA); Charybdotoxin was purchased from Research Biochemicals Inc. (Natick, MA, USA); and 1H-[1,2,4]oxadiazolo[4,3-a]quinoxalin-1-one (ODQ) was purchased from Tocris (Ballwin, MO, USA); A23187 was purchased from Molecular Probes (Eugene, OR, USA). UTP and L-NAME were dissolved in distilled water; L-NA was dissolved in hot distilled water; indomethacin was dissolved in 15 mM Na_2CO_3; ODQ was dissolved in ethanol; and A23187 was dissolved in dimethyl sulfoxide. Charybdotoxin and ODQ were added to the extraluminal bath. UTP and A23187 were added to the PSS perfusing the lumen. L-NAME, L-NA, and indomethacin were added to both luminal and extraluminal compartments. The physiological saline solution had the following composition (mM): NaCl 119, KCl 4.7, $NaHCO_3$ 24, KH_2PO_4 1.18, $MgSO_4$ 1.17, EDTA 0.026, $CaCl_2$ 1.6 and glucose 5.5 (Bryan Jr. *et al.*, 1996).

1.6. Statistical analysis

All data are presented as means ± SEM. For concentration–response curves, the results are presented as percent of the maximal diameter of the vessel and calculated by the following equation:

$$\% \text{ maximal diameter} = [(D_{\text{drug}} - D_{\text{base}})/(D_{\text{max}} - D_{\text{base}})] * 100,$$

where D_{max} is the maximal diameter of the vessel at a luminal pressure of 85 mmHg, D_{base} is the baseline diameter of the vessel before addition of dilator (or agonist), and D_{drug} is the diameter of the vessel after dilatation. D_{max} is the diameter of the vessel immediately after pressurization and before development of spontaneous tone.

Previous studies have shown that D_{max}, as determined above, is identical to the diameter in Ca-free buffer for a given pressure (personal observations).

For comparison of the concentration–response curves, the two-way repeated measures analysis of variance (2 way RM-ANOVA) was used followed by a post-hoc Student–Newman–Keuls test when appropriate. Maximal dilatations to UTP and $EC_{50}s$ (following log transformation) were compared using a one-way ANOVA. Changes in membrane potential and diameter after a single concentration of UTP were compared using Student's *t*-test for paired observations. The acceptable level of significance was defined as *p* was less than .05.

2. RESULTS

Brain lesions were verified for all animals by Triphenyltetrazolium chloride staining and quantified for a random sampling of animals. The mean lesion volume ($108 \pm 26 \, mm^3$; $n = 11$) represented approximately 13% of the right cerebral hemisphere. Sham brains showed no evidence of lesion by Triphenyltetrazolium chloride staining.

Transmission electron micrographs of the endothelium revealed tight junctions (zonulae occludentes) between endothelial cells in both sham and ischemia/reperfusion vessels (Figure 43.2). Protrusions of the endothelium (microvilli) were present in both sham and ischemia/reperfusion samples. The anatomical integrity of the endothelium appeared intact under both conditions.

The initial diameters for the sham and ischemia/reperfusion (reperfused) artery segments immediately following pressurization to 85 mmHg (before tone developed) were not significantly different and averaged 298 ± 6 ($n = 17$) and 303 ± 3 ($n = 33$) µm, respectively. During the 60 minutes following pressurization, the arteries spontaneously constricted by 27 ± 1 (sham, $n = 8$) and $28 \pm 1\%$ (reperfused, $n = 16$).

The dilitation to $10^{-7} M$ UTP was significantly more pronounced in reperfused vessels than in sham arteries (Figures 43.3 and 43.4). Oscillations in artery diameter occurred for both sham and reperfused vessels and diminished in amplitude as the arteries approached maximal dilatation (Figure 43.4). The $EC_{50}s$ for UTP in sham and reperfused vessels were significantly different and averaged 86 ± 24 and $344 \pm 187 \, \eta M$, respectively. However, maximal dilatations elicited by UTP in the sham and reperfused arteries were not significantly different.

In sham arteries, L-NAME ($10^{-5} M$) completely blocked the dilatation to $10^{-7} M$ UTP and attenuated that to $10^{-6} M$ by 89% without suppressing the maximal dilatation occurring at $10^{-5} M$ (Figures 43.4 and 43.5). The concentration–response curve to UTP in the presence of L-NAME was consistent with data from naïve animals (You *et al.*, 1997). L-NAME had no effect on the dilatation elicited by $10^{-6} M$ UTP in the reperfused segments but attenuated that to $10^{-7} M$ UTP (Figures 43.4 and 43.5). In the presence of L-NAME, the concentration–response curve obtained in reperfused arteries was significantly shifted to the left of that obtained in sham preparations. Increasing the L-NAME concentration from 10^{-5} to $10^{-3} M$ (Figure 43.4, mean data not shown, $n = 3$), combined L-NAME ($5 \times 10^{-5} M$) plus ODQ ($10^{-6} M$), an inhibitor of guanylate cyclase ($n = 4$), L-NAME ($10^{-5} M$) plus indomethacin ($10^{-5} M$, $n = 4$), or administration of L-NA ($5 \times 10^{-5} M$, $n = 3$) did not significantly affect the UTP mediated dilatations in reperfused arteries more than $10^{-5} M$

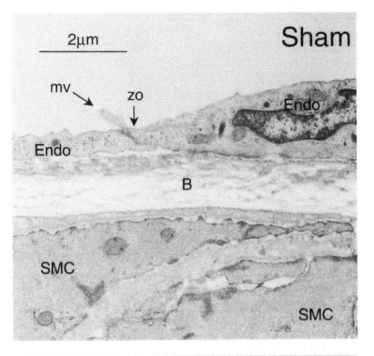

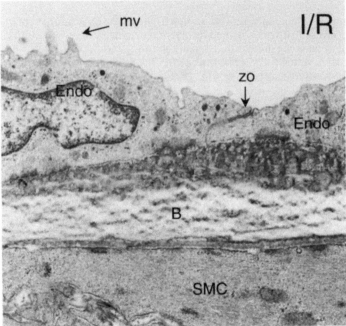

Figure 43.2 Transmission electron microscopy photographs of sections from the right middle cerebral artery from a sham (top) and ischemia/reperfusion (I/R) rat (bottom). Zonulae occludente = zo; Endo = endothelial cells; mv = microvilli; B = basement membrane; SMC = smooth muscle cell.

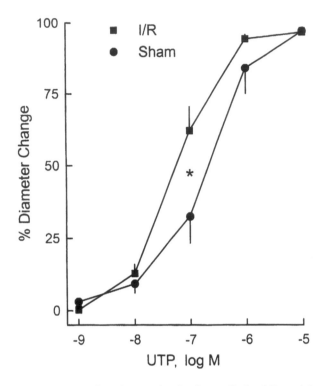

Figure 43.3 Dilatations to luminally applied uridine triphosphate (UTP) for sham ($n = 5$) and reperfused (I/R; $n = 8$) middle cerebral arteries. Curves are plotted as a percent of maximal dilatation. Data are shown as means ± SEM. The asterisk indicates a statistically significant ($p < .05$) difference between sham and reperfused arteries at 10^{-7} M UTP. (Redrawn from Marrelli *et al.* (1999) with permission.)

L-NAME alone (data not shown). Removal of the endothelium abolished the dilatations to UTP (data not shown, $n = 6$).

Dilatations to luminal application of A23187 in the presence of L-NAME (10^{-5} M) were potentiated in reperfused vessels (Figure 43.5). Charybdotoxin (10^{-7} M) abolished the L-NAME insensitive dilatations to UTP and A23187 in reperfused arteries (Figure 43.6).

In the studies where diameter and membrane potential were simultaneously measured for sham and I/R vessels in the presence of L-NAME (5×10^{-5} M), the diameter of sham arteries was significantly less than that of reperfused arteries (Figure 43.7). The significantly smaller diameter in sham arteries corresponded to the more depolarized vascular smooth muscle. In sham arteries, 10^{-6} M UTP had no significant effect on the diameter or membrane potential. However, the same concentration of UTP dilated and significantly hyperpolarized the reperfused arteries (Figure 43.7). This dilation corresponded to a near-maximal dilatation of the artery. Sham arteries dilated maximally to 10^{-5} M UTP. This dilatation at a higher concentration of UTP was accompanied by a significant hyperpolarization.

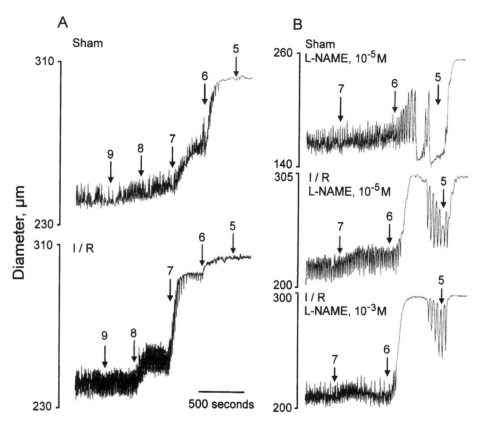

Figure 43.4 Continuous diameter tracings of individual sham and reperfused (I/R) arteries to the luminal application of increasing molar concentrations of uridine triphosphate (UTP) without (A) and with inhibition of nitric oxide synthase (B). The absolute diameter is plotted on the y-axis in microns. Note the greater response to 10^{-7} M UTP following ischemia/reperfusion. L-NAME N^{ω}-nitro-L-arginine methyl ester.

3. DISCUSSION

Two hours of cerebral ischemia followed by 24 hours of reperfusion enhanced EDHF-mediated dilatations in the rat middle cerebral artery. The enhanced responses were apparent when the dilatations were elicited by either luminally applied UTP or A23187. The upregulation of EDHF may be an important mechanism that provides cerebral protection during ischemia/reperfusion. In fact, the upregulated response may be a general protective mechanism in a number of diverse pathological conditions where there is a diminished capacity of NO/cyclic GMP pathway (Hecker, 2000).

EDHF is defined as a relaxing factor which (a) is released from the endothelium; (b) is distinct from NO and prostacyclin; and (c) hyperpolarizes vascular smooth muscle by opening a potassium conductance. In rat cerebral vessels, the latter is a calcium-activated potassium channel or a closely related channel, which is sensitive to charybdotoxin (You *et al.*, 1998; You *et al.*, 1999). Applications of UTP or ATP to the

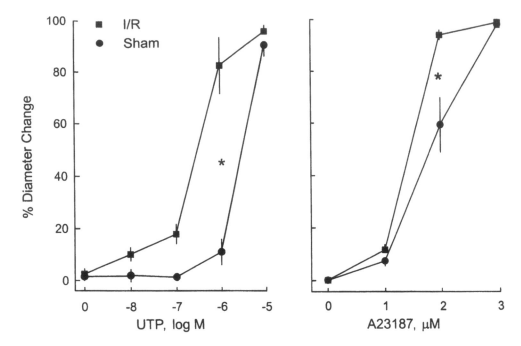

Figure 43.5 Dilatations to UTP and A23187 in the presence of N^{ω}-nitro-L-arginine methyl
ester (L-NAME, 10^{-5} M) in sham and reperfused (I/R) arteries. For UTP
responses, $n = 5$ and 8 for sham and reperfused arteries, respectively. For
A23187 responses, $n = 4$ and 7 for sham and reperfused arteries, respectively.
Data are shown as means ± SEM. The asterisk indicates a statistically significant
($p < .05$) difference between sham and reperfused arteries at corresponding concentrations of UTP or A23187. (The graph on the left was redrawn from Marrelli
et al. (1999) with permission.)

lumen of cerebral arteries and arterioles from naïve rats elicited dilatations (You *et al.*,
1997; You *et al.*, 1998; You *et al.*, 1999). A major portion of this response persisted
following inhibition of nitric oxide synthase and cyclooxygenase. This remaining
component can be attributed to EDHF (You *et al.*, 1998; You *et al.*, 1999). Thus,
EDHF was responsible for the dilatation when nitric oxide synthase was inhibited.

In the present study, isolated rat middle cerebral arteries studied following 2 hours
of focal ischemia and 24 hours of reperfusion, showed an enhanced sensitivity to
luminally applied UTP. The EC_{50} following ischemia/reperfusion was approximately
25% of the EC_{50} derived from sham arteries. The difference between sham and
reperfused arteries was accentuated following inhibition of nitric oxide synthase alone
or in combination with inhibition of cycloxygenase (data not shown). The component remaining after inhibition of nitric oxide synthase hyperpolarized the vascular
smooth muscle and was prevented by charybdotoxin. Thus, EDHF could totally
account for the dilatation following nitric oxide synthase inhibition. Presumably, it
was this EDHF-mediated component that was responsible for the potentiated dilatation in reperfused arteries when inhibitors of nitric oxide were absent.

There are a several of possibilities that could account for the enhanced EDHF
component of UTP-mediated dilations in reperfused arteries. First, more EDHF

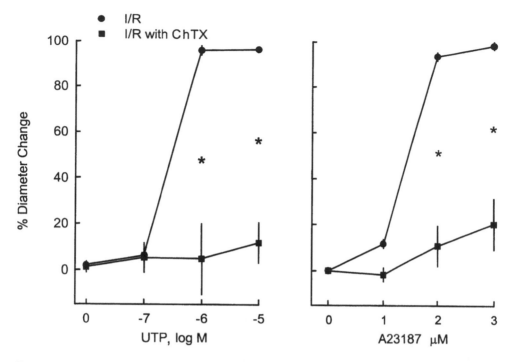

Figure 43.6 UTP- or A23187-mediated dilatations ($n = 3$ and 6, respectively) in the presence of charybdotoxin (CHTX, 10^{-7} M) in middle cerebral arteries from ischemia/reperfusion (I/R) rats. All studies were conducted in the presence of N^{ω}-nitro-L-arginine methyl ester (L-NAME, 5×10^{-5} M). Data are shown as means $\pm$ SEM. The asterisk indicates a statistically significant ($p < .05$) difference between reperfused (I/R) arteries with and without charybdotoxin at corresponding concentrations of UTP or A23187. (The graph on the left was redrawn from Marrelli *et al.* (1999) with permission.)

could have been released for a given concentration of UTP as a result of (a) increased receptor number; (b) increased affinity of the receptor for UTP; (c) dis-inhibition of EDHF synthesis due to reduced NO concentration (Olmos *et al.*, 1995; Bauersachs *et al.*, 1996); or (d) amplification along the signal transduction pathway for EDHF release. Alternatively, the vascular smooth muscle in reperfused arteries may have been more sensitive to EDHF.

The present studies provide limited insight into the mechanism for the enhanced EDHF response in reperfused arteries. Since Ca^{2+} is the presumed second messenger for EDHF release (or possibly the synthesis and release), a Ca^{2+} ionophore (A23187) was used to circumvent the P2Y$_2$-like receptors and directly increase Ca^{2+}. Similar to the response with UTP, the EDHF-mediated component was enhanced in reperfused arteries upon exposure to A23187. It appears, therefore, that a potentiation of the response in reperfused arteries occurs at the Ca^{2+} step or downstream from Ca^{2+}. Likewise, an increased receptor density or increased affinities of the receptors for UTP are not responsible for the potentiated EDHF component in I/R vessels.

EDHF or the actions of EDHF are enhanced during pathological conditions. Although circumstantial in some instances, there appears to be an enhanced

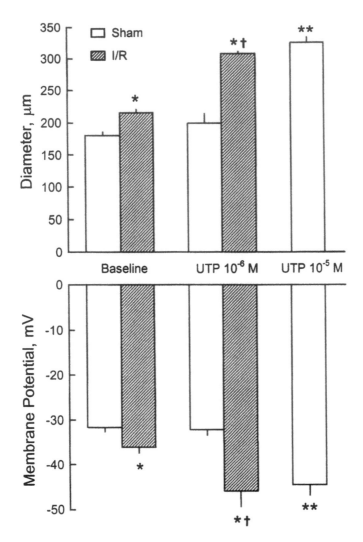

Figure 43.7 Change in diameter (top) and smooth muscle membrane potential (bottom) in sham ($n = 5$) and reperfused (I/R, $n = 5$) middle cerebral arteries. All values for diameter and membrane potential are in the presence of N^{ω}-nitro-L-arginine methyl ester (L-NAME, 5×10^{-5} M). Data are shown as means $\pm$ SEM. The single asterisk indicates a statistically significant ($p < .05$) difference between sham and reperfused arteries. The double asterisk indicates a statistically significant ($p < .05$) difference between 10^{-6} and 10^{-5} M UTP for sham arteries. The dagger indicates a statistically significant ($p < .05$) difference between 10^{-6} M UTP and baseline for reperfused arteries. (Redrawn from Marrelli *et al.* (1999) with permission.)

EDHF-mediated component in certain peripheral arteries following endothelial regeneration, during congestive heart failure, hypercholesterolemia, or coronary ischemia/reperfusion (Thollon *et al.*, 1999; Najibi *et al.*, 1994; Brandes *et al.*, 1997; Malmsjo *et al.*, 1999; Chan and Woodman, 1999). Since each of these pathological conditions is associated with decreased activity of the NO/cyclic GMP pathway, a reciprocal relationship may exist between the NO pathway and the EDHF pathway (Olmos *et al.*, 1995; Bauersachs *et al.*, 1996; Bauersachs *et al.*, 1997; Hecker, 2000). When the NO/cyclic GMP pathway is suppressed, the EDHF-mediated pathway may become enhanced in order to take over the role of NO.

ACKNOWLEDGMENTS

This study was supported by PHS grants PO1 NS 27616 and NS 37250. Drs Marrelli and Bryan dedicate this publication to Dr William F. Childres who passed away during the writing of this manuscript.

44 The EDHF-dependent but not the NO-dependent component of the acetylcholine-induced relaxation of the rabbit aorta is resistant to ionized radiation

Anatoly I. Soloviev, Sergey M. Tishkin,
Alexander V. Parshikov, Irina V. Mosse,
Alexander V. Stefanov, Oleg N. Osipenko
and Alison M. Gurney

The contribution of endothelium-derived relaxing factor (EDRF/NO) and endothelium-derived hyperpolarizing factor (EDHF) to the impairment of endothelium-dependent relaxation caused by acetylcholine was examined in the rabbit thoracic aorta after irradiation. The changes in membrane potential and contractile force in response to acetylcholine were recorded during contractions to phenylephrine in the presence or absence of N^ω-nitro-L-arginine and indomethacin. The acetylcholine-induced relaxations were smaller in tissues obtained from irradiated animals than in those from healthy rabbits. Aortic rings from irradiated animals showed enhanced responses to authentic NO compared with non-irradiated animals. The acetylcholine-stimulated release of NO, detected by chemiluminescence, was not different in irradiated and non-irradiated vascular tissues. The relaxation to acetylcholine in non-irradiated animals was only partly reduced in the presence of N^ω-nitro-L-arginine and indomethacin, indicating a sizable EDHF-mediated component. A similar experiment in aortas from irradiated animals showed that the EDHF-dependent component of the acetylcholine-induced relaxation was unchanged while the EDRF/NO component was decreased. The EDRF/NO-dependent component, but not the EDHF-dependent component of the acetylcholine-induced relaxation was restored by the treatment of irradiated animals with the antioxidant α-tocopherol acetate. Electrophysiological studies demonstrated that application of acetylcholine hyperpolarized both healthy and irradiated rabbit aortas but that the peak amplitude of hyperpolarization was smaller after irradiation. In the presence of N^G-nitro-L-arginine and indomethacin the amplitudes of hyperpolarization were similar in healthy and irradiated tissues. In the presence of N^ω-nitro-L-arginine and indomethacin, the acetylcholine-induced relaxations and hyperpolarizations in both tissues were unaffected by glibenclamide but reduced by apamin combined with charybdotoxin. They were almost completely blocked by tetraethylammonium, a non-selective inhibitor of calcium-dependent potassium channels, or when the tissues were contracted with potassium chloride instead of phenylephrine. These results are consistent with the hypothesis that the depression of endothelial function following ionized irradiation are due mainly to an alteration in EDRF/NO metabolism but not to a decrease in EDHF. Since the release and/or action of EDHF are relatively resistant to radiation-induced oxidative stress, EDHF seems unlikely to be a metabolite of arachidonic acid formed by cytochrome P450 monoxygenase or generated by other oxygen-dependent enzymes.

The most common health problems in the Ukrainian population exposed to radiation as a result of the 1986 Chernobyl nuclear accident are diseases of the cardiovascular system. Cardiovascular disease is also prevalent among survivors of the Nagasaki and Hiroshima atomic bombs. It is likely that blood vessels are the major target for ionizing radiation. Exposure of vascular tissue to ionizing radiation leads to formation of reactive oxygen species that are associated with radiation-induced cytotoxicity. Endothelial injury is one of the common effects of ionizing irradiation. As endothelium is the most vulnerable component of the vascular wall, vascular injury under ionized irradiation first appears as an endothelial dysfunction (Menendez *et al.*, 1998; Oi *et al.*, 1998; Sugihara *et al.*, 1999).

A number of endothelium-derived factors contribute to the regulation of vascular tone in health and disease. Among those endothelium-derived relaxing factor identified as nitric oxide (EDRF/NO), and endothelium-derived hyperpolarizing factor (EDHF) play a main role. The chemical nature of EDHF is uncertain. A cytochrome P450-derived epoxide could represent EDHF, at least in some vascular beds (Fisslthaler *et al.*, 1999). The term EDHF should be restricted to describe phenomena in which endothelium-dependent hyperpolarizations and relaxations are resistant to inhibitors of nitric oxide synthase and cyclooxygenase, insensitive to glibenclamide and sensitive to charybdotoxin plus apamin (Vanhoutte and Félétou, 1999). The depression of endothelium-dependent relaxations in irradiated animals could be due to decreases in the synthesis or release of either EDRF/NO or EDHF, to alterations in their metabolism, or to changes in sensitivity of smooth muscle cells to these endothelial relaxing factors. The present study was designed to evaluate the relative contribution of EDRF/NO and EDHF in the endothelial dysfunction after irradiation.

1. METHODS

The study was performed on white rabbits weighing 2.5–3.0 kg. Whole body irradiation was performed with gamma rays from a cobalt-60 source (TGT ROCUS M, Russia).

1.1. Tension measurements

Rings (1–2 mm width) of thoracic aorta were suspended isometrically in an organ chamber between a stationary stainless steel hook and an isometric force transducer (AE 801, SensoNor A/S, Norten, Norway) that was coupled to a chart recorder (Model 202, Cole-Parmer Instrument Company, USA). The rings were equilibrated for one hour with a resting tension of 25 mN. Experiments were performed at 37 °C in modified Krebs bicarbonate buffer of the following composition (in mM): NaCl 133, KCl 4.7, NaHCO$_3$ 16.3, NaH$_2$PO$_4$ 1.38, CaCl$_2$ 2.5, MgCl$_2$ 1.2, glucose 7.8 and pH 7.4. All experiments were performed in the presence of indomethacin (10^{-5} M).

1.2. Microelectrode studies

Aortic rings were inverted and suspended between two stainless steel hooks for the recording of membrane potential. Glass electrodes filled with 3 M KCl (tip resistance

$60-80\,\text{M}\Omega$) were inserted into smooth muscle cells from the intimal side. A micro-electrode amplifier MZ-4 (Nihon, Cohden, Japan) was used for the measurement of transmembrane potentials. Membrane potentials were displayed continuously on an oscilloscope (ATAC-250, Nihon, Cohden, Japan) and recorded on a chart recorder (Model 202, Cole-Parmer Instrument Company, USA).

1.3. Chemiluminescence

The detection of nitric oxide was based upon chemiluminescence reaction between NO and the luminol (5-amino-2,3-dihydro-1,4-phthalazinedione) – H_2O_2 system. The reaction solution contained 0.2 mM luminol, 250 µM 1,10-phenanthroline, 50 mM H_2O_2 and 4 mM potassium carbonate. For the chemiluminescence assay the effluent (2 ml/min, flow rate) of the organ chamber was mixed with a luminol-containing solution (0.8 ml/min) in a special reactor cell connected to a flow cell-type chemiluminescence detector with a photomultiplier tube (Model R 2693, Hamamatsu). The limit of NO determination was approximately $5 \times 10^{-11}\,\text{M}$ (linear range of $10^{-10} - 3 \times 10^{-9}\,\text{M}$). NO concentrations were detected within five seconds after the superfusate exited from the organ chamber.

Standard aqueous NO solution (authentic NO) was prepared according to the following procedure. At first, NO was prepared by flushing 99% NO gas through a sealed bottle for 30 min. Further, deoxygenated water was prepared by flushing O_2-free argon for 3 h through a sealed bottle containing HPLS-grade H_2O. Then NO gas was injected into the deoxygenated water. The saturated solution of NO (3 mM) was obtained by adding 5 ml NO gas to 20 ml deoxygenated water.

1.4. Chemicals

Luminol sodium salt, phenylephrine, acetylcholine chloride, glibenclamide, charybdotoxin, tetraethylammonium, indomethacin, N^{ω}-nitro-L-arginine were obtained from Sigma (St. Louis, MO, USA). 1,10-Phenanthroline was from Serva (Heidelberg, Germany).

1.5. Statistical analysis

All values are reported as Means ± SEM. The data were analysed statistically using analysis of variance and Student's t-test. p values of less than .05 were considered to indicate statistically significant difference.

2. RESULTS

2.1. Relaxations

While the amplitude of relaxations to large concentrations $(1.3 \times 10^{-7} - 10^{-5}\,\text{M})$ of acetylcholine were decreased after irradiation, the response to low concentrations $(10^{-8} - 1.3 \times 10^{-7}\,\text{M})$ were significantly increased (Figure 44.1). A significant leftward shift dose–response curve to acetylcholine was noted in irradiated tissues, indicating that the sensitivity of vascular wall to acetylcholine had increased (Figure 44.1).

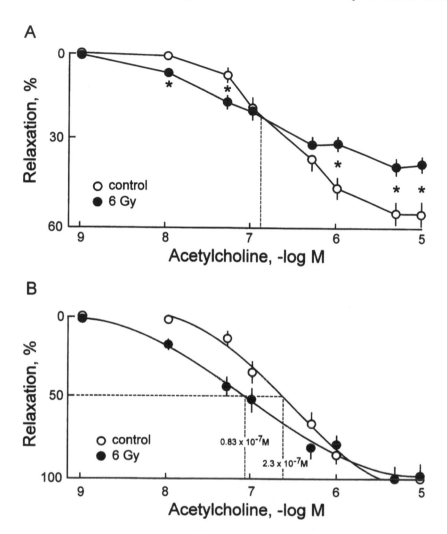

Figure 44.1 Concentration–relaxation curves to acetylcholine obtained in thoracic aortas from healthy (open circles) and irradiated (6 Gy, closed circles) rabbits. (Upper) Curves were normalized relatively to the maximal amplitude of phenylephrine-induced contraction. (Lower) Curves were normalized relatively to the maximal acetylcholine-induced relaxation. The dotted lines indicate the EC_{50}. Data shown as means $\pm$ SEM. The asterisks indicate statistically significant differences ($p < .05$).

The sensitivity of aortic tissues from irradiated animals to authentic NO was also significantly greater compared to healthy rabbits (EC_{50} $4.3 \pm 1.1 \times 10^{-7}$ M and $1.4 \pm 0.49 \times 10^{-6}$ M, respectively, $n = 14$; Figure 44.2).

A positive correlation was found between the acetylcholine-stimulated increment of NO concentration in the buffer solution and the corresponding relaxation in thoracic aortas from healthy rabbits. In contrast, irradiated aortic tissues yielded a negative correlation (Figure 44.3). Calculations showed no significant difference in the two groups between NO released by 1 mg aortic tissue per minute under acetylcholine

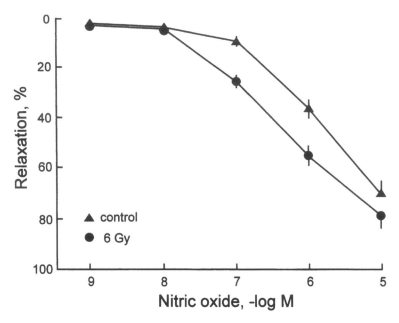

Figure 44.2 Concentration–response curves to authentic nitric oxide in thoracic aortas from healthy (triangles) and irradiated (6 Gy, circles) rabbits.

treatment ($2.75 \pm 0.97 \times 10^{-11}$ M and $3.4 \pm 0.8 \times 10^{-11}$ M for healthy and irradiated rabbits respectively, $n = 11$).

Acetylcholine at a maximal concentration of 10^{-5} M relaxed the aortas by $54.4 \pm 2.7\%$ in the absence of N^{ω}-nitro-L-arginine, and by $40.3 \pm 2.3\%$ of developed force ($n = 12$) when N^{ω}-nitro-L-arginine was added. The difference was statistically significant. When the data were expressed as percent relatively to the maximal acetylcholine-induced relaxation in the absence of N^{ω}-nitro-L-arginine, the remaining, EDHF-dependent component averaged $74.1 \pm 4.2\%$ of the total acetylcholine-induced relaxation (Figure 44.4). When added to the bath solution alone, indomethacin had no effect on acetylcholine-induced relaxation (data not shown).

After radiation, the total acetylcholine relaxation decreased two fold and EDHF-dependent component by 32% only (Figure 44.4). α-Tocopherol acetate, orally administered 1 h after irradiation in dose 50 mg/kg, significantly restored the EDRF/NO component but had no effect on the EDHF component of the acetylcholine-induced relaxation (Figure 44.4).

In the presence of both apamin (10^{-6} M) plus charybdotoxin (10^{-8} M), the relaxation to acetylcholine was significantly reduced and reduced additionally (two fold) when N^{ω}-nitro-L-arginine was added to this mixture (Figure 44.4). Similar effects were seen when tetraethylammonium (10^{-3} M), a non-selective inhibitor of calcium-dependent potassium channels, was used or when the tissues were constricted with potassium chloride (50 mM) instead of phenyleprine. The EDHF component was unaffected by glibenclamide at a concentration of 10^{-5} M (not shown).

In irradiated tissue, the acetylcholine-induced relaxation was absent in the presence of a mixture of apamin plus charybdotoxin, alone or in combination with N^{ω}-nitro-L-arginine (Figure 44.4).

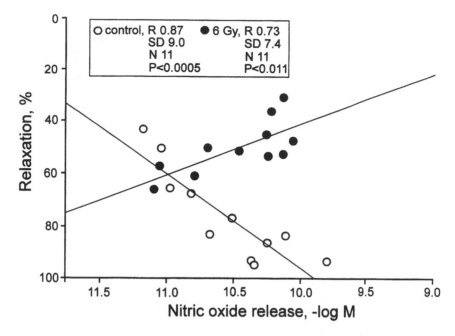

Figure 44.3 Relationship between acetylcholine-stimulated increments of NO concentration in the bath solution and the amplitude of the corresponding relaxations in thoracic aortas from healthy (open circles) and irradiated (6 Gy, closed circles) rabbits.

2.2. Microelectrode studies

The resting membrane potential of aortas with endothelium averaged $-53.6 \pm$ 3.1 mV ($n = 12$). Acetylcholine, at a maximal concentration of 10^{-5} M, hyperpolarized the cell membrane. N^ω-nitro-L-arginine plus indomethacin significantly reduced the hyperpolarization induced by acetylcholine. As a rule, the membrane responses to acetylcholine were monophasic and transient (Figure 44.5).

Hyperpolarization upon exposure to acetylcholine, was also observed in aortas of irradiated rabbits. However, it was significantly lower than that seen in healthy rabbits and was similar to the value observed in healthy tissues in the presence of N^ω-nitro-L-arginine and indomethacin. The treatment with N^G-nitro-L-arginine and indomethacin did not reduce the hyperpolarization in irradiated tissues (Figure 44.5).

The hyperpolarization induced by acetylcholine in both types of tissue in the presence of N^ω-nitro-L-arginine and indomethacin (5×10^{-6} M) was nearly abolished by tetraethylammonium (10^{-3} M) or by a mixture of charybdotoxin (10^{-8} M) plus apamin (10^{-6} M) (data not shown).

3. DISCUSSION

The main finding of the present study is the resistance of the EDHF-dependent component of acetylcholine-induced relaxation to ionized radiation.

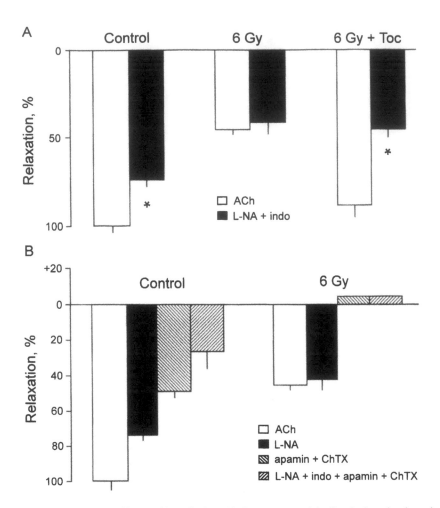

Figure 44.4 (A) Effects of irradiation (6 Gy) on acetylcholine-induced relaxations in the absence and presence of N^{ω}-nitro-L-arginine (L-NA, 10^{-5} M), and with the addition of the antioxidant α-tocopherol acetate orally administrated 1 h after irradiation (50 mg/kg). (B) Effect of potassium channels blockers added to the organ chamber. Apamin (10^{-6} M), charybdotoxin (ChTX, 10^{-8} M), N^{ω}-nitro-L-arginine (L-NA, 10^{-5} M). Relaxations are expressed as percent relatively to the maximal acetylcholine-induced relaxation in healthy tissue in the absence of N^{ω}-nitro-L-arginine. All experiments were performed in the presence of indomethacin (5×10^{-6} M). Data shown as means $\pm$ SEM. The asterisks indicate statistically significant differences ($p < .05$).

Acetylcholine-induced hyperpolarization and related relaxation can be attributed to the release of three main compounds: nitric oxide (NO), prostacyclin and EDHF. Removal of NO and prostacyclin-dependent components can be achieved using combination of N^{ω}-nitro-L-arginine and indomethacin.

In isolated rabbit thoracic aortas contracted with phenylephrine, acetylcholine elicits endothelium-dependent relaxations, which involve the action of both NO and EDHF. The prostanoid component seems to be negligible in this preparation since the

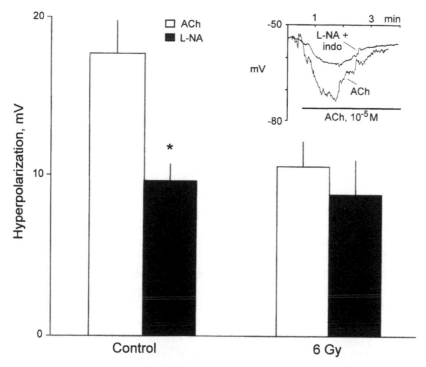

Figure 44.5 Effect of N^{ω}-nitro-L-arginine, (L-NA, 10^{-5} M) on acetylcholine (Ach, 10^{-5} M)-induced hyperpolarization in aortas from healthy and irradiated (6 Gy) rabbits. The inset shows original recordings of hyperpolarization to acetylcholine in the presence and absence of N^{ω}-nitro-L-arginine in a control aorta. All experiments were performed in the presence of indomethacin (5×10^{-6} M). Data shown as means $\pm$ SEM. The asterisk indicates a statistically significant difference ($p < .05$).

addition of indomethacin alone to the buffer solution had no significant effect on acetylcholine-induced relaxations.

Experiments with N^{ω}-nitro-L-arginine (and indomethacin) showed that NO (and prostacyclin) cannot entirely account for the acetylcholine-induced endothelium-dependent relaxation of the rabbit thoracic aorta, since the vasodilator response was not completely suppressed by these inhibitors. EDHF appeared to contribute mainly to the acetylcholine-induced relaxation in this blood vessels. EDHF appears to play an important role in the maintenance of vascular tone both in health and disease. For example, alterations in EDHF-mediated responses have been reported in hypertension (Fuji *et al.*, 1996; Soloviev *et al.*, 1999) and diabetes (Fukao *et al.*, 1999).

The present data demonstrate that radiation attenuates the relaxation to acetyl-choline mainly by inhibition of the NO-dependent component of the response. Indeed, the N^{ω}-nitro-L-arginine and indomethacin-resistant, EDHF-dependent component of the acetylcholine-induced relaxation demonstrated surprising stability after radiation. The hyperpolarization caused by acetylcholine in healthy and irradiated thoracic aorta in the presence of N^{ω}-nitro-L-arginine and indomethacin was insensitive to glibenclamide but was inhibited by the combination of charybdotoxin plus apamin or by tetraethylammonium, indicating that EDHF and its target, calcium-dependent potassium channels, are involved in this radiation-resistant response. This seems to be a general characteristic of EDHF, since in contrast to NO and prostacyclin, the release, and presumably also the action of EDHF is resistant to an increase in local concentration of superoxide anions and peroxynitrite (Kaw and Hecker, 1999).

It is likely that irradiated vascular cells suffer first of all of oxidative attacks. One of the chemical groups, the content of which increases significantly in living tissues and biological liquids in response to irradiation, are the oxygen-derived free radicals (superoxide anion, hydroxyl anions and others) and hydrogen peroxide (Serkiz, 1997). Superoxide anions are of particular importance as their chemical activity is higher in hydrophobic than in water phase, which explains their damaging effect to the hydrophobic zones of the cell membrane complex close to ionic channels. Hydroxyl radicals are generated in living systems in large quantities also by ionizing radiation. These radicals are one of the main agents in the radiation-induced lipid peroxidation (Sidoryk *et al.*, 1997). Hydrogen peroxide diffuses for large distances and actively participates in the oxidation of organic molecules. Hydrogen peroxide and the formed free radicals cause lesions in all biological molecules such as breaks in DNA, oxidation of SH-groups and enzyme inactivation. But the most dangerous for the cells is an initiation by these molecules of the chain of events leading to lipid peroxidation (Baraboy, 1997). Multiple processes lead to endothelial damage during irradiation but the generation of oxygen derived free radicals and the subsequent lipid peroxidation may be one of the key components in this cascade of events. The probable targets for oxygen derived free radicals in endothelial cells are ionic channels in the plasma membrane. Thus, a harmful effect of radiation may be related to damage of phospholipid environment of the ionic channels and subsequent disturbance in calcium and/or potassium transport. Another possible reason for depression of EDRF/NO-dependent responses after irradiation is a fast interaction between NO and superoxide anions (Rubanyi and Vanhoutte, 1986) an formation of less potent vasodilator, peroxynitrite, which, in turn, possesses the ability to initiate lipid peroxidation (Radi *et al.*, 1991).

Experiments with the measurement of NO release and the administration of antioxidant, α-tocopherol acetate, support the view that the loss of availability of endothelium-derived NO after irradiation may be due to its accelerated degradation by the excess production of superoxide anions and subsequent formation of peroxynitrite. By contrast, the resistance of the EDHF-component to irradiation, seems to make it unlikely that membrane phospholipid metabolism or the formation of cytochrome P450-generated epoxy-metabolites of arachidonic acid contribute mainly to the generation of EDHF.

The increased sensitivity of vascular smooth muscle to authentic NO after irradiation may represent a compensatory phenomenon. Thus, suppression of endothelial function, with the consequent upregulation of the NO receptor, soluble guanylyl cyclase, results in an increased sensitivity to exogenous NO (Moncada *et al.*, 1991).

4. CONCLUSION

The present data suggest that EDHF does not contribute significantly to the impairment of endothelium-dependent vascular function after ionized irradiation.

The loss of endothelial function after irradiation is mainly due to an alteration in EDRF/NO. EDHF may constitute a reserve mechanism for the maintenance of blood flow during radiation attack. Since the release and the mechanisms of EDHF action are relatively resistant to irradiation-induced oxidative stress, it is unlikely that EDHF is a metabolite of arachidonic acid formed by cytochrome P450 monoxygenase or generated by other oxygen-dependent enzymes.

ACKNOWLEDGEMENT

This study was supported by Wellcome Trust grant 055168/Z/98/Z.

45 Inhibition of converting enzyme prevents the age-related decline in endothelium-dependent hyperpolarization

Koji Fujii, Kenichi Goto
and Isao Abe

The studies summarized here tested whether or not endothelium-dependent hyperpolarization and relaxation caused by endothelium-derived hyperpolarizing factor (EDHF) decline with aging, and, if so, whether or not chronic treatment with a converting enzyme inhibitor improves the age-related endothelial dysfunction. EDHF-mediated hyperpolarization and relaxation were examined in mesenteric arteries obtained from 3-, 6-, 12-, and 24-month-old, normotensive Wistar Kyoto rats (WKY). In addition, a number of the rats were treated for 3 months with either enalapril or a combination of hydralazine and hydrochlorothiazide from 9- to 12-month-old. EDHF-mediated hyperpolarization to acetylcholine was impaired in arteries from 12- and 24-month-old rats compared with younger rats, with the response tending to be further impaired in 24-month-old rats than in 12-month-old rats. EDHF-mediated relaxations also exhibited an age-related impairment. The EDHF-mediated hyperpolarizations and relaxations in 12-month-old rats improved by 3 months of treatment with enalapril but not with a combination of hydralazine and hydrochlorothiazide, despite a similar reduction in blood pressure by both treatments. These findings suggest that: (a) endothelium-dependent hyperpolarization and relaxation via EDHF decline with aging in rat arteries; and (b) chronic treatment with converting enzyme inhibitor enalapril, but not a conventional therapy with vasodilators and diuretics, improves the age-related impairment of EDHF-mediated responses. These findings raise the possibility that blockade of the renin-angiotensin system might prevent or retard the age-related endothelial dysfunction.

Endothelium-dependent relaxation is accounted for by several factors, such as nitric oxide (NO) (Furchgott and Zawadzki, 1980; Ignarro, 1989), prostacyclin, and endothelium-derived hyperpolarizing factor (EDHF) (Félétou and Vanhoutte, 1988; Chen *et al.*, 1988; Chen and Suzuki, 1989; Cohen and Vanhoutte, 1995). Endothelial dysfunction is associated with various cardiovascular risk factors, such as hypertension, hypercholesterolemia and aging. Although the mechanisms for endothelial dysfunction may differ depending on the types of risk factors, an impaired EDHF-mediated hyperpolarization accounts, at least in part, for the decreased endothelium-dependent relaxation associated with hypertension or aging (Fujii *et al.*, 1992; Fujii *et al.*, 1993).

Because endothelial dysfunction may work as an aggravating factor for cardiovascular disease (Vanhoutte, 1997), it is clinically relevant to prevent or reverse endothelial dysfunction. Several clinical and experimental studies have shown that antihypertensive treatment improves endothelial dysfunction in hypertension (Taddei *et al.*, 1998;

Tschudi *et al.*, 1994; Kähönen *et al.*, 1995; Onaka *et al.*, 1998). However, only limited information is available concerning as to effect of drug treatment on age-related endothelial dysfunction. The studies summarized in this chapter demonstrate an age-related decline in endothelium-dependent hyperpolarization and relaxation via EDHF, and an improvement with chronic treatment with a converting enzyme inhibitor.

1. METHODS

1.1. Animals

Three-, 6-, 12-, 24-month-old male Wistar Kyoto rats (WKY) were used in the first part of this study, which were referred to as WKY-3, WKY-6, WKY-12 and WKY-24, respectively. In the second part of this study, a part of 9-month-old WKY were assigned to either a control group (WKY-O) or to one of two treatment groups. The WKY were treated with either enalapril (20 mg/kg/day; WKY-E), or a combination of hydralazine (50 mg/kg/day) and hydrochlorothiazide (7.5 mg/kg/day) (WKY-H) for 3 months until the age of 12 months. All drugs were given in the drinking water. Untreated, 3-month-old WKY also served as young controls (WKY-Y). There were six to ten rats in each. In addition, a part of 3-month-old WKY had been treated with enalapril (20 mg/kg/day) from 8 to 12 weeks (WKY-Y-E) ($n = 4$).

Systolic blood pressure was measured in conscious rats by the tail-cuff method. The drugs were withdrawn two days prior to the experiments. The rats were anesthetized with ether and killed by decapitation. The main branch of the mesenteric artery was excised and bathed in cold Krebs solution having the following composition (in mmol/L): $Na^+ 137.4$, $K^+ 5.9$, $Mg^{2+} 1.2$, $Ca^{2+} 2.5$, $HCO_3^- 15.5$, $H_2PO_4^- 1.2$, $Cl^- 134$, and glucose 11.5. The artery was cut into rings of 3 mm and 1.2 mm width for the electrophysiological and tension experiments, respectively.

1.2. Membrane potential

Transverse strips cut along the longitudinal axis of the rings were placed in the experimental chamber with the endothelial layer up. Tissues were carefully pinned to the rubber base attached to the bottom of the 2 ml chamber and then superfused with 36 °C Krebs solution aerated with 95% O_2–5% CO_2 (pH 7.3–7.4) at a rate of 3 ml/min. After equilibration for at least 60 min, the membrane potentials of vascular smooth muscle cells were recorded using the conventional microelectrode technique. Briefly, conventional glass capillary microelectrodes filled with 3 mol/l KCl and with tip resistance of 50–80 MΩ were inserted into the smooth muscle cells from the endothelial side. Electrical signals were amplified through an amplifier (MEZ-7200, Nihon Koden, Tokyo, Japan), monitored on an oscilloscope (VC-11, Nihon Koden), and recorded with a pen recorder (RJG-4002, Nihon Koden).

1.3. Isometric tension

Rings with intact endothelium were placed in the 5 ml organ chambers filled with 36 °C Krebs solution aerated with 93% O_2–7% CO_2 (pH 7.4). Two fine, stainless steel wires were placed through the lumen of the ring; one was anchored, and the other was attached to the mechano-transducer (UM-203, Kishimoto, Kyoto, Japan). After the rings were allowed to equilibrate for 60 min at an optimal resting tension of 1.0 g, they were exposed to indomethacin, an inhibitor of cyclooxygenase, and N^G-nitro-L-arginine, an inhibitor of NO synthase. The rings were contracted with norepinephrine (10^{-5} M), and the relaxant effects of acetylcholine were studied by adding the drug in increasing concentrations, from 10^{-9} to 10^{-5} M.

In some preparations, the rings were contracted with 77 mmol/l KCl solution in the presence of indomethacin (10^{-5} M), and a relaxation to acetylcholine was obtained. Relaxations in response to levcromakalim, a direct activator of ATP-sensitive K^+ channels, and sodium nitroprusside were studied in rings contracted with norepinephrine (10^{-5} M) in the presence of indomethacin (10^{-5} M). The extent of the relaxation was expressed as the percentage of the initial contraction evoked by the contractile agonist.

1.4. Drugs and solutions

Drugs used in this study were acetylcholine chloride, norepinephrine, indomethacin, N^G-nitro-L-arginine, enalapril, hydralazine, hydrochlorothiazide, sodium nitroprusside (Sigma, St Louis, MO, USA), TCV-116 (a gift from Takeda Pharmaceuticals, Osaka, Japan), and levcromakalim (a gift from SmithKline Beecham Pharmaceuticals, Worthing, UK).

Indomethacin was dissolved in 10 mmol/l Na_2CO_3, N^G-nitro-L-arginine in 0.2 mol/l HCl, and levcromakalim in 90% ethanol. All other drugs were dissolved in distilled water. The solutions containing 20 mmol/l or 77 mmol/l KCl were obtained by equimolar replacement of NaCl by KCl in Krebs solution.

1.5. Statistics

Results are given as mean ± SEM. The concentration–response curves of hyperpolarization and relaxation were analyzed by two-way analysis of variance followed by Scheffé's test for multiple comparisons. Other variables were analyzed by one-way analysis of variance followed by Scheffé's test for multiple comparisons or paired Student's t-test. A level of p was less than .05 was considered to be statistically significant.

2. RESULTS

2.1. Age-related changes

Endothelium-dependent hyperpolarizations to acetylcholine, applied in the resting state of the membrane, were significantly smaller in WKY-12 and WKY-24 than in WKY-3 or WKY-6 (Figure 45.1). In addition, the hyperpolarization tended to be smaller, but not significantly so, in WKY-24 than in WKY-12.

Endothelium-dependent relaxations to acetylcholine in rings contracted with norepinephrine (10^{-5} M) in the presence of indomethacin (10^{-5} M) and N^G-nitro-L-arginine (10^{-4} M) were significantly smaller in WKY-12 and WKY-24 than in WKY-3 or WKY-6 (Figure 45.1). In addition, the relaxation was significantly smaller in WKY-24 than in WKY-12.

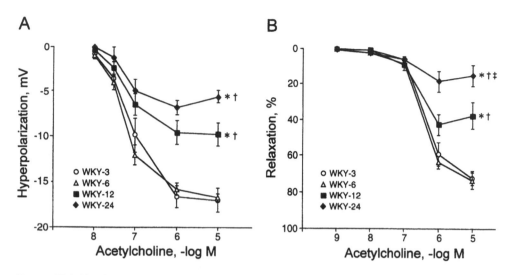

Figure 45.1 (A) Concentration–hyperpolarization curves to acetylcholine in mesenteric arteries with endothelium of 3- (WKY-3), 6- (WKY-6), 12- (WKY-12), and 24-month-old Wistar Kyoto rats (WKY-24). Acetylcholine was applied under resting conditions without treatment. (B) Concentration–relaxation curves to acetylcholine in mesenteric arterial rings with endothelium contracted with norepinephrine (10^{-5} M) in the presence of indomethacin (10^{-5} M) and N^G-nitro-L-arginine (10^{-4} M) of WKY-3, WKY-6, WKY-12, and WKY-24. Values are shown as means ± SEM. There were six to ten rats in each group. The asterisks indicate significant differences as compared to the values of WKY-3 ($p < .05$, by two-way analysis of variance); the daggers indicate significant differences as compared to the values of WKY-6 ($p < .05$); and the double daggers indicate significant differences as compared to the values of WKY-12 ($p < .05$).

2.2. Effects of chronic treatment with enalapril

Enalapril or a combination of hydralazine and hydrochlorothiazide lowered the blood pressure to a comparable extent. The systolic blood pressure at the end of the treatment period was 126 ± 5 mmHg for WKY-E, 124 ± 4 mmHg for WKY-H, and 155 ± 4 mmHg for WKY-O. The systolic blood pressure of WKY-Y was 148 ± 4 mmHg.

The resting membrane potential of smooth muscle cells of the mesenteric artery did not differ significantly among the study groups (WKY-O -49.6 ± 0.5; WKY-E -50.3 ± 1.3; WKY-H -50.3 ± 2.2; WKY-Y -48.8 ± 1.2 mV).

Enalapril treatment (WKY-E) but not the combination of hydralazine and hydrochlorothiazide (WKY-H) significantly improved acetylcholine-induced hyperpolarization compared with WKY-O, and the response attained in WKY-E was comparable to that in WKY-Y (Figure 45.2).

EDHF-mediated relaxation to acetylcholine, as assessed in rings contracted with norepinephrine in the presence of indomethacin and N^G-nitro-L-arginine, was significantly smaller in WKY-O than in WKY-Y (Figure 45.2). Enalapril (WKY-E) but not the combination of hydralazine and hydrochlorothiazide (WKY-H) significantly improved the N^G-nitro-L-arginine-resistant relaxations to acetylcholine to a level comparable to that observed in WKY-Y (Figure 45.2).

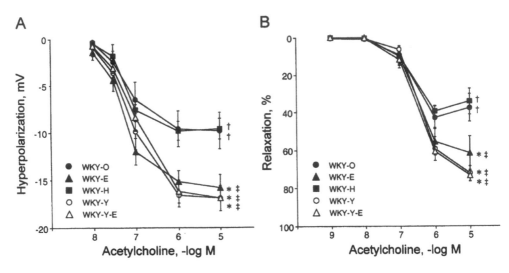

Figure 45.2 (A) Concentration–hyperpolarization curves to acetylcholine in mesenteric arteries with endothelium of 12-month-old, untreated Wistar Kyoto rats (WKY-O), enalapril-treated WKY (WKY-E), WKY treated with a combination of hydralazine and hydrochlorothiazide (WKY-H), 3-month-old, untreated WKY (WKY-Y), and 3-month-old, enalapril-treated WKY (WKY-Y-E). Acetylcholine was applied under the resting conditions without treatment. (B) Concentration–relaxation curves to acetylcholine in mesenteric arterial rings with endothelium contracted with norepinephrine (10^{-5} M) in the presence of indomethacin (10^{-5} M) and N^G-nitro-L-arginine (10^{-4} M) of WKY-O, WKY-E, WKY-H, WKY-Y, and WKY-Y-E. Values are shown as means $\pm$ SEM. There were six to ten rats in each group. The asterisks indicate significant differences as compared to the values of WKY-O ($p < .05$, by two-way analysis of variance); the daggers indicate significant differences as compared to the values of WKY-Y ($p < .05$); and the double daggers indicate significant differences as compared to the values of WKY-H ($p < .05$) (modified from Goto *et al.*, 2000b).

Four weeks treatment of 8-week-old WKY (WKY-Y-E) lowered systolic blood pressure from 148.0 ± 3.4 to 123.0 ± 5.0 mmHg. The acetylcholine-induced hyperpolarizations in mesenteric arteries were not different between WKY-Y-E and WKY-Y (Figure 45.2). Acetylcholine-induced relaxation in rings contracted with norepinephrine (10^{-5} M) in the presence of indomethacin and N^G-nitro-L-arginine also did not differ significantly in WKY-Y and WKY-Y-E (Figure 45.2).

When rings treated with indomethacin were contracted with KCl (77 mM), which eliminates EDHF-mediated hyperpolarization, no difference was found in acetylcholine-induced relaxations among the five groups of WKY-O, WKY-E, WKY-H, WKY-Y and WKY-Y-E (data not shown).

2.3. Endothelium-independent hyperpolarization and relaxation

Endothelium-independent hyperpolarizations and relaxations to levcromakalim, a direct activator of ATP-sensitive K^+-channels did not differ among the study groups (data not shown).

3. DISCUSSION

The studies summarized in this chapter have demonstrated that: (a) endothelium-dependent hyperpolarization, presumably mediated by EDHF, and its contribution to relaxation decline with aging; and (b) antihypertensive treatment with the converting enzyme inhibitor enalapril but not the combination of hydralazine and hydro-chlorothiazide improves the age-related impairment of EDHF-mediated responses.

Endothelium-dependent hyperpolarization and its contribution to relaxation are impaired with aging even in normotensive rats (Fujii *et al.*, 1993). The findings in this study suggest that such an impairment of EDHF-mediated responses may become evident at around the age of 12 months, and that thereafter the responses further decline with increasing age (Fujii *et al.*, 1993; Nakashima and Vanhoutte, 1996).

Antihypertensive therapy has in most cases led to an improvement of endothelial function (Taddei *et al.*, 1998; Tschudi *et al.*, 1994; Kähönen *et al.*, 1995; Onaka *et al.*, 1998). Although the mechanisms responsible for such improvement may vary depending on the species used, the vascular bed studied, or the etiology of hypertension, the restoration of EDHF-mediated hyperpolarization accounts, at least in part, for such an improvement (Onaka *et al.*, 1998). In that study, EDHF-mediated responses improved regardless of the types of antihypertensive drugs used, suggesting that blood pressure lowering may be primarily important for the improvement. However, the degree of improvement tended to be greater with converting enzyme inhibitors compared with a conventional antihypertensive therapy. In humans, antihypertensive treatment with the converting enzyme inhibitor lisinopril or the AT1 antagonist losartan, but not with the β-blocker atenolol corrected endothelial dysfunction of resistance arteries from patients with essential hypertension (Schiffrin and Deng, 1995; Schiffrin *et al.*, 2000). These findings raise the possibility that the renin-angiotensin system blockade *per se* may also play an important role in improving endothelial function.

In the present study, chronic treatment of rats with enalapril, from 9 to 12 months of age, improved EDHF-mediated hyperpolarization and relaxation, while the combination of hydralazine and hydrochlorothiazide failed to do so, despite achieving an identical reduction in blood pressure (Goto *et al.*, 2000b). Because treatment of younger rats with enalapril did not affect endothelial function, it is likely that the converting enzyme inhibitor prevents the age-related decline in EDHF-mediated hyperpolarization and relaxation, presumably through the blockade of the renin-angiotensin system. These findings further imply the importance of the renin-angiotensin system blockade in correcting endothelial dysfunction.

Underlying mechanisms for the age-related impairment of EDHF-mediated hyperpolarization and its improvement by converting enzyme inhibitors remain speculative. However, considering the accumulating evidence that endothelium-dependent hyperpolarization may involve myoendothelial gap junctional communications (Chaytor *et al.*, 1998; Edwards *et al.*, 1999; Yamamoto *et al.*, 1999), it can be speculated that structural changes of the vessel wall, such as subendothelial thickening, might be involved in such alterations. Converting enzyme inhibitors are most effective in reversing hypertensive target organ damages, such as left ventricular hypertrophy (Dahlöf *et al.*, 1992) and vascular remodeling (Schiffrin and Deng, 1995). Furthermore, in the SHR, the converting enzyme inhibitor lisinopril but not hydralazine reduced the subendothelial thickening of the aortic wall (Clozel *et al.*, 1990).

It remains to be tested whether or not the improvement of EDHF-mediated responses by the converting enzyme inhibitor is related to the reversal of the vascular structural changes associated with aging.

The converting enzyme inhibitor perindoprilat potentiates bradykinin-induced hyperpolarization mediated by EDHF in human coronary arteries (Nakashima *et al.*, 1993). Although acute treatment with the converting enzyme inhibitor captopril did not affect the acetylcholine-induced hyperpolarization in the rat mesenteric artery (Onaka *et al.*, 1998), it remains to be determined whether or not the enhanced action of bradykinin contributes to the chronic effects of converting enzyme inhibitors on the EDHF pathway.

The EDHF pathway exists in human arteries, and EDHF-mediated relaxations might also be compromised with aging in humans (Nakashima *et al.*, 1993; Urakami-Harasawa *et al.*, 1997).

4. CONCLUSION

The present study demonstrates that the treatment of normotensive rats with a converting enzyme inhibitor prevents the age-related decline in endothelium-dependent hyperpolarization and relaxation mediated by EDHF, presumably through the blockade of the renin-angiotensin system but not lowering the blood pressure alone. Thus, the possibility exists that the early, functional aging process of the endothelium can be modulated by the inhibitors of the renin-angiotensin system.

46 Effects of a converting enzyme inhibitor, an AT$_1$-receptor antagonist and their combination on endothelial dysfunction in hypertension

Kenichi Goto, Koji Fujii
and Isao Abe

Endothelium-dependent hyperpolarization and relaxation to acetylcholine mediated by endothelium-derived hyperpolarizing factor (EDHF) are impaired in arteries of spontaneously hypertensive rats (SHR). The studies summarized in this chapter tested: (a) whether or not antihypertensive treatment improves the impaired EDHF-mediated responses in SHR arteries; (b) whether or not there are any differences in the beneficial effects among different classes of antihypertensive drugs (the converting enzyme inhibitor enalapril, the AT$_1$-receptor antagonist TCV-116, and a conventional therapy with hydralazine and hydrochlorothiazide); and (c) whether or not the combination of AT$_1$-receptor blockade and converting enzyme inhibition exerts additional effects compared with each intervention alone. All antihypertensive treatments improved EDHF-mediated hyperpolarization and relaxation in mesenteric arteries from SHR. The improvement achieved with enalapril or TCV-116 tended to be greater than that with a conventional therapy with hydralazine and hydrochlorothiazide. The combination of enalapril and TCV-116 exerted similar effects to those of each intervention, although EDHF-mediated hyperpolarization tended to be greater in the former. These findings suggest that: (a) antihypertensive treatment restores the impaired EDHF-mediated responses in SHR; (b) blockers of the renin-angiotensin system may be more efficacious in improving endothelial function; and (c) combined AT$_1$-receptor blockade and converting enzyme inhibition does not appear to have an additive or synergistic effect.

Endothelial cells contribute to the regulation of vascular tone through the release of relaxing factors such as nitric oxide (NO) (Furchgott and Zawadzki, 1980; Ignarro, 1989), prostacyclin, and endothelium-derived hyperpolarizing factor (EDHF) (Félétou and Vanhoutte, 1988; Chen *et al.*, 1988; Chen and Suzuki, 1989). EDHF hyperpolarizes the underlying smooth muscle cells, thereby causing relaxation (Chen and Suzuki, 1989; Kauser *et al.*, 1989; Cohen and Vanhoutte, 1995). Although the identity of EDHF is still debated (Campbell *et al.*, 1996; Fisslthaler *et al.*, 1999; Edwards *et al.*, 1998), possible involvement of myoendothelial gap junctions has been suggested in certain arteries (Chaytor *et al*, 1998; Yamamoto *et al*, 1999; Edwards *et al.*, 1999).

Endothelium-dependent relaxation is impaired in hypertension (Fujii *et al.*, 1992; Taddei *et al.*, 1998). Although the mechanisms underlying this dysfunction are heterogeneous, impaired EDHF-mediated hyperpolarization accounts, at least in part, for the decreased endothelium-dependent relaxation in arteries of spontaneously hypertensive rats (SHR) (Fujii *et al.*, 1992; Fujii *et al.*, 1993). Because endothelial dysfunction may work as an aggravating factor for cardiovascular diseases (Vanhoutte, 1997), it is of clinical importance to find effective treatment to restore endothelial function in hypertension.

1. METHODS

1.1. Animals

Male SHR and age-matched Wistar Kyoto rats (WKY) (the Disease Model Cooperative Research Association, Kyoto, Japan) were used. At the age of 8–9 months, SHR were assigned to one control (SHR-C) and four treatment groups. The SHR were treated with either a combination of hydralazine (25 mg/kg/day) and hydro-chlorothiazide (7.5 mg/kg/day) (SHR-H), TCV-116 (5 mg/kg/day, an AT_1-receptor antagonist; SHR-T), enalapril (40 mg/kg/day, a converting enzyme inhibitor; SHR-E), or their combination (SHR-T&E) for 3 months. All drugs were administered through drinking water. Untreated WKY served as normotensive controls. There were eight to twelve rats in each group.

Systolic blood pressure was measured in conscious rats by the tail-cuff method. The drugs were withdrawn two days prior to the experiments. The rats were anesthetized with ether and killed by decapitation. The main branch of the mesenteric artery was excised and bathed in cold Krebs solution having the following composition (in mmol/L): Na^+ 137.4, K^+ 5.9, Mg^{2+} 1.2, Ca^{2+} 2.5, HCO_3^- 15.5, $H_2PO_4^-$ 1.2, Cl^- 134, and glucose 11.5. The artery was cut into rings of 3 and 1.2 mm for the electro-physiological and tension experiments, respectively.

1.2. Membrane Potential

Transverse strips cut along the longitudinal axis of the rings were placed in the experimental chamber with the endothelial layer up. Tissues were carefully pinned to the rubber base attached to the bottom of the 2-ml chamber and superfused with 36 °C Krebs solution aerated with 95% O_2–5% CO_2 (pH 7.3–7.4) at the rate of 3 ml/minute. After equilibration for at least 60 minutes, the membrane potentials of vascular smooth muscle cells were recorded using conventional microelectrode technique. Briefly, conventional glass capillary microelectrodes filled with 3 mol/l KCl and with a tip resistance of 50–80 MΩ were inserted into the smooth muscle cell from the endothelial side. Electrical signals were amplified through an amplifier (MEZ-7200, Nihon Koden, Tokyo, Japan), monitored on an oscilloscope (VC-11, Nihon Koden), and recorded with a pen recorder (RJG-4002, Nihon Koden).

1.3. Isometric tension

Rings with endothelium were placed in the 5-ml organ chambers filled with 36 °C Krebs solution aerated with 93% O_2–7% CO_2 (pH 7.4). Two fine, stainless steel wires were placed through the lumen of the ring; one was anchored, and the other was attached to the mechano-transducer (UM-203, Kishimoto, Kyoto, Japan). After equilibration for 60 minutes at an optimal resting tension of 1.0 g, the rings were incubated with indomethacin (10^{-5} M) and N^G-nitro-L-arginine (10^{-4} M). The rings were contracted with norepinephrine (10^{-5} M), and relaxations to acetylcholine were studied by adding the drug cumulatively.

Some rings were contracted with KCl (77 mM) solution in the presence of indomethacin (10^{-5} M), and relaxations to acetylcholine were observed. Relaxations to levcromakalim (a direct activator of ATP-sensitive K^+ channels), and sodium nitroprusside were studied in rings contracted with norepinephrine (10^{-5} M) in the presence of indomethacin (10^{-5} M). The extent of the relaxation was expressed as the percentage of the initial contraction.

1.4. Drugs and solutions

Drugs used in this study were acetylcholine chloride, norepinephrine, indomethacin, N^G-nitro-L-arginine, enalapril, hydralazine, hydrochlorothiazide, sodium nitroprusside (Sigma, St Louis, USA), TCV-116 (a gift from Takeda Pharmaceuticals, Osaka, Japan), and levcromakalim (a gift from SmithKline Beecham Pharmaceuticals, Worthing, UK).

Indomethacin was dissolved in 10 mmol/l Na_2CO_3, N^G-nitro-L-arginine in 0.2 mol/l HCl, and levcromakalim in 90% ethanol. All other drugs were dissolved in distilled water. The solutions containing 20 mmol/l or 77 mmol/l KCl were obtained by equimolar replacement of NaCl by KCl in Krebs solution.

1.5. Statistics

Results are given as means ± SEM. Concentration–response curves of hyperpolarization and relaxation were analyzed by a two-way ANOVA followed by Scheffé's test for multiple comparisons. Other variables were analyzed by one-way ANOVA followed by Scheffé's test for multiple comparisons or a paired Student's t-test. A level of p was less than .05 was considered to be statistically significant.

2. RESULTS

2.1. Systolic blood pressure

A combination of hydralazine and hydrochlorothiazide, enalapril, TCV-116, and their combination significantly lowered the blood pressure of SHR. Systolic blood pressure after three months of treatment averaged 253 ± 6 mmHg for SHR-C, 163 ± 6 mmHg for SHR-H, 135 ± 6 mmHg for SHR-E, 120 ± 6 mmHg for SHR-T, and 111 ± 3 mmHg for SHR-T&E, and 155 ± 4 mmHg for WKY. The systolic blood pressure was significantly lower in SHR-T and SHR-T&E than in WKY or SHR-H after treatment.

2.2. Membrane potential

The resting membrane potential of the mesenteric artery was −45.7 ± 1.4 mV for SHR-C, −46.1 ± 1.3 mV for SHR-H, −49.8 ± 1.1 mV for SHR-E, −53.4 ± 0.8 mV for SHR-T, −53.7 ± 0.8 mV for SHR-T&E, and −49.6 ± 0.5 mV for WKY.

2.3. Endothelium-dependent hyperpolarization

Acetylcholine (10^{-5} M) induced hyperpolarizations in the presence of norepinephrine (10^{-5} M), which was attenuated significantly in SHR-C compared with WKY (Figure 46.1). All the treatments improved the acetylcholine-induced hyperpolarization, and the response in SHR-H, SHR-T and SHR-E was similar to that in WKY (Figure 46.1). Furthermore, the acetylcholine-induced hyperpolarization was significantly greater in SHR-T&E than in SHR-H, SHR-E or WKY, and was also greater in SHR-T than in SHR-H (Figure 46.1).

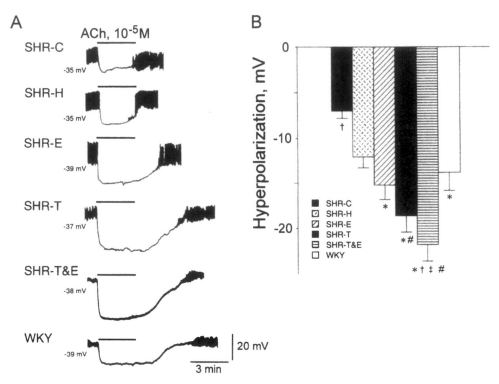

Figure 46.1 (A) Representative tracings showing hyperpolarizations to acetylcholine (10^{-5} M) under conditions of depolarization with norepinephrine (10^{-5} M) in the presence of indomethacin (10^{-5} M) in mesenteric arteries with endothelium of untreated spontaneously hypertensive rats (SHR-C), SHR treated with a combination of hydralazine and hydrochlorothiazide (SHR-H), enalapril-treated SHR (SHR-E), TCV-116-treated SHR (SHR-T), SHR treated with a combination of TCV-116 and enalapril (SHR-T&E), and untreated Wistar Kyoto rats (WKY). (B) Amplitudes of hyperpolarizations to acetylcholine (10^{-5} M) under conditions of depolarization with norepinephrine (10^{-5} M) in the presence of indomethacin (10^{-5} M) in mesenteric arteries with endothelium of SHR-C, SHR-H, SHR-E, SHR-T, SHR-T&E, and WKY. Values are shown as means ± SEM. There were eight to eleven rats in each group. The asterisks indicate significant differences as compared to the values of SHR-C ($p < .05$, by two-way analysis of variance); the daggers indicate significant differences as compared to the values of WKY ($p < .05$); the double daggers indicate significant differences as compared to the values of SHR-E ($p < .05$); and the sharps indicate significant differences as compared to the values of SHR-H ($p < .05$) (modified from Goto *et al.*, 2000a).

Hyperpolarizations to acetylcholine, obtained in quiescent preparations, were also attenuated in SHR-C compared with WKY. All treatments improved the acetylcholine-induced hyperpolarization to a comparable extent compared with SHR-C (data not shown).

2.4. Endothelium-dependent relaxation

EDHF-mediated relaxation was assessed in mesenteric rings contracted with norepinephrine (10^{-5} M) in the presence of indomethacin (10^{-5} M) and N^G-nitro-L-arginine (10^{-4} M). Under these conditions, acetylcholine produced a dose-dependent relaxation in WKY, but only negligible relaxations in SHR-C (Figure 46.2). The four treatments restored the N^G-nitro-L-arginine-resistant relaxation to acetylcholine in SHR, and the relaxation in SHR-H was comparable to that in WKY. The relaxations in SHR-E, SHR-T and SHR-T&E were more pronounced than those obtained in WKY or SHR-H (Figure 46.2).

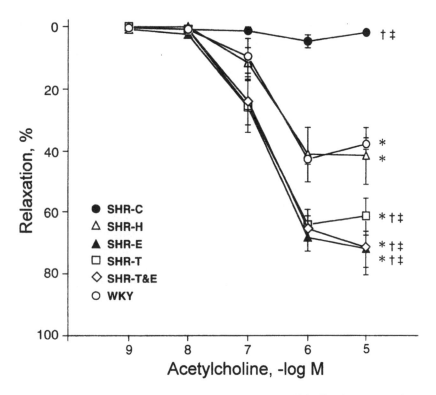

Figure 46.2 Concentration–relaxation curves to acetylcholine in mesenteric arterial rings with endothelium contracted with norepinephrine (10^{-5} M) in the presence of indomethacin (10^{-5} M) and nitro-L-arginine (10^{-4} M) in SHR-C, SHR-H, SHR-E, SHR-T, SHR-T&E, and WKY. There were eight to twelve rats in each group. The asterisks indicate significant differences as compared to the values of SHR-C ($p < .05$, by two-way analysis of variance); the daggers indicate significant differences as compared to the values of WKY ($p < .05$); and the double daggers indicate significant differences as compared to the values of SHR-H ($p < .05$).

When rings treated with indomethacin were contracted with KCl (77 mM), which eliminates EDHF-mediated hyperpolarization, no difference was found in acetylcholine-induced relaxations among the five groups (data not shown).

2.5. Endothelium-Independent hyperpolarizations and relaxations

Endothelium-independent hyperpolarizations and relaxations (assessed in rings contracted with norepinephrine) to levcromakalim, a direct opener of ATP-sensitive K^+ channels, were comparable among the five groups studied (data not shown).

Relaxations to sodium nitroprusside, a NO-donor, in rings contracted with norepinephrine (10^{-5} M) did not significantly differ among the five groups (data not shown).

3. DISCUSSION

The studies summarized in this chapter have demonstrated that: (a) antihypertensive treatment restores the impaired EDHF-mediated responses in SHR mesenteric arteries; (b) among the antihypertensive drugs tested, blockers of the renin-angiotensin system may be most efficacious in improving endothelial function; and (c) the beneficial effects of the combined AT_1-receptor blockade and ACE inhibition appear to be for the most part similar to those of each intervention alone.

Because all the antihypertensive drugs tested improved endothelial function in SHR, blood pressure lowering may primarily be important for this effect. However, blockers of the renin-angiotensin system tended to be more effective in improving EDHF-mediated responses than the conventional antihypertensive therapy, despite a similar, or only a slightly greater reduction in blood pressure. These findings suggest that in addition to blood pressure lowering, the renin-angiotensin system blockade may also play an important role in improving endothelial function (Schiffrin *et al.*, 1995; Onaka *et al.*, 1998; Schiffrin *et al.*, 2000; Goto *et al.*, 2000a).

The reason for the greater benefits of the renin-angiotensin system blockade remains speculative, partially because the underlying mechanism of the impaired EDHF-mediated responses in hypertension is unknown. The identity of EDHF is still elusive; however, an increasing number of studies suggest the critical importance of myoendothelial gap junctions in EDHF-mediated hyperpolarization (Chaytor *et al.*, 1998; Edwards *et al.*, 1999; Yamamoto *et al.*, 1999). If this were the case in the rat mesenteric artery (Edwards *et al.*, 1999), thickened subendothelial space in hypertension might alter myoendothelial gap junctional communications, possibly leading to an impaired endothelium-dependent hyperpolarization. Converting enzyme inhibitors are efficacious in reversing hypertensive target organ damages, such as left ventricular hypertrophy (Dahlöf *et al.*, 1992), and vascular structural changes (Schiffrin *et al.*, 1995). Indeed, lisinopril but not hydralazine corrects subendothelial thickenings of the aortic wall in the SHR (Clozel *et al.*, 1990). It is tempting to speculate that a greater restoration of EDHF-mediated responses by blockade of the renin-angiotensin system might be related to its greater effects on cardiovascular structural changes.

Several clinical studies have demonstrated possible benefits of a combination of converting enzyme inhibitors and AT_1-receptor antagonists in patients with heart failure (Baruch *et al.*, 1999; McKelvie *et al.*, 1999). Although both drugs inhibit the renin-angiotensin system, there are certain differences between them; e.g., converting enzyme inhibitors may increase bradykinin concentrations (Mombouli *et al.*, 1992), while AT_1-receptor antagonists block the action of angiotensin II regardless of its generation pathway (e.g., chymase; Urata *et al.*, 1996). When AT_1-receptors are blocked, angiotensin II may stimulate AT_2-receptors (Matsubara, 1998). However, in the present study, enalapril and TCV-116 improved the EDHF-mediated hyper-polarizations and relaxations to a similar extent, suggesting that their additional effects may not play a major role in improving endothelial function. Furthermore, although the acetylcholine-induced hyperpolarization in the presence of norepinephrine tended to be larger in SHR treated with a combination of the converting enzyme inhibitor and the AT_1-receptor antagonist, the difference was limited, and this combination does not seem to have definite advantages over each intervention regarding endo-thelial function.

The NO-mediated relaxations, as assessed by acetylcholine-mediated relaxations in rings contracted with high K solution, in which EDHF-mediated hyperpolarization is absent, were normal in the SHR. Thus, the NO system is preserved in SHR mesenteric arteries and is not modulated by antihypertensive therapy. These findings are con-sistent with those observed in the SHR aorta (Luscher and Vanhoutte, 1986).

Although only limited information is available concerning the role of EDHF in human hypertension, partially because of the difficulty in assessing the role of EDHF in human arteries, the EDHF pathway functions in human arteries (Nakashima *et al.*, 1993; Urakami-Harasawa *et al.*, 1997), and its role might be more important in resistance arteries (Urakami-Harasawa *et al.*, 1997). Considering the fact that the EDHF pathway may be more susceptible to high blood pressure than is the NO pathway, as demonstrated in this study, further studies on EDHF-mediated responses in human hypertension may be warranted.

4. CONCLUSION

Antihypertensive therapy restores the impaired EDHF-mediated hyperpolarization and relaxation in the SHR. Blockers of the renin-angiotensin system (converting enzyme inhibitors, AT_1-receptor antagonists, and their combination) may be most effective in improving the endothelial dysfunction.

47 EDHF: gap junction or chemical? and many other questions

Michel Félétou and Paul M. Vanhoutte

When reading the chapters from this monograph, one can only be impressed by the fact that the field of endothelium-derived hyperpolarizing factor (EDHF) has progressed considerably in the last few years. But as always in science, the acquisition of knowledge unavoidably opens new questions, or partially answers the existing ones.

1. Ca^{2+}-DEPENDENT K^+ CHANNELS: WHAT AND WHERE ARE THEY?

In the blood vessels studied *in vitro*, in bicarbonate-buffered solution, endothelium-dependent hyperpolarizations are prevented by the odd combination of two toxins apamin plus charybdotoxin but not by that of apamin plus iberiotoxin. The present consensus is that the small and intermediate conductance calcium-activated potassium channels, blocked by apamin and charybdotoxin, respectively, are not situated on the smooth muscle cells, as originally thought, but on the endothelial cells. This conclusion permits to clarify the series of events that lead to endothelium-dependent hyperpolarizations. Thus it appears that substances which produce endothelium-dependent hyperpolarizations increase the endothelial intracellular concentration of calcium. This activates calcium-dependent potassium channels sensitive to the mixture of the two toxins. The resulting hyperpolarization of the endothelial cells accelerates the entry of calcium into the endothelial cells and seems to be a prerequisite for the occurrence of endothelium-dependent hyperpolarization of the underlying vascular smooth muscle cells. But the question remains what is the exact role of endothelial hyperpolarization.

2. DIFFUSIBLE MEDIATORS: OF OLD AND NEW CANDIDATES?

Hypotheses to explain endothelium-dependent hyperpolarizations include metabolites of arachidonic acid, potassium ions and hydrogen peroxide. In the porcine coronary artery, the P450 isoform 2C9 has been proposed as an EDHF-synthase and 11,12 epoxyeicosatrienoic acid (EET) is supposed to be EDHF. However, although EETs are produced by porcine endothelial cells in response to mediators such as bradykinin, there is no evidence for a release of these cytochrome P450 metabolites. Furthermore, EETs hyperpolarize and relax vascular smooth muscle by activating large conductance calcium-activated potassium channels sensitive to iberiotoxin, a mechanism that is not associated with EDHF-mediated responses. Therefore, the hypothesis that endothelial cells release an epoxyeicosatrienoic acid (EET) which diffuses and produces hyperpolarization of the smooth muscle cells, is not really tenable. Nevertheless, in these blood vessels and possibly also in the arterioles of the hamster cheek pouch, EETs synthesis may be an essential step in the cascade of event leading to the endothelial increase in intracellular calcium and hyperpolarization. Endothelial cytochrome P450 produces superoxide anions and could also significantly contributes to the level of oxidative stress within the arterial wall. In the rat brain, EETs derived from cytochrome P450 2C11 located in the astrocytes could be involved in the functional hyperemia linked to neuronal activity.

In some blood vessels, such as the rabbit aorta, lipoxygenase metabolites of arachidonic acid can be considered as endothelium-derived hyperpolarizing factor. However, the production of these metabolites is unlikely to explain the EDHF-mediated responses in the various vascular beds mentioned earlier.

Whether or not potassium ion is EDHF is also a matter of intense debate. Potassium-induced relaxations and hyperpolarizations are not observed in all blood vessels. In those where such responses are recorded the inability to reproduce the relaxation or the hyperpolarization could be linked to differences in experimental conditions. For example, the level of vascular tone, the mean of administration of potassium (bolus or constant perfusion), whether or not the blood vessel is pressurized, the level of depolarization of the endothelial cells, linked to the level of activation chloride conductances, appear to be important parameters. Furthermore, the two targets of potassium ions (the Na^+/K^+ pump and the inward rectifying potassium channel) are not necessary located on the smooth muscle cells but may be on the endothelial cells. The release of potassium ions could act as an amplification mechanism participating in the hyperpolarization of the endothelial cells, that then propagates to adjacent smooth muscle cells (through gap junctions). Thus the role of potassium ion in EDHF-mediated responses alone or in concert with gap junctions is still uncertain.

Endothelium-dependent relaxations (or vasodilatations) sensitivite to the combination of charybdotoxin plus apamin, the hallmark of EDHF-mediated responses, have been demonstrated in eNOS knock-out mice. These observations definitively rule out the hypothesis that residual NO produced by an incomplete blockade of the endothelial NO-synthase accounts for all EDHF-mediated responses. In the mouse, but not in the rat or the pig, hydrogen peroxide derived from the endothelial NO-synthase could be an additional EDHF.

3. GAP JUNCTIONS: CONDUCTORS OF ELECTRICITY OR OF MEDIATORS?

In submucosal arterioles of the guinea-pig small intestine, acetylcholine induces outward currents in endothelial and smooth muscle cells. After the administration of blockers of gap junctions, acetylcholine elicits an outward current in endothelial cells but no longer in the smooth muscle cells suggesting that the two cell types are connected electrically and form a functional syncytium. In arterioles and feed arteries from the retractor muscle of the hamster, simultaneous measurements of the membrane potential in endothelial and smooth muscle cells show that electrical signals travel freely and bidirectionally between the two layers. These electrical signals were associated with vasomotor responses. In fact, in this tissue the myoendothelial coupling ensures that smooth muscle cells are electrically coupled because the coupling between the smooth muscle cells themselves, in contrast with that between endothelial cells, is rather poor. In this blood vessel, endothelio–endothelial and myo–endothelial gap junctions probably are the privileged pathways of communication between the cells. In contrast, in the arterioles from the cheek pouch of the same species, the smooth muscle cells are well coupled. The duration of the electrophysiological responses is longer in smooth muscle cells than those recorded in adjacent endothelial cells, suggesting an heterocellular signalling other than direct electrical coupling. In the presence of an inhibitor of cytochrome P450, the conducted vasodilatation and the hyperpolarization produced by acetylcholine are inhibited in the smooth muscle cells, but not in the endothelial cells. This suggests that, in this blood vessel either cytochrome P450 is an obligatory step in myo–endothelial coupling or that a metabolite of cytochrome P450 (in essence an EDHF) rapidly hyperpolarizes and relaxes surrounding smooth muscle cells. In larger blood vessels, inhibitors of gap junctions produce complete (guinea-pig carotid artery), partial (rat mesenteric artery) or minimal inhibition (rat hepatic artery) of the endothelium-dependent hyperpolarizations. These varying results raise the question of what do gap junctions do anyway. Another obvious question is whether or not the differences in EDHF-mediated responses, observed between vascular beds and between species, are linked to the differential expression of connexins subtypes. The various types of connexins expressed in the vascular wall and their precise cellular locations are still a matter of debate.

Gap junctions are the assembly of two hemichannels located on both cellular sides that are each composed of six proteins called connexins. More than fifteen different connexin genes have been described (in the mouse) leading to potential enormous structural diversity in gap junctions. In the endothelial and smooth muscle cell, connexins 37, 40 and 43 predominate, the proportion of each varying depending on the cell type and the species. Additionally, connexin45 is also expressed in vascular smooth muscle cells and plays a prominent role during development. The movement of charges through gap junctions, necessary for the propagation of action potentials in excitable cells is not the only function of such junctions. Connexin 43 for instance allows the diffusion of large molecules such as adenosine diphosphate and triphosphate or cyclic adenosine monophosphate. The permeability of a given gap junction is regulated by the voltage-dependent gating properties, the permselectivity of the hemichannel assembly, the phosphorylation state of the connexins, and their life cycle. Mice deficient for connexin40 are hypertensive and exhibit a reduced spread of dilatation in response to endothelium-dependent vasodilators. Whether or not this phenotype is linked to the deletion of connexin40 in the vascular wall itself is uncertain. In contrast, mice subjected to specific deletion of endothelial connexin43 do not present any alteration in blood pressure (general knock-out for this connexin is lethal). Therefore, one is forced to admit that the role of gap junctions in the vascular wall is far from being clear. And the question remains whether gap junctions are a privileged site for the transfer of electrical charges or to messenger molecules (EDHF). Again, a simple answer may not be possible. Indeed, in the arteries of the rabbit, relaxations attributed to EDHF in response to agonists and the calcium ionophore, A23187 appear to involve the same mechanisms. However the response to the former are sensitive to gap junctions blockers while those to the latter are not, suggesting that the calcium ionophore releases a factor across the endothelial surface while agonists provoke the preferential diffusion of this substance through gap junctions. Further-more, to inhibit gap junctions, the tools available are either poorly specific (carben-oxolone, 18-α-glycyrrhetininc acid, 18-β-glycyrrhetininc acid, ouabain, halothane, heptanol) or apparently specific of the connexin subtype targeted (gap peptides). From the non-peptidic inhibitors, 18-α-glycyrrhetininc acid may be the most selective. The mechanisms involved in the inhibition of gap junctions are different depending on the inhibitor studied and include disruption of gap junction plaques (glycyrrhetininc acids), the consequence of a possible secondary increase in intracellular calcium (ouabain), or undefined subtle alterations (gap peptides). The hepatic artery of the rat is the prototype artery where potassium ions account for EDHF-mediated responses. In this artery, in contrast to rabbit arteries, gap 27 (an inhibitor of connexins 37 and 43) and glycyrrhetininc acid do not affect endothelium-dependent hyperpolarizations. However, in this blood vessel, connexin40 can be expressed in both endothelial and smooth muscle cells, allowing the possible formation of homotypic connexin40 channels insensitive to gap 27. Thus, inhibitors of connexins 40 and 43 produce a partial inhibition of the relaxation attributed to EDHF, implying a potential role for gap junctions. One word of caution is required as although gap peptides are supposed to be very specific, the elevated concentration required to produce inhibition should temper the interpretation of the results obtained.

When considering the role of gap junctions in the spread of endothelium-dependent hyperpolarization, the location between the different cell type becomes crucial. In the small arteries from the retractor muscle of the hamster or the intestine of the guinea-pig, myo–endotelial junctions appear to play an essential role while in the hamster cheek pouch myo–myo junctions are an essential pathway. In both arteries, endothelial–endothelial junctions are required to observe conducted vasodilatation with acetylcholine. In the porcine coronary artery, endothelium-dependent hyper-polarization to substance P can be recorded with sharp microelectrodes in the smooth muscle cells situated close to the intimal layer or close to the adventitia. Gap junction blockers inhibit the hyperpolarization in the outer layer while the response remains unaffected in the intimal layer. Similarly, relaxation and hyperpolarization can be observed in porcine coronary smooth muscle cells in segments without endothelial lining (separated by a partition chamber from the rest of the artery) only if this area is not physically separated from the intact segment. These observations suggest that in large blood vessels, such as the porcine coronary artery, muscle–muscle gap junctions play a preponderant role in the spread of endothelium-dependent hyperpolarizations.

4. EDHF-MEDIATED RESPONSES: USEFUL OR EPIPHENOMENON?

The identification of apamin and charybdotoxin as rather specific inhibitors of the EDHF responses has allowed the demonstration of a physiological role for EDHF. Thus, in the canine coronary circulation, EDHF is involved in the increase in flow observed in response to pulsations. In mice, the vasodilatation of the hind limbs or the decrease in blood pressure in response to bradykinin or acetylcholine depends essentially on the EDHF-pathway. In humans, apamin plus charybdotoxin cannot be given but the role of EDHF is assessed using ouabain as a, albeit imperfect, tool to inhibit EDHF-mediated responses. Thus, in hypertensive patients this mechanism

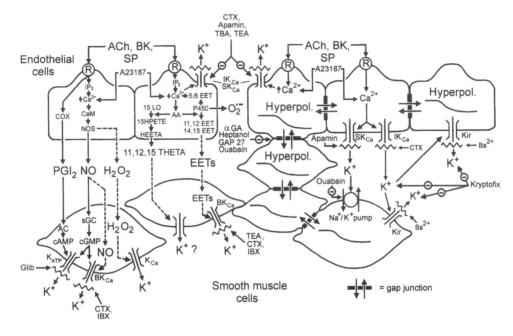

Figure 47.1 Possible mechanisms leading to endothelium-dependent hyperpolarizations Substances such as acetylcholine (ACh), bradykinin (BK) and substance P (SP),
through the activation of M_3 muscarinic, B_2 bradykinin and NK_1 neurokinin
receptor subtypes, respectively, and agents which increase intracellular calcium,
such as the calcium ionophore A23187, release endothelium-derived hyperpolarizing factors. R = receptor; NOS = nitric oxide synthase; COX = cycloxygenase;
15 LO=15-lipoxygenase; P450=cytochrome P450 monoxygenase; CaM=calmodulin;
NO=nitric oxide; O_2^-=superoxide anion; PGI_2=prostacyclin; H_2O_2=hydrogen
peroxide; 5,6 EET=5,6-epoxy-eicosatrienoic acid; 11,12 EET=11,12-epoxy-eico-
satrienoic acid; 14,15 EET=14,15-epoxy-eicosatrienoic acid; 15-HPETE=
15-hydroperoxy-eicosatetraenoic acid; HEETA = hydroxyepoxyeicosatrienoic
acid; 11,12,15 THETA=11,12,15-trihydroxyeicosatrienoic acid; GC= guanylate
cyclase, cGMP=cyclic guanosine monophosphate; cAMP=cyclic adenosine
monophosphate; ATP=adenosine trisphosphate; IP_3=inositol trisphosphate;
Hyperpol=hyperpolarization. Glibenclamide (Glib) is a selective inhibitor of
ATP sensitive potassium channels (K_{ATP}^+). Tetraethyl ammonium (TEA) is a non
specific inhibitors of potassium channels when used at high concentrations
(>5mM) while at lower concentrations (1–3 mM) these drugs are selective
for calcium-activated potassium channels ($K_{Ca^{2+}}^+$). Iberiotoxin (IBX) is a specific
inhibitor of large conductance $K_{Ca^{2+}}^+$. Charybdotoxin (CTX) is an inhibitor of
large conductance $K_{Ca^{2+}}^+$, intermediate conductance $K_{Ca^{2+}}^+$ ($IK_{Ca^{2+}}$) and voltage-
dependent potassium channels. Apamin is a specific inhibitor of small con-
ductance $K_{Ca^{2+}}^+$ ($SK_{Ca^{2+}}$). Barium (Ba^{2+}) in the micromolar range, is a specific inhibitor of the inward rectifier potassium channel (K_{ir}). Gap27, an eleven amino acid
peptide possessing conserved sequence homology to a portion of the second extracellular loop of connexin, 18-α-glycyrrhetinic acid (18αGA) and heptanol are gap junction uncouplers.

may compensate the impairment of the vasodilatation linked to the dysfunction of
NO-synthase. This observation performed on patients is consistent with reports that
show a compensatory role for EDHF in human isolated skeletal muscle resistance

arteries taken from ischemic limbs and in various animal models where NO synthase is affected (including angioplasty, ischemia-reperfusion, ionized irradiation). In general, EDHF-mediated responses appear to be more resistant to oxidative stress than the NO-dependent endothelium-dependent relaxations. However, the EDHF pathway is altered in human subcutaneous resistance arteries taken from patients suffering from critical limb ischemia, in animal models of diabetes, hypertension and aging.

The improvement of the EDHF response could contribute to the restoration of endothelial function during therapeutic interventions. This is suggested by the observation that angiotensin converting enzyme inhibitors, AT_1-receptor antagonists and estrogens augments endothelium-dependent hyperpolarizations. Interestingly, the up-regulation of the EDHF response by oestrogen could involve the over-expression of connexin43 in the vascular wall.

5. CONCLUSION

Gap junctions can play an important role in EDHF responses. However, the cellular location, the type of connexins involved, the nature of the signal transmitted, the occurrence of a regenerative mechanism as well as the presence of alternative or additional chemical pathways remain to be determined.

References

Abdul-Karim, R., Assali, N.S. (1961) Pressor response to angiotensin in pregnant and non-pregnant women. *Am. J. Obstet. Gynecol.*, **82**: 246–251.

Abiru, T., Watanabe, Y., Kamata, K., Kasuya, Y. (1993) Changes in endothelium-dependent relaxation and levels of cyclic nucleotides in the mesenteric arterial bed from streptozotocin-induced diabetic rats. *Life Sciences*, **53**: 7–12.

Abraham, N.G., Pinto, A., Mullane, K.M., Levere, R.D., Spokas, E. (1985) Presence of cytochrome P450-dependent monooxygenase in intimal cells of the hog aorta. *Hypertension*, **7**: 899–904.

Acar, C., Jebara, V.A., Portoghese, M., Beyssen, B., Pagny, J.Y., Grare, P., Chachques, J.C., Fabiani, J.-N., Deloche, A., Guermonprez, J.L., Carpentier, A.F. (1992) Revival of the radial artery for coronary artery bypass grafting. *Ann. Thorac. Surg.*, **54**: 652–660.

Ackermann, E.J., Conde-Frieboes, K., Dennis, E.A. (1995) Inhibition of macrophage Ca(2+)-independent phospholipase A2 by bromoenol lactone and trifluoromethyl ketones. *J. Biol. Chem.*, **270**: 445–450.

Adams, D.J. (1994) Ionic channels in vascular endothelial cells. *Trend. Cardiovasc. Med.*, **4**: 18–26.

Adeagbo, A.S.O. (1997) Endothelium-derived hyperpolarizing factor: characterization as a cytochrome P450 1A-linked metabolite of arachidonic acid in perfused rat mesenteric pre-arteriolar bed. *Am. J. Hypert.*, **10**: 763–771.

Adeagbo, A.S.O. (1999) 1-Ethyl-2-benzimidazolinone stimulates endothelial K_{Ca} channels and nitric oxide formation in rat mesenteric vessels. *Eur. J. Pharmacol.*, **379**: 151–159.

Adeagbo, A.S.O., Henzel, M.K. (1998) Calcium-dependent phospholipase A_2 mediates the production of endothelium-derived hyperpolarizing factor in perfused rat mesenteric prearteriolar bed. *J. Vasc. Res.*, **35**: 27–35.

Adeagbo, A.S.O., Malik, K.U. (1990) Endothelium-dependent and BRL 34915-induced vasodilatation in rat isolated perfused mesenteric arteries: role of G-proteins, K^+ and calcium channels. *Br. J. Pharmacol.*, **100**: 427–434.

Adeagbo, A.S.O., Malik, K.U. (1990) Mechanism of vascular actions of prostacyclin in the rat isolated perfused mesenteric arteries. *J. Pharmacol. Exp. Ther.*, **252**: 26–34.

Adeagbo, A.S.O., Triggle, C.R. (1993) Varying extracellular (K+): a functional approach to separating EDHF- and EDNO-related mechanisms in perfused rat mesenteric arterial bed. *J. Cardiovasc. Pharmacol.*, **21**: 423–429.

Akaike, T., Yoshida, M., Miyamoto, Y., Sato, K., Kohno, M., Sasamoto, K., Miyazaki, K., Ueda, S., Maeda, H. (1993) Antagonistic action of imidazolineoxyl N-oxides against endothelium-derived relaxing factor/NO through a radical reaction. *Biochemistry*, **32**: 827–832.

Alexander, S.P.H., Peters, J.A. (2000) TiPS receptor and ion channel nomenclature supplement, edited by S.P.H. Alexander, J.A. Peters, vol. 11, pp. 107, UK (Cambridge): Elsevier Science.

Alkayed, N.J., Birks, E.K., Narayanan, J., Petrie, K.A., Kohler-Cabot, A.E., Harder, D.R. (1997) Role of P-450 arachidonic acid epoxygenase in the response of cerebral blood flow to glutamate in rats. *Stroke*, **28**: 1066–1072.

Alkayed, N.J., Narayanan, J., Gebremedhin, D., Medhora, M., Roman, R.J., Harder, D.R. (1996) Molecular characterization of an arachidonic acid epoxygenase in rat brain astrocytes. *Stroke*, **27**: 971–979.

Alvarez, J., Montero, M., Garcia-Sancho, J. (1992) High affinty inhibition of Ca^{2+}-dependent K^+ channels by cytochrome P-450 inhibitors. *J. Biol. Chem.*, **267**: 11789–11793.

Amer, M.S., McKinney, G.R., Akcasu, A. (1974) Effect of glycyrrhetinic acid on the cyclic nucleotide system of the rat stomach. *Biochem. Pharmacol.*, **23**: 3085–3092.

Amezcua, J.L., Palmer, R.M.J., Souza, B.M., Moncada, S. (1989) Nitric oxide synthesized from L-arginine regulates vascular tone in the coronary circulation of the rabbit. *Br. J. Pharmacol.*, **97**: 1119–1124.

Amruthesh, S.C., Boerschel, M.F., McKinney, J.S., Willoughby, K.A., Ellis, E.F. (1993) Metabolism of arachidonic acid to epoxyeicosatrienoic acids, hydroxyeicosatetraenoic acids, and prostaglandins in cultured rat hippocampal astrocytes. *J. Neurochem.*, **61**: 150–159.

Amruthesh, S.C., Falck, J.R., Ellis, E.F. (1992) Brain synthesis and cerebrovascular action of epoxygenase metabolites of arachidonic acid. *J. Neurochem.*, **58**: 503–510.

Andersen, H.L., Weis, J.U., Fjalland, B., Korsgaard, N. (1999) Effect of acute and long-term treatment with 17-β-estradiol on the vasomotor responses in the rat aorta. *Br. J. Pharmacol.*, **126**: 159–168.

Andersson, D.A., Zygmunt, P.M., Movahed, P., Andersson, T.L.G., Högestätt, E.D. (2000) Effects of inhibitors of small- and intermediate-conductance calcium-activated potassium channels, inwardly-rectifying potassium channels and Na^+/K^+ ATPase on EDHF relaxations in the rat hepatic artery. *Br. J. Pharmacol.*, **129**: 1490–1496.

Aoki, H., Kobayashi, S., Nishimura, J., Kanaide, H. (1994) Sensitivity of G-protein involved in endothelin-1-induced Ca^{2+} influx to pertussis toxin in porcine endothelial cells *in situ*. *Br. J. Pharmacol.*, **111**: 989–996.

Archer, S.L., Huang, J.M.C., Hampl, V., Nelson, D.P., Shultz, P.J., Weir, E.K. (1994) Nitric oxide and cGMP cause vasorelaxation by activation of a charybdotoxin-sensitive K^+-channel by cGMP-dependent protein-kinase. *Proc. Natl. Acad. Sci. USA*, **91**: 7583–7587.

Arii, T., Ohyanagi, M., Shibuya, J., Iwasaki, T. (1999) Increased function of the voltage-dependent calcium channels, without increase of Ca^{2+} release from the sarcoplasmic reticulum in the arterioles of spontaneous hypertensive rats. *Am. J. Hypert.*, **12**: 1236–1242.

Ashida, Y., Saijo, T., Kuriki, H., Makino, H., Terao, S., Maki, Y. (1983) Pharmacological profile of AA-861, a 5-lipoxygenase inhibitor. *Prostaglandins*, **26**: 955–972.

Ashworth, J.R., Warren, A.Y., Baker, D.M., Johnson, I.R. (1996) A comparison of endothelium-dependent relaxation in omental and myometrial resistance arteries in pregnant and non-pregnant women. *Am. J. Obstet. Gynecol.*, **175**: 1307–1312.

Ayajiki, K., Okamura, T., Fujioka, H., Imaoka, S., Funae, Y., Toda, N. (1999) Involvement of CYP3A-derived arachidonic acid metabolite(s) in responses to endothelium-derived K^+ channel opening substance in monkey lingual artery. *Br. J. Pharmacol.*, **128**: 802–808.

Bakker, E.N., Sipkema, P. (1997) Components of acetylcholine-induced dilation in isolated rat arterioles. *Am. J. Physiol.*, **273**: H1848–1853.

Banach, K., Ramanan, S.V., Brink, P.R. (2000) The influence of surface charge on the conductance of the human connexin37 gap junction channel. *Biophys. J.*, **78**: 752–760.

Baraboy, V.A. (1997) Biological effects in animals Changes in biochemical indices of the organism vitally important systems. In *Chornobyl catastrophe*, edited by V. Baryakhtar, pp. 285–288, Ukraine: (Kiev): Editorial House of Annual Issue "Export of Ukraine".

Barlow, R.S., El-Mowafy, A.M., White, R.E. (2000) H_2O_2 opens BKCa channels via the PLA2-arachidonic acid signaling cascade in coronary artery smooth muscle. *Am. J. Physiol.*, **279**: H475–483.

Barlow, R.S., White, R.E. (1998) Hydrogen peroxide relaxes porcine coronary arteries by stimulating BKCa channel activity. *Am. J. Physiol.*, **275**: H1283–H1289.

Baron, A., Frieden, M., Bény, J.-L. (1997) Epoxyeicosatrienoic acids activate a high-conductance, Ca^{2+}-dependent K^+ channel on pig coronary artery endothelial cells. *J. Physiol.*, **504**: 537–543.

Baron, A., Frieden, M., Chabaud, F., Bény, J.-L. (1996) Ca^{2+}-dependent non-selective cation and K^+ channels activated by bradykinin in pig coronary artery endothelial cells. *J. Physiol.*, **493**: 691–706.

Barr, L. (1963) Propagation in vertebrate visceral smooth muscle. *Theoret. Biol.*, **4**: 73–85.

Bartlett, I.S., Segal, S.S. (2000) Resolution of smooth muscle and endothelial pathways for conduction along hamster cheek pouch arterioles. *Am. J. Physiol.*, **278**: H604–H612.

Baruch, L., Anand, I., Cohen, I.-S., Ziesche, S., Judd, D., Cohn, J.-N. (1999) Augmented short- and long-term hemodynamic and hormonal effects of an angiotensin receptor blocker added to angiotensin converting enzyme inhibitor therapy in patients with heart failure. *Circulation*, **99**: 2658–2664.

Bassenge, E., Heusch, G. (1990) Endothelial and neuro-humoral control of coronary blood flow in health and disease. *Rev. Physiol. Biochem. Pharmacol.*, **116**: 77–165.

Bauersachs, J., Fleming, I., Scholz, D., Popp, R., Busse, R. (1997) Endothelium-derived hyperpolarizing factor, but not nitric oxide, is reversibly inhibited by Brefeldin A. *Hypertension*, **30**: 1598–1605.

Bauersachs, J., Hecker, M., Busse, R. (1994) Display of the characteristics of endothelium-derived hyperpolarizing factor by a cytochrome P450-derived arachidonic acid metabolite in the coronary microcirculation, *Br. J. Pharmacol.*, **113**: 1548–1553.

Bauersachs, J., Popp, R., Fleming, I., Busse, R. (1997) Nitric oxide and endothelium-derived hyperpolarizing factor: formation and interactions. *Prostaglandins Leukot. Essent. Fatty Acids*, **57**: 439–446.

Bauersachs, J., Popp, R., Hecker, M., Sauer, E., Fleming, I., Busse, R. (1996) Nitric oxide attenuates the release of endothelium-derived hyperpolarizing factor. *Circulation*, **94**: 3341–3347.

Beblo, D.A., Veenstra, R.D. (1997) Monovalent cation permeation through Cx40 gap junction channels. *J. Gen. Physiol.*, **109**: 509–522.

Belardetti, F., Campbell, W.B., Falck, J.R., Demontis, G., Rosolowsky, M. (1989) Products of heme-catalyzed transformation of the arachidonate derivative 12-HpETE open S-type K^+ channels in Aplysia. *Neuron.*, **3**: 497–505.

Belevich, A.E., Zima, A.V., Kharkhun, M.I., Shuba, M.F. (1998) Role of cAMP, cGMP, and protein kinase C in regulation of calcium current through the L-type calcium channels in the electroexcitable membrane of smooth muscle cells. *Neurophysiol.*, **30**: 63–71.

Bennett, B.M., McDonald, B.J., Nigam, R., Long, P.G., Simon, W.C. (1992) Inhibition of nitrovasodilator- and acetylcholine-induced relaxation and cyclic GMP accumulation by the cytochrome P450 substrate, 7-ethoxyresorufin. *Can. J. Physiol. Pharmacol.*, **70**: 1297–1303.

Bény, J., Zhu, P., Haefliger, I.O. (1997) Lack of bradykinin-induced smooth muscle hyperpolarization despite heterocellular dye coupling and endothelial cell hyperpolarization in porcine ciliary artery. *J. Vasc. Res.*, **34**: 344–350.

Bény, J.L. (1997) Electrical coupling between smooth muscle cells and endothelial cells in pig coronary arteries. *Pflügers Archiv.*, **433**: 364–367.

Bény, J.L. (1999) Information networks in the arterial wall. *News in Physiological Sciences*, **14**: 68–73.

Bény, J.L., Brunet, P.C. (1988) Neither nitric oxide nor nitroglycerin accounts for all the characteristics of endothelially mediated vasodilatation of pig coronary arteries. *Blood Vessels*, **25**: 308–311.

Beny, J.-L., Conat, J.L. (1992) An electron microscopy study of smooth muscle cell dye coupling in the pig coronary arteries. Role of gap junctions. *Circ. Res.*, **70**: 49–55.

Bény, J.-L., Haefliger, I.O. (1999) Endothelium-dependent hyperpolarization cannot be explained by electrical coupling between the endothelial and the smooth muscle cells in muscular arteries. In *Endothelium-derived hyperpolarizing factor*, edited by P.M. Vanhoutte, vol. 1, pp. 1–9, The Netherlands: Harwood Academic Publishers.

Bény, J.-L., Pacicca, C. (1994) Bidirectional electrical communication between smooth muscle and endothelial cells in the pig coronary artery. *Am. J. Physiol.*, **266**: H1465–H1472.

Bény, J.-L., Schaad, O. (2000) An evaluation of potassium ions as endothelium-derived hyperpolarizing factor in porcine coronary arteries. *Br. J. Pharmacol.*, **131**: 965–973.

Bény, J.-L., von der Weid, P.Y. (1991) Hydrogen peroxide: an endogenous smooth muscle cell hyperpolarizing factor. *Biochem. Biophys. Res. Commun.*, **176**: 378–384.

Berman, R.S., Griffith, T.M. (1998) Spatial heterogeneity in the mechanisms contributing to acetylcholine-induced dilatation in the rabbit isolated ear. *Br. J. Pharmacol.*, **124**: 1245–1253.

Berman, R.S., Griffith, T.M. (1997) Differential actions of charybdotoxin on central and daughter branch arteries of the rabbit isolated ear. *Br. J. Pharmacol.*, **120**: 639–646.

Berry, C., Hamilton, C.A., Brosnan, M.J., Magill, F.G., Berg, G.A., McMurray, J.J.V., Dominiczak, A.F. (2000) An investigation into the sources of superoxide in human blood vessels: Angiotensin II increases superoxide production in human internal mammary arteries. *Circulation*, **101**: 2206–2212.

Beven, J.A., Torok, J. (1978) Movement of norepinephrine through the media of rabbit aorta. *Circ. Res.*, **27**: 325–331.

Beyer, E.C. (1993) Gap junctions Inten. *Rev. of Cyto.*, **137**: 1–37.

Beyer, E.C., Gemel, J., Seul, K.H., Larson, D.M., Banach, K., Brink, P.R. (2000) Modulation of intercellular communication by differential regulation of heteromeric mixing of co-expressed connexins. *Brz. J. Med. and Biol. Res.*, **33**: 391–397.

Beyer, E.C., Paul, D.L., Goodenough, D.A. (1987) Connexin43 – a protein from rat-heart homologous to a gap junction protein from liver. *J. Cell Biol.*, **105**: 2621–2629.

Blanco, G., Mercer, R.W. (1998) Isoenzymes of the Na-K-ATPase: heterogeneity in structure, diversity in function. *Am. J. Physiol.*, **275**: F633–F650.

Bobadilla, R.A., Nenkel, C.C., Henkel, E.V.C., Escalante, B., Hong, E. (1997) Possible involvement of endothelium-derived hyperpolarizing factor in vascular responses of abdominal aorta from pregnant rats. *Hypertension*, **30**: 96–602.

Bolotina, V.M., Najibi, S., Palacino, J.J., Pagano, P.J., Cohen, R.A. (1994) Nitric oxide directly activates calcium-dependent potassium channels in vascular smooth muscle. *Nature*, **368**: 850–853.

Bolz, S.B., Fisslthaler, B., Pieperhoff, S., De Wit, C., Fleming, I., Busse, R., Pohl, U. (2000) Antisense oligonucleotide against cytochrome P450 2C8 attenuates EDHF-mediated Ca^{2+} changes and dilation in isolated resistance arteries. *FASEB J.*, **14**: 255–260.

Bolz, S.S., De Wit, C., Pohl, U. (1999) Endothelium-derived hyperpolarizing factor but not NO reduces smooth muscle Ca^{2+} during acetylcholine-induced dilation of microvessels. *Br. J. Pharmacol.*, **128**: 124–134.

Bondy, S.C., Naderi, S. (1994) Contribution of hepatic cytochrome P450 systems to the generation of reactive oxygen species. *Biochem. Pharmacol.*, **48**: 155–159.

Borda, E.S., Sterin-Borda, L., Gimeno, M.F., Lazzari, M.A., Gimeno, A.C. (1983) The stimulatory effect of prostacyclin (PGI_2) on isolated rabbit and rat aorta is probably associated to the generation of a thromboxane A_2 (TXA_2) "like material". *Arch. Int. Pharmacodyn. Ther.*, **261**: 79–89.

Borg-Capra, C., Fournet-Bourguignon, M.P., Janiak, P., Villeneuve, N., Bidouard, J.P., Vilaine, J.P., Vanhoutte, P.M. (1997) Morphological heterogeneity with normal expression but altered function of G proteins in porcine cultured regenerated coronary endothelial cells. *Br. J. Pharmacol.*, **122**: 999–1008.

Bradley, K.K., Jaggar, J.H., Bonev, A.D., Heppner, T.J., Flynn, E.R.M., Nelson, M.T., Horowitz, B. (1999) $K_{ir}2.1$ encodes the inward rectifier potassium channel in rat arterial smooth muscle cells. *J. Physiol.*, **513**: 639–651.

Brandes, R.P., Behra, A., Lebherz, C., Böger, R.H., Bode-Böger, S.M., Phivthong-Ngam, L., Mügge, A. (1997) N$^{\omega}$-nitro-L-arginine- and indomethacin-resistant endothelium-dependent relaxation in the rabbit renal artery: effect of hypercholesterolemia. *Atherosclerosis*, **135**: 49–55.

Brayden, J.E., Nelson, M.T. (1992) Regulation of arterial tone by activation of calcium-dependent potassium channels. *Science*, **256**: 532–535.

Brink, P.R. (1998) Gap junctions in vascular smooth muscle. *Acta Physiol. Scand.*, **164**: 349–356.

Brink, P.R., Barr, L. (2000) The path of intercellular communication. In *A functional view of smooth muscle*, edited by Barr and Christ, pp. 397–423, JAI Press.

Brink, P.R., Cronin, K., Banach, K., Peterson, E., Westphale, E.M., Seul, K.H., Ramanan, S.V., Beyer, E.C. (1997) Evidence for heteromeric gap junction channels composed of hCx37 and rCx43. *Am. J. Physiol.*, **273**: C1386–C1396.

Brink, P.R., Cronin, K., Ramanan, S.V. (1996) Gap junctions in excitable cells *J. BioEnergetics BioMembranes*, **28**: 351–358.

Brink, P.R., Ramaman, S.V., Christ, G.J. (1996) Human connexin43 gap junction channel gating: evidence for mode shifts and/or heterogeneity. *Am. J. Physiol.*, **271**: C321–C331.

Brink, P.R., Ricotta, J., Christ, G.J. (2000) Biophysical characteristics of gap junctions in vascular wall cells: implications for vascular biology and disease. *Brazil. J. Med. Biol. Res.*, **33**: 415–422.

Brink, P.R., Valiunas, V., Christ, G.J. (2000) Homotypic, heterotypic and heteromeric gap junction channels. In *Gap Junctions*, edited by C. Perracchia., vol. 49, pp. 131–142. Current Topics in Membranes.

Brugnara, C., Armsby, C.C., De Franceschi, L., Crest, M., Martin Euclaire, M.F., Alper, S.L. (1995) Ca^{2+}-activated K^{+} channels of human and rabbit erythrocytes display distinctive patterns of inhibition by venom peptide toxins. *J. Membr. Biol.*, **147**: 71–82.

Brunet, P.C., Bény, J.-L. (1989) Substance P and bradykinin hyperpolarize pig coronary artery endothelial cells in primary culture. *Blood Vessels*, **26**: 228–234.

Bryan, R.M., Jr., Eichler, M.Y., Swafford, M.W., Johnson, T.D., Suresh, M.S., Childres, W.F. (1996) Stimulation of α_2 adrenoceptors dilates the rat middle cerebral artery. *Anesthesiology*, **85**: 82–90.

Bryan, R.M., Jr., Steenberg, M.L., Eichler, M.Y., Johnson, T.D., Swafford, M.W.G., Suresh, M.S. (1995) Permissive role of NO in α_2-adrenoceptor-mediated dilations in rat cerebral arteries. *Am. J. Physiol.*, **269**: H1171–H1174.

Bucala, R., Tracy, K.J., Cerami, A. (1991) Advanced glycosylation end products quench nitric oxide and mediate defective endothelial-dependent vasodilatation in experimental diabetes. *J. Clin. Invest.*, **87**: 432–438.

Budunova, I.V., Mittelman, L.A., Miloszewska, J. (1994) Role of protein kinase C in the regulation of gap junctional communication. *Teratogenesis Carcinogenesis & Mutagenesis*, **14**: 259–270.

Bukauskas, F.F., Jordan, K., Bukauskiene, A., Bennett, M.V., Lampe, P.D., Laird, D.W., Verselis, V.K. (2000) Clustering of connexin43-enhanced green fluorescent protein gap junction channels and functional coupling in living cells1. *Proc. Natl. Acad. Sci. USA*, **97**: 2556–2561.

Burns, K.D., Capdevila, J., Wei, S., Breyer, M.D., Homma, T., Harris, R.C. (1995) Role of cytochrome P-450 epoxygenase metabolites in EGF signaling in renal proximal tubule. *Am. J. Physiol.*, **269**: C831–C840.

Burt, J., Frank, J.S., Berns, M.W. (1982) Permeability and structural studies of heart cell gap junctions under normal and altered ionic conditions. *J. Mem. Biol.*, **68**: 227–238.

Burt, J.M., Spray D.C. (1988) Inotropic agents modulate gap junction conductance between cardiac myocytes. *Am. J. Physiol.*, **254**: H1206.

Buss, N.H., Simonsen, U., Pilegaard, H.K., Mulvany, M.J. (2000) Nitric oxide, prostanoid and non-NO, non-prostanoid involvement in acetylcholine relaxation of isolated human arteries. *Br. J. Pharmacol.*, **129**: 184–192.

Busse, R., Fichtner, H., Luckhoff, A., Kohlhardt, M. (1988) Hyperpolarization and increased free calcium in acetylcholine-stimulated endothelial cells. *Am. J. Physiol.*, **255**: H965–H969.

Buttner, N., Siegelbaum, S.A., Volterra, A. (1989) Direct modulation of Aplysia S-K+ channels by a 12-lipoxygenase metabolite of arachidonic acid. *Nature*, **342**: 553–555.

Buus, N.H., Simonsen, U., Pilegaard, H.K., Mulvany, M.J. (1998) Limited role of nitric oxide and prostanoids in acetylcholine relaxation of human small arteries. *J. Vasc. Res.*, **35**: S1–S4.

Buus, N.H., Simonsen, U., Pilegaard, H.K., Mulvany, M.J. (2000) Nitric oxide, prostanoid and non-NO, non-prostanoid involvement in acetylcholine relaxation of isolated human small arteries. *Br. J. Pharmacol.*, **129**: 184–192.

Cai, S., Garneau, L., Sauve, R. (1998) Single-channel characterization of the pharmacological properties of the $K(Ca^{2+})$ channel of intermediate conductance in bovine aortic endothelial cells. *J. Memb. Biol.*, **163**: 147–158.

Calver, A., Collier, J., Vallence, P. (1992) Inhibition and stimulation of nitric oxide synthesis in the human forearm bed of patients with insulin-dependent diabetes mellitus. *J. Clin. Invest.*, **90**: 2548–2554.

Cameron, N.E., Cotter, M.A. (1992) Impaired contraction and relaxation in aorta from streptozotocin-diabetic rats: role of the polyol pathway. *Diabetologia*, **35**: 1011–1019.

Campbell, W.B., Gebremedhin D., Pratt P.F., Harder D.R. (1996) Identification of epoxy-eicosatrienoic acids as endothelium-derived hyperpolarizing factors. *Circ. Res.*, **78**: 415–423.

Campbell, W.B., Harder D.R. (1999) Endothelium-derived hyperpolarizing factors and vascular cytochrome P450 metabolites of arachidonic acid in the regulation of tone. *Circ. Res.*, **84**: 484–488.

Capdevila, J.H., Falck, J.R., Estabrook, R.W. (1992) Cytochrome P450 and the arachidonic acid cascade. *FASEB J.*, **6**: 731–736.

Carrier, G.O., Fuchs, L.C., Winecoff, A.P., Giulumian, A.D., White, R.E. (1997) Nitro-vasodilators relax mesenteric microvessels by cGMP-induced stimulation of Ca-activated K channels. *Am. J. Physiol.*, **42**: H76–H84.

Carter, T.D., Chen, X.Y., Carlile, G., Kalapothakis, E., Ogden, D., Evans, W.H. (1996) Porcine aortic endothelial gap junctions: identification and permeation by caged InsP3. *J. Cell Sci.*, **109**: 1765–1773.

Chan, E.C., Woodman, O.L. (1999) Enhanced role for the opening of potassium channels in relaxant responses to acetylcholine after myocardial ischaemia and reperfusion in dog coronary arteries. *Br. J. Pharmacol.*, **126**: 925–932.

Chataigneau, T., Félétou, M., Duhault, J., Vanhoutte, P.M. (1998) Epoxyeicosatrienoic acids, potassium channel blockers and endothelium-dependent hyperpolarization in the guinea-pig carotid artery. *Br. J. Pharmacol.*, **123**: 574–580.

Chataigneau, T., Félétou, M., Huang, P.L., Fishman, M.C., Duhault, J., Vanhoutte, P.M. (1999) Acetylcholine-induced relaxation in blood vessels from endothelial nitric oxide synthase knockout mice. *Br. J. Pharmacol.*, **126**: 219–226.

Chataigneau, T., Félétou, M., Thollon, C., Villeneuve, N., Vilaine, J.-P., Duhault, J., Vanhoutte, P.M. (1998) Cannabinoid CB1 receptor and endothelium-dependent hyperpolarization in guinea-pig carotid, rat mesenteric and porcine coronary arteries. *Br. J. Pharmacol.*, **123**: 968–974.

Chaytor, A.T., Evans, W.H., Griffith, T.M. (1997) Peptides homologous to extracellular loop motifs of connexin43 reversibly abolish rhythmic contractile activity in rabbit arteries. *J. Physiol.*, **503**: 99–110.

Chaytor, A.T., Evans, W.H., Griffith, T.M. (1998) Central role of heterocellular gap junctional communication in endothelium-dependent relaxations of rabbit arteries. *J. Physiol.*, **508**: 561–573.

Chaytor, A.T., Martin, P.E.M., Evans, W.H., Randall, M.D., Griffith, T.M. (1999) The endothelial component of cannabinoid-induced relaxation in rabbit mesenteric artery depends on gap junctional communication. *J. Physiol.*, **520**: 539–550.

Chen, G., Cheng, D.W. (1996) Modulation of endothelium-dependent hyperpolarization and relaxation to acetylcholine in rat mesenteric artery by cytochrome P450 enzyme activity. *Circ. Res.*, **79**: 827–833.

Chen, G., Cheung, D.W. (1997) Effect of K^+-channel blockers on ACh-induced hyperpolarization and relaxation in mesenteric arteries. *Am. J. Physiol.*, **272**: H2306–H2312.

Chen, G., Suzuki, H. (1989) Some electrical properties of the endothelium-dependent hyperpolarization recorded from rat arterial smooth muscle cells. *J. Physiol.*, **410**: 91–106.

Chen, G., Suzuki, H. (1990) Calcium-dependency of the endothelium-dependent hyperpolarization in smooth muscle cells of the rabbit carotid artery. *J. Physiol.*, **421**: 521–534.

Chen, G., Suzuki, H., Weston, A.H. (1988) Acetylcholine releases endothelium-derived hyperpolarizing factor and EDRF from rat blood vessels. *Br. J. Pharmacol.*, **95**: 1165–1174.

Chen, G., Yamamoto, Y., Miwa, K., Suzuki, H. (1991) Hyperpolarization of arterial smooth muscle induced by endothelial humoral substances. *Am. J. Physiol.*, **260**: H1888–H1892.

Chen, J.K., Falck, J.R., Reddy, K.M., Capdevila, J., Harris, R.C. (1998) Epoxyeicosatrienoic acids and their sulfonimide derivatives stimulate tyrosine phosphorylation and induce mitogenesis in renal epithelial cells. *J. Biol. Chem.*, **273**: 29254–29261.

Chen, J.K, Wang, D.W., Falck, J.R., Capdevila, J., Harris, R.C. (1999) Transfection of an active cytochrome P450 arachidonic acid epoxygenase indicates that 14,15-epoxyeicosatrienoic acid functions as an intracellular second messenger in response to epidermal growth factor. *J. Biol. Chem.*, **274**: 4764–4769.

Chester, A.H., O'Neil, G.S., Moncada, S., Tadjkarimi, S., Yacoub, M.H. (1990) Low basal and stimulated release of nitric oxide in atherosclerotic epicardial coronary arteries. *Lancet*, **336**: 897–900.

Chi, E.Y., Henderson, W.R., Klebanoff, S.J. (1982) Phospholipase A2-induced rat mast cell secretion. Role of arachidonic acid metabolites. *Lab Invest Lab Invest.*, **47**: 579–585.

Cho, H., Ueda, M., Tamaoka, M., Hamaguchi, M., Aisaka, K., Kiso, Y., Inoue, T., Ogino, R., Tatsuoka, T., Ishihara, T., Noguchi, T., Morita, I., Murota, S.-I. (1991) Novel caffeic acid derivatives: extremely potent inhibitors of 12-lipoxygenase. *J. Med. Chem.*, **34**: 1503–1505.

Choi, S.H., Shin, K.H., Kang, S.W., Chun, Y.S., Chun, B.G. (1999) Guanosine 5′,3′-cyclic monophosphate enhances lipopolysaccharide-induced nitric oxide synthase expression in mixed glial cell cultures of rat. *Neuroscience Letters*, **276**: 29–32.

Choo, L.K., Malta, E., Mitchelson, F. (1986) Investigation of the antimuscarinic and other actions of proadifen *in vitro*. *J. Pharmacol. Exp. Ther.*, **38**: 898–901.

Christ, G.J., Barr. L. (2000) The Neural Control of smooth muscle. In *A functional view of smooth muscle*, edited by Barr and Christ, pp. 345–396, JAI Press.

Christ, G.J., Brink P.R., Ramanan, S.V. (1994) Dynamic gap junction communication: a delimiting model for tissue responses. *Biophys. J.*, **67**: 1335–1344.

Christ, G.J., Brink, P.R. (1999) Analysis of the presence and physiological relevance of subconducting states of connexin43-derived gap junction channels in cultured human corporal vascular smooth muscle cells. *Circ. Res.*, **84**: 797–803.

Christ, G.J., Moreno, A.P., Gondre, C.M., Roy, C., Campos de Carvalho, A.C., Melman, A., Spray, D.C. (1993) Gap junctions in human corpus cavernosum vascular smooth muscle: A test of functional significance. *Progress in Cell Res.*, **3**: 211–217.

Christ, G.J., Moreno, A.P., Melman, A., Spray, D.C. (1992) Gap junction-mediated intercellular diffusion of Ca^{2+} in cultured human corporal smooth muscle cells. *Am. J. Physiol.*, **263**: C373–C383.

Christ, G.J., Spektor, M., Brink, P.R., Barr, L. (1999) Further evidence for the selective disruption of intercellular communication by heptanol. *Am. J. Physiol.*, **276**: H1911–H1917.

Christ, G.J., Spray, D.C., el-Sabban, M., Moore, L.K., Brink, P.R. (1996) Gap junctions in vascular tissues. Evaluating the role of intercellular communication in the modulation of vasomotor tone. *Circ. Res.*, **79**: 631–646.

Christ, M., Bauersachs, J., Heck, M., Wehling, M. (1999) Glucocorticoids attenuate endothelial-dependent, NO-mediated vasodilation by modulation of receptor-dependent calcium-signaling. *Circulation*, **100**: I-416.

Christ, M., Wehling, M. (1998) Cardiovascular steroid actions: swift swallows or sluggish snails? *Cardiovasc. Res.*, **40**: 34–44.

Clozel, M., Kuhn, H., Hefti, F. (1990) Effects of angiotensin converting enzyme inhibitors and of hydralazine on endothelial function in hypertensive rats. *Hypertension*, **16**: 532–540.

Cockell, A.P., Poston, L. (1996) Isolated mesenteric arteries from pregnant rats show enhanced flow-mediated relaxation but normal myogenic tone. *J. Physiol.*, **495**: 545–551.

Cocks, T.M., Angus, J.A. (1983) Endothelium-dependent relaxation of coronary arteries by noradrenaline and serotonin. *Nature*, **305**: 627–630.

Cocks, T.M., King, S.J., Angus, J.A. (1990) Glibenclamide is a competitive inhibitor of the thromboxane A_2 receptor in dog coronary artery *in vitro*. *Br. J. Pharmacol.*, **100**: 375–378.

Cohen, R.A., Plane, F., Najibi, S., Huk, I., Malinski, T., Garland, C.J. (1997) Nitric oxide is the mediator of both endothelium-dependent relaxation and hyperpolarization of the rabbit carotid artery. *Proc. Natl. Acad. Sci. USA*, **94**: 4193–4198.

Cohen, R.A., Plane, F., Najibi, S., Huk, I., Malinski, T., Gollasch, M., Steinke, T., Ried, C., Luft, F.C., Haller, H. (1997) Nitric oxide is the mediator of both endothelium-dependent relaxation and hyperpolarization of the rabbit carotid artery. *Proc. Natl. Acad. Sci. USA*, **94**: 4193–4198.

Cohen, R.A., Shepherd, J.T., Vanhoutte, P.M. (1983) Inhibitory role of the endothelium in the response of isolated coronary arteries to platelets. *Science*, **221**: 273–274.

Cohen, R.A., Vanhoutte, P.M. (1995) Endothelium-dependent hyperpolarization. Beyond nitric oxide and cyclic GMP. *Circulation*, **92**: 3337–3349.

Cohen, R.A., Zitnay, K.M., Haudenschild, C.C., Cunningham, D. (1988) Loss of selective endothelial cell vasoactive functions caused by hypercholesterolemia in pig coronary arteries. *Circ. Res.*, **63**: 903–910.

Cole, W., Clement-Chomiene, O. (2000) Properties, regulation, and role of K^+ channels in smooth muscle. In *A functional view of smooth muscle*, edited by Barr and Christ, JAI Press.

Cole, W., Clement-Choniene, O., Aiello, E.A. (1996) Regulation of 4 aminopyridine-sensitive, delayed rectifier K^+ channels in vascular smooth muscle by phosphorylation. *Biochem. and Cell Biol.*, **74**: 439–447.

Coleman, H.A., Tare, M., Parkington, H.C. (2001) K^+ currents underlying the action of endothelium-derived hyperpolarizing factor in guinea-pig, rat and human blood vessels. *J. Physiol.*, **531**: 359–373.

Coles, J.A., Tsacopoulos, M. (1977) A method of making fine double-barreled potassium-sensitive micro-electrodes for intracellular recording. *J. Physiol.*, **270**: 13–14P.

Coles, J.A., Tsacopoulos, M. (1979) K^+ activity in photoreceptors, glial cells and extracellular space in the drone retina: changes during photostimulation. *J. Physiol.*, **290**: 525–549.

Conrad, M.C. (1968) Abnormalities of the digital vasculature as related to ulceration and gangrene. *Circ.*, **38**: 568–581.

Corriu, C., Félétou, M., Canet, E., Vanhoutte, P.M. (1996a) Endothelium-derived factors and hyperpolarization of the carotid artery of the guinea-pig. *Br. J. Pharmacol.*, **119**: 959–964.

Corriu, C., Félétou, M., Canet, E., Vanhoutte, P.M. (1996b) Inhibitors of the cytochrome P450-monooxygenase and endothelium-dependent hyperpolarisations in the guinea-pig isolated carotid artery. *Br. J. Pharmacol.*, **117**: 607–610.

Cosentino, F., Katusic, Z.S. (1995) Tetrahydrobiopterin and dysfunction of endothelial nitric oxide synthase in coronary arteries. *Circulation*, **91**: 139–144.

Cotter, M.A., Love, A., Watt, M.J., Cameron, N.E., Dines, K.C. (1995) Effects of natural free radical scavengers on peripheral nerve and neurovascular function in diabetic rats. *Diabetologia*, **38**: 1285–1294.

Cowan, C.L., Cohen, R.A. (1991) Two mechanisms mediate relaxation by bradykinin of pig coronary artery: NO-dependent and -independent responses. *Am. J. Physiol.*, **261**: H830–H835.

Cowan, C.L., Palacino, J.J., Najibi, S., Cohen, R.A. (1993) Potassium channel-mediated relaxation to acetylcholine in rabbit arteries. *J. Pharmacol. Exp. Ther.*, **266**: 1482–1489.

Cowan, D.B., Lye, S.J., Langille, B.L. (1998) Regulation of vascular connexin43 gene expression by mechanical loads. *Circ. Res.*, **82**: 786–793.

Creager, M.A., Cooke, J.P., Mendelsohn, M.E., Gallagher, S.J., Coleman, S.M., Loscalzo, J., Dzau, V.J. (1990) Impaired vasodilation of forearm resistance vessels in hypercholesterolemic humans. *J. Clin. Invest.*, **86**: 228–234.

Criqui, M.H., Fronek, A., Klauber, M.R., Barrett-Connor, E., Gabriel, S. (1985) The sensitivity, specificity and predictive value of traditional clinical evaluation of peripheral arterial disease: results from non-invasive testing in a defined population. *Circulation*, **71**: 516–522.

Cross, A.R., Jones, O.T. (1986) The effect of the inhibitor diphenylene iodonium on the superoxide-generating system of neutrophils. Specific labelling of a component polypeptide of the oxidase. *Biochem. J.*, **237**: 111–116.

Dahlöf, B., Pennert, K., Hansson, L. (1992) Reversal of left ventricular hypertrophy in hypertensive patients. A metaanalysis of 109 treatment studies. *Am. J. Hypert.*, **5**: 95–110.

Daut, J., Mehrke, G., Nees, S., Newman, W.H. (1988) Passive electrical properties and electrogenic sodium transport of cultured guinea-pig coronary endothelial cells. *J. Physiol.*, **402**: 237–254.

Daut, J., Standen, N.B., Nelson, M.T. (1994) The role of the membrane potential of endothelial and smooth muscle cells in the regulation of coronary blood flow. *J. Cardiovasc. Electrophysiol.*, **5**: 154–181.

Davidge, S., McLauphlin, M. (1992) Endogenous modulation of the blunted response in resistance sized mesenteric arteries from the pregnant rat. *Am. J. Obstet. Gynecol.*, **167**: 1691–1698.

Davidson, J.S., Baumgarten, I.M. (1988) Glycyrrhetinic acid derivatives: a novel class of inhibitors of gap-junctional intercellular communication. Structure-activity relationships. *J. Pharmacol. Exp. Ther.*, **246**: 1104–1107.

Davidson, J.S., Baumgarten, I.M., Harley, E.H. (1986) Reversible inhibition of intercellular junctional communication by glycyrrhetinic acid. *Biochem. Biophys. Res. Commun.*, **134**: 29–36.

Davies, P.F. (1995) Flow-mediated endothelial mechanotransduction. *Physiol. Rev.*, **75**: 519–560.

Davis, K., Grinsburg, R., Bristow, M., Harrison, D.C. (1980) Biphasic action of prostacyclin in the human coronary artery. *Clin. Res.*, **28**: 165A.

De Gaetano, G. (1992) The use of prostanoids in critical ischaemia. *Crit. Ischaemia*, **2**: 5–12.

De Mey, J.G., Claeys, M., Vanhoutte, P.M. (1982) Endothelium-dependent inhibitory effects of acetylcholine, adenosine triphosphate, thrombin and arachidonic acid in the canine femoral artery. *J. Pharmacol. Exp. Ther.*, **222**: 166–173.

De Tejada, I.S., Goldstein, I., Azadzoi, K., Krane, R.J., Cohen, R.A. (1989) Impaired neurogenic and endothelium-mediated relaxation of penile smooth muscle from diabetic men with impotence. *New Engl. J. Med.*, **320**: 1025–1030.

De Vriese, A.S., Endlich, K., Elger, M., Lameire, N.H., Atkins, R.C., Lan, H.Y., Rupin, A., Kriz, W., Steinhausen, M.W. (1999) The role of selectins in glomerular leukocyte recruitment in rat anti-glomerular basement membrane glomerulonephritis. *J. Am. Soc. Nephrol.*, **10**: 2510–2517.

De Vriese, A.S., Verbeuren, T.J., Vallez, M.O., Lameire, N.H., De Buyzere, M., Vanhoutte, P.M. (2000b) Off-line analysis of red blood cell velocity in renal arterioles. *J. Vasc. Res.*, **37**: 26–31.

De Vriese, A.S., Verbeuren, T.J., Van de Voorde, J., Lameire, N.H., Vanhoutte, P.M. (2000a) Endothelial dysfunction in diabetes. *Br. J. Pharmacol.*, **130**: 963–974.

De Wit, C., Roos, F., Bolz, S.-S., Kirchhoff, S., Krüger, O., Willecke, K., Pohl, U. (2000) Impaired conduction of vasodilatation along arterioles in connexin40-deficient mice. *Circ. Res.*, **86**: 649–655.

Declaration of Helsinki (1997) *Cardiovasc. Res.*, **35**: 2–3.

Delage, B., Deleze, J. (2000) Reexamination of calcium effects on gap junctions in heart myocytes. *Curr. Top. Memb.*, **49**: 189–203.

Dembinska-Kiec, A., Pallapies, D., Simmet, T., Peskar, B.M., Peskar, B.A. (1991) Effect of carbenoxolone on the biological activity of nitric oxide: relation to gastroprotection. *Br. J. Pharmacol.*, **104**: 811–816.

DeMello, W. (1988) Increase in junctional conductance caused by isoproterenol in heart cell pairs is suppressed by cAMP dependent protein-kinase inhibitor. *Biochem. Biophys. Res. Comm.*, **154**: 509.

Diamantopoulos, E., Grigoriadou, M. (1997) Epidemiological and demographical characteristics of chronic peripheral occlusive disease of the lower limbs. *Crit. Ischemia*, **7**: 5–13.

Diederich, D., Skopec, J., Diederich, A., Dai, F.X. (1994) Endothelial dysfunction in mesenteric resistance arteries of diabetic rats: role of free radicals. *Am. J. Physiol.*, **266**: H1153–1161.

Ding, H., Kubes, P., Triggle, C. (2000) Potassium- and acetylcholine-induced vasorelaxation in mice lacking endothelial nitric oxide synthase. *Br. J. Pharmacol.*, **129**: 1194–1200.

Domenighetti, A.A., Bény, J.-L., Chabaud, F., Frieden, M. (1998) An intercellular regenerative calcium wave in porcine coronary artery endothelial cells in primary culture. *J. Neurochem.*, **69**: 721–728.

Dong, H., Waldron, G.J., Galipeau, D., Cole, W.C., Triggle, C.R. (1997) NO/PGI$_2$-independent vasorelaxation and the cytochrome P450 pathway in rabbit carotid artery. *Br. J. Pharmacol.*, **120**: 695–701.

Dora, K.A., Doyle, M.P., Duling, B.R. (1997) Elevation of intracellular calcium in smooth muscle causes endothelial cell generation of NO in arterioles. *Proc. Natl. Acad. Sci.*, **94**: 6529–6534.

Dora, K.A., Martin, P.E.M., Chaytor, A.T., Evans, W.H., Garland, C.J., Griffith, T.M. (1999) Role of heterocellular gap junctional communication in endothelium-dependent smooth muscle hyperpolarization: inhibition by a connexin-mimetic peptide. *Biochem. Biophys. Res. Commun.*, **254**: 27–31.

Doughty, J.M., Boyle, J.P., Langton, P.D. (2000) Potassium does not mimic EDHF in rat mesenteric arteries. *Br. J. Pharmacol.*, **130**: 1174–1182.

Doughty, J.M., Langton, P.D. (1999) The effects of ouabain and barium on EDHF- and 10 mm K$^+$-induced dilations in pressurized rat mesenteric artery. *J. Physiol.*, **518**: 34.

Doughty, J.M., Miller, A.L., Langton, P.D. (1998) Non-specificity of chloride channel blockers in rat cerebral arteries: block of the L-type calcium channel. *J. Physiol.*, **507**: 433–439.

Doughty, J.M., Plane, F., Langton, P.D. (1999) Charybdotoxin and apamin block EDHF in rat mesenteric artery if selectively applied to the endothelium. *Am. J. Physiol.*, **276**: H1107–H1112.

Dowell, F.J., Hamilton, C.A., McMurray, J., Reid, J.L. (1993) Effects of a xanthine oxidase/hypoxanthine free radical and reactive oxygen species generating system on endothelial function in New Zealand white rabbit aortic rings. *J. Cardiovasc. Pharmacol.*, **22**: 792–797.

Drummond, G.R., Selemidis, S., Cocks, T.M. (2000) Apamin-sensitive, non-nitric oxide (NO) endothelium-dependent relaxations to bradykinin in the bovine isolated coronary artery: no role for cytochrome P450 and K$^+$. *Br. J. Pharmacol.*, **129**: 811–819.

Dudek, R.R., Conforto, A., Pinto, V., Wildhirt, S., Suzuki, H. (1995) Inhibition of endothelial nitric oxide synthase by cytochrome P450 reductase inhibitors. *Proc. Soc. Exp. Biol. Med.,* **209**: 60–64.

Eckman, D.M., Hopkins, N., McBride, C. Keef, K.D. (1998) Endothelium-dependent relaxation and hyperpolarization in guinea-pig coronary artery: role of epoxyeicosatrienoic acid. *Br. J. Pharmacol.,* **124**: 181–189.

Edwards, F.R., Hirst, G.D.S. (1988) Inward rectification in submucosal arterioles of guinea-pig ileum. *J. Physiol.,* **404**: 437–454.

Edwards, F.R., Hirst, G.D.S., Silverberg, G.D. (1988) Inward rectification in rat cerebral arterioles; Involvement of potassium ions in autoregulation. *J. Physiol.,* **404**: 455–466.

Edwards, G., Dora, K.A., Gardener, M.J., Garland, C.J., Weston, A.H. (1998) K^+ is an endothelium-derived hyperpolarizing factor in rat arteries. *Nature,* **396**: 269–272.

Edwards, G., Félétou, M., Gardener, M.J., Thollon, C., Vanhoutte, P.M., Weston, A.H (1999) Role of gap junctions in the responses to EDHF in rat and guinea-pig small arteries. *Br. J. Pharmacol.,* **128**: 1788–1794.

Edwards, G., Gardener, M.J., Félétou, M., Brady, G., Vanhoutte, P.M., Weston, A.H. (1999) Further investigation of endothelium-derived hyperpolarizing factor (EDHF) in rat hepatic artery: studies using 1-EBIO and ouabain. *Br. J. Pharmacol.,* **128**: 1064–1070.

Edwards, G., Niederste-Hollenberg, A., Schneider, J., Noack, T., Weston, A.H. (1994) Ion channel modulation by NS 1619, the putative BK_{Ca} channel opener, in vascular smooth muscle. *Br. J. Pharmacol.,* **113**: 1538–1547.

Edwards, G., Thollon, C., Gardener, M.J., Félétou, M., Vilaine, J.-P., Vanhoutte, P.M., Weston, A.H. (2000) Role of gap junctions and EETs in endothelium-dependent hyperpolarization of porcine coronary artery. *Br. J. Pharmacol.,* **129**: 1145–1154.

Edwards, G., Weston, A.H. (1998) Endothelium-derived hyperpolarizing factor-a critical appraisal. *Progress in Drug Research,* **50**: 107–133.

Edwards, G., Weston, A.H. (1998) Potassium channel openers and vascular smooth muscle relaxation. *Pharmacol. & Ther.,* **48**: 237–258.

Edwards, G., Zygmunt, P.M., Högestätt, E.D., Weston, A.H. (1996) Effects of cytochrome P450 inhibitors on potassium currents and mechanical activity in rat portal vein. *Br. J. Pharmacol.,* **119**: 691–701.

Elenes, S., Moreno, A.P. (2000) Heteromultimeric gap junction channels and cardiac disease. In Gap Junctions edited by C. Perracchia. *Current Topics in Membranes,* **49**: 61–92.

Elfgang, C., Eckert, R., Lichtenberg-Frate, H., Butterweck, A., Traub, O., Klein, R.A., Hulser, D.F., Willecke, K. (1995) Specific permeability and selective formation of gap junction channels in connexin-transfected HeLa cells. *J. Cell. Biol.,* **129**: 805–817.

Elliott, T.G., Cockcroft, J.R., Gropp, P.H., Viberti, G.C., Ritter, J.M. (1993) Inhibition of nitric oxide synthesis in forearm vasculature of insulin-dependent diabetic patients: blunted vasconstriction in patients with microalbuminuria. *Clin. Sci.,* **85**: 687–693.

Ellis, E.F., Police, R.J., Yancey, L., McKinney, J.S., Amruthesh, S.C. (1990) Dilation of cerebral arterioles by cytochrome P-450 metabolites of arachidonic acid. *Am. J. Physiol.,* **259**: H1171–H1177.

Emerson, G.G., Segal, S.S. (2000a) Endothelial cell pathway for conduction of hyperpolarization and vasodilation along hamster feed artery. *Circ. Res.,* **86**: 94–100.

Emerson, G.G., Segal, S.S. (2000b) Electrical coupling between endothelial cells and smooth muscle cells in hamster feed arteries: Role in vasomotor control. *Circ. Res.,* **87**: 474–479.

Endo, K., Abiru, T., Machida, H., Kasuya, Y., Kamata, K. (1995) Endothelium-derived hyperpolarizing factor does not contribute to the decrease in endothelium-dependent relaxation in the aorta of streptozotocin-induced diabetic rats. *Gen. Pharmacol.,* **26**: 149–153.

European Consensus Document (1991) *Circulation,* **84**: 1–26.

Evans, A.T., Formukong, E., Evans, F.J. (1987) Activation of phospholipase A_2 by cannabinoids. Lack of correlation with CNS effects. *FEBS Lett.,* **211**: 119–122.

Evans, W.H., Ahmad, S., Diez, J., George, D.H., Kendall, J.M., Martin, P.E.M. (1999) Trafficking pathways leading to the formation of gap junctions, Novartis Foundation Symposium, vol. 219, pp. 44–54. Chichester: Wiley.

Fagrell, B. (1977) The skin microcirculation and the pathogenesis of ischemic necrosis and gangrene. *Scand. J. Clin. Lab. Invest.*, **37**: 473–476.

Fagrell, B., Lundberg, G. (1984) A simplified evaluation of vital capillary microscopy for predicting skin viability in patients with severe arterial insufficiency. *Clin. Physiol.*, **4**: 403–411.

Falk, M.M., Kumar, N.M., Gilula, N.B. (1994) Membrane insertion of gap junction connexins: polytopic channel forming membrane proteins. *J. Cell Biol.*, **127**: 343–355.

Faraci, F.M., Sigmund, C.D., Shesely, E.G., Maeda, N., Heistad, D.D. (1998) Responses of carotid artery in mice deficient in expression of the gene for endothelial NO synthase. *Am. J. Physiol.*, **274**: H564–H570.

Félétou M., Vanhoutte P.M. (1999) Endothelium-derived hyperpolarizing Factor. *Drugs News Perspectives*, **12**: 217–222.

Félétou, M., Vanhoutte, P.M. (1999) The third pathway: endothelium-dependent hyperpolarization. *J. Physiol. Pharmacol.*, **50**: 525–534.

Félétou, M., Vanhoutte, P.M. (1988) Endothelium-dependent hyperpolarization of canine coronary smooth muscle. *Br. J. Pharmacol.*, **93**: 515–524.

Félétou, M., Vanhoutte, P.M. (1999) The alternative: EDHF. *J. Mol. Cell. Cardiol.*, **31**: 15–22.

Ferris, T.F. (1983) The pathophysiology of toxemia and hypertension during pregnancy. *Drugs*, **25**: 198–205.

Ferris, T.F., Conrad, K.P., Barrera, S.A., Friedman, P.A., Schmidt, V.M. (1991) Evidence for attenuation of myoinositol uptake, phosphoinositide turnover and inositol phosphate production in aortic vasculature of rat during pregnancy. *J. Clin. Invest.*, **87**: 1700–1709.

Field, L., Dilts, R.V., Ravichandran, R., Lenhert, P.G., Carnahan, G.E. (1978) An unusually stable thionitrite from *N*-acetyl-D,L-penicillamine; X-ray crystal and molecular structure of 2-(acetylamino)-2-carboxy-1,1-dimethylethyl thionitrite. *J. Chem. Soci. Chem. Comm.*, **6**: 249–250.

Fisslthaler, B., Hinsch, N., Chataigneau, T., Popp, R., Kiss, L., Busse, R., Fleming, I. (2000) Nifedipine increases cytochrome P450 2C expression and EDHF-mediated responses in coronary arteries. *Hypertension*, **36**: 270–275.

Fisslthaler, B., Popp, R., Kiss, L., Potente, M., Harder, D.R., Fleming, I., Busse, R. (1999) Cytochrome P450 2C is an EDHF synthase in coronary arteries. *Nature*, **401**: 493–497.

Fleming, I. (2000) Myoendothelial gap junctions: The gap is there, but does EDHF go through it? *Circ. Res.*, **86**: 249–250.

Förstermann, U., Mügge, A., Alheid, U., Haverich, A., Frölich, J.C. (1988) Selective attenuation of endothelium-mediated vasodilation in atherosclerotic human coronary arteries. *Circ. Res.*, **62**: 185–190.

Förstermann, U., Neufang, B. (1984) The endothelium-dependent relaxation of rabbit aorta: effects of antioxidants and hydroxylated eicosatetraenoic acids. *Br. J. Pharmacol.*, **82**: 765–767.

Foschi, M., Chari, S., Dunn, M.J., Sorokin, A. (1997) Biphasic activation of p21[ras] by endothelin-1 sequentially activates the ERK cascade and phosphatidylinositol 3-kinase. *EMBO J.*, **16**: 6439–6451.

Fournet-Bourguignon, M.P., Castedo-Delrieu, M., Bidouard, J.P., Leonce, S., Saboureau, D., Delescluse, I., Vilaine, J.-P., Vanhoutte, P.M. (2000) Phenotypic and functional changes in regenerated porcine coronary endothelial cells. Increased uptake of modified LDL and reduced production of NO. *Circ. Res.*, **86**: 854–861.

Franzeck, U.K., Talke, P., Bernstein, E.F., Golbranson, F.L., Fronek, A. (1982) Transcutaneous oxygen tension measurements in health and peripheral occlusive disease. *Surgery*, **91**: 156–163.

Frei, B., England, L., Ames, B.N. (1989) Ascorbate is an outstanding antioxidant in human blood plasma. *Proc. Natl. Acad. Sci. USA*, **86**: 6377–6381.

Frieden, M., Sollini, M., Bény, J.-L. (1999) Substance P and bradykinin activate different types of KCa currents to hyperpolarize cultured porcine coronary artery endothelial cells. *J. Physiol.*, **519**: 361–371.

Fuji, K., Tominaga, M., Ohmori, S., Abe, I., Fujishima, M. (1996) Impaired endothelium-dependent hyperpolarization in the mesenteric artery of spontaneously hypertensive rats. In *Endothelim-derived hyperpolarizing factors*, edited by P.M. Vanhoutte, vol. 1, pp. 247–254. The Netherlands: Harwood Academic Publishers.

Fujii, K., Ohmori, S., Tominaga, M., Abe, I., Takata, Y., Ohya, Y., Kobayashi, K., Fujishima, M. (1993) Age-related changes in endothelium-dependent hyperpolarization in the rat mesenteric artery. *Am. J. Physiol.*, **265**: H509–H516.

Fujii, K., Tominaga, M., Ohmori, S., Kobayashi, K., Koga, T., Takata, Y., Fujishima, M. (1992) Decreased endothelium-dependent hyperpolarization to acetylcholine in smooth muscle of the mesenteric artery of spontaneously hypertensive rats. *Circ. Res.*, **70**: 660–669.

Fujimoto, S., Ikegami, Y., Isaka, M., Kato, T., Nishimura, K., Itoh, T. (1999) K(+) channel blockers and cytochrome P450 inhibitors on acetylcholine-induced, endothelium-dependent relaxation in rabbit mesenteric artery. *Eur. J. Pharmacol.*, **384**: 7–15.

Fukao, M., Hattori, Y., Kanno, M., Sakuma, I., Kitabatake, A. (1997a) Alterations in endothelium-dependent hyperpolarization and relaxation in mesenteric arteries from streptozotocin-induced diabetic rats. *Br. J. Pharmacol.*, **121**: 1383–1391.

Fukao, M., Hattori, Y., Kanno, M., Sakuma, I., Kitabatake, A. (1997b) Evidence against a role of cytochrome P450-derived arachidonic acid metabolites in endothelium-dependent hyperpolarization by acetylcholine in rat isolated mesenteric artery. *Br. J. Pharmacol.*, **120**: 439–446.

Fukao, M., Hattori, Y., Kanno, M., Sakuma, I., Kitabatake, A. (1996) Endothelium-dependent hyperpolarizations in arteries from diabetic rats. In *Endothelim-derived hyperpolarizing factor*, edited by P.M. Vanhoutte, vol. 1, pp. 263–270. The Netherlands: Harwood Academic Publishers.

Fukao, M., Mason, H.S., Britton, F.C., Kenyon, J.L., Horowitz, B., Keef, K.C. (1999) Cyclic GMP-dependent protein kinase activates cloned BKCa channels expressed in mammalian cells by direct phosphorylation at serine 1072. *J. Biol. Chem.*, **274**: 10927–10935.

Fukuta, H., Hashitani, H., Yamamoto, Y., Suzuki, H. (1999) Calcium responses induced by acetylcholine in submucosal arterioles of the guinea-pig small intestine. *J. Physiol.*, **515**: 489–499.

Fukuta, H., Koshita, M., Yamamoto, Y., Suzuki, H. (1999) Inhibition of the endothelium-dependent relaxation by 18β-glycyrrhetinic acid in the guinea-pig aorta. *Jpn. J. Physiol.*, **49**: 267–274.

Fulton, D., Mahboubi, K., McGiff, J.C., Quilley, J. (1995) Cytochrome P450-dependent effects of bradykinin in the rat heart. *Br. J. Pharmacol.*, **114**: 99–102.

Fulton, D., McGiff, J.C., Quilley, J. (1994) Role of K$^+$ channels in the vasodilator response to bradykinin in the rat heart. *Br. J. Pharmacol.*, **113**: 954–958.

Fulton, D., McGiff, J.C., Quilley, J. (1996) Cytochrome P450 arachidonate metabolites: deficit in diabetes mellitus? *FASEB J.*, **9**: A113.

Fulton, D., McGiff, J.C., Wolin, M.S., Kaminski, P., Quilley, J. (1997) Evidence against a cytochrome P450-derived reactive oxygen species as the mediator of the nitric oxide-independent vasodilator effect of bradykinin in the perfused heart of the rat. *J. Pharmacol. Exp. Ther.*, **280**: 702–709.

Furchgott, R.F., Vanhoutte, P.M. (1989) Endothelium-derived relaxing and contracting factors. *FASEB J.*, **3**: 2007–2018.

Furchgott, R.F., Zawadzki, J.W. (1980) The obligatory role of endothelial cells in the relaxation of arterial smooth muscle by acetylcholine. *Nature*, **288**: 373–376.

Gabriels, J.E., Paul, D.L. (1998) Connexin43 is highly localized to sites of disturbed flow in rat aortic endothelium but connexin37 and connexin40 are more uniformly distributed. *Circ. Res.*, **83**: 636–643.

Galvez, A., Gimenez-Gallego, G., Reuben, J.P., Roy-Contancin, L., Feigenbaum, P., Kaczorowski, G.J., Garcia, M.L. (1990) Purification and characterization of a unique, potent, peptidyl probe for the high conductance calcium-activated potassium channel from venom of the scorpion Buthus tamulus. *J. Biol. Chem.*, **265**: 11083–11090.

Gant, N.F., Worley, R.J.M., Everett, R.B., MacDonald, P.C. (1980) Control of vascular responsiveness during human pregnancy. *Kidney Int.*, **18**: 253–258.

Garland, C.J., Plane, F., Kemp, B.K., Cocks, T.M. (1995) Endothelium-dependent hyperpolarization: a role in the control of vascular tone. *Trends Pharmacol. Sci.*, **16**: 23–30.

Garland, C.J., Plane, F. (1996) Relative importance of endothelium-derived hyperpolarizing factor for the relaxation of vascular smooth muscle in different arterial beds. In *Endothelium-Derived Hyperpolarizing Factor*, edited by P.M. Vanhoutte, vol. 1, pp. 173–179. The Netherlands: Harwood Academic Publishers.

Garland, C.J., Plane, F., Kemp, B.K., Cocks, T.M. (1995) Endothelium-dependent hyperpolarization: a role in the control of vascular tone. *Trends Pharmacol. Sci.*, **16**: 23–30.

Garthwaite, J., Charles, S.L., Chess-Williams, R. (1988) Endothelium derived relaxing factor release on activation of NMDA receptors suggest role as intercellular messenger in the brain. *Nature*, **336**: 385–388.

Gauthier-Rein, K.M., Rusch, N.J. (1997) Distinct endothelial impairment in coronary microvessels from hypertensive Dahl rats. *Hypertension*, **31**: 328–334.

Gaziano, J.M., Manson, J.E., Ridker, P.M., Buring, J.E., Hennekens, C.H. (1990) β-carotene therapy for chronic stable angina. *Circulation*, **82**: III-201.

Gebremedhin, D., Harder, D., Pratt, P.F., Campbell, W.B. (1998) Bioassay of an endothelium-derived hyperpolarizing factor from bovine coronary arteries: role of a cytochrome P450 metabolite. *J. Vasc. Res.*, **35**: 274–284.

Gebremedhin, D., Lange, A., Lowry, T., Taheri, M., Birks, E., Hudetz, A., Narayanan, J., Falck, J., Okamoto, H., Roman, R., Nithipatikom, K., Campbell, W., Harder, D.R. (2000) Production of 20-HETE and its role in autoregulation of cerebral blood flow. *Circ. Res.*, **87**: 60–65.

Gebremedhin, D., Lange, A., Narayanan, J., Aebly, M., Jacobs, E., Harder, D.R. (1998b) Cat cerebral arterial smooth muscle cells express cytochrome P450 4A2 enzyme and produce the vasoconstrictor 20-HETE which enhances L-type Ca^{2+} current. *J. Physiol.*, **507**: 771–781.

Gebremedhin, D., Ma, Y., Falck, J., Roman, R.J., VanRollins, M., Harder, D.R. (1992) Mechanism of action of cerebral epoxyeicosatrienoic acids on cerebral arterial smooth muscle. *Am. J. Physiol.*, **263**: H519–H525.

Ged, C., Beaune, P. (1991) Isolation of the human cytochrome P-450 IIC8 gene: multiple glucocorticoid responsive elements in the 5' region. *Biochem. Biophys. Acta*, **1088**: 433–435.

Gelband, C.H., Hume, J.R. (1992) Ionic currents in single smooth-muscle cells of the canine renal-artery. *Circ. Res.*, **71**: 745–758.

George, C.H., Kendall, J.M., Campbell, A.K., Evans, W.H. (1998a) Connexin-aequorin chimerae report cytoplasmic calcium environments along trafficking pathways leading to gap junction biogenesis in living COS-7 cells. *J. Biol. Chem.*, **273**: 29822–29829.

George, C.H., Martin, P.E.M., Evans, W.H. (1998) Rapid determination of gap junction formation using HeLa cells microinjected with cDNAs encoding wild-type and chimeric connexins. *Biochem. Biophys. Res. Comm.*, **247**: 785–789.

Gerber, R.T., Anwar, M.A., Poston, L. (1998) Enhanced acetylcholine-induced relaxation in small mesenteric arteries from pregnant rats: an important role for endothelium-derived hyperpolarizing factor (EDHF). *Br. J. Pharmacol.*, **125**: 455–460.

Giaume, C., Venance, L. (1998) Intercellular calcium signalling and gap junctional communication in astrocytes. *Glia*, **24**: 50–64.

Gilligan, D.M., Badar, D.M., Panza, J.A., Quyyumi, A.A., Cannon, R.O.III (1994) Acute vascular effects of estrogen in postmenopausal women. *Circulation*, **90**: 786–791.

Gisclard, V., Miller, V.M., Vanhoutte, P.M. (1988) Effect of 17β estradiol on endothelial responses in the rabbit. *J. Pharmacol. Exp. Ther.*, **244**: 19–22.

Giulumian, A.D., Clark, S.G., Fuchs, L.C. (1999) Effect of behavioral stress on coronary artery relaxation altered with aging in BHR. *Am. J. Physiol.*, **45**: R435–R440.

Godecke, A., Decking, U.K., Ding, Z., Hirchenhain, J., Bidmon, H.J., Godecke, S., Schrader, J. (1998) Coronary hemodynamics in endothelial NO synthase knockout mice. *Circ. Res.*, **82**: 186–194.

Goldberg, G.S., Bechberger, J.F., Naus, C.C. (1995) A pre-loading method of evaluating gap junctional communication by fluorescent dye transfer. *Biotechniques*, **3**: 490–497.

Goldberg, G.S., Lampe, P.D., Sheedy, D., Stewart, C.C., Nicholson, B.J., Naus, C.C. (1998) Direct isolation and analysis of endogenous transjunctional ADP from Cx43 transfected C6 glioma cells. *Exp. Cell Res.*, **239**: 82–92.

Goldberg, G.S., Moreno, A.P., Bechberger, J.F., Hearn, S.S., Shivers, R.R., MacPhee, D.J., Zhang, Y.C., Naus, C.C. (1996) Evidence that disruption of connexon particle arrangements in gap junction plaques is associated with inhibition of gap junctional communication by a glycyrrhetinic acid derivative. *Exper. Cell Res.*, **222**: 48–53.

Goodenough, D.A., Goliger, J.A., Paul, D.L. (1996) Connexins, connexons, and intercellular communication. *Ann. Rev. Biochem.*, **65**: 475–502.

Gordon, J.L., Martin, W. (1983) Endothelium-dependent relaxation of the pig aorta: relationship to stimulation of ^{86}RB efflux from isolated endothelial cells. *Br. J. Pharmacol.*, **79**: 531–541.

Goto, K., Fujii, K., Onaka, U., Abe, I., Fujishima, M. (2000) Renin-angiotensin system blockade improves endothelial dysfunction in hypertension. *Hypertension*, **36**: 575–580.

Goto, K., Fujii, K., Onaka, U., Abe, I., Fujishima, M. (2000) Angiotensin converting enzyme inhibitor prevents age-related endothelial dysfunction. *Hypertension*, **36**: 581–587.

Goto, M., Van Bavel, E., Giezeman, M.J., Spaan, J.A. (1996) Vasodilatatory effect of pulsatile pressure on coronary resistance. *Circ. Res.*, **79**: 1039–1045.

Graham-Lorence, S., Truan, G., Peterson, J.A., Falck, J.R., Wei, S., Helvig, C., Capdevila, J.H. (1997) An active site substitution, F87V, converts cytochrome P450 BM-3 into a regio- and stereoselective (14S, 15R)-arachidonic acid epoxygenase. *J. Biol. Chem.*, **272**: 1127–1135.

Graier, W.F., Holzmann, S., Hoebel, B.G., Kukovetz, W.R., Kostner, G.M. (1996) Mechanisms of L-N^G-nitroarginine/indomethacin-resistant relaxation in bovine and porcine coronary arteries. *Br. J. Pharmacol.*, **119**: 1177–1186.

Graier, W.F., Simecek, S., Sturek, M. (1995) Cytochrome P450 mono-monooxygenase-regulated signalling of Ca^{2+} entry in human and bovine endothelial cells. *J. Physiol.*, **482**: 259–274.

Grasby, D.J., Morris, J.L., Segal, S.S. (1999) Heterogeneity of vascular innervation in hamster cheek pouch and retractor muscle. *J. Vasc. Res.*, **36**: 465–476.

Green, S., Walter, P., Kumar, V., Krust, A., Bornert, J.M., Argos, P., Chambon, P. (1986) Human oestrogen receptor cDNA: sequence, expression and homology to v-erb-A. *Nature*, **320**: 134–139.

Greenwald, J.E., Bianchine, J.R., Wong, L.K. (1979) The production of the arachidonate metabolite HETE in vascular tissue. *Nature*, **281**: 588–589.

Griffin, K.L., Laughlin, M.H., Parker, J.L. (1999) Exercise training improves endothelium-mediated vasorelaxation after chronic coronary occlusion. *J. Appl. Physiol.*, **87**: 1948–1956.

Griffith, T.M., Taylor, H.J. (1999) Cyclic AMP mediates EDHF-type relaxations of rabbit jugular vein. *Biochem. Biophys. Res. Commun.*, **263**: 52–57.

Griffith, T.M., Chaytor, A.T., Evans, W.H. (1998) Role of gap junctions and Ca^{2+} stores in endothelium-dependent relaxations. *Pharmacol. Toxicol.*, **83**: 57–59

Grodstein, F., Stampfer, M.J., Colditz, G.A., Willett, W.C., Manson, J.E., Joffe, M., Rosner, B., Fuchs, C., Hankinson, S.E., Hunter, D.J., Hennekens, C.H., Speizer, F.E. (1997) Postmenopausal hormone therapy and mortality. *New Engl. J. Med.*, **336**: 1769–1775.

Gryglewski, R.J., Botting, R.M., Vane, J.R. (1991) Prostacyclin: from discovery to clinical application. In *cardiovascular significance of Endothelium-Derived Vasoactive Factors*, edited by G.M. Rubanyi, pp. 3–37, Mount Kisco, NY: Futura.

Gu, H., Ek-Vitorin, J.F., Taffet, S.M., Delmar, M. (2000) Coexpression of connexins40 and 43 enhances the pH sensitivity of gap junctions: A model for synergistic interactions among connexins. *Circ. Res.*, **86**: e98–e103.

Guan, K., Rohwedel, J., Wobus, A.M. (1999) Embryonic stem cell differentiation models: cardiogenesis, myogenesis, neurogenesis, epithelial and vascular smooth muscle cell differentiation *in vitro*. *Cytotechnology*, **30**: 211–226.

Guan, X., Wilson, S., Schlender, K.K., Ruch, R.J. (1996) Gap-junction disassembly and connexin43 dephosphorylation induced by 18β-glycyrrhetinic acid. *Mol. Carcinogenesis*, **16**: 157–164.

Guo, Y., Martinez-Williams, C., Gilbert, K.A., Rannels, D.E. (1999) Inhibition of gap junction communication in alveolar epithelial cells by 18α-glycyrrhetinic acid. *Am. J. Physiol.*, **276**: L1018–L1026.

Haas, T.L., Duling, B.R. (1997) Morphology favors an endothelial cell pathway for longitudinal conduction within arterioles. *Microvasc. Res.*, **53**: 113–120.

Haefliger, J.A., Castillo, E., Waeber, G., Aubert, J.F., Nicod, P., Waeber, B., Meda, P. (1997) Hypertension differentially affects the expression of the gap junction protein connexin43 in cardiac myocytes and aortic smooth muscle cells. *Hypert. and the Heart*, **432**: 71–82.

Hagendorff, A., Schumacher, B., Kirchhoff, S., Lüderitz, B., Willecke, K. (1999) Conduction disturbances and increased atrial vulnerability in connexin40-deficient mice analyzed by transesophageal stimulation. *Circulation*, **99**: 1508–1515.

Hall, E.D., McCall, J.M., Chase, R.L., Yonkers, P.A., Braughler, J.M. (1987) A non-glucocorticoid steroid analog of methylprednisolone duplicates its high-dose pharmacology in models of central nervous system trauma and neuronal membrane damage. *J. Pharmacol. Exp. Ther.*, **242**: 137–142.

Halliwell, B. (1992) Production of superoxide hydrogen peroxide and hydroxyl radicals by phagocytic cells: a cause of chronic inflammatory disease? *Cell Biol. Int.*, **6**: 529–542.

Hamill, O.P., Marty, A., Neher, E., Sackmann, B., Sigworth, F.J. (1981) Improved patch-clamp techniques for the high-resolution current recording from cells and cell-free membrane patches. *Pflügers Arch.*, **391**: 85–100.

Hamilton, C.A., Williams, R., Pathi, V., Berg, G., McArthur, K., McPhaden, A.R., Reid, J.L., Dominiczak, A.F. (1999) Pharmacological characterisation of endothelium-dependent relaxation in human radial artery: comparison with internal thoracic artery. *Cardiovasc. Res.*, **42**: 214–223.

Haq, I., Yeo, W., Jackson, P., Ramsay, L. (1997) The case for cholesterol reduction in peripheral arterial disease. *Crit. Ischemia*, **7**: 15–23.

Harder, D.R. (1984) Pressure dependent membrane depolarization in cat middle cerebral artery. *Circ. Res.*, **55**: 197–202.

Harder, D.R., Alkayed, N., Lange, A., Gebremedhin, D., Roman R.J. (1998a) Functional hyperemia in the brain: Hypothesis for astrocyte-derived vasodilator metabolites. *Stroke*, **28**: 229–234.

Harder, D.R., Campbell, W.B., Roman, R.J. (1995) Role of cytochrome P-450 enzymes and metabolites of arachidonic acid in the control of vascular tone. *J. Vasc. Res.*, **32**: 79–92.

Harder, D.R., Gebremedhin, D., Narayanan, J., Jefcoat, C., Falck, J.R., Campbell, W.B., Roman, R.J. (1994) Formation and action of a P450 4A metabolite of arachidonic acid in cat cerebral microvessels. *Am. J. Physiol.*, **266**: H2098–H2107.

Harder, D.R., Lange, A., Gebremedhin, D., Birks, E.K., Roman, R.J. (1997) Cytochrome P450 metabolites of arachidonic acid as intracellular signaling molecules in vascular tissue. *J. Vasc. Res.*, **34**: 237–243.

Harder, D.R., Roman, R.J., Gebremedhin, D. (2000) Molecular mechanisms controlling nutritive blood flow: role of cytochrome P450 enzymes. *Acta Physiol. Scand.*, **168**: 543–549.

Harder, D.R., Roman, R.J., Gebremedhin, D., Birks, E., Lange, A. (1998b) A common pathway for regulation of nutritive blood flow to the brain: arterial muscle membrane potential and cytochrome P450 metabolites. *Acta Physiol. Scand.*, **164**: 527–532.

Harris, D., Martin, P.E.M., Evans, W.H., Kendall, D.A., Griffith, T.M., Randall, M.D. (2000) Role of gap junctions in endothelium-derived hyperpolarizing factor responses and mechanisms of K^+-relaxation. *Eur. J. Pharmacol.*, **402**: 119–128.

Hasan, A.A.K., Cines, D.B., Ngaiza, J.R., Jaffe, E.A., Schmaier, A.H. (1995) High-molecular-weight kininogen is exclusively membrane bound on endothelial cells to influence activation of vascular endothelium. *Blood*, **85**: 3134–3143.

Hashitani, H., Suzuki, H. (1997) K^+ channels which contribute to the acetylcholine-induced hyperpolarization in smooth muscle of the guinea-pig submucosal arteriole. *J. Physiol.*, **501**: 319–329.

Hatton, C.J., Peers, C. (1997) Multiple effects of nordihydroguaiaretic acid on ionic currents in rat isolated type I carotid body cells. *Br. J. Pharmacol.*, **122**: 923–929.

Hattori, Y., Kawasaki, H., Abe, K., Kanno, M. (1991) Superoxide dismutase recovers altered endothelium dependent relaxation in diabetic rat aorta. *Am. J. Physiol.*, **261**: H1086–H1094.

Hayabuchi, Y., Nakaya, Y., Matsuoka, S., Kuroda, Y. (1998) Endothelium-derived hyperpolarizing factor activates Ca^{2+}-activated K^+ channels in porcine coronary artery smooth muscle cells. *J. Cardiovasc. Pharmacol.*, **32**: 642–649.

Hayabuchi, Y., Nakaya, Y., Matsuoka, S., Kuroda, Y. (1998) Hydrogen peroxide-induced vascular relaxation in porcine coronary arteries is mediated by Ca^{2+}-activated K^+ channels. *Heart Vessels*, **13**: 9–17.

He, D.S., Burt, J.M. (2000) Mechanism and selectivity of the effects of halothane on gap junction channel function. *Circ. Res.*, **86**: E104–E109.

He, D.S., Jiang, J.X., Taffet, S.M., Burt, J.M. (1999) Formation of heteromeric gap junction channels by connexins40 and 43 vascular smooth muscle cells. *Proc. Natl. Acad. Sci.*, **96**: 6495–6500.

Hecker, M. (2000) Endothelium-derived hyperpolarizing factor – fact or fiction? *News Physiol. Sci.*, **15**: 1–5.

Hecker, M., Bara, A., Bauersachs, J., Busse, R. (1994) Characterization of endothelium-derived hyperpolarizing factor as a cytochrome P450-derived arachidonic acid metabolite in mammals. *J. Physiol.*, **481**: 407–414.

Heesh, M., Roger, R.C. (1995) Effects of pregnancy and progesterone metabolites on regulation of sympathetic outflow. *Clin. Exper. Pharmacol. Physiol.*, **22**: 136–142.

Heistad, D.D., Faraci, F.M. (1996) Gene therapy for cerebral vascular disease. *Stroke*, **27**: 1688–1693.

Hendrickx, H., Casteels, R. (1974) Electrogenic sodium pump in arterial smooth muscle cells. *Pflügers Arch.*, **346**: 299–306.

Heygate, K.M., Davies, J., Holmes, M., James, R.F.L., Thurston, H. (1996) The effect of insulin treatment and of islet cell transplantation on the resistance artery function in the STZ-induced diabetic rat. *Br. J. Pharmacol.*, **119**: 495–504.

Hille, B., Schwarz, G. (1978) Potassium channels as multi-ion single-file pores. *J. Gener. Physiol.*, **72**: 409–442.

Hillier, C., McGee, A., McGrath, J.C. (1998) Bradykinin-induced vasorelaxation in both diabetic and non-diabetic human resistance arteries does not involve prostacyclin. *J. Vasc. Res.*, **35**: S1:6.

Hillier, C., Sayers, R.D., Watt, P.A.C., Naylor, R., Bell, P.F. (1999) Altered small artery morphology and reactivity in critical ischemia. *Clin. Sci.*, **96**: 155–163.

Hirano, K., Hirano, M., Kanaide, H. (1993) Enhancement by captopril of bradykinin-induced calcium transients in cultured endothelial cells of the bovine aorta. *Eur. J. Pharmacol.*, **244**: 133–137.

Hirst, G.D.S. (1977) Neuromuscular transmission in arterioles of guinea-pig submucosa. *J. Physiol.*, **273**: 263–275.

Hirst, G.D.S., Neild, T.O. (1978) An analysis of excitatory junctional potentials recorded from arterioles. *J. Physiol.*, **280**: 87–104.

Hirst, G.D.S., Neild, T.O. (1980) Some properties of spontaneous excitatory junction potentials recorded from arterioles of guinea-pigs. *J. Physiol.*, **303**: 43–60.

Hoebel, B.G., Kostner, G.M., Graier, W.F. (1997) Activation of microsomal cytochrome P450 mono-oxygenase by Ca^{2+} store depletion and its contribution to Ca^{2+} entry in porcine aortic endothelial cells. *Br. J. Pharmacol.*, **121**: 1579–1588.

Hoebel, B.G., Steyrer, E., Graier, W.F. (1998) Origin and function of epoxyeicosatrienoic acids in vascular endothelial cells: more than just endothelium-derived hyperpolarizing factor? *Clin. Exp. Pharmacol. Physiol.*, **10**: 826–830.

Holland, M., Langton, P.D., Standen, N.B., Boyle, J.P. (1996) Effects of the BK_{Ca} channel activator, NS 1619, on rat cerebral artery smooth muscle. *Br. J. Pharmacol.*, **117**: 119–129.

Holm, I., Mikhailov, A., Jillson, T., Rose, B. (1999) Dynamics of gap junctions observed in living cells with connexin43-GFP chimeric protein. *Eur. J. Cell Biol.*, **78**: 856–866.

Hong, T., Hill, C.E. (1998) Restricted expression of the gap junctional protein connexin43 in the arterial system of the rat. *J. Anatomy*, **193**: 583–593.

Houston, D.S., Vanhoutte, P.M. (1988) Platelets and endothelium-dependent responses. In *Relaxing and contracting factors*, edited by P.M. Vanhoutte, pp. 425–449, New Jersey: Humana Press.

Hu, S., Kim, H.S. (1993) Activation of K^+ channel in vascular smooth muscles by cytochrome P450 metabolites of arachidonic acid. *Eur. J. Pharmacol.*, **230**: 215–221.

Huang, A.H., Busse, R., Bassenge, E. (1988) Endothelium-dependent hyperpolarization of smooth muscle cells in rabbit femoral arteries is not mediated by EDRF (nitric oxide). *Naunyn Schmiedebergs Arch. Pharmacol.*, **338**: 438–442.

Huang, A.H., Sun, D., Smith, C.J., Connetta, J.A., Shesely, E.G., Koller, A., Kaley, G. (2000) In eNOS knockout mice skeletal muscle arteriolar dilation to acetylcholine is mediated by EDHF. *Am. J. Physiol.*, **278**: H762-H768.

Huang, G.Y., Cooper, E.S., Waldo, K., Kirby, M.L., Gilula, N.B., Lo, C.W. (1998) Gap junction-mediated cell–cell communication modulates mouse neural crest migration. *J. Cell Biol.*, **143**: 1725–1734.

Huang, P.L., Huang, Z., Mashimo, H., Bloch, K.D., Moskowitz, M.A., Bevan, J.A., Fishman, M.C. (1995) Hypertension in mice lacking the gene for endothelial nitric oxide synthase. *Nature*, **377**: 239–242.

Hui, J.Y., Taylor, S.L. (1985) Inhibition of *in vivo* histamine metabolism in rats by foodborne and pharmacologic inhibitors of diamine oxidase, histamine *N*-methyltransferase, and monoamine oxidase. *Toxicol. Appl. Pharmacol.*, **81**: 241–249.

Hutcheson, I.R., Chaytor, A.T., Evans, W.H., Griffith, T.M. (1999) Nitric oxide-independent relaxations to acetylcholine and A23187 involve different routes of heterocellular communication. Role of gap junctions and phospholipase A_2. *Circ. Res.*, **84**: 53–63.

Hwa, J.J., Ghibaudi, L., Williams, P., Chaterjee, M. (1994) Comparison of acetylcholine-dependent relaxation in large and small arteries of rat mesenteric vascular bed. *Am. J. Physiol.*, **266**: H952–H958.

Hwan Seul, K., Beyer, E.C. (2000) Heterogeneous localization of connexin40 in the renal vasculature. *Microvasc. Res.*, **59**: 140–148.

Ido, Y., Chang, K., Ostrow, E., Allison, W., Kilo, C., Tilton, R.G. (1990) Aminoguanidine prevents regional blood flow increases in streptozotocin-diabetic rats (abstract). *Diabetes*, **39**: 93A.

Ignarro, L.J. (1989) Biological actions and properties of endothelium-derived nitric oxide formed and released from artery and vein. *Circ. Res.*, **65**: 1–21.

Ignarro, L.J., Buga, G.M., Wood, K.D., Byrns, R.E., Chaudhuri, G. (1987) Endothelium-derived relaxing factor produced and released from artery and vein is nitric oxide. *Proc. Natl. Acad. Sci. USA*, **84**: 9265–9269.

Ikeda, U., Ikeda, M., Kano, S., Kanbe, T., Shimada, K. (1996) Effects of cilostazol, a cAMP phosphodiesterase inhibitor, on nitric oxide production by vascular smooth muscle cells. *Eur. J. Pharmacol.*, **24**: 197–202.

Imaoka, S., Enomoto, K., Oda, Y., Asada, A., Fujimori, M., Shimada, T., Fujita, S., Guengerich, F.P., Funae, Y. (1990) Lidocaine metabolism by human cytochrome P-450s purified from hepatic microsomes: comparison of those with rat hepatic cytochrome P-450s. *J. Pharmacol. Exp. Ther.*, **255**: 1385–1391.

Imaoka, S., Yamada, T., Hiroi, T., Hayashi, K., Sakaki, Y., Yabusaki, Y., Funae, Y. (1996) Multiple forms of human P450 expressed in *Saccharomyces cerevisiae*: Systematic characterization and comparison with those of the rat. *Biochem. Pharmacol.*, **51**: 1041–1050.

Ishibashi, Y., Duncker, D.J., Zhang, J., Bache, R.J. (1998) ATP-sensitive K^+ channels, adenosine, and nitric oxide-mediated mechanisms account for coronary vasodilation during exercise. *Circ. Res.*, **82**: 346–359.

Ishii, T.M., Silvia, C., Hirschberg, B., Bond, C.T., Adelman, J.P., Maylie, J. (1997) A human intermediate conductance calcium-activated potassium channel. *Proc. Natl. Acad. Sci. USA*, **94**: 11651–11656.

Ismail, N., Becker, B., Strzelczyk, P., Ritz, E. (1999) Renal disease and hypertension in non-insulin-dependent diabetes mellitus. *Kidney Int.*, **55**: 1–28.

Jackson, W.F. (2000) Ion channels and vascular tone. *Hypertension*, **35**: 173–178.

Jackson, W.F., König, A., Dambacher, T., Busse, R. (1993) Prostacyclin-induced vasodilation in rabbit heart is mediated by ATP-sensitive potassium channels. *Am. J. Physiol.*, **264**: H238–H243.

Jacobs, R.L., House, J.D., Brosnan, M.E., Brosnan, J.T. (1998) Effects of streptozotocin-induced diabetes and of insulin treatment on homocysteine metabolism in the rat. *Diabetes*, **47**: 1967–1970

Jaggar, J.H., Porter, V.A., Lederer, W.J., Nelson, M.T. (2000) Calcium sparks in smooth muscle. *Am. J. Physiol.*, **278**: C235–C256.

Jang, G.R., Wrighton, S.A., Benet, L.Z. (1996) Identification of CYP3A4 as the principal enzyme catalyzing mifepristone (RU 486) oxidation in human liver microsomes. *Biochem. Pharmacol.*, **52**: 753–761.

Javid, P.J., Watts, S.W., Webb, R.C. (1996) Inhibition of nitric oxide-induced vasodilation by gap junction inhibitors: a potential role for a cGMP-independent nitric oxide pathway. *J. Vasc. Res.*, **33**: 395–404.

Jensen, B.S., Strøbaek, D., Christophersen, P., Dyhring Jørgensen, T.D., Hansen, C., Silahtaroglu, A., Olesen, S.-P., Ahring, P.K. (1998) Characterization of the cloned human intermediate-conductance Ca^{2+}-activated K^+ channel. *Am. J. Physiol.*, **275**: C848–C856.

Joannides, R., Haefeli, W.E., Linder, L., Richard, V., Bakkali, E.H., Thuillez, C., Lüscher, T.F. (1995) Nitric oxide is responsible for flow-dependent dilation of human peripheral conduit arteries *in vivo*. *Circulation*, **91**: 1314–1319.

Jones, C.J.H., Kuo, L., Davis, M.J., DeFily, D.V., Chilian, W.M. (1995) Role of nitric oxide in the coronary microvascular responses to adenosine and increased metabolic demand. *Circulation*, **91**: 1807–1813.

Jongsma, H.J., van Rijen, H.V.M., Twak, B.K., Chanson, M. (2000) Phosphorylation of connexins: Consequences of permeability, conductance and kinetics of gap junction channels. In *Gap Junctions*, edited by C. Perracchia., vol. 49, pp. 131–142. Current Topics in Membranes.

Jordan, K., Solan, J.L., Dominguez, M., Sia, M., Hand, A., Lampe, P.D., Laird, D.W. (1999) Trafficking, assembly, and function of a connexin43-green fluorescent protein chimera in live mammalian cells. *Mol. Biol. Cell*, **10**: 2033–2050.

Juncos, L.A., Ito, S., Carretero, O.A., Garvin, J.L. (1994) Removal of endothelium-dependent relaxation by antibody and complement in afferent arterioles. *Hypertension*, **23**: 154–159.

Juneja, S.C., Barr, K.J., Enders, G.C., Kidder, G.M. (1999) Defects in the germ line and gonads of mice lacking connexin43. *Biol. Reprod.*, **60**: 1263–1270.

Kaapa, P., Raj, J.U., Ibe, B.O., Anderson J. (1991) Vasoconstrictor response to prostacyclin in rabbit pulmonary circulation. *Respir. Physiol.*, **85**: 193–204.

Kaczorowski, G.J., Garcia, M. (1999) Pharmacology of voltage-gated and calcium-activated potassium channels. *Curr. Opin. Chem. Biol.*, **3**: 448–458.

Kaczorowski, G.J., Knaus, H.G., Leonard, D.R.J., McManus, O.B., Garcia, M.L. (1996) High-conductance calcium-activated potassium channels; structure, pharmacology, and function. *J. Bioenerg. Biomembr.*, **28**: 255–267.

Kadowitz, P.J., Chapnick, B.M., Feigen, L.P., Hyman, A.L., Nelson, P.K., Spannhake, E.W. (1978) Pulmonary and systemic vasodilator effects of the newly discovered prostaglandin PGI_2. *J. Applied Physiol.*, **45**: 408–413.

Kagota, S., Yamaguchi, Y., Nakamura, K. Kunitomo, M. (1999) Characterization of nitric oxide- and prostaglandin-independent relaxation in response to acetylcholine in rabbit renal artery. *Clin. Exp. Pharmacol. Physiol.*, **26**: 790–796.

Kähönen, M., Mäkynen, H., Wu, X., Arvola, P., Pörsti, I. (1995) Endothelial function in spontaneously hypertensive rats: Influence of quinapril treatment. *Br. J. Pharmacol.*, **115**: 859–867.

Kalsner, S. (1985) Coronary artery reactivity in human vessels: some questions and some answers. *Federation Proc.*, **44**: 321–325.

Kamata, K., Miyata, N., Kasuya, Y. (1989) Impairment of endothelium-dependent relaxation and changes in levels of cyclic GMP in aorta from streptozotocin-induced diabetic rats. *Br. J. Pharmacol.*, **97**: 614–618.

Kanamaru, K., Waga, S., Fujimoto, K., Itoh, H., Kubo, Y. (1989) Endothelium-dependent relaxation of human basilar arteries. *Stroke*, **20**: 1208–1211.

Kanamaru, K., Waga, S., Kojima, T., Fujimoto, K., Itoh, H. (1987) Endothelium-dependent relaxation of canine basilar arteries. Part 1: Difference between acetylcholine- and A23187-induced relaxation and involvement of lipoxygenase metabolite(s). *Stroke*, **18**: 932–937.

Kato, K., Evans, A.M., Kozlowski, R.Z. (1999) Relaxation of endothelin-1-induced pulmonary arterial constriction by niflumic acid and NPPB: mechanism(s) independent of chloride channel block. *J. Pharmacol. Exp. Ther.*, **288**: 1242–1250.

Kauser, K., Stekiel, W.J., Rubanyi, G., Harder, D.R. (1989) Mechanism of action of EDRF on pressurized arteries: effect on K^+ conductance. *Circ. Res.*, **65**: 199–204.

Kaw, S., Hecker, M. (1999) Endothelium-derived hyperpolarising factor, but not nitric oxide or prostacyclin release, is resistant to menadione-induced oxidative stress in the bovine coronary artery. *Naunyn-Schmiedeberg's Arch. Pharmacol.*, **359**: 133–139.

Keegan, A., Walbank, H., Cotter, M.A., Cameron, N.E. (1995) Chronic vitamin E treatment prevents defective endothelium-dependent relaxation in diabetic rat aorta. *Diabetologia*, **38**: 1475–1478.

Kemp, B.K., Cocks, T.M. (1997) Evidence that mechanisms dependent and independent of nitric oxide mediate endothelium-dependent relaxation to bradykinin in human small resistance-like coronary arteries. *Br. J. Pharmacol.*, **120**: 757–762.

Kemp, B.K., Smolich, J.J., Ritchie, B.C., Cocks, T.M. (1995) Endothelium-dependent relaxations in sheep pulmonary arteries and veins: resistance to block by N^G-nitro-L-arginine in pulmonary hypertension. *Br. J. Pharmacol.*, **116**: 2457–2467.

Kempermann, G., Knoth, R., Gebicke-Haerter, P.J., Stolz, B.-J., Volk, B. (1994) Cytochrome P450 in rat astrocytes *in vivo* and *in vitro*: Intracellular localization and induction by phenytoin. *J. Neuroscience Res.*, **39**: 576–588.

Kerr, S., Brosnan, M.J., McIntyre, M., Reid, J.L., Dominiczak, A.F., Hamilton, C.A. (1999) Superoxide anion production is increased in a model of genetic hypertension: the role of endothelium. *Hypertension*, **33**: 1353–1358.

Kessler, P., Popp, R., Busse, R., Schini-Kerth, V.B. (1999) Proinflammatory mediators chronically downregulate the formation of the endothelium-derived hyperpolarizing factor in arteries via a nitric oxide/cyclic GMP dependent mechanism. *Circulation*, **99**: 1878–1884.

Kihara, M., Schmelzer, J.D., Poduslo, J.F., Curran, G.L., Nickander, K.K., Low, P.A. (1991) Aminoguanidine effects on nerve blood flow, vascular permeability, electrophysiology, and oxygen free radicals. *Proc. Natl. Acad. Sci. USA*, **88**: 6107–6111.

Kilpatrick, E.V., Cocks, T.M. (1994) Evidence for differential roles of nitric oxide (NO) and hyperpolarisation in endothelium-dependent relaxation of pig isolated coronary artery. *Br. J. Pharmacol.*, **112**: 557–565.

Kirchhoff, S., Kim, J.-S., Hagendorff, A., Thönissen, E., Krueger, O., Lamers, W.H., Willecke, K. (2000) Abnormal cardiac conduction and morphogenesis in connexin40 and connexin43 double-deficient mice. *Circ. Res.*, **87**: 399–405.

Kirchhoff, S., Nelles, E., Hagendorff, A., Krüger, O., Traub, O., Willecke, K. (1998) Reduced cardiac conduction velocity and predisposition to arrhythmias in connexin40-deficient mice. *Current Biology*, **8**: 299–302.

Klein-Hitpass, L., Schorpp, M., Wagner, U., Ryffel, G.U. (1986) An estrogen-responsive element derived from the 5′ flanking region of the Xenopus vitellogenin A2 gene functions in transfected human cells. *Cell*, **46**: 1053–1061.

Knot, H.J., Zimmermann, P.A., Nelson, M.T. (1996) Extracellular K^+-induced hyperpolarizations and dilatations of rat coronary and cerebral arteries involve inward rectifier K^+ channels. *J. Physiol.*, **492**: 419–430.

Koh, K.K., Mincemoyer, R., Bui, M.N., Csako, G., Pucino, F., Guetta, V., Waclawiw, M., Cannon, R.O.III. (1997) Effects of hormone-replacement therapy on fibrinolysis in postmenopausal women. *New Engl. J. Med.*, **336**: 683–690.

Koller, A., Messina, E.J., Wolin, M.S., Kaley, G. (1989) Endothelial impairment inhibits prostaglandin and EDRF-mediated arteriolar dilation *in vivo*. *Am. J. Physiol.*, **257**: H1966–H1970.

Kolodny, G.M. (1971) Evidence for transfer of macromolecular RNA between mammalian cells in culture. *Exp. Cell Res.*, **65**: 113.

Komori, K, Lorenz, R.R., Vanhoutte, P.M. (1988) Nitric oxide, ACh, and electrical and mechanical properties of canine arterial smooth muscle. *Am. J. Physiol.*, **255**: H207–H212.

Komori, K., Vanhoutte, P.M. (1990) Endothelium-Derived Hyperpolarizing Factor. *Blood Vessels*, **27**: 238–245.

Komori, M.A. (1993) A novel P450 expressed at high level in rat brain. *Biochem. Biophys. Res. Commun.*, **196**: 721–728.

Kronbach, T., Larabee, T.M., Johnson, E.F. (1989) Hybrid cytochromes P450 identify a substrate binding domain in P-450 IIC5 and P-450 IIC4. *Proc. Natl. Acad. Sci. USA*, **86**: 8262–8265.

Krueger, O., Plum, A., Kim, J.-S., Winterhager, E., Maxeiner, S., Hallas, G., Kirchhoff, S., Traub, O., Lamers, W.H., Willecke, K. (2000) Defective vascular development in connexin45-deficient mice. *Development*, **127**: 4179–4193.

Kublickiene, K.-R., Kubliukas, M., Lindblom, B., Lunell, N.-O., Nisell, H.A (1997) Comparison of myogenic and endothelial properties of myometrial and omental resistance vessels in late pregnancy. *Am. J. Obstet. Gynecol.*, **176**: 560–566.

Kuga, T., Egashira, K., Mohri, M., Tsutsui, H., Harasawa, Y., Urabe, Y., Ando, S., Shimokawa, H., Takeshita, A. (1995) Bradykinin-induced vasodilatation is impaired at the atherosclerotic site but is preserved at the spastic site of human coronary arteries *in vivo*. *Circulation*, **92**: 183–189.

Kühberger, E., Groschner, K., Kukovetz, W.R., Brunner, F. (1994) The role of myoendothelial cell contact in non-nitric oxide-, non-prostanoid-mediated endothelium-dependent relaxation of porcine coronary artery. *Br. J. Pharmacol.*, **113**: 1289–1294.

Kumai, M., Nishii, K., Nakamura, K., Takeda, N., Suzuki, M., Shibata, Y. (2000) Loss of connexin45 causes a cushion defect in early cardiogenesis. *Development*, **127**: 3501–3512.

Kumar, N.M., Gilula, N.B. (1996) The gap junction communication channel. *Cell*, **84**: 381–388.

Kumari, K., Umar, S., Bansal, V., Sahib, M.K. (1991) Monoaminoguanididne inhibits aldose reductase. *Biochem. Pharmacol.*, **4**: 1527–1528.

Kuo, L., Chilian, W.M., Davis, M.J. (1991) Interaction of pressure- and flow-induced responses in porcine coronary resistance vessels. *Am. J. Physiol.*, **261**: H1706–H1715.

Kuriyama, H., Kitamura, K., Nabata, H. (1995) Pharmacological and physiological significance of ion channels and factors that modulate then in vascular tissues. *Pharmacol. Rev.*, **47**: 387–573.

Kuroiwa, M., Aoki, H., Kobayashi, S., Nishimura, J., Kanaide, H. (1995) Mechanism of endothelium-dependent relaxation induced by substance P in the coronary artery of the pig. *Br. J. Pharmacol.*, **116**: 2040–2047.

Kwak, B.R., Hermans, M.M., Dejonge, H.R., Lohmann, S.M., Jongsma, H.J., Chanson, M. (1995) Differential regulation of distinct types of gap junction channels by similar phosphorylating conditions. *Mol. Biol. Cell*, **6**: 1707–1719.

Kwak, B.R., Jongsma, H.J. (1996) Regulation of cardiac gap junction channel permeability and conductance by several phosphorylating conditions. *Mol. & Cellular Biochem.*, **157**: 93–99.

Kwak, B.R., Saez, J.C., Wilders, R., Chanson, M., Fishman, G.I., Hertzberg, E.L., Spray, D.C., Jongsma, H.J. (1995) Effects of CGMP dependent phosphorylation of rat and human connexin43 gap junction channels. *Pflügers Arch. Eur. J. Physiol.*, **430**: 770–778.

Kwak, B.R., Vanveen, T.A., Analbers, L.J., Jongsma, H.J. (1995) TPA increases conductance but decreases permeability in neonatal rat cardiomyocyte gap junction channels. *Exp. Cell Res.*, **220**: 456–463.

Lacy, P.S., Pilkington, G., Hanvesakul, R., Fish, H.J., Boyle, J.P., Thurston, H. (2000) Evidence against potassium as an endothelium-derived hyperpolarizing factor in rat mesenteric small arteries. *Br. J. Pharmacol.*, **129**: 605–611.

Laing, J.G., Beyer, E.C. (1995) The gap junction protein connexin43 is degraded via ubiquitin proteasome pathway. *J. Biol. Chem.*, **270**: 26399–26403.

Laing, J.G., Beyer, E.C. (2000) Degradation of gap junctions and connexins. *Cur. Top. Memb.*, **49**: 23–41.

Laing, J.G., Tadros, P.N., Westphale, E.M., Beyer, E.C. (1997) Degradation of connexin43 gap junctions involves both the proteasome and the lysosome. *Exp. Cell Res.*, **236**: 482–492.

Laird, D. (1996) The life cycte of a connexin, Gap Junction formation, removal and degradation. *J. Bioener. and Biomembr.*, **28**: 311–317.

Lamontage, D., Pohl, U., Busse, R. (1991) N^G-Nitro-L-arginine antagonizes endothelium-depentent dilator responses by inhibiting endothelium-derived relaxing factor release in the isolated rabbit heart. *Pflügers Arch.*, **418**: 255–270.

Lange, A., Gebremedhin, D., Narayanan, J., Harder, D.R. (1997) 20-Hydroxyeicosatetraenoic acid-induced vasoconstriction and inhibition of potassium current in cerebral vascular smooth muscle is dependent on activation of protein kinase C. *J. Biol. Chem.*, **272**: 27345–27352.

Langer, B., Barthelemebs, M., Grima, M., Coquard, C., Imbs, J.-L. (1993) *In vitro* vascular reactivity of rat utero-feto-placental unit. *Obstet. Gynecol.*, **82**: 380–386.

Larson, D.M., Laing, J.G., Seul, K.H., Beyer, E.C. (1997) Synthesis, assembly, and degradation of human connexin37-FLAG in BWEM and NRK cells. *Molecular Biology of the Cell*, **8**: 418a.

Laskey, R.E., Adams, D.J., Johns, A., Rubanyi, G.M., Van Breemen, C. (1990) Membrane potential and Na^+-K^+ pump activity modulate resting and bradykinin-stimulated changes in cytosolic free calcium in cultured endothelial cells from bovine atria. *J. Biol. Chem.*, **265**: 2613–2619.

Latorre, R., Oberhauser, A., Labarca, P., Alvarez, O. (1989) Varieties of calcium-activated potassium channels. *Ann. Rev. Physiol.*, **51**: 385–399.

Lau, A.F., Warn-Cramer, B., Lin, R. (2000) Regulation of connexin43 tyrosine protein kinases. In *Gap Junctions – Current Topics in Membranes*, edited by C. Perracchia., vol. 49, pp. 131–142.

Lawson, T.A. (1991) Involvement of lauric acid hydroxylase in the activation of β-substituted nitrosamines. *Cancer Lett.*, **59**: 177–182.

Lazrak, A., Peracchia, C. (1993) Gap junction gating sensitivity to physiological internal calcium regardless of pH in Novikoff hepatoma-cells. *Biophs. J.*, **65**: 2002–2012.

Leffler, C.W., Fedinec, A.L. (1997) Newborn piglet cerebral microvascular responses to epoxyeicosatrienoic acids. *Am. J. Physiol.*, **273**: H333–H338.

Lew, A.S., Laramee, P., Cerek, B., Rodriguez, L., Shah, P.K., Ganz, W. (1985) The effects of the rate of intravenous infusion of streptokinase and the duration of symptoms on the time interval to reperfusion in patients with acute myocardial infarction. *Circulation*, **72**: 1053–1058.

Li, P.L., Campbell, W.B. (1997) Epoxyeicosatrienoic acids activate K^+ channels in coronary smooth muscle through a guanine nucleotide binding protein. *Circ. Res.*, **80**: 877–884.

Li, P.L., Zou, A.P., Campbell, W.B. (1997) Regulation of potassium channels in coronary arterial smooth muscle by endothelium-derived vasodilators. *Hypertension*, **29**: 262–267.

Li, X., Simard, J.M. (1999) Multiple connexins form gap junction channels in rat basilar artery smooth muscle cells. *Circ. Res.*, **84**: 1277–1284.

Lijnen, H.R., Collen, D. (1995) Mechanisms of physiological fibrinolysis. *Bailieres Clin. Haematol.*, **8**: 277–282.

Lijnen, H.R., Collen, D. (1997) Endothelium in hemostasis and thrombosis. *Prog. Cardiovasc. Dis.*, **39**: 343–350.

Lin, J.H.C., Kobari,Y., Zhu,Y., Stemerman, M.B., Pritchard, K.A., Jr. (1996) Human umbilical vein endothelial cells express P450 2C8 mRNA: cloning of endothelial P450 epoxygenase. *Endothelium*, **4**: 219–229.

Linder, L., Kiowski, W., Bühler, F.R., Lüscher, T.F. (1990) Indirect evidence for the release of endothelium-derived relaxing factor in the human forearm circulation *in vivo*: Blunted response in essential hypertension. *Circulation*, **81**: 1762–1767.

Lischke, V., Busse, R., Hecker M. (1995) Selective inhibition by barbiturates of the synthesis of endothelium-derived hyperpolarizing factor in the rabbit carotid artery. *Br. J. Pharmacol.*, **115**: 969–974.

Little, T.L., Beyer, E.C., Duling, B.R. (1995a) Connexin43 and connexin40 gap junctional proteins are present in arteriolar smooth muscle and endothelium *in vivo*. *Am. J. Physiol.*, **268**: H729–H739.

Little, T.L., Xia, J., Duling, B.R. (1995b) Dye tracers define differential endothelial and smooth muscle coupling patterns within the arteriolar wall. *Circ. Res.*, **76**: 498–504.

Longa, E.Z., Weinstein, P.R., Carlson, S., Cummins, R. (1989) Reversible middle cerebral artery occlusion without craniectomy in rats. *Stroke*, **20**: 84–91.

Losonczy, G., Mucha, I., Muller, V., Kriston, T., Ungvari, Z., Tornoci, L., Rosivall, L., Venuto, R. (1996) The vasoconstrictor effect of L-NAME, a nitric oxide synthase inhibitor, in pregnant rabbits. *Br. J. Pharmacol.*, **118**: 1012–1018.

Lowry, O.H., Rosebrough, N.J., Farr, A.L., Randall, R.J. (1951) Protein measurement with the folin phenol reagent. *J. Biol. Chem.*, **193**: 265–275.

Lu, C., McMahon, D.G. (1997) Modulation of hybrid bass retinal gap junctional channel gating by nitric oxide. *J. Physiol.*, **499**: 689–699.

Lüscher, T.F., Vanhoutte, P.M. (1986) Endothelium-dependent contractions to acetylcholine in the aorta of the spontaneously hypertensive rat. *Hypertension*, **8**: 344–348.

Lüscher, T.F., Vanhoutte, P.M. (1990) The endothelium: modulator of cardiovascular function. pp. 1–228, Boca Raton, Fla, CRC Press, Inc.

Maier, K.G., Henderson, L., Narayanan, J., Alonso-Galicia, M., Falck, J.R., Roman, R.J. (2000) Fluorescent HPLC assay for 20-HETE and other P450 metabolites of arachidonic acid. *Am. J. Physiol.*, **279**: H863–H871.

Maier, K.G., Henderson, L., Narayanan, J., Falck, J.R., Harder, D.R., Roman, R.J. (2000) A rapid, sensitive fluorescent HPLC assay for HETES and EETS. *FASEB J.*, **14**: A140.

Makino, A., Ohuchi, K., Kamata, K. (2000) Mechanisms underlying the attenuation of endothelium-dependent vasodilatation in the mesenteric arterial bed of the streptozotocin-induced diabetic rat. *Br. J. Pharmacol.*, **130**: 549–556.

Malmsjö, M., Berghahl, A., Zhao, X.-H., Sun, X.-Y., Hedner, T., Edvinsson, L., Erlinge, D. (1999) Enhanced acetylcholine and P2Y-receptor stimulated vascular EDHF-dilatation in congestive heart failure. *Cardiovasc. Res.*, **43**: 200–209.

Manasse, E., Sperti, G., Suma, H., Canosa, C., Kol, A., Martinelli, L., Schiavello, R., Crea, F., Maseri, A., Possati, G.F. (1996) Use of the radial artery for myocardial revascularization. *Ann. Thorac. Surg.*, **62**: 1076–1083.

Manivannan, K., Ramanan, S.V., Mathias, R.T., Brink, P.R. (1992) Multichannel recordings from membranes which contain gap junctions. *Biophys. J.*, **61**: 216–227.

Manthey, D., Bukauskas, F., Lee, C.G., Kozak, C.A., Willecke, K. (1999) Molecular clones and functional expression of the mouse gap junction gene connexin57 in human HeLa cells. *J. Biol. Chem.*, **274**: 14716–14723.

Marchenko, S.M., Sage, S.O. (1994a) Mechanism of acetylcholine action on membrane potential of endothelium of intact rat aorta. *Am. J. Physiol.*, **266**: H2388–H2395.

Marchenko, S.M., Sage, S.O. (1994b) Smooth muscle cells affect endothelial membrane potential in rat aorta. *Am. J. Physiol.*, **267**: H804–H811.

Marchenko, S.M., Sage, S.O. (1996) Calcium-activated potassium channels in the endothelium of intact rat aorta. *J. Physiol.*, **492**: 53–60.

Marre, F., Fabre, G., Lacarelle, B., Bourrie, M., Catalin, J., Berger, Y., Rahmani, R., Cano, J.P. (1992) Involvement of the cytochrome P-450 IID subfamily in minaprine 4-hydroxylation by human hepatic microsomes. *Drug Metab. Dispos.*, **20**: 316–321.

Marrelli, S.P., Khorovets, A., Johnson, T.D., Childres, W.F., Bryan, R.M., Jr. (1999) P2 purinoceptor-mediated dilations in the rat middle cerebral artery after ischemia/reperfusion. *Am. J. Physiol.*, **276**: H33–H41.

Martens, J.R., Gelband, C.H. (1998) Ion channels in vascular smooth muscle: Alterations in essential hypertension. *Proc. Soc. for Exper. Bio. & Med.*, **218**: 192–203.

Martin, P.E.M., Steggles, J., Wilson, C., Ahmad, S., Evans, W.H. (2000) Targeting motifs and functional parameters governing the assembly of connexins into gap junctions. *Biochem. J.*, **349**: 281–287.

Masferrer, J., Mullane, K.M. (1988) Modulation of vascular tone by 12(R)-, but not 12(S)-, hydroxyeicosatetraenoic acid. *Eur. J. Pharmacol.*, **151**: 487–490.

Matesic, D.F., Rupp, H.L., Bonney, W.J., Ruch, R.J., Trosko, J.E. (1994) Changes in gap-junction permeability, phosphorylation, and number mediated by phorbol ester and non-phorbol-ester tumor promoters in rat liver epithelial cells. *Molecular Carcinogenesis*, **10**: 226–236.

Matoba, T., Shimokawa, H., Nakashima, M., Hirakawa, Y., Mukai, Y., Hirano, K., Kanaide, H., Takeshita, A. (2000) Hydrogen peroxide is an endothelium-derived hyperpolarizing factor in mice. *J. Clin. Invest.*, **106**: 1521–1530.

Matsubara, H. (1998) Pathophysiological role of angiotensin II type 2 receptor in cardiovascular and renal diseases. *Circ. Res.*, **83**: 1182–1191.

Matsumoto, T., Kanamaru, K., Sugiyama, Y., Murata, Y. (1992) Endothelium-derived relaxation of the pregnant and nonpregnant canine uterine artery. *J. Reprod. Med.*, **37**: 529–533.

Maurer, P., Weingart, R. (1987) Cell pairs isolated from adult guinea pig and rat hearts: effects of (Ca^{2+})i on nexal membrane resistance. *Pflüg. Arch. – Eur. J. Physiol.*, **409**: 394–402.

Maurice, M., Pichard, L., Daujat, M., Fabre, I., Joyeux, H., Domergue, J., Maurel, P. (1992) Effects of imidazole derivatives on cytochromes P450 from human hepatocytes in primary culture. *FASEB J.*, **6**: 752–758.

McCarron, J.G., Halpern, W. (1990) Potassium dilates rat cerebral arteries by two independent mechanisms. *Am. J. Physiol.*, **259**: H902–H908.

McCulloch, A.I., Bottrill, F.E., Randall, M.D., Hiley, C.R. (1997) Characterization and modulation of EDHF-mediated relaxations in the rat isolated superior mesenteric artery. *Br. J. Pharmacol.*, **20**: 1431–1438.

McEwan, A.J., Ledingham, J.M. (1971) Blood flow characteristics and tissue nutrition in apparently ischemic feet. *Br. Med. J.*, **24**: 220–224.

McGiff, J.C., Steinberg, M., Quilley, J. (1996) Missing links: cytochrome P450 arachidonate products – a new class of lipid mediators. *Trends Cardiovasc. Med.*, **6**: 4–10.

McIntyre, M., Bohr, D.F., Dominiczak, A.F. (1999) Endothelial function in hypertension: the role of superoxide anion. *Hypertension*, **34**: 539–545.

McKelvie, R.S., Yusuf, S., Pericak, D., Avezum, A., Burns, R.J., Probstfield, J., Tsuyuki, R.T., White, M., Rouleau, J., Latini, R., Maggioni, A., Young, J., Pogue, J. (1999) Comparison of candesartan, enalapril, and their combination in congestive heart failure: Randomized Evaluation of Strategies for Left Ventricular Dysfunction (RESOLVED) Pilot Study. *Circulation*, **100**: 1056–1064.

McLean, I.W., Nakane, P.K. (1974) Periodate-lysine-paraformaldehyde fixative. A new fixation for immunoelectron microscopy. *J. Histochem. Cytochem.*, **22**: 1077–1083.

McNally, P.G., Watt, P., Rimmer, T., Burden, A.C., Hearnshaw, J.R., Thurston, H. (1994) Impaired contraction and endothelium-dependent relaxation in isolated resistance vessels from patients with insulin-dependent diabetes mellitus. *Clin. Sci.*, **87**: 31–36.

Medhora, M., Harder, D.R. (1998) Functional role of epoxyeicosatrienoic acids and their production in astrocytes: Approaches for gene transfer and therapy. *Int. J. Mol. Med.*, **2**: 661–669.

Menendez, J.C., Casanova, D., Amado, J.A., Salas, E., Garsia-Unzueta, M.T., Fernandez, F., Perez de la Lastra, M., Berrazueta, J.R. (1998) Effects of radiation on endothelial function. *Int. J. Radiation Oncology Biol. Phys.*, **41**: 905–913.

Meng, W., Ayata, C., Waeber, C., Huang, P.L., Moskowitz, M.A. (1998) Neuronal NOS-cGMP-dependent ACh-induced relaxation in pial arterioles of endothelial NOS knockout mice. *Am. J. Physiol.*, **274**: H411–H415.

Meng, W., Ma, J., Ayata, C., Hara, H., Huang, P.L., Fishman, M.C., Moskowitz, M.A. (1996) ACh dilates pial arterioles in endothelial and neuronal NOS knockout mice by NO-dependent mechanisms. *Am. J. Physiol.*, **271**: H1145–H1150.

Meyer, M.C., Brayden, J.E., Maclaughlin, M.K. (1993) Characteristics of vascular smooth muscle in the maternal resistance circulation during pregnancy in the rat. *Am. J. Obstet. Gynecol.*, **169**: 1510–1516.

Mian, K.B., Martin, W. (1997) Hydrogen peroxide-induced impairment of reactivity in rat isolated aorta: potentiation by 3-amino-1,2,4-triazole. *Br. J. Pharmacol.*, **121**: 813–819.

Minamiyama, Y., Tamemura, S., Akiyama, T., Imaoka, S., Inoue, M., Funae, Y., Okada S. (1999) Isoforms of cytochrome P450 on organic nitrate-derived nitric oxide release in human vessels. *FEBS Lett.*, **452**: 165–169.

Miura, H., Gutterman, D.D. (1998) Human coronary arteriolar dilation to arachidonic acid depends on cytochrome P450 monooxygenase and Ca^{2+}-activated K^+ channels. *Cir. Res.*, **83**: 501–507.

Miura, H., Liu, Y., Gutterman, D.D. (1999) Human coronary arteriolar dilation to bradykinin depends on membrane hyperpolarization: contribution of nitric oxide and Ca^{2+}-activated K^+ channels. *Circulation*, **99**: 3132–3138.

Mombouli, J.-V., Bissiriou, I., Agboton, V.D., Vanhoutte, P.M. (1996) Bioassay of endothelium-derived hyperpolarizing factor. *Biochem. and Biophys. Res. Comm.*, **221**: 484–488.

Mombouli, J.-V., Holzmann, S., Kostner, G.M., Graier, W.F. (1999) Potentiation of Ca^{2+} signaling in endothelial cells by 11,12-epoxyeicosatrienoic acid. *J. Cardiovasc. Pharmacol.*, **33**: 779–784.

Mombouli, J.-V., Illiano, S., Nagao, T., Scott-Burden, T., Vanhoutte, P.M. (1992) Potentiation of endothelium-dependent relaxations to bradykinin by angiotensin I converting enzyme inhibitors in canine coronary artery involves both endothelium-derived relaxing and hyperpolarizing factors. *Circ. Res.*, **71**: 137–144.

Mombouli, J.-V., Vanhoutte, P.M. (1997) Endothelium-derived hyperpolarizing factor(s): updating the unknown. *Trends Pharmacol. Sci.*, **18**: 252–256.

Moncada, S., Gryglewski, R.J., Bunting, S., Vane, J.R. (1976) An enzyme isolated from arteries transforms prostaglandin endoperoxides to an unstable substance that inhibits platelet aggregation. *Nature*, **263**: 663–665.

Moncada, S., Herman, A.G., Higgs, E.A., Vane, J.R. (1977) Differential formation of prostacyclin (PGX or PGI2) by layers of the arterial wall. An explanation for the anti-thrombotic properties of vascular endothelium. *Thromb. Res.*, **11**: 323–344.

Moncada, S., Palmer, R.J.M., Higgs, E.A. (1991) Nitric oxide: Physiology, Pathophysiology, and Pharmacology. *Pharmacol. Rev.*, **43**: 109–142.

Moncada, S., Rees, D.D., Schultz, R., Palmer, R.M.J. (1991) Development and mechanism of a specific supersensitivity to nitrovasodilators after inhibition of vascular nitric oxide synthase. *Proc. Natl. Acad. Sci. USA*, **88**: 2166–2170.

Moncada, S., Vane, J.R. (1979) Pharmacology and endogenous role of prostaglandins, endoperoxides, thromboxane A_2 and prostacyclin. *Pharmacol. Rev.*, **30**: 293–331.

Monnier, V.M., Vishwanatah, V., Frank, E., Elmets, C.A., Dauchot, P., Kohn, R.R. (1986) Relation between complications of type 1 diabetes mellitus and collagen linked fluorescence. *New Engl. J. Med.*, **314**: 403–408.

Montoliu, C., Sancho-Tello, M., Azorin, I., Burgal, M., Valles, S., Renau-Piqueras, J., Guerri, C. (1995) Ethanol increases cytochrome P450 2E1 and induces oxidative stress in astrocytes. *J. Neurochem.*, **65**: 2561–2570.

Moore, L.K., Beyer, E.C., Burt, J.M. (1991) Characterization of gap junction channels in A7R5 vascular smooth-muscle cells. *Am. J. Physiol.*, **260**: C975–C981.

Morais, S.M., Schweikl, H., Blaisdell, J., Goldstein, J.A. (1993) Gene structure and upstream regulatory regions of human CYP2C9 and CYP2C18. *Biochem. Biophys. Res. Commun.*, **194**: 194–201.

Moreno, A.P., Campos de Carvalho, A.C., Christ, G., Melman, A., Spray, D.C. (1993) Gap junctions between human corpus cavernosum smooth muscle cells: gating properties and unitary conductance. *Am. J. Physiol.*, **263**: C80–C92.

Moreno, A.P., Saez, J.C., Fishman, G.I., Spray, D.C. (1994) Human Cx43 gap junction channels Regulation of unitary conductance by phosphorylation. *Circ. Res.*, **74**: 1051–1057.

Morley, G.E., Vaidya, D., Samie, F.H., Lo, C., Delmar, M., Jalife, J. (1999) Characterization of conduction in the ventricles of normal and heterozygous Cx43 knockout mice using optical mapping. *J. Cardiovasc. Electrophysiol.*, **10**: 1361–1375.

Mosselman, S., Polman, J., Dijkema, R. (1996) ER BETA: identification and characterization of a novel human estrogen receptor. *FEBS Lett.*, **392**: 49–53.

Mügge, A., Brandes, R.P., Böger, R.H., Dwenger, A., Bode-Böger, S., Kienke, S., Frölich, J.C., Lichtlen, P.R. (1994) Vascular release of superoxide radicals is enhanced in hypercholesterolemic rabbits. *J. Cardiovasc. Pharmacol.*, **24**: 994–998.

Mügge, A., Lopez, J.A.G., Piegors, D.J., Breese, K.R., Heistad, D.D. (1991) Acetylcholine-induced vasodilatation in rabbit hindlimb *in vivo* is not inhibited by analogues of L-arginine. *Am. J. Physiol.*, **260**: H242–H247.

Muhonen, M.G., Ooboshi, H., Welsh, M.J., Davidson, B.L., Heistad, D.L. (1997) Gene transfer to cerebral blood vessels after subarachnoid hemorrhage. *Stroke*, **28**: 822–829.

Mulvany, M.J., Halpern, W. (1977) Contractile properties of small arterial resistance vessels in spontaneously hypertensive and normotensive rats. *Circ. Res.*, **41**: 19–26.

Munoz, J.-L., Deyhimi, F., Coles, J.A. (1983) Silanization of glass in making of ion-sensitive microelectrodes. *J. Neurosc. Methods*, **8**: 231–247.

Münzel, T., Harrison, D.G. (1999) Increased superoxide in heart failure: a biochemical baroreflex Gone Awry. *Circulation*, **100**: 216–218.

Munzenmaier, D.H., Harder D.R. (2000) Cerebral microvascular endothelial cell tube formation: role of astrocytic epoxyeicosatrienoic acid release. *Am. J. Physiol.*, **278**: H1163–H1167.

Murai, T., Muraki, K., Imaizumi, Y., Watanabe, M. (1999) Levcromakalim causes indirect endothelial hyperpolarization via a myoendothelial pathway. *Br. J. Pharmacol.*, **128**: 1491–1496.

Muraki, K., Imaizumi, Y., Ohya, S., Sato, K., Takii, T., Onozaki, K., Watanabe, M. (1997) Apamin-sensitive Ca^{2+}-dependent K^+ current and hyperpolarization in human endothelial cells. *Biochem. Biophys. Res. Commun.*, **236**: 340–353.

Murphy, M.E., Brayden, J.E. (1995) Nitric oxide hyperpolarization of rabbit mesenteric arteries via ATP-sensitive potassium channels. *J. Physiol. (London)* **86**: 47–58.

Murphy, M.E., Brayden, J.E. (1995) Apamin-sensitive K^+ channels mediate an endothelium-dependent hyperpolarization in rabbit mesenteric arteries. *J. Physiol.*, **489**: 723–734.

Musil, L., Goodenough, D.A. (1993) Multisubunit assembly of an internal membrane protein, gap junction Cx43, occurs after exit from the ER. *Cell*, **74**: 1065–1077.

Nagao, T., Illiano, S., Vanhoutte, P.M. (1992) Calmodulin antagonists inhibit endothelium-dependent hyperpolarization in the canine coronary artery. *Br. J. Pharmacol.*, **107**: 382–386.

Nagao, T., Illiano, S., Vanhoutte, P.M. (1992) Heterogeneous distribution of endothelium-dependent relaxations resistant to N^G-nitro-L-arginine in rats. *Am. J. Physiol.*, **263**: H1090–1094.

Nagao, T., Vanhoutte, P.M. (1991) Hyperpolariation contributes to endothelium-dependent relaxations to acetylcholine in femoral veins of rats. *Am. J. Physiol.*, **261**: H1034–H1037.

Nagao, T., Vanhoutte, P.M. (1992) Hyperpolarization as a mechanism for endothelium-dependent relaxations in the porcine coronary artery. *J. Physiol.*, **445**: 355–367.

Nagao, T., Vanhoutte, P.M. (1993) Endothelium-derived hyperpolarizing factor and endothelium-dependent relaxations. *Am. J. Respir. Cell Mol. Biol.*, **8**: 1–6.

Najibi, S., Cowan, C.L., Palacino, J.J., Cohen, R.A. (1994) Enhanced role of potassium channels in relaxations to acetylcholine in hypercholesterolemic rabbit carotid artery. *Am. J. Physiol.*, **266**: H2061–H2067.

Nakamura, K., Inai, T., Nakamura, K., Shibata, Y. (1999) Distribution of gap junction protein connexin37 in smooth muscle cells of the rat trachea and pulmonary artery. *Arch. Histol. Cytol.*, **62**: 27–37.

Nakashima, M., Mombouli, J.-V., Taylor, A.A., Vanhoutte, P.M. (1993) Endothelium-dependent hyperpolarization caused by bradykinin in human coronary arteries. *J. Clin. Invest.*, **92**: 2867–2871.

Nakashima, M., Vanhoutte, P.M. (1996) Decreased endothelium-dependent hyperpolarization with aging and hypertension in the rat mesenteric artery. In *Endothelium-Derived Hyperpolarizing Factor*, edited by P.M. Vanhoutte, vol. 1, pp. 227–233. The Netherlands: Harwood Academic Publishers.

Narayanan, J., Medhora, M., Kraemer, R., Capdevila, J.H., Harder, D.R. (2000) Functional expression of recombinant adenovirus carrying bacterial cP450 epoxygenase in rat hippocampal astrocytes. *FASEB J.*, **14**: A152.

Narumiya, S., Sugimoto, Y., Ushikubi, F. (1999) Prostanoid receptors: Structures, properties and functions. *Physiol. Rev.*, **79**: 1193–1226.

Negishi, M., Irie, A., Nagata, N., Ichikawa, A. (1991) Specific binding of glycyrrhetinic acid to the rat liver membrane. *Biochimica Biophysica Acta*, **1066**: 77–82.

Nelson, M.T., Conway, M.A., Knot, H.J., Brayden, J.E. (1997) Chloride channel blockers inhibit myogenic tone in rat cerebral arteries. *J. Physiol.*, **502**: 259–264.

Nelson, M.T., Quayle, J.M. (1995) Physiological roles and properties of potassium channels in arterial smooth muscle. *Am. J. Physiol.*, **268**: C799–C822.

Neylon, C.B., Lang, R.J., Fu, L.Y., Bobik, A., Reinhart, P.T. (1999) Molecular cloning and characterization of the intermediate-conductance Ca^{2+}-activated K^+ channel in vascular smooth muscle. Relationship between K^{Ca} channel diversity and smooth muscle cell function. *Circ. Res.*, **85**: e33–e43.

Neyton, J., Trautmann, A. (1986) Acetylcholine modulation of the conductance of intercellular junctions between rat lacrimal cells. *J. Physiol.*, **377**: 283–293.

Ni, Y., Meyer, M., Osol, G. (1997) Gestation increases a nitric oxide-mediated vasodilation in rat uterine arteries. *Am. J. Obstet. Gynecol.*, **176**: 856–864.

Nilius, B., Viana, F., Droogmans, G. (1997) Ion channels in vascular endothelium. *Annu. Rev. Physiol.*, **59**: 145–170.

Nishikawa, K., Shibayama, Y., Kuna, P., Calcaterra, E., Kaplan, A.P., Reddigari, S.R. (1992) Generation of vasoactive peptide bradykinin from human umbilical vein endothelium-bound high molecular weight kininogen by plasma kallikrein. *Blood*, **80**: 1980–1988.

Nishikawa, Y., Stepp, D.W., Chilian, W.M. (1999) *In vivo* location and mechanism of EDHF-mediated vasodilation in canine coronary microcirculation. *Am. J. Physiol.*, **277**: H1252–H1259.

Nishiyama, M., Hashitani, H., Fukuta, H., Yamamoto, Y., Suzuki, H. (1998) Potassium channels activated in the endothelium-dependent hyperpolarization in guinea-pig coronary artery. *J. Physiol.*, **510**: 455–465.

Nithipatikom, K., Pratt, P.F., Campbell, W.B. (2000) Determination of EETs using microbore liquid chromatography with fluorescence detection. *Am. J. Physiol.*, **279**: H857–H862.

Nobiling, R., Bührle, C.P., Hackenthal, E., Helmchen, U., Steinhausen, M., Whalley, A., Taugner, R. (1986) Ultrastructure, renin status, contractile and electrophysiological properties of the afferent glomerular arteriole in the rat hydronephrotic kidney. *Virchows Arch.*, **410**: 31–42.

Node, K., Huo, Y., Ruan, X., Yang, B., Spiecker, M., Ley, K., Zeldin, D.C., Liao, J.K. (1999) Anti-inflammatory properties of cytochrome P450 epoxygenase-derived eicosanoids. *Science*, **285**: 1276–1279.

Node, K., Kitakaze, M., Kosaka, H., Minamino, T., Hori, M. (1997) Bradykinin mediation of Ca^{2+}-activated K^+ channels regulates coronary blood flow in ischemic myocardium. *Circulation*, **95**: 1560–1567.

Noel, F., Godfraind, T. (1984) Heterogeneity of ouabain specific binding sites and ($Na^+ + K^+$)-ATPase inhibition in microsomes from rat heart. *Biochem. Pharmacol.*, **33**: 47–53.

O'Brien, R., Timmins, K. (1994) The role of oxidation and glycation in the pathogenesis of diabetic atherosclerosis. *Trends Endocrinol. Metab.*, **1194**: 1–6.

Obejero-Paz, C.A., Auslender, M., Scarpa, A. (1998) PKC activity modulates availability and long openings of L-type Ca^{2+} channels in A7r5 cells. *Am. J. Physiol.*, **44**: C535–C543.

Obi, T., Miyamoto, A., Matumoto, M., Ishiguro, S., Nishio, A. (1991) Participation of H1-receptors in histamine-induced contraction and relaxation of horse coronary artery *in vitro*. *J. Vet. Med. Sci.*, **53**: 789–795.

Oh, W.C., Harris, D., Randall, M.D. (2000) Mechanisms of potassium-induced vasorelaxation in the rat aorta. *Br. J. Pharmacol.*, **131**: 77P.

Ohashi, M., Satoh, K., Itoh, T. (1999) Acetylcholine-induced membrane potential changes in endothelial cells of rabbit aortic valve. *Br. J. Pharmacol.*, **126**: 19–26.

Ohba, M., Shibanuma, M., Kuroki, T., Nose, K. (1994) Production of hydrogen peroxide by transforming growth factor-β1 and its involvement in induction of egr-1 in mouse osteoblastic cells. *J. Cell Biol.*, **126**: 1079–1088.

Ohlmann, P., Martinez, M.C., Schneider, F., Stoclet, J.C., Andriantsitohaina, R. (1997) Characterization of endothelium-derived relaxing factors released by bradykinin in human resistance arteries. *Br. J. Pharmacol.*, **121**: 657–664.

Ohno, M., Gibbons, G.H., Dzau, V.J., Cooke, J.P. (1993) Shear stress elevates endothelial cGMP. Role of a potassium channel and G protein coupling. *Circulation*, **88**: 193–197.

Okamoto, H., Wang, X., Harder, D.R., Roman, R.J. (2000) Regional differences in cytochrome P450 4A1, 2, 8 and 2C11 mRNA expression in the rat cerebral microcirculation. *FASEB J.*, **14**: A152.

Okazaki, K., Endou, M., Okumura, F. (1998) Involvement of barium-sensitive K^+ channels in endothelium-dependent vasodilation produced by hypercapnia in rat mesenteric vascular beds. *Br. J. Pharmacol.*, **125**: 168–174.

O'Leary, D.S., Rowell, L.B., Scher, A.M. (1991) Baroreflex-induced vasoconstriction in active skeletal muscle of conscious dogs. *Am. J. Physiol.*, **260**: H37–H41.

Olesen, S.P., Munch, E., Moldt, P., Drejer, J. (1994) Selective activation of Ca^{2+} dependent K^+ channels by novel benzimidazolone. *Eur. J. Pharmacol.*, **251**: 53–59.

Olmos, L., Mombouli, J.-V., Illiano, S., Vanhoutte, P.M. (1995) cGMP mediates the desensitization to bradykinin in isolated canine coronary arteries. *Am. J. Physiol.*, **268**: H865–H870.

Oltman, C.L., Weintraub, N.L., VanRollins, M., Dellsperger, K.C. (1998) Epoxyeicosatrienoic acids and dihydroxyeicosatrienoic acids are potent vasodilators in the canine coronary microcirculation. *Circ. Res.*, **83**: 932–939.

Onaka, U., Fujii, K., Abe, I., Fujishima, M. (1998) Antihypertensive treatment improves endothelium-dependent hyperpolarization in the mesenteric artery of spontaneously hypertensive rats. *Circulation*, **98**: 175–182.

Ooboshi, H., Welsh, M.J., Rios, C.D., Davidson, B.L., Heistad, D.D. (1995) Adenovirus-mediated gene transfer *in vivo* to cerebral blood vessels and perivascular tissue. *Circ. Res.*, **77**: 7–13.

Pacicca, C., Schaad, O., Bény, J.-L. (1996) Electrotonic propagation of kinin-induced, endothelium-dependent hyperpolarizations in pig coronary smooth muscles. *J. Vasc. Res.*, **33**: 380–385.

Pacicca, C.,Von der Weid, P.-Y., Bény, J.-L. (1992) Effect of Nitro-L-Arginine on endothelium-dependent hyperpolarizations and relaxations of pig coronary arteries. *J. Physiol.*, **457**: 247–256.

Paemeleire, K., Martin, P.E.M., Coleman, S.L., Fogarty, K.E., Carrington, W.A., Leybaert, L., Tuft, R.A., Evans, W.H., Sanderson, M.J. (2000) Intercellular calcium waves in HeLa cells expressing GFP-labelled connexin43, 32 or 26. *Mol. Biol. Cell*, **11**: 1815–1827.

Pagliaro, P., Senzaki, H., Paolocci, N., Isoda, T., Sunagawa, G., Recchia, F.A., Kass, D.A. (1999) Specificity of synergistic coronary flow enhancement by adenosine and pulsatile perfusion in the dog. *J. Physiol.*, **520**: 271–280.

Palmer, A.M., Thomas, C.R., Gopaul, N., Dhir, S., Anggard, E.E., Poston, L., Tribe, R.M. (1998) Dietary antioxidant supplementation reduces lipid peroxidation but impairs vascular function in small mesenteric arteries of the streptozotocin-diabetic rat. *Diabetologia*, **41**: 148–156.

Palmer, R.M.J., Ferrige, A.G., Moncada, S. (1987) Nitric oxide release accounts for the biological activity of endothelium-derived relaxing factor. *Nature*, **327**: 524–526.

Panza, J.A., Garcìa, C.E., Kilcoyne, C.M., Quyyumi, A., Cannon III, R.O. (1995) Impaired endothelium-dependent vasodilatation in patients with essential hypertension. Evidence that nitric oxide abnormality is not localised to a single signal transduction pathway. *Circulation*, **91**: 1732–1738.

Panza, J.A., Quyyumi, A.A., Brush, J.E., Jr., Epstein, S.E. (1990) Abnormal endothelium dependent vascular relaxation in patients with essential hypertension. *New Engl. J. Med.*, **323**: 22–27.

Parkington, H.C., Tare, M., Tonta, M.A., Coleman, H.A. (1993) Stretch revealed three components in the hyperpolarization of guinea-pig coronary artery in response to acetylcholine. *J. Physiol.*, **465**: 459–476.

Parkington, H.C., Tonta, M.A., Coleman, H.A., Tare, M. (1995) Role of membrane potential in endothelium-dependent relaxation of guinea-pig coronary arterial smooth muscle. *J. Physiol.*, **484**: 469–480.

Perkins, G.A., Goodenough, D.A., Sosinsky, G.E. (1998) Formation of the gap junction intercellular channel requires a 30 degree rotation for interdigitating two apposing connexins. *J. Molec. Biol.*, **277**: 171–177.

Petersson, J., Zygmunt, P.M., Brandt, L., Högestätt, E.D. (1995) Substance P-induced relaxation and hyperpolarization in human cerebral arteries. *Br. J. Pharmacol.*, **115**: 889–894.

Petersson, J., Zygmunt, P.M., Högestätt, E.D. (1997) Characterization of the potassium channels involved in EDHF-mediated relaxation in cerebral arteries. *Br. J. Pharmacol.*, **120**: 1344–1350.

Pfister, S.L., Campbell, W.B. (1992) Arachidonic acid- and acetylcholine-induced relaxations of rabbit aorta. *Hypertension*, **20**: 682–689.

Pfister, S.L., Schmitz, J.M., Willerson, J.T., Campbell, W.B. (1988) Characterization of arachidonic acid metabolism in Watanabe Heritable Hyperlipidemic (WHHL) and New Zealand White (NZW) rabbit aortas. *Prostaglandins*, **36**: 515–531.

Pfister, S.L., Spitzbarth, N., Nithipatikom, K., Edgemond, W.S., Falck, J.R., Campbell, W.B. (1998) Identification of 11,14,15- and 11,12,15-trihydroxyeicosatrienoic acids as endothelium-derived relaxing factors of rabbit aorta. *J. Biol. Chem.*, **273**: 30879–30887.

Pfister, S.L., Falck, J.R., Campbell, W.B. (1991) Enhanced synthesis of epoxyeicosatrienoic acids by cholesterol-fed rabbit aorta. *Am. J. Physiol.*, **261**: H843–H852.

Pfister, S.L., Spitzbarth, N., Edgemond, W., Campbell, W.B. (1996) Vasorelaxation by an endothelium-derived metabolite of arachidonic acid. *Am. J. Physiol.*, **270**: H1021–H1030.

Pfister, S.L., Spitzbarth, N., Nithipatikom, K., Edgemond, W.S., Campbell, W.B. (1999) Endothelium-derived eicosanoids from lipoxygenase relax the rabbit aorta by opening the potassium channel. In *Endothelium-Dependent Hyperpolarizations*, edited by P.M. Vanhoutte, vol. 2, pp. 17–28. The Netherlands: Harwood Academic Publishers.

Picard, S., Parthasarathy, S., Fruebis, J., Witztum, J.L. (1992) Aminoguanidine inhibits oxidative modification of low density lipoprotein protein and the subsequent increase in uptake by macrophage scavenger receptors. *Proc. Natl. Acad. Sci. USA*, **89**: 6876–6880.

Pinto, A., Abraham, N.G., Mullane K.M. (1986) Cytochrome P-450-dependent mono-oxygenase activity and endothelial-dependent relaxations induced by arachidonic acid. *J. Pharmacol. Exp. Ther.*, **236**: 445–451.

Piomelli, D., Volterra, A., Dale, N., Siegelbaum, S.A., Kandel, E.R., Schwartz, J.H., Belardetti F. (1987) Lipoxygenase metabolites of arachidonic acid as second messengers for presynaptic inhibition of Aplysia sensory cells. *Nature*, **328**: 38–43.

Plane, F., Holland, M, Waldron, G.J., Garland, C.J., Boyle, J.P. (1997) Evidence that anandamide and EDHF act via different mechanisms in rat isolated mesenteric arteries. *Br. J. Pharmacol.* **121**: 1509–1511.

Plum, A., Hallas, G., Magin,T., Dombrowski, F., Hagendorff, A., Schumacher, B., Wolpert, C., Kim, J.-S., Lamers, W., Evert, M., Meda, P., Traub, O., Willecke, K. (2000) Specialization among gap junction proteins: unique and shared functions of different connexins in mice. *Current Biology*, **10**: 1083–1091.

Pomerantz, K., Sintetos, A., Ramwell, P. (1978) The effect of prostacyclin on the human umbilical artery. *Prostaglandins*, **15**: 1035–1044.

Popp, R., Bauersachs, J., Hecker, M., Fleming, I., Busse R. (1996) A transferable, β-naph-thoflavone-inducible, hyperpolarizing factor is synthesized by native and cultured porcine coronary endothelial cells. *J. Physiol.*, **497**: 699–709.

Popp, R., Fleming, I., Busse, R. (1998) Pulsatile stretch in coronary arteries elicits release of endothelium-derived hyperpolarizing factor. *Circ. Res.*, **82**: 696–703.

Pozzi, A., Risek, B., Kiang, D.T., Gilula, N.B., Kumar, N.M. (1995) Analysis of multiple gap junction gene products in the rodent and human mammary gland. *Exp. Cell Res.*, **220**: 212–219.

Prior, H.M., Webster, N., Quinn, K., Beech, D.J., Yates, M.S. (1998) K^+ induced dilation of a small renal artery: no role for inward rectifier K^+ channels. *Cardiovasc. Res.*, **37**: 780–790.

Puntarulo, S., Cederbaum, A.I. (1998) Production of reactive oxygen species by microsomes enriched in specific human cytochrome P450 enzymes. *Free Radical Biol. Med.*, **24**: 1324–1330.

Qi, F.Z., Sugihara, T., Hattori, Y., Yamamoto, Y., Kanno, M., Abe, K. (1998) Functional and morphological damage of endothelium in rabbit ear artery following irradiation with cobalt[60]. *Br. J. Pharmacol.*, **123**: 653–660.

Quayle, J.M., Dart, C., Standen, N.B. (1996) The properties and distribution of inward rectifier potassium currents in pig coronary arterial smooth muscle. *J. Physiol.*, **494**: 715–726.

Quayle, J.M., McCarron, J.G., Brayden, J.E., Nelson, M.T. (1993) Inward rectifier K^+ currents in smooth muscle cells from rat resistance-sized cerebral arteries. *Am. J. Physiol.*, **265**: C1363-C1370.

Quayle, J.M., Nelson, M.T., Standen, N.B. (1997) ATP-sensitive and inwardly rectifying potassium channels in smooth muscle. *Physiological Reviews*, **77**: 1165–1232.

Quignard, J.-F., Félétou, M., Edwards, G., Duhault, J., Weston, A.H., Vanhoutte, P.M. (2000) Role of endothelial cells hyperpolarization in EDHF-mediated responses in the guinea-pig carotid artery. *Br. J. Pharmacol.*, **129**: 1103–1112.

Quignard, J.-F., Félétou, M., Thollon, C., Vilaine, J.-P., Duhault, J., Vanhoutte, P.M. (1999) Potassium ions and endothelium-derived hyperpolarizing factor in guinea-pig carotid and porcine coronary arteries. *Br. J. Pharmacol.*, **127**: 27–34.

Quilley, J., Fulton, D., McGiff, J.C. (1997) Hyperpolarizing factors. *Biochem. Pharmacol.*, **54**: 1059–1070.

Quilley, J., McGiff, J.C. (2000) Is EDHF an epoxyeicosatrienoic acid? *Trends Pharmacol. Sci.*, **21**: 121–124.

Quilley, J., McGiff, J.C., Mieyal, P., Rapacon, M., Fulton, D. (1996) NO-independent coronary vasodilation to bradykinin in diabetes. *Hypertension*, **28**: P178.

Radi, R., Beckman, J., Bush, K., Freeman, B. (1991) Peroxynitrite-induced membrane lipid peroxydation: the cytotoxic potential of superoxide and nitric oxide. *Arch. of Biophys. and Biochem.*, **288**: 481–487.

Radomski, M.W., Palmer, R.M., Moncada, S. (1990) Glucocorticoids inhibit the expression of an inducible, but not the constitutive, nitric oxide synthase in vascular endothelial cells. *Proc. Natl. Acad. Sci. USA*, **87**: 10043–10047.

Ralevic, V., Belai, A., Burnstock, G. (1993) Impaired sensory-motor nerve function in the isolated mesenteric arterial bed of streptozotocin-diabetic and ganglioside-treated streptozotocin-diabetic rats. *Br. J. Pharmacol.*, **110**: 1105–1111.

Ramanan, S.V., Brink, P.R., Christ, G. (1998) Neuronal Innervation, Intracellular Signal Transduction and Intercellular Coupling: a Model for syncytial Tissue Responses in the Steady state. *J. Theor. Biol.*, **193**: 69–84.

Ramanan, S.V., Brink, P.R., Varadaraj, K., Peterson, E., Schirrmacher, K., Banach, K. (1999) A three-state model for Connexin37 gating kinetics. *Biophys. J.*, **76**: 2520–2529.

Randall, M.D., Alexander, S.P.H., Bennett, T., Boyd, E.A., Fry, J.R., Gardiner, S.M., Kemp, P.A., McCullock, A.L., Kendall, D.A. (1996) An endogenous cannabinoid as an endothelium-derived vasorelaxant. *Biochem. Biophys. Res. Commun.*, **229**: 114–120.

Randall, M.D., Kendall, D.A. (1998) Endocannabinoids: a new class of vasoactive substances. *Trends Pharmacol. Sci.*, **19**: 55–58.

Rapacon, M., Mieyal, P., McGiff, J.C., Fulton, D., Quilley, J. (1996) Contribution of calcium-activated potassium channels to the vasodilator effect of bradykinin in the isolated, perfused kidney of the rat. *Br. J. Pharmacol.*, **118**: 1504–1508.

Rapoport, R.M., Williams, S.P. (1996) Role of prostaglandins in acetylcholine-induced contraction of aorta from spontaneously hypertensive and Wistar-Kyoto rats. *Hypertension*, **28**: 64–75.

Ravelic, V., Burnstock, G. (1996) Mesenteric arterial function in the rat in pregnancy: role of sympathetic and sensory-motor perivascular nerves, endothelium, smooth muscle, nitric oxide and prostaglandins. *Br. J. Pharmacol.*, **117**: 1463–1470.

Reaume, A.G., de Sousa, P.A., Kulkarni, S., Langille, B.C., Zhu, D., Davies, T.C., Juneja, S.C., Kidder, G.M., Rossant, J. (1995) Cardiac malformation in neonatal mice lacking connexin43. *Science*, **267**: 1831–1834.

Reavan, P.D., Witzum, J.L. (1993) Comparison of supplementation of RRR-α-tocopherol and racemic α-tocopherol in humans: effect on lipid levels and lipoprotein susceptibility to oxidation. *Arteriosler. Thromb.*, **13**: 601.

Recchia, F.A., Byrne, B.J., Kass, D.A. (1999) Sustained vessel dilation induced by increased pulsatile perfusion of porcine carotid arteries *in vitro*. *Acta Physiol. Scand.*, **166**: 15–21.

Recchia, F.A., Senzaki, H., Saeki, A., Byrne, B.J., Kass, D.A. (1996) Pulse-pressure related changes in coronary flow *in vivo* are modulated by nitric oxide and adenosine. *Circ Res.*, **79**: 849–856.

Rees, D.D., Palmer, R.M., Schulz, R., Hodson, H.F., Moncada, S. (1990) Characterization of three inhibitors of endothelial nitric oxide synthase *in vitro* and *in vivo*. *Br. J. Pharmacol.*, **101**: 746–752.

Richard, V., Tanner, F.C., Tschudi, M., Lüscher, T.F. (1990) Different activation of L-arginine pathway by bradykinin, serotonin, and clonidine in coronary arteries. *Am. J. Physiol.*, **259**: H1433–H1439.

Robertson, B.E., Schubert, R., Hescheler, J., Nelson, M.T. (1993) cGMP-dependent protein kinase activates Ca-activated K channels in cerebral artery smooth muscle cells. *Am. J. Physiol.*, **265**: C299–C303.

Rosenblum, W.I. (1986) Endothelial dependent relaxation demonstrated *in vivo* in cerebral arterioles. *Stroke*, **17**: 494–497.

Rosentreter, U., Boshagen, H., Seuter, F., Perzborn, E., Fiedler, V.B. (1989) Synthesis and absolute configuration of the new thromboxane antagonist (3R)-3-(4-flurophenylsulfonamido)-1,2,3,4-tetrahydro-9carbazolepropanoic acid and comparison with its enantiomer. *Arzneimittelforschung*, **39**: 1519–1521.

Rosolowsky, M., Campbell, W.B. (1993) Role of PGI_2 and epoxyeicosatrienic acids in relaxation of bovine coronary arteries to arachidonic acid. *Am. J. Physiol.*, **264**: H327-H335

Rosolowsky, M., Campbell, W.B. (1996) Synthesis of hydroxyeicosatetraenoic (HETEs) and epoxyeicosatrienoic acids (EETs) by cultured bovine coronary artery endothelial cells. *Biochem. Biophys. Acta*, **1299**: 267–277.

Rosolowsky, M., Falck, J.R., Willerson, J.T., Campbell, W.B. (1990) Synthesis of lipoxygenase and epoxygenase products of arachidonic acid by normal and stenosed canine coronary arteries. *Circ. Res.* **66**: 608–621.

Ross, G., Stinson, E., Schroeder, J., Ginsburg, R. (1980) Spontaneous phasic activity of isolated human coronary arteries. *Cardiovasc. Res.*, **14**: 613–618.

Rubanyi, G.M., Romero, J.C., Vanhoutte, P.M. (1986) Flow-induced release of endothelium-derived relaxing factor. *Am. J. Physiol.*, **250**: H1145–H1149.

Rubanyi, G.M., Vanhoutte, P.M. (1985) Ouabain inhibits endothelium-dependent relaxations to arachidonic acid in canine coronary arteries. *J. Pharm. Exper. Ther.*, **235**: 81–86.

Rubanyi, G.M., Vanhoutte, P.M. (1986a) Oxygen-derived free radicals, endothelium, and responsiveness of vascular smooth muscle. *Am. J. Physiol.*, **250**: H815–821.

Rubanyi, G.M., Vanhoutte, P.M. (1986b) Superoxide anions and hyperoxia inactivate endothelium-derived relaxing factor. *Am. J. Physiol.*, **250**: H822–827.

Rubanyi, G.M., Vanhoutte, P.M. (1987) Nature of endothelium-derived relaxing factor: Are there two relaxing mediators? *Circ. Res.*, **61**: II61–II67.

Rumbaut, R.E., Sial, A.J. (1999) Differential phototoxicity of fluorescent dye-labeled albumin conjugates. *Microcirculation*, **6**: 205–213.

Sack, M.N., Rader, D.J., Cannon, R.O.III. (1994) Oestrogen and inhibition of oxidation of low-density lipoproteins in postmenopausal women. *Lancet*, **343**: 269–270.

Sai, Y., Dai, R., Yang, T.J., Krausz, K.W., Gonzalez, F.J., Gelboin, H.V., Shou, M. (2000) Assessment of specificity of eight chemical inhibitors using cDNA-expressed cytochromes P450. *Xenobiotica*, **30**: 327–343.

Salari, H., Braquet, P., Borgeat, P. (1984) Comparative effects of indomethacin, acetylenic acids, 15-HETE, nordihydroguaiaretic acid and BW755C on the metabolism of arachidonic acid in human leukocytes and platelets. *Prostaglandins Leukot Med.*, **13**: 53–60.

Sanders, S.A., Eisenthal, R., Harrison, R. (1997) NADH oxidase activity of human xanthine oxidoreductase – Generation of superoxide anion. *Eur. J. Biochem.*, **245**: 541–548.

Sandow, S.L., Hill, C.E. (2000) Incidence of myoendothelial gap junctions in the proximal and distal mesenteric arteries of the rat is suggestive of a role in endothelium-derived hyperpolarizing factor-mediated responses. *Circ. Res.*, **86**: 341–346.

Satake, N., Shibata, M., Shibata, S. (1997) The involvement of KCa, KATP and KV channels in vasorelaxing responses to acetylcholine in rat aortic rings. *Gen. Pharmacol.*, **28**: 453–457.

Schiffrin, E.L., Deng, L.Y. (1995) Comparison of effects of angiotensin I-converting enzyme inhibition and β-blockade for 2 years on function of small arteries from hypertensive patients. *Hypertension*, **25**: 699–703.

Schiffrin, E.L., Park, J.B., Intengan, H.D., Touyz, R.M. (2000) Correction of arterial structure and endothelial dysfunction in human essential hypertension by the angiotensin receptor antagonist losartan. *Circulation*, **101**: 1653–1659.

Schilling, W.P. Elliott, S.J. (1992) Ca^{2+} signaling mechanisms of vascular endothelial cells and their role in oxidant-induced endothelial cell dysfunction. *Am. J. Physiol.*, **262**: H1617–H1630.

Schirrmacher, K., Nonhoff, D., Wiemann, M., Peterson-Grine, E., Brink, P.R., Bingmann, D., (1996) Effects of calcium on gap junctions between osteoblast-like cells in culture. *Calcif. Tissue Int.*, **59**: 259–264.

Schultz, K.D., Schultz, K., Schultz, G. (1997) Sodium nitroprusside and other smooth muscle relaxants increase cyclic GMP levels in rat ductus deferens. *Nature*, **265**: 750–751.

Seeds, M.C., Bass, D.A. (1999) Regulation and metabolism of arachidonic acid. *Clin. Rev. Allergy Immunol.*, **17**: 5–26.

Segal, S.S., Duling, B.R. (1986) Flow control among microvessels coordinated by intercellular conduction. *Science*, **234**: 868–870.

Segal, S.S., Neild, T.O. (1996) Conducted depolarization in arteriole networks of the guinea-pig small intestine: effect of branching on signal dissipation. *J. Physiol.*, **496**: 229–244.

Segal, S.S., Welsh, D.G., Kurjiaka, D.T. (1999) Spread of vasodilatation and vasoconstriction along feed arteries and arterioles of hamster skeletal muscle. *J. Physiol.*, **516**: 283–291.

Seiden, J.E., Platoshyn, O., Bakst, A.E., McDaniel, S.S., Yuan, J.X. (2000) High K^+-induced membrane depolarization attenuates endothelium-dependent pulmonary vasodilation. *Am. J. Physiol.*, **278**: L261–L267.

Seifert, H., Jager, K., Bollinger, A. (1988) Analysis of flow motion by the Laser Doppler technique in patients with peripheral arterial occlusive disease. *Int. J. Microcirc.*, **7**: 223–236.

Selemidis, S., Ziogas, J., Cocks, T.M. (1998) Apamin- and nitric oxide-sensitive biphasic non-adrenergic non-cholinergic inhibitory junction potentials in the rat anococcygeus muscle. *J. Physiol.*, **513**: 835–844.

Selwyn, A.P., Ganz, P. (1990) Coronary vasomotor response to acetylcholine relates to risk factors for coronary artery disease. *Circulation*, **81**: 491–497.

Serkiz, Y.I. (1997) Peculiarities of the low efficiency radiation biological effects. In *Chornobyl catastrophe*, edited by V.Baryakhtar, pp. 279–281. Ukraine (Kiev): Editorial House of Annual Issue "Export of Ukraine".

Shan, J., Resnick, L.M., Liu, Q.Y., Wu, X.C., Barbagallo, M., Pang, P.K. (1994) Vascular effects of 17 β-estradiol in male Sprague-Dawley rats. *Am. J. Physiol.*, **266**: H967–H973.

Shatara, R.K., Quest, D.W., Wilson, T.W. (2000) Fenofibrate lowers blood pressure in two genetic models of hypertension. *Canad. J. Physiol. & Pharmacol.*, **78**: 367–371.

Shimokawa, H. (1999) Primary endothelial dysfunction: atherosclerosis. *J. Mol. Cell Cardiol.*, **31**: 23–37.

Shimokawa, H., Aarhus, L.L., Vanhoutte, P.M. (1987) Porcine coronary arteries with regenerated endothelium have a reduced endothelium-dependent responsiveness to aggregating platelets and serotonin. *Circ. Res.*, **61**: 256–270.

Shimokawa, H., Flavahan, N.A., Vanhoutte, P.M. (1989) Natural course of the impairment of endothelium-dependent relaxations after balloon endothelium removal in porcine coronary arteries. *Circ. Res.*, **65**: 740–753.

Shimokawa, H., Urakami-Harasawa, L., Nakashima, M., Tagawa, H., Hirooka, Y., Takeshita, A. (1999) Importance of endothelium-derived hyperpolarizing factor in human arteries. In *Endothelium-derived Hyperpolarizing Factor*, edited by P.M. Vanhoutte, vol. 2, pp. 391–398. The Netherlands: Harwood Academic Publishers.

Shimokawa, H., Yasutake, H., Fujii, K., Owada, M.K., Nakaike, R., Fukumoto, Y., Takayanagi, T., Nagao, T., Egashira, K., Fujishima, M., Takeshita, A. (1996) The importance of the hyperpolarizing mechanism increases as the vessel size decreases in endothelium-dependent relaxations in rat mesenteric circulation. *J. Cardiovasc. Pharmacol.*, **28**: 703–711.

Shivachar, A.C., Willoughby, K.A., Ellis, E.F. (1995) Effect of protein kinase C modulators on 14,15-epoxyeicosatrienoic acid incorporation into astroglial phospholipids. *J. Neurochem*, **65**: 338–346.

Siegel, G., Stock, G., Schnalke, F., Litza, B. (1987) Electrical and mechanical effects of prostacyclin in canine carotid artery. In *Prostacyclin and its stable analogue iloprost*, edited by R.J. Gryglewski & G. Stock, pp. 143–149. Berlin Heidelberg: Springer-Verlag.

Simon, A.M., Goodenough, D.A. (1998) Diverse functions of vertebrate gap junctions. *Trends in Cell Biol.*, **8**: 477–483.

Simon, A.M., Goodenough, D.A., Paul, D.L. (1998) Mice lacking connexin40 have cardiac conduction abnormalities characteristics of atrioventrivular block and bundle brunch block. *Current Biology*, **8**: 295–298.

Simonsen, U., Wadsworth, R.M., Buus, N.H., Mulvany, M.J. (1999) *In vitro* simultaneous measurements of relaxation and nitric oxide concentration in rat superior mesenteric artery. *J. Physiol.*, **516**: 271–282.

Singer, H.A., Peach, M.J. (1983) Endothelium-dependent relaxation of rabbit aorta. I. Relaxation stimulated by arachidonic acid. *J. Pharmacol. Exp. Ther.*, **226**: 790–795.

Skyrme-Jones, A., O'Brien, R., Berry, K., Meredith, I. (2000) Vitamin E supplementation improves endothelial function in Type 1 Diabetes Mellitus: a randomized, placebo controlled study. *J. Am. Coll. Cardiol.*, **36**: 94–102.

Sladek, S.M., Magness, R.R., Conrad, K.P. (1997) Nitric oxide and pregnancy. *Am. J. Physiol.*, **272**: 441–463.

Smiley, R.M., Finster, M. (1996) Do receptors get pregnant too? Adrenergic receptor alterations in human pregnancy. *J. Maternal Fetal Medicine*, **5**: 106–114.

Sneyd, J., Wetton, B.T., Charles, A.C., Sanderson, M.J. (1995) Intercellular calcium waves mediated by diffusion of IP3: a two dimensional model. *Am. J. Physiol.*, **268**: C1537–C1545.

Soloviev, A., Tishkin, S., Parshikov, A., Stefanov, A., Mosse, I. (1999) Depression of endothelium-dependent relaxation despite normal release of nitric oxide in the aorta of spontaneously hypertensive rats: possible role of protein kinase C. In *Endothelium-dependent hyperpolarizations*, edited by P.M.Vanhoutte, vol. 2, pp. 289–296. The Netherlands: Harwood Academic Publishers.

Solzbach, U., Hornig, B., Jeserich, M., Just, H. (1997) Vitamin C improves endothelial dysfunction of epicardial coronary arteries in hypertensive patients. *Circulation*, **96**: 1513–1519.

Soulis, T., Cooper, M.E., Vranes, D., Bucala, R., Jerums, G. (1996) Effects of aminoguanidine in preventing experimental diabetic nephropathy are related to the duration of treatment. *Kidney International*, **50**: 627–634.

Soulis-Liparota, T., Cooper, M., Papazoglou, D., Clarke, B., Jerums, G. (1991) Retardation by aminoguanidine of development of albuminuria, mesangial expansion, and tissue fluorescence in streptozotocin-induced diabetic rat. *Diabetes*, **40**: 1328–1334.

Spagnoli, L.G., Villaschi, S., Neri, L., Palmeri, G. (1982) Gap junctions in myoendothelial bridges of rabbit carotid arteries. *Experimentia*, **38**: 124–125.

Spray, D.C., Bennett, M.V.L. (1985) Physiology and pharmacology of gap junctions. *Ann. Rev. Physiol.*, **47**: 281–303.

Spray, D.C., Burt, J.M. (1990) Structure–activity relations of the cardiac gap junction channel. *Am. J. Physiol.*, **258**: C195–C205.

Srinivas, M., Costa, M., Gao, Y., Fort, A., Fishman, G.I., Spray, D.C. (1999) Voltage dependence of macroscopic and unitary currents of gap junction channels formed by mouse connexin50 expressed in rat neuroblastoma cells. *J. Physiol.*, **517**: 673–689.

Standen, N.B., Quayle, J.M. (1998) K channel modulation in arterial smooth muscle. *Acta Scand.*, **164**: 549–558.

Standen, N.B., Quayle, J.M., Davies, N.W., Brayden, J.E., Huang, Y., Nelson, M.T. (1989) Hyperpolarizing vasodilators activate ATP-sensitive K^+ channels in arterial smooth muscle. *Science*, **245**: 177–180.

Steinhausen, M., Endlich, K. (1993) The hydronephrotic kidney: a model to study renal microcirculation. In *Experimental and genetic rat models of chronic renal failure*, edited by N. Gretz, M. Strauch, pp 169–183, Basel: Karger.

Steinhausen, M., Snoei, H., Parekh, N., Baker, R., Johnson, P.C. (1983) Hydronephrosis: a new method to visualize vas afferens, efferens and glomerular network. *Kidney Int.*, **23**: 794–806.

Stephens, N.G., Parsons, A., Schofield, P.M., Kelly, F., Cheeseman, K., Mitchinson, M.J. (1996) Randomized controlled trial of vitamin E in patients with coronary disease: Cambridge Heart Antioxidant Study (CHAOS). *Lancet*, **347**: 781–786.

Stroes, E., Hijmering, M., van Zandvoort, M., Wever, R., Rabelink, T.J., van Faassen, E.E. (1998) Origin of superoxide production by endothelial nitric oxide synthase. *FEBS. Lett.*, **438**: 161–164.

Sugihara, T., Hattori, Y., Yamamoto, Y., Qi, F.Z., Ichikawa, R., Sato, A., Liu, M.Y., Abe, K., Canno, M. (1999) Preferential impairment of nitric oxide-dependent relaxation in human cervical arteries after irradiation. *Circulation*, **100**: 635–641.

Suwaidi, J.A., Hamasaki, S., Higano, S.T., Nishimura, R.A., Holmes, D.R., Lerman, A. (2000) Long-term follow-up of patients with mild coronary artery disease and endothelial dysfunction. *Circulation*, **101**: 948–954.

Suzuki, H., Nakano, N., Ito, M., Yamashita, N., Sugiyama, E., Maruyama, M., Yano, S. (1983) Effect of glycyrrhizin and glycyrrhetinic acid on production of O_2^-, H_2O_2 by macrophages. *Igaku no Ayumi.*, **124**: 109–111.

Svendsen, E., Austarheim, A.-M.S., Haugen, B., Dalen, H., Dregelid, E. (1990) Myoendothelial junctions in human saphenous veins. *Acta Anat.*, **138**: 150–153.

Sydoryk, Ye., P., Druzhina, M.O., Burlaka, A.P., Puknova, G.G. (1997) Biological effects in animals. Changes of biophysical characteristics in the organs and in the blood. In *Chornobyl catastrophe*, edited by V. Baryakhtar, pp. 282–284. Ukraine (Kiev): Editorial House of Annual Issue "Export of Ukraine".

Taddei, S., Virdis, A., Ghiadoni, L., Magagna, A., Salvetti, A. (1998) Vitamin C improves endothelium-dependent vasodilatation by restoring nitric oxide activity in essential hypertension. *Circulation*, **97**: 2222–2229.

Taddei, S., Virdis, A., Mattei, P., Ghiadoni, L., Gennari, A., Fasolo, C.B., Sudano, I., Salvetti, A. (1995) Aging and endothelial function in normotensive subjects and patients with essential hypertension. *Circulation*, **91**: 1981–1987.

Taddei, S., Virdis, A., Mattei, P., Salvetti, A. (1993) Vasodilatation to acetylcholine in primary and secondary forms of human hypertension. *Hypertension*, **21**: 929–933.

Takamura, Y., Shimokawa, H., Zhao, H., Igarashi, H., Egashira, K., Takeshita, A. (1999) Important role of endothelium-derived hyperpolarizing factor in shear stress-induced endothelium-dependent vasorelaxations in the rat mesenteric artery. *J. Cardiovasc. Pharmacol.*, **34**: 381–387.

Takens-Kwak, B.R., Jongsma, H.J. (1992) Cardiac gap-junctions-3 distinct single channel conductances and their modulation by phosphorylating treatments. *Pflügers Arch. Eur. J. Physiol.*, **422**: 198–200.

Takens-Kwak, B.R., Jongsma, H.J., Rook, M.B., Vanginneken, A.C. (1992) Mechanism of heptanol-induced uncoupling of cardiac gap-junctions – A perforated patch-clamp study. *Am. J. Physiol.*, **262**: C1531–C1538.

Taylor, H.J., Chaytor, A.T., Evan, W.H., Griffith, T.M. (1998) Inhibition of the gap junctional component of endothelium-dependent relaxation in rabbit iliac artery by 18-α glycyrrhetinic acid. *Br. J. Pharmacol.*, **125**: 1–3.

Taylor, P.D., McCarthy, A.L., Thomas, C.R., Poston, L. (1992) Endothelium-dependent relaxation and noradrenaline sensitivity in mesenteric resistance arteries of streptozotocin-induced diabetic rats. *Br. J. Pharmacol.*, **107**: 393–399.

Taylor, P.D., Graves, J.E., Poston, L. (1995) Selective impairment of acetylcholine-mediated endothelium-dependent relaxation in isolated resistance arteries of the streptozotocin-induced diabetic rat. *Clin. Sci.*, **88**: 519–524.

Taylor, S.G., Weston, A.H. (1988) Endothelial-derived hyperpolarizing factor; a new endogenous inhibitor from the vascular endothelium. *Trends Pharmacol. Sci.*, **9**: 272–274.

Terasawa, T., Okada, T., Nishino, H. (1992) Antitumor-promoter activity of modified glycyrrhetinic acid derivatives – synthesis and structure-activity relationships. *Eur. J. Med. Chem.*, **27**: 689–692.

The Diabetes Control and Complications Trial Research Group/Epidemiology of Diabetes Interventions and Complications Research Group (2000) Retinopathy and nephropathy in patients with type 1 diabetes four years after a trial of intensive therapy. *New Engl. J. Med.*, **342**: 381–389.

Theis, M., de Wit, C., Schlaeger, T., Eckardt, D., Krueger, O., Doering, B., Risau, W., Deutsch, U., Pohl, U., Willecke, K. (2001) Endothelium specific replacement of the connexin43 coding region by a LacZ reporter gene. *Genesis*, **29**: 1–13.

Theis, M., Magin, T.M., Plum, A., Willecke, K. (2000) General or cell type-specific deletion and replacement of connexin-coding DNA in the mouse. *Methods*, **20**: 205–218.

Thollon, C., Bidouard, J.P., Cambarrat, C., Delescluse, I., Villeneuve, N., Vanhoutte, P.M., Vilaine, J.-P. (1999a) Alteration of endothelium-dependent hyperpolarizations in porcine coronary arteries with regenerated endothelium. *Circ. Res.*, **84**: 371–377.

Thollon, C., Fournet-Bourguignon, M.P., Cambarrat, C., Saboureau, D., Delescluse, I., Vanhoutte, P.M., Vilaine, J.-P. (1999b) Contribution of nitric oxide and endothelium-derived hyperpolarizing factor to the relaxation evoked by bradykinin in porcine coronary arteries four weeks after removal of the endothelium. In *Endothelium-derived hyperpolarizing factor*, edited by P.M. Vanhoutte, vol. 2, pp. 335–341. The Netherlands: Harwood academic publishers.

Thomas, S.A., Schuessler, R.B., Berul, C.I., Beardslee, M.A., Beyer, E.C., Medelsohn, M.E., Saffitz, J.E. (1998) Disparate effects of deficient expression of connexin43 on atrial and ventricular conduction. *Circulation*, **97**: 686–691.

Thompson, L., Trujillo, M., Telleri, R., Redi, R. (1995) Kinetics of cytochrome C 2+ oxidation by peroxynitrite: implications for superoxide measurements in nitric oxide producing biological systems. *Arch. Biochem. Biophys.*, **319**: 491–497.

Tilton, R.G., Chang, K., Ostrow, E., Allison, W., Williamson, J.R. (1990) Aminoguanidine reduces increased 131I-albumin permeation of retinal and uveal vessels in streptozotocin-diabetic rats. *Invest. Ophthalmol. Vis. Sci.*, **31**: 342.

Tilton, R.G., Faller, A.M., Allison, W. (1992) Aminoguanidine prevents capillary basement membrane thickening but not vascular 125I-albumin permeation in retinas of chronically diabetic rats (abstract). *Diabetes*, **41**: 21A.

Ting, H.H., Timimi, F.K., Boles, K.S., Creager, S.J., Ganz, P., Creager, M.A. (1996). Vitamin C improves endothelium-dependent vasodilatation in patients with non-insulin dependent diabetes mellitus. *J. Clin. Invest.*, **97**: 22–28.

Toda, N. (1974) Responsiveness to potassium and calcium ions isolated cerebral arteries. *Am. J. Physiol.*, **227**: 1206–1211.

Tomioka, H., Hattori, Y., Fukao, M., Sato, A., Liu, M., Sakuma, I., Kitabatake, A., Kanno, M. (1999) Relaxation in different-sized rat blood vessels mediated by endothelium-derived hyperpolarizing factor: importance of processes mediating precontractions. *J. Vasc. Res.*, **36**: 311–320.

Tonumura, Y. (1986) (Na$^+$, K$^+$) ATPase in the plasma membrane. In *Energy-transducing ATPase: structure and kinetics*, pp. 240–281. UK (Cambridge): Cambridge Univ. Press.

Traverse, J.H., Wang, Y.L., Du, R., Nelson, D., Lindstrom, P., Archer, S.L., Gong, G., Bache, R.J. (2000) Coronary nitric oxide production in response to exercise and endothelium-dependent agonists. *Circulation*, **101**: 2526–2531.

Triggle, C.R. (2000) Endothelial cell K$^+$ channels, membrane potential and the release of vasoactive factors from the vascular endothelium. In *Potassium Channels in Cardiovascular Biology*, edited by S.L. Archer and N.J. Rusch. New York: Plenum Press.

Tschudi, M.R., Criscione, L., Novosel, D., Pfeiffer, K., Lüscher, T.F. (1994) Antihypertensive therapy augments endothelium-dependent relaxations in coronary arteries of spontaneously hypertensive rats. *Circulation*, **89**: 2212–2218.

Tsein, R., Weingart, R. (1976) Inotropic effect of cAMP in calf ventricular muscle studied by cut end methods. *J. Physiol.*, **260**: 117–140.

UK Prospective Diabetes Study Group (1998) Tight blood pressure control and risk of macrovascular and microvascular complications in type 2 diabetes: UKPDS 38. *B.M.J.*, **317**: 703–713.

Urakami-Harasawa, L., Shimokawa, H., Nakashima, M., Egashira, K., Takeshita, A. (1997) Importance of endothelium-derived hyperpolarizing factor in human arteries. *J. Clin. Invest.*, **100**: 2793–2799.

Urata, H., Nishimura, H., Ganten, D. (1996) Chymase-dependent angiotensin II forming systems in humans. *Am. J. Hypert.*, **9**: 277–284.

Usui, M., Matsuoka, H., Miyazaki, H., Ueda, S., Okuda, S., Imaizumi, T. (1999) Endothelial dysfunction by acute hyperhomocyst(e)inaemia: restoration by folic acid. *Clin. Sci.*, **96**: 235–239.

Vaca, L., Licea, A., Possani, L.D. (1996) Modulation of cell membrane potential in cultured vascular endothelium. *Am. J. Physiol.*, **270**: C819–824.

Valiunas, V., Bukauskas, F.F., Weingart, R. (1997) Conductances and selective permeability of Cx43 gap junction channels examined in neonatal rat heart cells. *Cir. Res.*, **80**: 708–719.

Valiunas, V.R., Weingart, Brink, P.R. (2000) Formation of heterotypic gap junction channels by Cx40 and Cx43. *Cir. Res.*, **86e**: 42–49.

Vallance, P., Coller, J., Moncada, S. (1989) Effects of endothelium-derived nitric oxide on peripheral arteriolar tone in man. *Lancet*, **2**: 997–1000.

Van de Voorde, J., Vanheel, B. (1997) Influence of cytochrome P-450 inhibitors on endothelium-dependent nitro-L-arginine-resistant relaxation and cromakalim-induced relaxation in rat mesenteric arteries. *J. Cardiovasc. Pharmacol.*, **29**: 827–832.

Van de Voorde, J., Vanheel, B. (2000) EDHF-mediated relaxation in rat gastric small arteries: influence of ouabain/Ba^{2+} and relation to potassium ions. *J. Cardiovasc. Pharmacol.*, **35**: 543–548.

Van Iwaarden, F., De Groot, P.G., Bouma, B.N. (1988) The binding of high molecular weight kininogen to cultured human endothelial cells. *J. Biol. Chem.*, **263**: 4698–4703.

van Kempen, M.J.A., Jongsma, H.J. (1999) Distribution of connexin37, connexin40 and connexin43 in the aorta and coronary artery of several mammals. *Histochem. Cell Biol.*, **112**: 479–486.

Van Rijen, H.V.M., van Veen, T.A.B., van Kempen, M.J.A., Wilms-Schopman, F.J.G., Potse, M., Krueger, O., Willecke, K., Jongsma, H.J. (2001) Impaired conduction in the bundle branches of mouse hearts lacking the gap junction protein connexin40. *Circulation*, in press.

Vanheel, B., de Hemptinne, A. (1992) Influence of K_{ATP} channel modulation on net potassium efflux from ischaemic mammalian cardiac tissue. *Cardiovasc. Res.*, **26**: 1030–1039.

Vanheel, B., de Hemptinne, A., Leusen, I. (1990) Acidification and intracellular sodium ion activity during simulated myocardial ischemia. *Am. J. Physiol.*, **259**: C169–C179.

Vanheel, B., Van de Voorde, J. (1995) Membrane potential responses to endothelium-dependent and -independent vasodilators in rat aorta and mesenteric arteries (Abstract). *Pflügers Arch. Eur. J. Physiol.*, **430**: R140.

Vanheel, B., Van de Voorde, J. (1997) Evidence against the involvement of cytochrome P450 metabolites in endothelium-dependent hyperpolarization in the rat main mesenteric artery. *J. Physiol.*, **501**: 331–341.

Vanheel, B., Van de Voorde, J. (1999) Barium decreases endothelium-dependent smooth muscle responses to transient but not to more prolonged acetylcholine applications. *Pflügers Arch. Eur. J. Physiol.*, **439**: 123–129.

Vanheel, B., Van de Voorde, J., Leusen, I. (1994) Contribution of nitric oxide to the endothelium-dependent hyperpolarization in rat aorta. *J. Physiol.*, **475**: 277–284.

Vanhoutte, P.M. (1997) Endothelial dysfunction and atherosclerosis. *Eur. Heart. J.*, **18**: E19–E29.

Vanhoutte, P.M. (1998) Old-timer makes a comeback. *Nature*, **396**: 213–216.

Vanhoutte, P.M., Félétou, M. (1999) Concluding remarks: identified and unidentified endothelium-derived hyperpolarizing factors. In *Endothelium-dependent hyperpolarizations*, edited by P.M. Vanhoutte, vol. 2, pp. 399–403. The Netherlands: Harwood Academic Publishers.

Vanhoutte, P.M., Félétou, M., Boulanger, C.M., Höffner, U., Rubanyi, G.M. (1996) Existence of multiple endothelium-derived relaxing factors. In *Endothelium-derived Hyperpolarizing factor*, edited by P.M. Vanhoutte, vol. 1, pp. 1–10. The Netherlands: Harwood Academic Publishers.

Vanhoutte, P.M., Mombouli, J.-V. (1996) Vascular endothelium: vasoactive mediators. *Prog. Cardiovasc. Dis.*, **39**: 229–238.

Vapaatalo, H., Linden, I., Metsa-Ketela, T., Kangasaho, M., Laustiola, K. (1977) Effect of carbenoxolone on phosphodiesterase and prostaglandin synthetase activities. *Experimentia*, **34**: 384–385.

Vedernikov, Y.P., Belfort, M.A., Saade, G., Wen, T. (1996) Endothelial hyperpolarizing factor is important in bradykinin-induced relaxation of isolated pregnant human omental artery. *J. Soc. Gynecol. Invest.*, **3**: 286A.

Vedernikov, Y.P., Belfort, M.A., Saade, G.R., Garfield, R.E. (1999) Endothelium-derived hyperpolarizing factor in omental arteries from normotensive pregnant women. In *Endothelium-Dependent Hyperpolarizations*, edited by P.M Vanhoutte, vol. 2, pp. 363–369. The Netherlands: Harwood Academic Publishers.

Vedernikov, Y.P., Liao, Q.P., Jain, V., Saade, G.R., Chwalisz, K., Garfield, R.E. (1997) Effect of chronic treatment with 17β-estradiol and progesterone on endothelium-dependent and endothelium-independent relaxation in isolated aortic rings from ovariectomized rats. *Am. J. Obstet. Gynecol.*, **176**: 603–608.

Veenstra, R.D., Wang, H.-Z., Beblo, D.A., Chilton, M.G., Harris, A.L., Beyer, E.C., Brink, P.R. (1995) Selectivity of connexin-specific gap junctions does not correlate with channel conductance. *Cir. Res.*, **77**: 1156–1165.

Veenstra, R.D., Wang, Z., Beyer, E.C., Brink, P.R. (1994) Selective dye and ionic permeability of gap junction channels form by connexin45 Channels. *Cir. Res.*, **268**: 706–712.

Verbeke, M., Van de Voorde, J., de Ridder, L., Lameire, N. (1999) Beneficial effect of serotonin 5-HT2-receptor antagonism on renal blood flow autoregulation in cyclosporin-treated rats. *J. Am. Soc. Nephrol.*, **10**: 28–34.

Verhaar, M.C., Wever, R.M., Kastelein, J.J., van Dam, T., Koomans, H.A., Rabelink, T.J. (1998) 5-methyltetrahydrofolate, the active form of folic acid, restores endothelial function in familial hypercholesterolemia. *Circulation*, **97**: 237–241.

Verhaar, M.C., Wever, R.M., Kastelein, J.J., van Loon, D., Milstien, S., Koomans, H.A., Rabelink, T.J. (1999) Effects of oral folic acid supplementation on endothelial function in familial hypercholesterolemia: a randomized placebo-controlled trial. *Circulation*, **100**: 335–338.

Verheule, S., van Batenburg, C.A.J.A.C., Coenjaerts, F.E.J., Kirchhoff, S., Willecke, K., Jongsma, H.J. (1999) Cardiac conduction abnormalities in mice lacking the gap junction protein connexin40. *J. Cardiovasc. Electrophysiol.*, **10**: 1380–1389.

Vita, J.A., Treasure, C.B., Nabel, E.G., Mclenacham, J.M., Fish, R.D., Yeung, A.C., Vekshtein, V.I., Rees, D.D., Palmer, R.M.J., Hodson, H.F., Moncada, S. (1989) A specific inhibitor of nitric oxide formation from L-arginine attenuates endothelium-dependent relaxation. *Br. J. Pharmacol.*, **96**: 418–424.

Voets, T., Droogmans, G., Nilius, B. (1996) Membrane currents and the resting membrane potential in cultured bovine pulmonary artery endothelial cells. *J. Physiol.*, **497**: 95–107.

Vogalis, F., Goyal, R.K. (1997) Activation of small conductance Ca^{2+}-dependent K^+ channels by purinergic agonists in smooth muscle cells of the mouse ileum. *J. Physiol.*, **502**: 497–508.

Von der Weid, P.-Y., Bény, J.-L. (1993) Simultaneous oscillations in the membrane potential of pig coronary artery endothelial and smooth muscle cells. *J. Physiol.*, **471**: 13–24.

Wagner, J.A., Varga, K., Jarai, Z., Kunos, G. (1999) Mesenteric vasodilation mediated by endothelial anandamide receptors. *Hypertension*, **33**: 429–434.

Waldron, G.J., Cole, W.C. (1999) Activation of vascular smooth muscle K^+ channels by endothelium-derived relaxing factors. *Clin. Exp. Pharmacol. Physiol.*, **26**: 180–184.

Waldron, G.J., Ding, H., Cole, W.C., Kubes, P., Triggle, C.R. (1999) Acetylcholine-induced relaxation of peripheral arteries isolated from mice lacking endothelial nitric oxide synthase. *Br. J. Pharmacol.*, **128**: 653–658.

Wallerath, T., Witte, K., Schafer, S.C., Schwarz, P.M., Prellwitz, W., Wohlfahrt, P., Kleinert, H., Lehr, H.A., Lemmer, B., Förstermann, U. (1999) Down-regulation of the expression of endothelial NO synthase is likely to contribute to glucocorticoid-mediated hypertension. *Proc. Natl. Acad. Sci. USA*, **96**: 13357–13362.

Walsh, B.W., Schiff, I., Rosner, B., Greenberg, L., Ravnikar, V., Sacks, F.M. (1991) Effects of postmenopausal estrogen replacement on the concentrations and metabolism of plasma lipoproteins. *New Engl. J. Med.*, **325**: 1196–1204.

Wang, H.Z., Jian, L., Lemanski, L.F., Veenstra, R.D. (1992) Gating of mammalian cardiac gap junction channels by transjunction voltage. *Biophys. J.*, **63**: 139–151.

Wang, Q., Hogg, R.C., Large, W.A. (1993) A monovalent ion-sensitive cation current activated by noradrenaline in smooth muscle cells of rabbit ear artery. *Pflügers Arch.*, **423**: 28–33.

Watsky, M.A., McCartney, M.D., McLaughlin, B.J., Edelhauser, H.F. (1990) Corneal endothelial junctions and the effect of ouabain. *Invest. Ophthalmol. Vis. Sci.*, **31**: 933–941.

Wautier, J.L., Zoukourian, C., Chappey, O., Wautier, M.P., Guillausseau, P.J., Cao, R., Hori, O., Stern, D., Schmidt, A.M. (1996) Receptor-mediated endothelial cell dysfunction in diabetic vasculopathy: Soluble receptor for advanced glycation end products blocks hyperpermeability in diabetic rats. *J. Clin. Invest.*, **97**: 238–243.

Waxman, D.J. (1984) Rat hepatic cytochrome P-450 isoenzyme 2C. Identification as a male-specific developmentally induced steroid 16α-hydroxylase and comparison to a female-specific cytochrome P-450 isoenzyme. *J. Biol. Chem.*, **259**: 15481–15490.

Waxman, D.J., Lapenson, D.P., Aoyama, T., Gelboin, H.V., Gonzalez, F.J., Korzekwa, K. (1991) Steroid hormone hydroxylase specificities of eleven cDNA-expressed human cytochrome P450s. *Arch. Biochem. Biophys.*, **290**: 160–166.

Weidmann, S. (1966) The diffusion of radiopotassium across intercalated disks of mammalian heart. *J. Physiol.*, **187**: 323–342.

Weidmann, S. (1970) Electrical constants of trabecular muscle from mammalian heart *J. Physiol.*, **210**: 1041–1054.

Weiner, C.P., Lizasoain, I., Baylis, S.A., Knowles, R.G., Charles, I.G., Moncada, S. (1994) Induction of calcium-dependent nitric oxide synthase by sex hormones. *Proc. Natl. Acad. Sci. USA*, **91**: 5212–5216.

Weintraub, N.L., Stephenson, A.H., Sprague, R.S., Lonigro, A.J. (1999) Role of phospholipase A2 in EDHF-mediated relaxation of the porcine coronary artery. In *Endothelium dependent hyperpolarizations*, edited by P.M. Vanhoutte, vol. 2, pp. 97–108. The Netherlands: Harwood academic publishers.

Welsh, D.G., Segal, S.S. (1998) Endothelial and smooth muscle cell conduction in arterioles controlling blood flow. *Am. J. Physiol.*, **274**: H178–H186.

Welsh, D.G., Segal, S.S. (2000) Role of EDHF in conduction of vasodilation along hamster cheek pouch arterioles *in vivo*. *Am. J. Physiol.*, **278**: H1832–H1839.

White, R., Hiley, C.R. (1997) A comparison of EDHF-mediated and anandamide-induced relaxations in the rat isolated mesenteric artery. *Br. J. Pharmacol.*, **122**: 1573–1584.

White, T., Bruzzone, R. (1996) Multiple connexin proteins in single intercellular channels connexin compatibility and functional consequences. *J. Bioenerg. BioMembr.*, **28**: 339–350.

Whitney, R.J. (1953) The measurement of volume changes in human limbs. *J. Physiol.*, **121**: 1–27.

Wigg, S.J., Tare, M., O'Brien, R.C., Meredith, I.T., Parkington, H.C. (2000) Reduced endothelium-derived hyperpolarizing factor accounts for impaired endothelial vasodilator function in diabetic rats. *Clin. Exper. Pharm. Physiol.*, **27**: A19.

Willecke, K., Haubrich, S. (1996) Connexin expression systems: to what extent do they reflect the situation in the animal? *J. Bioenerg. Biomembr.*, **28**: 319–326.

Williams, D.A., Segal, S.S. (1993) Feed artery role in blood flow control to rat hindlimb skeletal muscles. *J. Physiol.*, **463**: 631–646.

Williams, S.B., Cusco, J.A., Roddy, M.A., Johnstone, M.T., Creager, M.A. (1996) Impaired nitric oxide-mediated vasodilatation in patients with non-insulin dependent diabetes mellitus. *J. Am. Coll. Cardiol.*, **27**: 567–574.

Williams, S.P., Dorn, G.W., Rapoport, R.M. (1994) Prostaglandin I_2 mediates contractions and relaxation of vascular smooth muscle. *Am. J. Physiol.*, **267**: H796–H803.

Williams, S.P., Shackelford, D.P., Iams, S.G., Mustafa, S.J. (1988) Endothelium-dependent relaxation in estrogen-treated spontaneous hypertensive rats. *Eur. J. Pharmacol.*, 145: 205–207.

Wise, H., Jones, R.L. (1996) Focus on prostacyclin and its novel mimetics, *Trends Pharmacol. Sci.*, **17**: 17–21.

Wolff, D.J., Datto, G.A., Samatovicz, R.A., Tempsick, R.A. (1993) Calmodulin-dependent nitric oxide synthase. Mechanism of inhibition by imidazole and phenylimidazoles. *J. Biol. Chem.*, **268**: 9425–9429.

Wolff, D.J., Lubeskie, A. (1995) Aminoguanidine is an isoform-selective, mechanism-based inactivator of nitric oxide synthase. *Arch. Biochem. Biophys.*, **316**: 290–301.

Wolin, M.S. (2000) Interactions of oxidants with vascular signalling systems. *Arterioscler. Thromb. Vasc. Biol.*, **20**: 1430–1442.

Woodman, O. (1995) Modulation of vasoconstriction by endothelium-derived nitric oxide: the influence of vascular disease. *Clin. Exp. Pharmacol. Physiol.*, **22**: 585–593.

Wu, K.K., Thiagarajan, P. (1996) Role of endothelium in thrombosis and hemostasis. *Ann. Rev. Med.*, **47**: 315–331.

Xia, J., Duling, B.R. (1995a) Electromechanical coupling and the conducted vasomotor response. *Am. J. Physiol.*, **269**: H2022–H2030.

Xia, J., Little, T.L., Duling, B.R. (1995b) Cellular pathways of the conducted electrical response in arterioles of hamster cheek pouch *in vitro*. *Am. J. Physiol.*, **269**: H2031–H2038.

Xia, Y., Tsai, A.L., Berka, V., Zweier, J.L. (1998) Superoxide generation from endothelial nitric oxide synthase. *J. Biol. Chem.*, **273**: 25804–25808.

Yajima, K., Nishiyama, M., Yamamoto, Y., Suzuki, H. (1999) Inhibition of endothelium-dependent hyperpolarization by endothelial prostanoids in guinea-pig coronary artery. *Br. J. Pharmacol.*, **126**: 1–10.

Yamamoto, K.R. (1985) Steroid receptor regulated transcription of specific genes and gene networks. *Annu. Rev. Genet.*, **19**: 209–252.

Yamamoto, Y., Fukuta, H., Nakahira, Y, Suzuki, H. (1998) Blockade by 18β-glycyrrhetinic acid of intercellular electrical coupling in guinea-pig arterioles. *J. Physiol.*, **511**: 501–508.

Yamamoto, Y., Imaeda, K., Suzuki, H. (1999) Endothelium-dependent hyperpolarization and intercellular electrical coupling in guinea-pig mesenteric arterioles. *J. Physiol.*, **514**: 505–513.

Yamamoto, Y., Tomoike, H., Egashira, K., Nakamura, M. (1987) Attenuation of endothelium-related relaxation and enhanced responsiveness of vascular smooth muscle to histamine in spastic coronary arterial segments from miniature pigs. *Circ. Res.*, **61**: 772–778.

Yamamura, H., Nagano, N., Hirano, M., Muraki, K., Watanabe, M., Imaizumi, Y. (1999) Activation of Ca(2+)-dependent K(+) current by nordihydroguaiaretic acid in porcine coronary arterial smooth muscle cells. *J. Pharmacol. Exp. Ther.*, **291**: 140–146.

Yamanaka, A., Ishikawa, T., Goto, K. (1998) Characterization of endothelium-dependent relaxation independent of NO and prostaglandins in guinea-pig coronary artery. *J. Pharmacol. Exp. Ther.*, **285**: 480–489.

Yamazaki, M., Ito, Y., Kuze, S., Shibuya, N., Momose, Y. (1992) Effects of ketamine on voltage-dependent CA-2+ currents in single smooth-muscle cells from rabbit portal-vein. *Pharmacol.*, **45**: 162–169.

Yang, Z., Lüscher, T.F. (1991) Endothelium-dependent responses in human blood vessels in health and cardiovascular disease. *Coron. Artery. Dis.*, **2**: 338–348.

Yeager, M., Nicholson, B.J. (1996) Structure of gap junction intercellular channels. *Current Opinion in Structural Biology*, **6**: 183–192.

Yeh, H.-I., Rothery, S., Dupont, E., Coppen, S.R., Severs, N.J. (1998) Individual gap junction plaques contain multiple connexins in arterial endothelium. *Circ. Res.*, **83**: 1248–1263.

You, J., Johnson, T.D., Childres W.F., Bryan, R.M. (1997) Endothelial-mediated dilations of rat middle cerebral arteries by ATP and ADP. *Am. J. Physiol.*, **273**: H1472–H1477.

You, J., Johnson, T.D., Marrelli, S.P., Bryan, R.M., Jr. (1999) Functional heterogeneity of endothelial P2 purinoceptors in the cerebrovascular tree of the rat. *Am. J. Physiol.*, **277**: H893–H900.

You, J., Johnson, T.D., Marrelli, S.P., Mombouli, J.-V., Bryan, R.M., Jr. (1998) P2u-receptor mediated release of endothelium-derived relaxing factor/nitric oxide and endothelium-derived hyperpolarizing factor from cerebrovascular endothelium in rats. *Stroke*, **30**: 1125–1133.

Young, S.H., Ennes, H.S., Mayer, E.A. (1996) Propagation of calcium waves between colonic smooth muscle cells in culture. *Cell Calcium*, **20**: 257–271.

Yu, W., Dahl, G., Werner, R. (1994) The connexin43 gene is responsive to oestrogen. *Proc. R. Soc. Lond. B. Biol. Sci.*, **255**: 125–132.

Yusuf, S., Sleight, P., Pogue, J., Bosch, J., Davies, R., Dagenais, G. (2000) Vitamin E supplementation and cardiovascular events in high risk patients. The Heart Outcomes Prevention Evaluation Study Investigators. *New Engl. J. Med.*, **342**: 154–160.

Zeldin, D.C., DuBois, R.N., Falck, J.R., Capdevila, J.H. (1995) Molecular cloning, expression and characterization of an endogenous human cytochrome P450 arachidonic acid epoxygenase isoform. *Arch. Biochem. Biophys.*, **322**: 76–86.

Zhang, G., Niwa, H., Masaoka, A., Yamamoto, Y., Suzuki, H. (1996) Endothelial prostanoids involved in the relaxation produced by acetylcholine in the human pulmonary artery. *Jpn. J. Physiol.*, **46**: 403–409.

Zhang, H., Stockbridge, N., Weir, B., Krueger, C., Cook, D. (1991) Glibenclamide relaxes vascular smooth muscle contraction produced by prostaglandin F$_2$. *Eur. J. Pharmacol.*, **195**: 27–35.

Zhang, Y.W., Morita, I., Nishida, M., Murota, S.I. (1999) Involvement of tyrosine kinase in the hypoxia/reoxygenation-induced gap junctional intercellular communication abnormality in cultured human umbilical vein endothelial cells. *J. Cell Physiol.*, **180**: 305–313.

Zhao, Y.J., Wang, J., Tod, M.L., Rubin, L.J., Yuan X.J. (1996) Pulmonary vasoconstrictor effects of prostacyclin in rats: potential role of thromboxane receptors. *J. Appl. Physiol.*, **81**: 2595–2603.

Zygmunt, P.M., Edwards, G., Weston, A.H., Davis, S.C., Högestätt, E.D. (1996) Effects of cytochrome P450 inhibitors on EDHF-mediated relaxation in the rat hepatic artery. *Br. J. Pharmacol.*, **118**: 1147–1152.

Zygmunt, P.M., Edwards, G., Weston, A.H., Larsson B., Högestätt, E.D. (1997) Involvement of voltage-dependent potassium channels in the EDHF-mediated relaxation of rat hepatic artery. *Br. J. Pharmacol.*, **121**: 141–149.

Zygmunt, P.M., Högestätt, E.D. (1996) Role of potassium channels in endothelium-dependent relaxation resistant to nitroarginine in the rat hepatic artery. *Br. J. Pharmacol.*, **117**: 1600–1606.

Zygmunt, P.M., Plane, F., Paulsson, M., Garland, C.J., Högestätt, E.D. (1998) Interactions between endothelium-derived relaxing factors in the rat hepatic artery: focus on regulation of EDHF. *Br. J. Pharmacol.*, **124**: 992–1000.

Zygmunt, P.M., Ryman, T., Högestätt, E.D. (1995) Regional differences in endothelium-dependent relaxation in the rat – contribution of nitric oxide and nitric oxide-independent mechanisms. *Acta. Physiol. Scand.*, **155**: 257–266.

Zygmunt, P.M., Sorgard, M., Petersson, J., Johansson, R., Högestätt, E.D. (2000) Differential actions of anandamide, potassium ions and endothelium-derived hyperpolarizing factor in guinea-pig basilar artery. *Naunyn-Schmiedeberg's Arch. Pharmacol.*, **361**: 535–542.

Index

Authors' articles appear where page numbers are **bold**.